Kidney Inflammation, Injury and Regeneration

Kidney Inflammation, Injury and Regeneration

Special Issue Editors

Patrick C. Baer
Benjamin Koch
Helmut Geiger

MDPI • Basel • Beijing • Wuhan • Barcelona • Belgrade • Manchester • Tokyo • Cluj • Tianjin

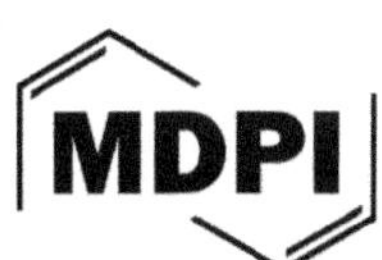

Special Issue Editors
Patrick C. Baer
Goethe-Universitat
Frankfurt am Main
Germany

Benjamin Koch
Goethe-Universitat
Frankfurt am Main
Germany

Helmut Geiger
Goethe-Universitat
Frankfurt am Main
Germany

Editorial Office
MDPI
St. Alban-Anlage 66
4052 Basel, Switzerland

This is a reprint of articles from the Special Issue published online in the open access journal *International Journal of Molecular Sciences* (ISSN 1422-0067) (available at: https://www.mdpi.com/journal/ijms/special_issues/kidney_ijms).

For citation purposes, cite each article independently as indicated on the article page online and as indicated below:

LastName, A.A.; LastName, B.B.; LastName, C.C. Article Title. *Journal Name* **Year**, *Article Number*, Page Range.

ISBN 978-3-03928-538-9 (Pbk)
ISBN 978-3-03928-539-6 (PDF)

Cover image courtesy of Patrick C. Baer.

Contents

About the Special Issue Editors

Patrick C. Baer is a Cell Biologist and Associate Professor of Experimental Medicine at the Hospital of the Goethe University in Frankfurt/M. He completed his studies in Biochemistry at the Technical University of Darmstadt and received his doctorate at the Goethe University of Frankfurt/M. P.C.B. has published 92 research articles, including three book chapters and three patents. P.C.B. has been working with cell culture models of proximal and distal tubular epithelial cells of the kidney for 25 years. His research also focuses on the isolation, culture and differentiation of mesenchymal stroma/stem cells (MSCs), and the transplantation of MSCs or their derivatives to improve renal regeneration.

Benjamin Koch earned a MD with Prof. W. Wels at the Georg-Speyer-Haus, Institute for Tumor Biology and Experimental Therapy, Frankfurt/M., Germany. His thesis work was establishing RNAseq in it's early days and integration with ChIPseq in order to identify novel target genes of an important transcription factor in leukemia. He then performed clinical training at the Goethe University Hospital (Division of Nephrology, Prof. Helmut Geiger). Besides his clinical work in nephrology he coordinates research projects in the lab of Prof. Patrick C. Baer and is directly involved researching athogen induced acute and chronic kidney injury as well as novel blood filtration devices in inflammation and sepsis. His research tools include RNAseq, proteomics, translatomics based on general molecular biology.

Helmut Geiger is Professor of Medicine and head of the department of nephrology at the University Hospital Frankfurt/M. He has worked as a physician since 1983 in Würzburg, Budapest, Nuremberg-Erlangen and Frankfurt/M. During this time he has written more than 250 scientific publications and has received funding from the DFG, BMBF, BMWi and several foundations. His main research interests are renal diseases, kidney transplantation and hypertension. H.G. has been awarded the Nils-Alwall Prize of the German Working Group for Clinical Nephrology and the Franz Gross Science Prize of the German High Pressure League.

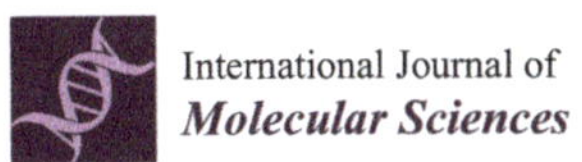 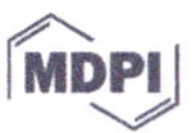

International Journal of
Molecular Sciences

Editorial

Kidney Inflammation, Injury and Regeneration

Patrick C. Baer *, Benjamin Koch and Helmut Geiger

Division of Nephrology, Department of Internal Medicine III, University Hospital, Goethe-University,
60596 Frankfurt, Germany; b.koch@med.uni-frankfurt.de (B.K.); h.geiger@em.uni-frankfurt.de (H.G.)
* Correspondence: p.baer@em.uni-frankfurt.de; Tel.: +49-69-6301-5554; Fax: +49-69-6301-4749

Received: 31 January 2020; Accepted: 6 February 2020; Published: 10 February 2020

Damage to kidney cells can occur due to a variety of ischemic and toxic insults and leads to inflammation and cell death, which can result in acute kidney injury (AKI). Inflammation plays a key role in the injury of renal cells, as well as subsequent cellular regeneration processes. However, persistent chronic inflammation may trigger renal fibrosis. The investigation of the molecular mechanisms involved in each individual injury is currently insufficiently elucidated. Whereas the kidney has a remarkable capacity for regeneration after injury and may completely recover depending on the type of renal lesions, the options for clinical intervention are restricted to fluid management and extracorporeal kidney support. AKI is still associated with high morbidity and mortality incidence rates, and it also bears an elevated risk of subsequent chronic kidney disease. Therefore, the development of novel therapies to improve renal regeneration capacity after AKI, to preserve renal function, and to prevent AKI is urgently needed. In this context, we wanted to offer a forum for the publication of new results on renal inflammation, injury and regeneration, as well as for the review and discussion of existing studies from this interesting research field.

This Special Issue covers research articles that investigated the molecular mechanisms of inflammation [1–3] and injury [4,5] during different renal pathologies and renal regeneration [6], diagnostics using new biomarkers [7–9], and the effects of different stimuli like medication or bacterial components on isolated renal cells or in vivo models [10–12], all of which were summarized in a very simplified manner. Furthermore, this Special Issue contains important reviews that dealt with the current knowledge of cell death and regeneration [13,14], inflammation [15–18], and the molecular mechanisms of kidney diseases [19–22]. In addition, the potential of cell-based therapy approaches that use mesenchymal stromal/stem cells (MSCs) or their derivates is summarized [23–25]. This edition is complemented by a series of reviews that deal with the current data situation on other very specific topics like diabetes and diabetic nephropathy [26–28], as well as new therapeutic targets [29].

In this Special Issue, twelve original research articles are presented that dealt with different questions and the research models used within. The findings of Mocker and co-workers demonstrate that renal chemerin expression, a chemoattractant adipokine, is associated with processes of inflammation and fibrosis during renal damage [2]. The protection of kidney function by attenuating induced renal inflammation was shown with the use of Farnesiferol B, an agonist of a receptor that is expressed by renal tubular epithelial cells [1]. The xanthin oxidase inhibitor febuxostat is shown to exert anti-inflammatory action and protect against diabetic nephropathy development [3]. Kidney injury leading to focal segmental glomerulosclerosis was shown by variants in the collagen 4A5 gene, demonstrating that the molecular genetics of different players in the glomerular filtration barrier can be used to evaluate the causes of kidney injury [5]. In addition, another study suggested that renal disease in colitis mice might be associated with changes in glomerular collagens and glomerular filtration barrier-related proteins [4].

No injury or inflammatory effects of two anti-diabetically used gliflozins on proximal tubular epithelial cells that were cultured in hyperglycemic conditions were found [10]. Stimulations with bacterial lipopolysaccharide were used to investigate acute renal fibrosis in a model of sepsis-induced

AKI [11] and the inflammatory cascade of obese kidney fibrosis in a metabolic endotoxemia mouse model [12].

A very interesting approach investigated the regeneration potential of MSC-derived extracellular vesicles that were transfected with specific miRNA mimics [6]. Furthermore, others introduced a kidney injury test for the noninvasive monitoring of IgA nephropathy progression [9]. Schiffer and co-workers described CXCL13 blood levels as a biomarker in T-cell-mediated rejection [8]. The marker correlates with B-cell involvement and might help to identify patients with a more severe clinical course of rejection [8]. Others demonstrated that that specific IL-18 genotypes may play a role in the etiology and progression of renal cell carcinoma and serve as useful early detection biomarkers.

Priante and co-workers reviewed the different modalities of apoptosis, necrosis, and regulated necrosis in kidney injuries in order to find evidence for the role of cell death, which may pave the way for new therapeutic opportunities [14]. Others discussed the molecular basis of injury and repair in distinct cell types of the kidney during arterial hypertension [21]. In this context, the main mechanisms of kidney regeneration, while focusing on epithelial cell dedifferentiation and the activation of progenitor cells with special attention on the potential niches of kidney progenitor cells, were also lighted [13]. Three reviews by Yun [25], Bochon [23] and Lee [24] summarized the therapeutic potential and efficacy of MSCs, which are primarily associated with their capability to inhibit inflammation and initiate renal regeneration. MSCs predominantly act through secreted factors, including microRNAs that are contained within extracellular vesicles, cytoprotective effects anti-inflammatory effects, anti-apoptotic effects, and the suppression of oxidative stress. In addition, further reviews summarized the inflammation-mediated mechanisms or the inflammasome in various renal diseases [15–18,26,27]. Very interesting and new approaches shed a light on the role of non-coding RNAs, either in the progression of glomerular or tubulointerstitial kidney diseases [20] or as new therapeutic targets or biomarkers for fibrotic changes [29]. Another interesting work reviewed the involvement of salt-inducible signal transduction pathways in AKI and discussed the possibility of new therapy options [22].

Author Contributions: Writing, review, and editing, P.C.B., B.K., H.G. All authors have read and agreed to the published version of the manuscript.

Funding: The authors received no funding for this editorial.

Conflicts of Interest: The authors declare no conflict of interest.

References

1. Zhang, L.; Fu, X.; Gui, T.; Wang, T.; Wang, Z.; Kullak-Ublick, G.A.; Gai, Z. Effects of farnesiferol B on ischemia-reperfusion-induced renal damage, inflammation, and NF-κB signaling. *Int. J. Mol. Sci.* **2019**, *20*, 2680. [CrossRef] [PubMed]

2. Mocker, A.; Hilgers, K.F.; Cordasic, N.; Wachtveitl, R.; Menendez-Castro, C.; Woelfle, J.; Hartner, A.; Fahlbusch, F.B. Renal chemerin expression is induced in models of hypertensive nephropathy and glomerulonephritis and correlates with markers of inflammation and fibrosis. *Int. J. Mol. Sci.* **2019**, *20*, 6240. [CrossRef] [PubMed]

3. Mizuno, Y.; Yamamotoya, T.; Nakatsu, Y.; Ueda, K.; Matsunaga, Y.; Inoue, M.-K.; Sakoda, H.; Fujishiro, M.; Ono, H.; Kikuchi, T.; et al. Xanthine oxidase inhibitor febuxostat exerts an anti-inflammatory action and protects against diabetic nephropathy development in KK-Ay obese diabetic mice. *Int. J. Mol. Sci.* **2019**, *20*, 4680. [CrossRef] [PubMed]

4. Chang, C.-J.; Wang, P.-C.; Huang, T.-C.; Taniguchi, A. Change in renal glomerular collagens and glomerular filtration barrier-related proteins in a dextran sulfate sodium-induced colitis mouse model. *Int. J. Mol. Sci.* **2019**, *20*, 1458. [CrossRef]

5. Frese, J.; Kettwig, M.; Zappel, H.; Hofer, J.; Gröne, H.-J.; Nagel, M.; Sunder-Plassmann, G.; Kain, R.; Neuweiler, J.; Gross, O. Kidney injury by variants in the COL4A5 gene aggravated by polymorphisms in slit diaphragm genes causes focal segmental glomerulosclerosis. *Int. J. Mol. Sci.* **2019**, *20*, 519. [CrossRef]

6. Tapparo, M.; Bruno, S.; Collino, F.; Togliatto, G.; Deregibus, M.C.; Provero, P.; Wen, S.; Quesenberry, P.J.; Camussi, G. Renal regenerative potential of extracellular vesicles derived from miRNA-engineered mesenchymal stromal cells. *Int. J. Mol. Sci.* **2019**, *20*, 2381. [CrossRef]

7. Chang, W.-S.; Shen, T.-C.; Yeh, W.-L.; Yu, C.-C.; Lin, H.-Y.; Wu, H.-C.; Tsai, C.-W.; Bau, D.-T. Contribution of inflammatory cytokine interleukin-18 genotypes to renal cell carcinoma. *Int. J. Mol. Sci.* **2019**, *20*, 1563. [CrossRef]

8. Schiffer, L.; Wiehler, F.; Bräsen, J.H.; Gwinner, W.; Greite, R.; Kreimann, K.; Thorenz, A.; Derlin, K.; Teng, B.; Rong, S.; et al. Chemokine CXCL13 as a new systemic biomarker for B-cell involvement in acute T cell-mediated kidney allograft rejection. *Int. J. Mol. Sci.* **2019**, *20*, 2552. [CrossRef]

9. Yang, J.Y.C.; Sarwal, R.D.; Fervenza, F.C.; Sarwal, M.M.; Lafayette, R.A. Noninvasive urinary monitoring of progression in IgA nephropathy. *Int. J. Mol. Sci.* **2019**, *20*, 4463. [CrossRef]

10. Baer, P.C.; Koch, B.; Freitag, J.; Schubert, R.; Geiger, H. No Cytotoxic and inflammatory effects of empagliflozin and dapagliflozin on primary renal proximal tubular epithelial cells under diabetic conditions in vitro. *Int. J. Mol. Sci.* **2020**, *21*, 391. [CrossRef]

11. Castellano, G.; Stasi, A.; Franzin, R.; Sallustio, F.; Divella, C.; Spinelli, A.; Netti, G.S.; Fiaccadori, E.; Cantaluppi, V.; Crovace, A.; et al. LPS-binding protein modulates acute renal fibrosis by inducing pericyte-to-myofibroblast trans-differentiation through TLR-4 signaling. *Int. J. Mol. Sci.* **2019**, *20*, 3682. [CrossRef]

12. Chang, J.-F.; Yeh, J.-C.; Ho, C.-T.; Liu, S.-H.; Hsieh, C.-Y.; Wang, T.-M.; Chang, S.-W.; Lee, I.-T.; Huang, K.-Y.; Wang, J.-Y.; et al. Targeting ROS and cPLA2/COX2 expressions ameliorated renal damage in obese mice with endotoxemia. *Int. J. Mol. Sci.* **2019**, *20*, 4393. [CrossRef] [PubMed]

13. Andrianova, N.V.; Buyan, M.I.; Zorova, L.D.; Pevzner, I.B.; Popkov, V.A.; Babenko, V.A.; Silachev, D.N.; Plotnikov, E.Y.; Zorov, D.B. Kidney cells regeneration: Dedifferentiation of tubular epithelium, resident stem cells and possible niches for renal progenitors. *Int. J. Mol. Sci.* **2019**, *20*, 6326. [CrossRef] [PubMed]

14. Priante, G.; Gianesello, L.; Ceol, M.; Del Prete, D.; Anglani, F. Cell death in the kidney. *Int. J. Mol. Sci.* **2019**, *20*, 3598. [CrossRef] [PubMed]

15. Giuliani, K.T.K.; Kassianos, A.J.; Healy, H.; Gois, P.H.F. Pigment nephropathy: Novel insights into inflammasome-mediated pathogenesis. *Int. J. Mol. Sci.* **2019**, *20*, 1997. [CrossRef]

16. Moreno, J.A.; Sevillano, Á.; Gutiérrez, E.; Guerrero-Hue, M.; Vázquez-Carballo, C.; Yuste, C.; Herencia, C.; García-Caballero, C.; Praga, M.; Egido, J. Glomerular hematuria: Cause or consequence of renal inflammation? *Int. J. Mol. Sci.* **2019**, *20*, 2205. [CrossRef]

17. Wang, T.; Fu, X.; Chen, Q.; Patra, J.K.; Wang, D.; Wang, Z.; Gai, Z. Arachidonic acid metabolism and kidney inflammation. *Int. J. Mol. Sci.* **2019**, *20*, 3683. [CrossRef]

18. Wu, P.-K.; Yeh, S.-C.; Li, S.-J.; Kang, Y.-N. Efficacy of polyunsaturated fatty acids on inflammatory markers in patients undergoing dialysis: A systematic review with network meta-analysis of randomized clinical trials. *Int. J. Mol. Sci.* **2019**, *20*, 3645. [CrossRef]

19. Guzzi, F.; Cirillo, L.; Roperto, R.M.; Romagnani, P.; Lazzeri, E. Molecular mechanisms of the acute kidney injury to chronic kidney disease transition: An updated view. *Int. J. Mol. Sci.* **2019**, *20*, 4941. [CrossRef]

20. Ignarski, M.; Islam, R.; Müller, R.-U. Long non-coding RNAs in kidney disease. *Int. J. Mol. Sci.* **2019**, *20*, 3276. [CrossRef] [PubMed]

21. Sievers, L.K.; Eckardt, K.-U. Molecular mechanisms of kidney injury and repair in arterial hypertension. *Int. J. Mol. Sci.* **2019**, *20*, 2138. [CrossRef]

22. Taub, M. Salt inducible kinase signaling networks: Implications for acute kidney injury and therapeutic potential. *Int. J. Mol. Sci.* **2019**, *20*, 3219. [CrossRef] [PubMed]

23. Bochon, B.; Kozubska, M.; Surygała, G.; Witkowska, A.; Kuźniewicz, R.; Grzeszczak, W.; Wystrychowski, G. Mesenchymal stem cells-potential applications in kidney diseases. *Int. J. Mol. Sci.* **2019**, *20*, 2426. [CrossRef]

24. Lee, K.-H.; Tseng, W.-C.; Yang, C.-Y.; Tarng, D.-C. The anti-inflammatory, anti-oxidative, and anti-apoptotic benefits of stem cells in acute ischemic kidney injury. *Int. J. Mol. Sci.* **2019**, *20*, 3529. [CrossRef] [PubMed]

25. Yun, C.W.; Lee, S.H. Potential and therapeutic efficacy of cell-based therapy using mesenchymal stem cells for acute/chronic kidney disease. *Int. J. Mol. Sci.* **2019**, *20*, 1619. [CrossRef]

26. Lee, J.H.; Kim, D.; Oh, Y.S.; Jun, H.-S. Lysophosphatidic acid signaling in diabetic nephropathy. *Int. J. Mol. Sci.* **2019**, *20*, 2850. [CrossRef]

27. Matoba, K.; Takeda, Y.; Nagai, Y.; Kawanami, D.; Utsunomiya, K.; Nishimura, R. Unraveling the role of inflammation in the pathogenesis of diabetic kidney disease. *Int. J. Mol. Sci.* **2019**, *20*, 3393. [CrossRef]

28. Ninčević, V.; Omanović Kolarić, T.; Roguljić, H.; Kizivat, T.; Smolić, M.; Bilić Ćurčić, I. Renal benefits of SGLT 2 inhibitors and GLP-1 receptor agonists: Evidence supporting a paradigm shift in the medical management of type 2 diabetes. *Int. J. Mol. Sci.* **2019**, *20*, 5831. [CrossRef]
29. Van der Hauwaert, C.; Glowacki, F.; Pottier, N.; Cauffiez, C. Non-coding RNAs as new therapeutic targets in the context of renal fibrosis. *Int. J. Mol. Sci.* **2019**, *20*, 1977. [CrossRef]

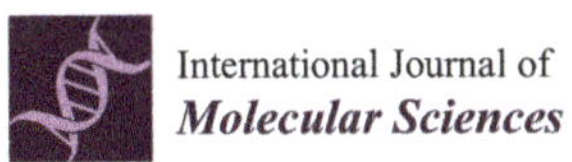

International Journal of
Molecular Sciences

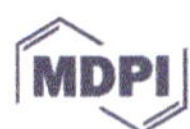

Article

Effects of Farnesiferol B on Ischemia-Reperfusion-Induced Renal Damage, Inflammation, and NF-κB Signaling

Lu Zhang [1,2,†], Xianjun Fu [1,†], Ting Gui [1], Tianqi Wang [1], Zhenguo Wang [1], Gerd A. Kullak-Ublick [2,3,*] and Zhibo Gai [1,2,*]

[1] College of Traditional Chinese Medicine; Shandong Co-Innovation Center of TCM Formula; Institute for Literature and Culture of Chinese Medicine; Key Laboratory of Traditional Chinese Medicine for Classical Theory, Ministry of Education, Shandong University of Traditional Chinese Medicine, Jinan 250355, China; Lu.zhang@usz.ch (L.Z.); xianxiu@hotmail.com (X.F.); stefina1982@gmail.com (T.G.); wangtianqi9292@gmail.com (T.W.); zhenguo.wang0101@gmail.com (Z.W.)

[2] Department of Clinical Pharmacology and Toxicology, University Hospital Zurich, University of Zurich, 8006 Zurich, Switzerland

[3] Mechanistic Safety, CMO & Patient Safety, Global Drug Development, Novartis Pharma, 4056 Basel, Switzerland

* Correspondence: gerd.kullak@usz.ch (G.A.K.-U.); gaizhibo@gmail.com (Z.G.); Tel.: +43-253-31-45

† These authors contributed equally to this work.

Received: 31 October 2019; Accepted: 10 December 2019; Published: 12 December 2019

Abstract: Background: G-protein-coupled bile acid receptor (TGR5), a membrane bile acid receptor, regulates macrophage reactivity, and attenuates inflammation in different disease models. However, the regulatory effects of TGR5 in ischemia/reperfusion (I/R)-induced kidney injury and inflammation have not yet been extensively studied. Therefore, we hypothesize that Farnesiferol B, a natural TGR5 agonist, could alleviate renal I/R injury by reducing inflammation and macrophage migration through activating TGR5. Methods: Mice were treated with Farnesiferol B before I/R or sham procedures. Renal function, pathological analysis, and inflammatory mediators were examined. In vitro, the regulatory effects of Farnesiferol B on the Nuclear Factor kappa-light-chain-enhancer of activated B cells (NF-κB) pathway in macrophages were investigated. Results: After I/R, Farnesiferol B-treated mice displayed better renal function and less tubular damage. Farnesiferol B reduced renal oxidative stress and inflammation significantly. In vitro, Farnesiferol B treatment alleviated lipopolysaccharide (LPS)-induced macrophage migration and activation, as well as LPS-induced NF-κB activation through TGR5. Conclusions: Farnesiferol B could protect kidney function from I/R-induced damage by attenuating inflammation though activating TGR5 in macrophages. Farnesiferol B might be a potent TGR5 ligand for the treatment of I/R-induced renal inflammation.

Keywords: inflammation; ischemia/reperfusion injury; Farnesiferol B; Nuclear Factor kappa-light-chain-enhancer of activated B cells (NF-κB); G-protein-coupled bile acid receptor (TGR5)

---

1. Introduction

Ischemia/reperfusion (I/R) is a common complication in patients undergoing major cardiac surgery, kidney transplantation, and those experiencing hemorrhage and dehydration [1]. Ischemia/reperfusion injury (I/RI) after renal transplantation is a well-recognized and prevalent postoperative complication, which has been thought as a risk factor for the loss of tubular epithelial cell function, leading to acute kidney injury (AKI), delayed graft function, as well as acute or chronic organ rejection [2,3]. The process of renal ischemia reperfusion (RIR) is exceedingly complex, including a series of intricate and related events that lead to renal cell injury and ultimately give rise to cell death via apoptosis and necrosis [4]. Even though reperfusion is critically paramount for the repair of ischemic tissue and the survival of patients, the additional cellular damage by itself has provoked much attention, largely due to the production of reactive oxygen species (ROS) and infiltration of neutrophils [5,6].

The mechanism and treatment of I/R on kidney injury is still under exploration. During I/R, toxic products of kidney cells and cytokine release cause damage to renal epithelial tubular cells [7]. Besides, several studies have suggested that I/R leads rise to neutrophil infiltration of kidney tissue and stimulates the oxidative stress processes producing ROS [8]. Oxidative stress directly or indirectly affects all aspects of the kidney damage by the pathway lead to apoptosis, necrosis, fibrosis, tissue damage progression, and renal dysfunction [9]. ROS is considered as both the mediator or a signaling molecule during acute kidney inflammatory diseases [10]. The oxidase activity is elevated soon after ischemic injury, which is may originate from macrophages and/or neutrophils [11]. Moreover, inflammatory cells can also induce post-hypoxic cellular damage by ROS, which in turn gives rise to tubular epithelial cell damage or death by triggering apoptosis and necrosis pathways [12,13].

Early in a classic pharmacopoeia of traditional Chinese medicine book, Ferulae Resina is recorded as widely used for its effects on removing stagnancy (Xiao Ji), dissolving hard mass (Hua Jia), dissipating obstruction (San Pi), and as having anthelmintic properties (Sha Chong). Previous research reported the isolation of Farnesiferol B, a new sesquiterpene that is highly produced in the Apiaceae family, from the roots of Ferula [14,15]. Farnesiferol B has shown anti-plasmodial activity and anti-cytotoxicity effects in rat skeletal fibroblasts, a L6-cell line [16]. In a recent in silico work, Farnesiferol B was confirmed as a TGR5 agonist, also known as a G-protein-coupled bile acid receptor 1 (GPBAR1) activator, which denotes a regulatory effect of Farnesiferol B on inflammation [17].

TGR5 is expressed in several types of cells, including hepatic non-parenchymal cells [18–20]. The renal tubular cells, and immune cells including monocytes and macrophages [21,22]. Recently, it was demonstrated that TGR5 activation could be exploited to confer protection from diabetic nephropathy [23]. Considering that TGR5 activation possesses anti-oxidant and anti-inflammatory roles [23,24] in the kidney, we hypothesized that Farnesiferol B would alleviate renal I/R injury by reducing inflammation and ROS through regulating renal tubular cells and macrophages over TGR5.

In this study, the protective effect of Farnesiferol B was examined in a mouse model of AKI induced by I/R. We investigated the regulatory effects of Farnesiferol B on pro-inflammatory pathways in LPS-treated macrophages.

2. Results

2.1. Farnesiferol B Protection for Kidney Damage in I/R Kidney

The overall effect of Farnesiferol B on kidney injury was first explored by histological assessment and creatinine quantification. Haemotoxylin and Eosin (HE) staining and kidney injury marker Kim-1 (kidney injury molecule-1) immunohistochemical staining analysis results show that I/R kidneys are characterized by tubular basal membrane rupture, nuclear infiltration, tubular vacuolization, higher Kim-1 expression, and a higher renal tubular injury score (Figure 1A,B,E). Levels of proximal tubular cell death and cell proliferation were assessed. In the TUNEL assay, the nuclei of TUNEL-positive cells were stained red (Figure 1C), and the levels of cell death were indicated as the percentage of TUNEL-positive cells (Figure 1F). TUNEL-positive cells were observed mainly in the tubular area of the renal cortex. I/R group displayed more TUNEL-positive cells that the sham group (Figure 1C(b) vs. (a)). PCNA expression was observed in proliferating cell nuclei, and was significantly increased in AKI compared with the sham group (Figure 1D,G). Serum creatinine levels in I/R mice were significantly elevated in comparison to sham-operated mice (Figure 1H). The treatment with Farnesiferol B prior to I/R decreased serum creatinine level, attenuating the I/R-induced kidney injury (Figure 1A,C,H). However, Farnesiferol B treatment did not change the I/R-induced cell proliferation (Figure 1D(c) vs. (b)). The above results suggest that, in general, Farnesiferol B treatment protects against the kidney damage caused by I/R.

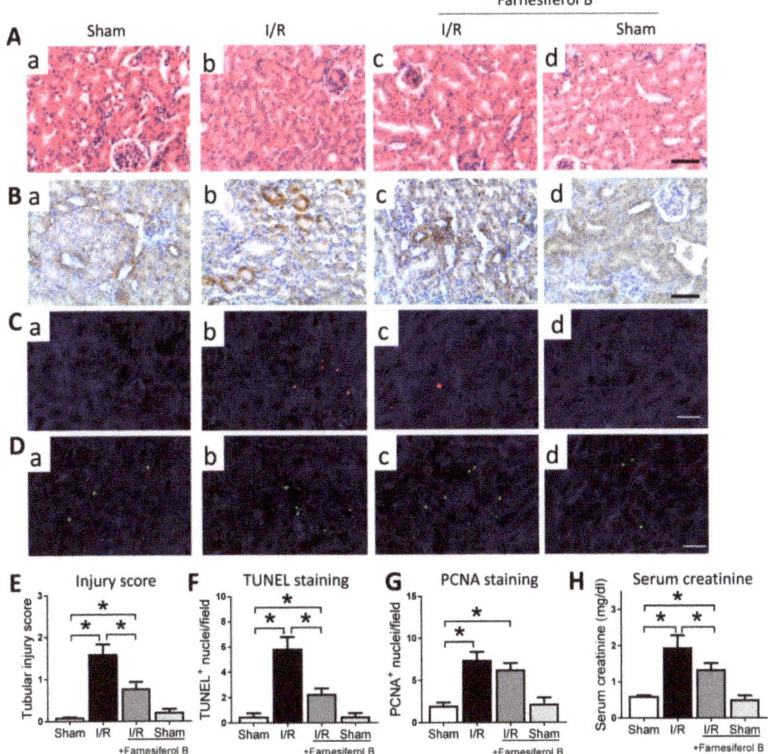

Figure 1. Farnesiferol B protects kidney from I/R-induced kidney damage. Representative images showing (**A**) Haemotoxylin and Eosin (HE) staining and (**B**) Kim1, (**C**) TUNEL, (**D**) PCNA immunostaining on renal sections from (**a**) sham, (**b**) I/R, (**c**) I/R + Farnesiferol B and (**d**) sham + Farnesiferol B groups (scale bar 50 μm). Quantitative analysis of (**E**) tubular injury scores, (**F**) TUNEL staining, (**G**) PCNA staining, and (**H**) serum creatinine from different groups. $n = 6$ mice/group. Data are means ± SD, one-way ANOVA with Bonferroni's test. * $p < 0.05$.

2.2. Farnesiferol B Reduces Oxidative Stress and Lipid Oxidative Signaling Pathways in I/R Kidney

I/R is often associated with oxidative stress, with existing evidence suggesting that oxidative stress is a paramount contributor in causing kidney damage [25]. Therefore, the effect of Farnesiferol B on oxidative stress in the kidney after I/R was evaluated. Immunohistochemical staining for NGAL neutrophil gelatinase-associated lipocalin (NGAL), an oxidative stress risk factor, showed that I/R may induced significant increases of oxidative stress in I/R kidneys (Figure 2A(b),B). The level of NGAL was reduced in mice treated with Farnesiferol B (Figure 2A(c),B). The potential mechanisms involved in the inhibitory effects of Farnesiferol B on I/R-induced oxidative stress were investigated. The I/R greatly increased the oxidative stress production and impaired antioxidant capacity in the injured kidney (Figure 2C–E). Farnesiferol B administration significantly diminished oxidative stress in the urine of injured group, namely H_2O_2 (hydrogen peroxide). Treatment with Farnesiferol B significantly increased the expression of Nrf2 and its downstream HO-1 (Figure 2D,E).

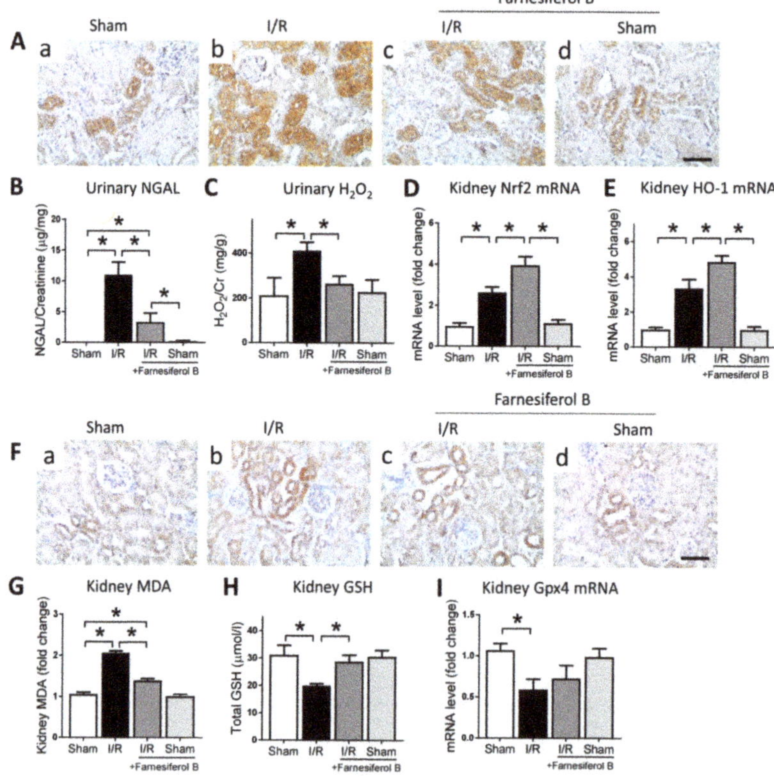

Figure 2. Farnesiferol B reduces oxidative stress in ischemia/reperfusion (I/R) kidney. (**A**) Representative images of immunostaining for NGAL on renal sections from (**a**) sham, (**b**) I/R, (**c**) I/R + Farnesiferol B and (**d**) sham + Farnesiferol B groups (scale bar 50 μm). (**B**) urinary neutrophil gelatinase-associated lipocalin (NGAL), (**C**) urinary H_2O_2, and kidney mRNA levels of (**D**) Nrf2 and (**E**) HO-1 were analyzed. $n = 6$ mice/group. Data are means ± SD, one-way ANOVA with Bonferroni's test. * $p < 0.05$. (**F**) Representative images of immunostaining for 4-HNE on renal sections from (**a**) sham, (**b**) I/R, (**c**) I/R + Farnesiferol B and (**d**) sham + Farnesiferol B groups (scale bar 50 μm). (**G**) kidney malondialdehyde (MDA), (**H**) kidney GSH, and kidney mRNA levels of (**I**) Gpx4 were analyzed. $n = 6$ mice/group. Data are means ± SD, one-way ANOVA with Bonferroni's test. * $p < 0.05$.

Reactive oxygen species accumulation can lead to lipid peroxidation and ferroptosis, a kind of regulated cell death [26]. The lipid peroxidation marker, 4-HNE (4-hydroxynonenal) and MDA (malondialdehyde), and markers related to ferroptosis were examined. The results show that 4-HNE and MDA levels were induced and GSH (glutathione) levels were reduced in the injured kidney (Figure 2F–H). Farnesiferol B administration reduced kidney lipid peroxidation and induced GSH level in the renal tissue homogenate. Furthermore, mRNA expression of Gpx4, the key ferroptosis regulator, was examined (Figure 2I). Gpx4 mRNA level was significantly down-regulated after I/R injury, whereas the expression seemed to be increased by Farnesiferol B treatment (not significantly). Taken together, the results indicated that anti-lipid peroxidation effects seen in Farnesiferol B treatment group could be an indirect result of its regulation on antioxidant pathways.

2.3. Farnesiferol B Protectes Kidney from I/R-Induced Inflammation and Inhibits NF-κB Signaling Pathway

The other oxidative stress-producer is the inflammatory cell such as monocytes and macrophages, which infiltrate into tissue, especially during acute inflammation [27]. Next, we analyzed the degree of kidney inflammation. I/R increased the positive stainings of macrophages and neutrophils in the kidney (Figure 3A–D). I/R also induced levels of TNFα and MCP-1 in mouse serum and kidney, as well as the proinflammatory mediator LTB$_4$ in the kidney (Figure 3E–I). The number of macrophages and neutrophils, as well as the serum and kidney levels of TNFα, MCP-1, and LTB4 were significantly reduced by Farnesiferol B treatment (Figure 3E–I). Inflammation-related genes expressed in the kidney were also measured. Quantitative analysis showed that I/R stimulated the expression of kidney TNFα, IL-6, and Icam mRNA levels, while levels of these mRNA decreased under treatment with Farnesiferol B (Figure 3J–L). The evidence presented here suggests a positive role of Farnesiferol B in attenuating renal inflammation.

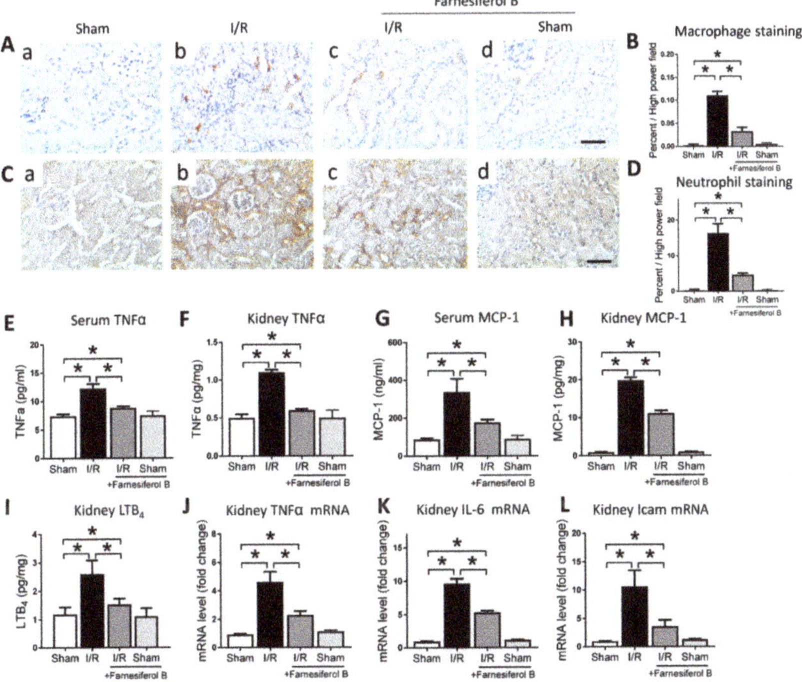

Figure 3. Farnesiferol B protects kidney from I/R-induced inflammation. (**A**) Representative images and (**B**) the quantitative analysis of positive immunostaining for macrophages on renal sections from (**a**) sham, (**b**) I/R, (**c**) I/R + Farnesiferol B, and (**d**) sham + Farnesiferol B groups (scale bar 50 μm). (**C**) Representative images and (**D**) the quantitative analysis of positive immunostaining for neutrophils on renal sections from (**a**) sham, (**b**) I/R, (**c**) I/R + Farnesiferol B, and (**d**) sham + Farnesiferol B groups (scale bar 50 μm). Levels of (**E**) serum TNFα, (**F**) kidney TNFα, (**G**) serum MCP-1, (**H**) kidney MCP-1, (**I**) kidney LTB$_4$, (**J**) kidney TNFα mRNA, (**K**) kidney IL-6 mRNA, and (**L**) kidney Icam mRNA from different treatment groups. $n = 6$ mice/group. Data are means ± SD, one-way ANOVA with Bonferroni's test. * $p < 0.05$.

NF-κB signaling pathway is one of the key inflammatory pathways during AKI. To examine the inhibitory effects of Farnesiferol B on I/R-induced inflammation, p65 levels from different treatment groups were evaluated. I/R induced increased tubulointerstitial staining of p65 in the kidney sections (Figure 4A(b)) and p65 translocation in the nuclei (Figure 4B). The I/R+Farnesiferol B group showed reduced levels of p65 immunostaining in kidney sections as well as nuclei translocation, indicating that part of anti-inflammatory effect is reacted on inflammatory cells.

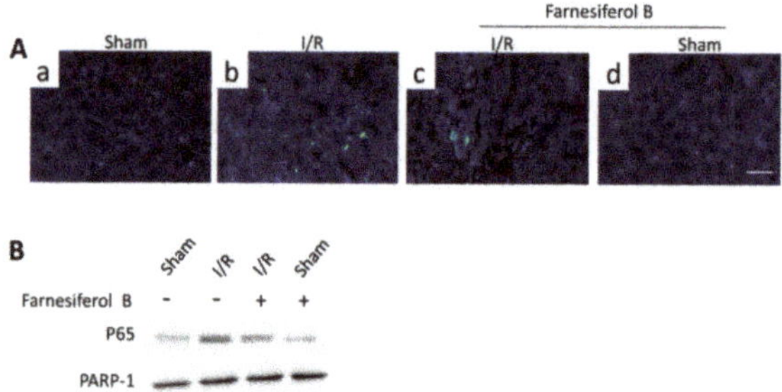

Figure 4. Farnesiferol B inhibits NF-κB signaling pathway in I/R kidney. (**A**) Representative images showing immunostaining of p65 on renal sections from (**a**) sham, (**b**) I/R, (**c**) I/R + Farnesiferol B and (**d**) sham + Farnesiferol B groups (scale bar 50 μm). (**B**) Representative immunoblotting image of nuclear protein for NF-κB p65 expression in kidney tissue. PARP-1 protein is used as the loading control.

2.4. Farnesiferol B Inhibits the Activity of Inflammatory Cells by Activating TGR5

To examine the direct effect of Farnesiferol B on macrophages, we conducted in vitro experiments using the J774 cell line. J774 macrophages were treated with LPS and/or Farnesiferol B and migration ability in a transwell system was monitored as a proxy for infiltration capability. Representative images show that migration induced by LPS was abolished by co-incubation with Farnesiferol B (Figure 5A). LPS-induced migration was associated with higher mRNA expression levels of TNFα, Ccl2, Ccl3 in macrophages, compared with that from the untreated cells. Treatment with Farnesiferol B lowered mRNA expression of these inflammatory cytokines significantly (Figure 5B–D).

Farnesiferol B was previously reported to be a TGR5 agonist, which can inhibit macrophage infiltration through inhibiting NF-κB activation [28]. Based on this, we speculated that the anti-inflammatory effect of Farnesiferol B may be related to its ability to activate TGR5. Therefore, we evaluated the regulatory effect of Farnesiferol B on LPS-induced NF-κB activation in J774 macrophages. Immunoblotting of nuclear protein for NF-κB p65 indicated an LPS-induced nuclear translocation in J774 macrophages (Figure 5E). Similar to INT777, a known TGR5 agonist, Farnesiferol B also significantly reduced p65 translocation in a dose-dependent way (Figure 5E). PARP-1 was stably expressed between groups as a nucleoprotein control (Figure 5E). An NF-κB binding assay also revealed that LPS-induced NF-κB binding activity was blocked by Farnesiferol B or INT777 co-incubation (Figure 5F), which was consistent with previous publications [29].

In order to further verify the target of Farnesiferol B in macrophages, RAW264.7 cells, which do not express TGR5 [30], were exposed to LPS with and without Farnesiferol B. As shown in Figure 6, Farnesiferol B could not inhibit LPS-induced cell migration, suggesting that Farnesiferol B suppresses LPS-mediated macrophage migration by activating TGR5. Benzoxathiole derivative (BOT), an NF-κB inhibitor, was used as a positive control to block LPS-induced migration (Figure 6c). Taken together, Farnesiferol B inhibits the LPS-induced NF-κB pathway by activating TGR5.

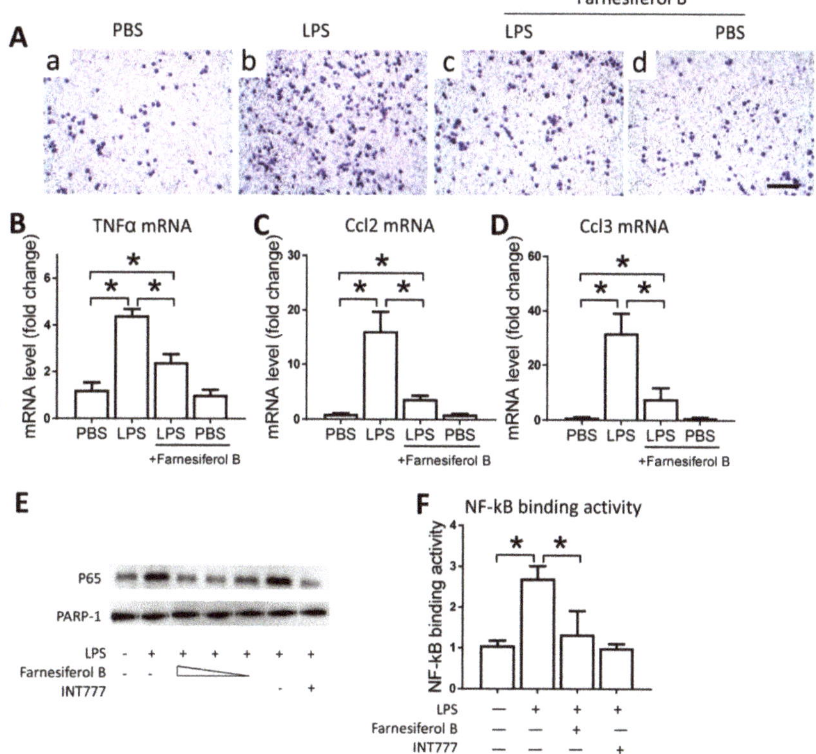

Figure 5. Farnesiferol B inhibits the activity of inflammatory cells by activating TGR5. (**A**) Representative images of J774 cells seeded in 3-μm pore polycarbonate membrane and stained with crystal violet for migration analysis (scale bar 100 μm) after treatment with (a) PBS, (b) LPS, (c) LPS+Farnesiferol B, or (d) PBS+Farnesiferol B. Level of mRNA for (**B**) TNFα, (**C**) Ccl2 and (**D**) Ccl3 with different treatments. (**E**) Representative immunoblotting image of nuclear protein for NF-κB p65 expression. J774 cells were treated with 100 ng/mL LPS with or without co-incubation with Farnesiferol B at 5 μM, 10 μM and 20 μM, or INT777 for 2 h. (**F**) NF-κB DNA binding activity. Data are means ± SD of at least three independent experiments, one-way ANOVA with Bonferroni's test. * $p < 0.05$.

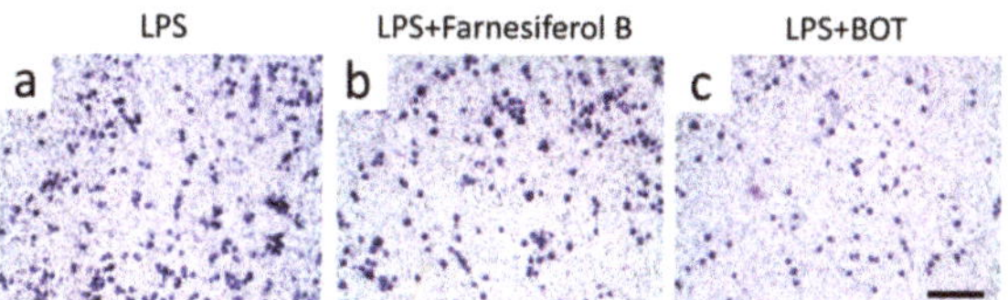

Figure 6. Farnesiferol does not inhibit migration of inflammatory cells not expressing TGR5. Representative images of RAW 264.7 macrophages seeded in 3-μm pore polycarbonate membrane with different treatment for 2 h, and stained with crystal violet for migration assay (scale bar 100 μm). Cells were treated with (**a**) 100 ng/mL LPS, (**b**) LPS with 20 μM Farnesiferol co-incubation, and (**c**) LPS with a NF-κB inhibitor, benzoxathiole derivative (BOT).

3. Discussion

In the current study, our results point out that Farnesiferol B treatment play a beneficial role in renal I/R injury. Compared with I/R treated mice, Farnesiferol B-treated mice showed lower score of renal injury, while significantly decreased levels of histological tubular injury, oxidative stress, and inflammation (Figure 7). In line with and based on our experiments in mice, the in vitro analysis show that Farnesiferol B reduces LPS-induced macrophage migration. Moreover, Farnesiferol B can inhibit NF-κB nuclear translocation through activating TGR5 in macrophages. Thus, Farnesiferol B might represent a novel natural compound against I/R-induced kidney damage.

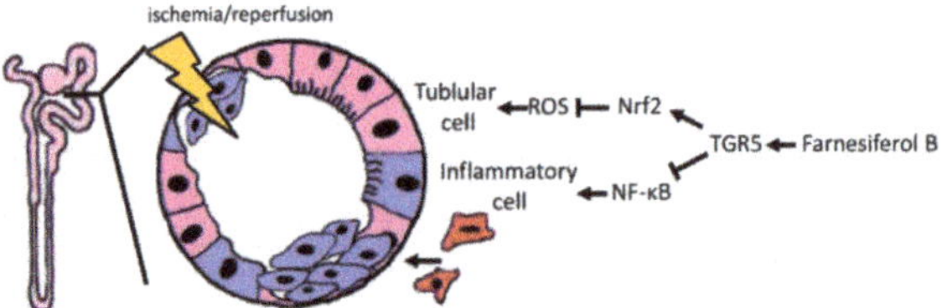

Figure 7. Model of the Farnesiferol B-mediated protection against ischemia/reperfusion-induced AKI. I/R induces ROS generation that causes tubular cell damage (shown in purple-blue). In parallel, inflammatory cell infiltration (shown in red) also promotes oxidative stress and post-hypoxic kidney damage after I/R. Farnesiferol B-mediated TGR5 activation induces the antioxidant Nrf2 pathway and inhibits the proinflammatory NF-κB signaling pathway, which in turn protects the kidney from tubular damage and inflammation.

Ischaemia-reperfusion (I/R) injury is the main cause of AKI under common clinical conditions [31,32]. Nowadays, the pathogenesis of AKI is characterized by renal tubular damage, inflammation, and vascular dysfunction [33,34]. In vivo experiment, we examined the kidney of AKI mice and found that Farnesiferol B effectively reduced the regulated cell death and oxidative stress. Although it was hard to identify the exact type of cell death, both results of TUNEL assay and ferroptosis marker Gxp4 showed that Farnesiferol B have protective effects on tubular cell damage during AKI. NGAL is an early biomarker of AKI which is produced in the distal nephron and its synthesis is upregulated in response to kidney injury [35]. Recent evidence demonstrates that high NGAL level is a risk factor for oxidative stress in patients [36]. In our case, I/R increased highly expression of NGAL in mice. Furthermore, Farnesiferol B reduced the NGAL level both in kidney and in urine, as well as the other oxidative stress marker MDA. Furthermore, with treatment of Farnesiferol B, GSH levels was increased and Nrf2 and HO-1 expression were restored in the I/R injured kidney, while at the same time, reduced oxidative stress (H_2O_2) and lipid peroxidation (4-HNE and MDA). These data indicated that antioxidant related pathways may be regulated by Farnesiferol B-TGR5 signaling pathway. Nrf2 and its target gene, HO-1, has generally been considered to be an adaptive cellular response to oxidative stress [26]. Recently, Nrf2/HO-1 has also been shown to be protective in AKI and diabetic nephropathy [37–39]. It has been reported that treatment with either FXR/TGR5 dual agonist INT-767 or TGR5 specific agonist INT-777 could prevent diabetic nephropathy through inducing Nrf2-mediated antioxidant generation, and reducing renal expression of oxidative stress [23,40]. We have seen similar effects in the I/R-induced mouse AKI model with treatment with FXR/TGR5 dual agonist [25]. In the study, treatment with 6alpha-ethyl-chenodeoxycholic acid (6-ECDCA), a potent dual FXR/TGR5 agonist [41], significantly improved Nrf2-mediated antioxidant capacity. Silencing of Nrf2 blocked the antioxidant effect of 6-ECDCA in proximal tubule cells exposed to hypoxia. Based on these findings, TGR5 could be a potent target to induce antioxidant pathways. However, to identify the renal signaling pathways regulated by FXR and TGR5 respectively and specify the regulatory effects of TGR5 on antioxidant pathways need to be further studied.

Renal inflammation after I/R is directly related to monocyte infiltration and macrophage activation [25,42]. TGR5, also called GPBAR1 or GPR131, is a bile acid–responsive G protein-coupled receptor, which plays a crucial role in protection against diet-induced diabetes through different cellular mechanisms [43]. The role of TGF5 activation in modulating inflammatory pathways was confirmed in experiments on mice and immune cells [21,28]. Recent evidence suggests that activation of TGR5 regulates inflammatory cell signaling pathways such as NF-κB, AKT and extracellular signal-regulated kinase (ERK) [44,45]. Macrophages play a pivotal role in kidney injury, inflammation, and fibrosis [46]. In the present study, we can clearly notice that, after I/R, the mice shown an increased inflammation level on renal tissue (e.g., the infiltration of macrophages and neutrophils in Figure 3 and high expression of p65 in Figure 5), as well as high level of proinflammatory factors (TNFα, MCP-1, IL-6) both in serum and kidney tissue. While the treatment with Farnesiferol B demonstrated a critical anti-inflammatory effects by reducing those inflammatory factors or NF-κB activation. However, NF-κB signaling can be activated in all cell types during AKI, thereby immunostaining or immunoblotting providing only limited information about cell-specific NF-κB functions in the kidney during AKI [47]. Therefore, we employed the in vitro experiments. Our results shown that Farnesiferol B effectively inhibited the expression of inflammatory cytokines, such as MCP-1, LTB4, and TNFα. Farnesiferol B inhibited LPS-induced NF-κB activation and decreased p65 translocation in J774 macrophages, possessing similar effects as other TGR5 agonists [40]. Moreover, the anti-inflammatory effect of Farnesiferol B was blocked in RAW264.7 cells, which do not express TGR5 [21,30]. Taken together, these results indicate that Farnesiferol B inhibits LPS-induced NF-κB activation through activating TGR5, which is consistent with previous predictive results [17].

Ferula species from the family Apiaceae are rich sources of biologically active natural products including sesquiterpene coumarins (SCs) and sesquiterpenes [48]. Some studies have shown that SCs are able to enhance the cytotoxicity of anticancer compounds [49]. Recently Kasaian et al. showed enhancement of doxorubicin cytotoxicity in MCF-7/Adr cells (doxorubicin resistant derivatives of MCF-7 cells overexpressing P-gp) when combined with non-toxic concentrations of farnesiferols, proving the significant activity of Farnesiferol B on multi-drug resistant cells [50]. Previous studies show that sesquiterpene coumarins and their derivative from *Ferula fukanensis* reduces IL-6 and TNFα, while inducing nitric oxide synthase in RAW264.7 cells, possessing inhibitory effects on LPS and IFN-γ induced pro-inflammatory cytokine release and nitric oxide production [51,52]. A recent study also showed the anti-inflammatory effect of *Ferula szowitsiana* in vitro, which indicates that Farnesiferol B might inhibit neuroinflammation via reducing the generation of inflammatory cytokines [53]. In this study, we show the active effect of Farnesiferol B on TGR5, which suppresses the NF-κB p65 binding activity and inhibits macrophage migration.

4. Materials and Methods

4.1. Animals Study Approval and Tissue Samples

All animal experiments conformed to both Swiss and Chinese animal protection laws and were approved (May, 2015) by the Scientific Animal Study Committee of Shandong University, Jinan, China (study number 2015064).

Six-week-old female C57/BJ mice were randomly assigned to I/R or sham procedures. They were divided into four groups with six animals each: sham, I/R, I/R + Farnesiferol B and sham + Farnesiferol B. AKI was induced by unilateral nephrectomy and contralateral ischemia and reperfusion, as previously described [25]. For Farnesiferol B treatment, mice were injected intraperitoneally (i.p.) with Farnesiferol B (10 mg/kg, Golexir Pars Co., Mashhad, Iran) 2 h before the procedure. All mice were killed under anesthesia 24 h after surgery. Kidneys were harvested for further analysis.

4.2. Measurements in Serum, Urine, and Kidney Samples

Urinary H_2O_2 and NGAL levels were measured in the resulting urine samples with the Amplex Red H_2O_2 assay kit (A12214, Invitrogen, Carlsbad, CA, USA) and Mouse Lipocalin-2/NGAL ELISA Kit (ab119601, Abcam, Cambridge, UK). Serum creatinine, MCP-1, TNFα, and LTB4 levels were measured with a creatinine assay kit (ab65340, Abcam, Cambridge, UK), Mouse MCP1 ELISA Kit (ab100721, Abcam), Mouse TNF alpha ELISA Kit (ab46105, Abcam), and LTB4 Parameter Assay Kit (KGE006B; R&D Systems, Minneapolis, MN, USA), respectively. Kidney malondialdehyde (MDA) levels were measured by a Lipid Peroxidation (MDA) Assay Kit (ab118970, Abcam).

4.3. Renal Pathological Assessments and Immunostaining

Tissue sections were stained with hematoxylin and eosin (HE) using standard protocols. TUNEL staining was performed with an ApopTag kit (Millipore, Billerica, MA, USA) based on the manufacturer's instructions. The antibodies for immunohistochemistry used in this study were those against Kim-1 (ab78494, Abcam), 4-hydroxynonenal (4-HNE, ab46545, Abcam), neutrophil gelatinase-associated lipocalin (NGAL, ab63929, Abcam), Ly-6B (NBP2-13077), NFκB p65 (sc-372, Santa Cruz, CA, USA), and MAC387 (ab22506, Abcam). Sections were treated with the Envision+ DAB kit (Dako, Basel, Switzerland) according to the manufacturer's instructions.

4.4. Cell Culture and Migration Assay

J774 cells were grown in Dulbecco's modified Eagle's medium and RAW264.7 macrophages were maintained in RPMI 1640 medium. Both cell culture media were supplemented with 10% FCS, 100 U/mL penicillin, and 100 mg/mL streptomycin. Cells were cultured at 37 °C in a humidified atmosphere with 5% CO_2.

For LPS treatment, J774 or RAW cells were treated with 100 ng/mL LPS with or without co-incubation of 20 μM Farnesiferol B for 2 h. Afterwards, RNA and protein were extracted for further analysis. For the migration assay, cells were seeded in 3-μm pore polycarbonate membrane inserts (Costar Corning, Darmstadt, Germany) on 12-well plates and treated with 100 ng/mL LPS (L3254, Sigma, St. Louis, MO, USA) or 20 μM Farnesiferol for 2 h at 37 °C. The inserts were washed, fixed, and stained with crystal violet for analysis.

4.5. NF-κB DNA Binding Assay

The assay was performed with a NF-κB p65 Transcription Factor Assay kit (ab133112, Abcam). Briefly, nuclear extracts from cells were incubated with a double stranded DNA sequence containing the NF-κB response element overnight. After washing, an NF-κB antibody was added and incubated for 1 h. Then an HRP-conjugated secondary antibody was added for 1 h and washed twice. After incubation with developing solution for 30 min, stop solution was added and the results were analyzed with a microplate reader (Glomax, Promega, Madison, WI, USA).

4.6. Isolation of RNA from Kidney Tissue and Quantitative Real-Time Polymerase Chain Reaction (qRT-PCR)

Total RNA was prepared using Trizol (Invitrogen, Carlsbad, CA, USA). The mRNA was quantified based on absorbance at 260 nm. After DNAse (Promega) treatment, 2 μg total RNA was reverse transcribed using oligo-dT priming and Superscript II (Invitrogen). First-strand complementary DNA was used as the template for real-time polymerase chain reaction analysis with TaqMan master mix and primers (Life Technologies, Carlsbad, CA, USA). Primers used were TNFα (No. Mm00443258-m1), Icam1 (No. Mm00516023_m1), IL-6 (No. Mm00446190_m1), Ccl2 (No. Mm00441242_m1), Ccl3 (No. Mm00441259_g1), Gpx4 (No. Mm00515041_m1), Nrf2 (No. Mm00477784_m1), HO-1 (No. Mm00516005_m1). Transcript levels, determined in two independent complementary DNA preparations, were calculated and expressed relative to levels of RNA for the housekeeping gene beta-actin (No. Mm00607939-s1) or GAPDH (No. Mm99999915-g1).

4.7. Western Blotting

Protein lysates (20 μg protein) from cells nuclear were separated by SDS-PAGE and blotted on polyvinylidene difluoride membranes (Millipore, Burlingtob, MA, USA). The membranes were incubated overnight at 4 °C with the respective primary antibodies and secondary antibodies accordingly. Staining was then developed using the ECL Plus detection system (Amersham Biosciences, Little Chalfont, UK). The antibodies used were anti-p65 (sc-372, Santa Cruz, Recife, Pernambuco) and PARP-1 (AV33754, Sigma-Aldrich).

4.8. Statistics

Data are expressed as means ± SD. For data relating to baseline characteristics and histological analysis, groups were compared by one-way ANOVA followed by Bonferroni's test. Statistical analyses were performed using GraphPad software (GraphPad Software Inc., San Diego, CA, USA).

5. Conclusions

In vivo, the present study clearly demonstrates that Farnesiferol B protects kidney from I/R-induced damage by reducing oxidative stress and inflammation. In vitro, Farnesiferol B ameliorates macrophage migration by activating TGR5.

Author Contributions: All authors (L.Z., X.F., T.G., T.W., Z.W., G.A.K.-U. and Z.G.) were responsible for: acquisition of data, or analysis and interpretation of data, final approval of the version to be published. Additionally, L.Z., X.F., T.W. and Z.G. were responsible for substantial contributions to conception and design and drafting the manuscript. Especially, L.Z., T.G., and Z.G. were responsible for revising the manuscript critically for important intellectual content.

Funding: This study was financially supported by the Swiss National Science foundation (grant No. 310030_175639) to G.A.K.-U., the National Natural Science foundation of China (grant Nos. 81530097, 81473369 and 81222051), the National Key Research and Development Program of China (No. 2017YFC1702703), and "Taishan Scholar" program.

Acknowledgments: We thank Sophia Samodelov for proofreading of the manuscript.

Conflicts of Interest: The authors declare no conflict of interest.

Abbreviations

4-HNE	4-hydroxynonenal
AKI	Acute kidney injury
ERK	Extracellular signal-regulated kinase
GPBAR1	G protein–coupled bile acid receptor 1
H_2O_2	Hydrogen peroxide
Icam	Intercellular adhesion molecule
IL-6	Interleukin-6
i.p.	Intraperitoneally
I/R	Ischemia/reperfusion
IRI	Ischemia/reperfusion injury
Kim1	Kidney injury molecule-1
MDA	Malondialdehyde
NF-κB	Nuclear factor-kappa B
NGAL	Neutrophil gelatinase-associated lipocalin
RIR	Renal ischemia reperfusion
ROS	Reactive oxygen species
TNFα	Tumor necrosis factor alpha

References

1. Bonventre, J.V. Pathophysiology of AKI: Injury and normal and abnormal repair. *Contrib. Nephrol.* **2010**, *165*, 9–17. [PubMed]
2. Saat, T.C.; van den Akker, E.K.; JN, I.J.; Dor, F.J.; de Bruin, R.W. Improving the outcome of kidney transplantation by ameliorating renal ischemia reperfusion injury: Lost in translation? *J. Transl. Med.* **2016**, *14*, 20. [CrossRef] [PubMed]
3. Smith, S.F.; Hosgood, S.A.; Nicholson, M.L. Ischemia-reperfusion injury in renal transplantation: 3 key signaling pathways in tubular epithelial cells. *Kidney Int.* **2019**, *95*, 50–56. [CrossRef] [PubMed]
4. Yang, B.; Lan, S.; Dieude, M.; Sabo-Vatasescu, J.P.; Karakeussian-Rimbaud, A.; Turgeon, J.; Qi, S.; Gunaratnam, L.; Patey, N.; Hebert, M.J. Caspase-3 Is a Pivotal Regulator of Microvascular Rarefaction and Renal Fibrosis after Ischemia-Reperfusion Injury. *J. Am. Soc. Nephrol.* **2018**, *29*, 1900–1916. [CrossRef]

5. Minutoli, L.; Puzzolo, D.; Rinaldi, M.; Irrera, N.; Marini, H.; Arcoraci, V.; Bitto, A.; Crea, G.; Pisani, A.; Squadrito, F.; et al. ROS-Mediated NLRP3 Inflammasome Activation in Brain, Heart, Kidney, and Testis Ischemia/Reperfusion Injury. *Oxid Med. Cell Longev.* **2016**, *2016*, 2183026. [CrossRef]

6. Raup-Konsavage, W.M.; Wang, Y.; Wang, W.W.; Feliers, D.; Ruan, H.; Reeves, W.B. Neutrophil peptidyl arginine deiminase-4 has a pivotal role in ischemia/reperfusion-induced acute kidney injury. *Kidney Int.* **2018**, *93*, 365–374. [CrossRef]

7. Masola, V.; Zaza, G.; Bellin, G.; Dall'Olmo, L.; Granata, S.; Vischini, G.; Secchi, M.F.; Lupo, A.; Gambaro, G.; Onisto, M. Heparanase regulates the M1 polarization of renal macrophages and their crosstalk with renal epithelial tubular cells after ischemia/reperfusion injury. *FASEB J.* **2018**, *32*, 742–756. [CrossRef]

8. Bonventre, J.V.; Weinberg, J.M. Recent advances in the pathophysiology of ischemic acute renal failure. *J. Am. Soc. Nephrol.* **2003**, *14*, 2199–2210. [CrossRef]

9. Ratliff, B.B.; Abdulmahdi, W.; Pawar, R.; Wolin, M.S. Oxidant Mechanisms in Renal Injury and Disease. *Antioxid. Redox Signal.* **2016**, *25*, 119–146. [CrossRef]

10. Mittal, M.; Siddiqui, M.R.; Tran, K.; Reddy, S.P.; Malik, A.B. Reactive oxygen species in inflammation and tissue injury. *Antioxid. Redox Signal.* **2014**, *20*, 1126–1167. [CrossRef]

11. Paller, M.S. Effect of neutrophil depletion on ischemic renal injury in the rat. *J. Lab. Clin. Med.* **1989**, *113*, 379–386. [PubMed]

12. Lever, J.M.; Boddu, R.; George, J.F.; Agarwal, A. Heme Oxygenase-1 in Kidney Health and Disease. *Antioxid. Redox Signal.* **2016**, *25*, 165–183. [CrossRef] [PubMed]

13. Li, C.; Jackson, R.M. Reactive species mechanisms of cellular hypoxia-reoxygenation injury. *Am. J. Physiol. Cell Physiol.* **2002**, *282*, C227–C241. [CrossRef] [PubMed]

14. Abd El-Razek, M.H.; Ohta, S.; Ahmed, A.A.; Hirata, T. Sesquiterpene coumarins from the roots of Ferula assa-foetida. *Phytochemistry* **2001**, *58*, 1289–1295. [CrossRef]

15. Ahmed, A.A.; Hegazy, M.E.; Zellagui, A.; Rhouati, S.; Mohamed, T.A.; Sayed, A.A.; Abdella, M.A.; Ohta, S.; Hirata, T. Ferulsinaic acid, a sesquiterpene coumarin with a rare carbon skeleton from Ferula species. *Phytochemistry* **2007**, *68*, 680–686. [CrossRef]

16. Dastan, D.; Salehi, P.; Reza Gohari, A.; Zimmermann, S.; Kaiser, M.; Hamburger, M.; Reza Khavasi, H.; Ebrahimi, S.N. Disesquiterpene and sesquiterpene coumarins from Ferula pseudalliacea, and determination of their absolute configurations. *Phytochemistry* **2012**, *78*, 170–178. [CrossRef]

17. Kirchweger, B.; Kratz, J.M.; Ladurner, A.; Grienke, U.; Langer, T.; Dirsch, V.M.; Rollinger, J.M. In Silico Workflow for the Discovery of Natural Products Activating the G Protein-Coupled Bile Acid Receptor 1. *Front. Chem.* **2018**, *6*, 242. [CrossRef]

18. Porez, G.; Prawitt, J.; Gross, B.; Staels, B. Bile acid receptors as targets for the treatment of dyslipidemia and cardiovascular disease. *J. Lipid Res.* **2012**, *53*, 1723–1737. [CrossRef]

19. Pols, T.W.; Noriega, L.G.; Nomura, M.; Auwerx, J.; Schoonjans, K. The bile acid membrane receptor TGR5 as an emerging target in metabolism and inflammation. *J. Hepatol.* **2011**, *54*, 1263–1272. [CrossRef]

20. Keitel, V.; Reinehr, R.; Gatsios, P.; Rupprecht, C.; Gorg, B.; Selbach, O.; Haussinger, D.; Kubitz, R. The G-protein coupled bile salt receptor TGR5 is expressed in liver sinusoidal endothelial cells. *Hepatology* **2007**, *45*, 695–704. [CrossRef]

21. Kawamata, Y.; Fujii, R.; Hosoya, M.; Harada, M.; Yoshida, H.; Miwa, M.; Fukusumi, S.; Habata, Y.; Itoh, T.; Shintani, Y.; et al. A G protein-coupled receptor responsive to bile acids. *J. Biol. Chem.* **2003**, *278*, 9435–9440. [CrossRef] [PubMed]

22. Keitel, V.; Donner, M.; Winandy, S.; Kubitz, R.; Haussinger, D. Expression and function of the bile acid receptor TGR5 in Kupffer cells. *Biochem. Biophys. Res. Commun.* **2008**, *372*, 78–84. [CrossRef] [PubMed]

23. Wang, X.X.; Edelstein, M.H.; Gafter, U.; Qiu, L.; Luo, Y.; Dobrinskikh, E.; Lucia, S.; Adorini, L.; D'Agati, V.D.; Levi, J.; et al. G Protein-Coupled Bile Acid Receptor TGR5 Activation Inhibits Kidney Disease in Obesity and Diabetes. *J. Am. Soc. Nephrol.* **2016**, *27*, 1362–1378. [CrossRef] [PubMed]

24. Su, J.; Zhang, Q.; Qi, H.; Wu, L.; Li, Y.; Yu, D.; Huang, W.; Chen, W.D.; Wang, Y.D. The G-protein-coupled bile acid receptor Gpbar1 (TGR5) protects against renal inflammation and renal cancer cell proliferation and migration through antagonizing NF-kappaB and STAT3 signaling pathways. *Oncotarget* **2017**, *8*, 54378–54387. [CrossRef]

25. Gai, Z.; Chu, L.; Xu, Z.; Song, X.; Sun, D.; Kullak-Ublick, G.A. Farnesoid X receptor activation protects the kidney from ischemia-reperfusion damage. *Sci. Rep.* **2017**, *7*, 9815. [CrossRef]

26. Dixon, S.J.; Stockwell, B.R. The role of iron and reactive oxygen species in cell death. *Nat. Chem. Biol.* **2014**, *10*, 9–17. [CrossRef]

27. Scindia, Y.; Dey, P.; Thirunagari, A.; Liping, H.; Rosin, D.L.; Floris, M.; Okusa, M.D.; Swaminathan, S. Hepcidin Mitigates Renal Ischemia-Reperfusion Injury by Modulating Systemic Iron Homeostasis. *J. Am. Soc. Nephrol.* **2015**, *26*, 2800–2814. [CrossRef]

28. Perino, A.; Pols, T.W.; Nomura, M.; Stein, S.; Pellicciari, R.; Schoonjans, K. TGR5 reduces macrophage migration through mTOR-induced C/EBPbeta differential translation. *J. Clin. Investig.* **2014**, *124*, 5424–5436. [CrossRef]

29. Pols, T.W.; Nomura, M.; Harach, T.; Lo Sasso, G.; Oosterveer, M.H.; Thomas, C.; Rizzo, G.; Gioiello, A.; Adorini, L.; Pellicciari, R.; et al. TGR5 activation inhibits atherosclerosis by reducing macrophage inflammation and lipid loading. *Cell Metab.* **2011**, *14*, 747–757. [CrossRef]

30. Miyazaki-Anzai, S.; Masuda, M.; Levi, M.; Keenan, A.L.; Miyazaki, M. Dual activation of the bile acid nuclear receptor FXR and G-protein-coupled receptor TGR5 protects mice against atherosclerosis. *PLoS ONE* **2014**, *9*, e108270. [CrossRef]

31. Verma, S.K.; Molitoris, B.A. Renal endothelial injury and microvascular dysfunction in acute kidney injury. *Semin. Nephrol.* **2015**, *35*, 96–107. [CrossRef] [PubMed]

32. Liano, F.; Pascual, J. Epidemiology of acute renal failure: A prospective, multicenter, community-based study. Madrid Acute Renal Failure Study Group. *Kidney Int.* **1996**, *50*, 811–818. [CrossRef] [PubMed]

33. Martin-Sanchez, D.; Fontecha-Barriuso, M.; Carrasco, S.; Sanchez-Nino, M.D.; Massenhausen, A.V.; Linkermann, A.; Cannata-Ortiz, P.; Ruiz-Ortega, M.; Egido, J.; Ortiz, A.; et al. TWEAK and RIPK1 mediate a second wave of cell death during AKI. *Proc. Natl. Acad. Sci. USA* **2018**, *115*, 4182–4187. [CrossRef]

34. Linkermann, A.; Stockwell, B.R.; Krautwald, S.; Anders, H.J. Regulated cell death and inflammation: An auto-amplification loop causes organ failure. *Nat. Rev. Immunol.* **2014**, *14*, 759–767. [CrossRef]

35. Devarajan, P. Neutrophil gelatinase-associated lipocalin (NGAL): A new marker of kidney disease. *Scand. J. Clin. Lab. Invest.* **2008**, *68* (Suppl. 241), 89–94. [CrossRef]

36. Nevo, A.; Armaly, Z.; Abd El Kadir, A.; Douvdevani, A.; Tovbin, D. Elevated Neutrophil Gelatinase Lipocalin Levels Are Associated with Increased Oxidative Stress in Hemodialysis Patients. *J. Clin. Med. Res.* **2018**, *10*, 461–465. [CrossRef]

37. Ibrahim, Z.S.; Alkafafy, M.E.; Ahmed, M.M.; Soliman, M.M. Renoprotective effect of curcumin against the combined oxidative stress of diabetes and nicotine in rats. *Mol. Med. Rep.* **2016**, *13*, 3017–3026. [CrossRef]

38. Sun, Q.; Meng, Q.T.; Jiang, Y.; Liu, H.M.; Lei, S.Q.; Su, W.T.; Duan, W.N.; Wu, Y.; Xia, Z.Y.; Xia, Z.Y. Protective effect of ginsenoside Rb1 against intestinal ischemia-reperfusion induced acute renal injury in mice. *PLoS ONE* **2013**, *8*, e80859. [CrossRef]

39. Shalaby, R.H.; Rashed, L.A.; Ismaail, A.E.; Madkour, N.K.; Elwakeel, S.H. Hematopoietic stem cells derived from human umbilical cord ameliorate cisplatin-induced acute renal failure in rats. *Am. J. Stem. Cells* **2014**, *3*, 83–96.

40. Wang, X.X.; Wang, D.; Luo, Y.; Myakala, K.; Dobrinskikh, E.; Rosenberg, A.Z.; Levi, J.; Kopp, J.B.; Field, A.; Hill, A.; et al. FXR/TGR5 Dual Agonist Prevents Progression of Nephropathy in Diabetes and Obesity. *J. Am. Soc. Nephrol.* **2018**, *29*, 118–137. [CrossRef]

41. Gioiello, A.; Rosatelli, E.; Nuti, R.; Macchiarulo, A.; Pellicciari, R. Patented TGR5 modulators: A review (2006–present). *Expert Opin. Pat.* **2012**, *22*, 1399–1414. [CrossRef] [PubMed]

42. Zhang, R.; He, G.; Wang, Y.; Wang, J.; Chen, W.; Xu, Y. The effect of different treatments of lymph after intestinal ischemia-reperfusion in rats on macrophages in vitro. *PLoS ONE* **2019**, *14*, e0211195. [CrossRef] [PubMed]

43. Harach, T.; Pols, T.W.; Nomura, M.; Maida, A.; Watanabe, M.; Auwerx, J.; Schoonjans, K. TGR5 potentiates GLP-1 secretion in response to anionic exchange resins. *Sci. Rep.* **2012**, *2*, 430. [CrossRef] [PubMed]

44. Kida, T.; Tsubosaka, Y.; Hori, M.; Ozaki, H.; Murata, T. Bile acid receptor TGR5 agonism induces NO production and reduces monocyte adhesion in vascular endothelial cells. *Arter. Thromb. Vasc. Biol.* **2013**, *33*, 1663–1669. [CrossRef] [PubMed]

45. Masyuk, A.I.; Huang, B.Q.; Radtke, B.N.; Gajdos, G.B.; Splinter, P.L.; Masyuk, T.V.; Gradilone, S.A.; LaRusso, N.F. Ciliary subcellular localization of TGR5 determines the cholangiocyte functional response to bile acid signaling. *Am. J. Physiol. Gastrointest. Liver Physiol.* **2013**, *304*, G1013–G1024. [CrossRef]

46. Cao, Q.; Harris, D.C.; Wang, Y. Macrophages in kidney injury, inflammation, and fibrosis. *Physiology* **2015**, *30*, 183–194. [CrossRef]

47. Marko, L.; Vigolo, E.; Hinze, C.; Park, J.K.; Roel, G.; Balogh, A.; Choi, M.; Wubken, A.; Cording, J.; Blasig, I.E.; et al. Tubular Epithelial NF-kappaB Activity Regulates Ischemic AKI. *J. Am. Soc. Nephrol.* **2016**, *27*, 2658–2669. [CrossRef]

48. Sattar, Z.; Iranshahi, M. Phytochemistry and pharmacology of Ferula persica Boiss.: A review. *Iran. J. Basic Med. Sci.* **2017**, *20*, 1–8.

49. Behnam Rassouli, F.; Matin, M.M.; Iranshahi, M.; Bahrami, A.R.; Neshati, V.; Mollazadeh, S.; Neshati, Z. Mogoltacin enhances vincristine cytotoxicity in human transitional cell carcinoma (TCC) cell line. *Phytomedicine* **2009**, *16*, 181–187. [CrossRef]

50. Kasaian, J.; Mosaffa, F.; Behravan, J.; Masullo, M.; Piacente, S.; Ghandadi, M.; Iranshahi, M. Reversal of P-glycoprotein-mediated multidrug resistance in MCF-7/Adr cancer cells by sesquiterpene coumarins. *Fitoterapia* **2015**, *103*, 149–154. [CrossRef]

51. Motai, T.; Daikonya, A.; Kitanaka, S. Sesquiterpene coumarins from Ferula fukanensis and their pro-inflammatory cytokine gene expression inhibitory effects. *Chem. Pharm. Bull.* **2013**, *61*, 618–623. [CrossRef] [PubMed]

52. Motai, T.; Kitanaka, S. Sesquiterpene coumarins from Ferula fukanensis and nitric oxide production inhibitory effects. *Chem. Pharm. Bull.* **2004**, *52*, 1215–1518. [CrossRef] [PubMed]

53. Xing, Y.; Li, N.; Zhou, D.; Chen, G.; Jiao, K.; Wang, W.; Si, Y.; Hou, Y. Sesquiterpene Coumarins from Ferula sinkiangensis Act as Neuroinflammation Inhibitors. *Planta Med.* **2017**, *83*, 135–142. [CrossRef]

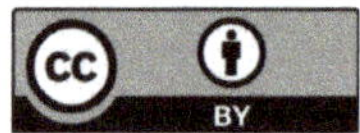

International Journal of
Molecular Sciences

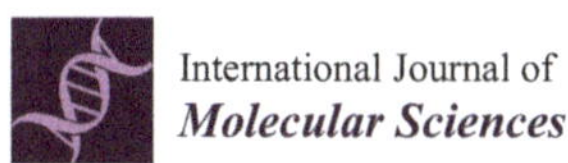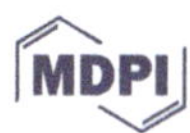

Article

Renal Chemerin Expression is Induced in Models of Hypertensive Nephropathy and Glomerulonephritis and Correlates with Markers of Inflammation and Fibrosis

Alexander Mocker [1], Karl F. Hilgers [2], Nada Cordasic [2], Rainer Wachtveitl [2], Carlos Menendez-Castro [1], Joachim Woelfle [1], Andrea Hartner [1,†] and Fabian B. Fahlbusch [1,*,†]

1   Department of Pediatrics and Adolescent Medicine, University Hospital of Erlangen, 91054 Erlangen, Germany; alexmocker@t-online.de (A.M.); Carlos.Menendez-Castro@uk-erlangen.de (C.M.-C.); joachim.woelfle@uk-erlangen.de (J.W.); andrea.hartner@uk-erlangen.de (A.H.)
2   Department of Nephrology and Hypertension, University Hospital of Erlangen, 91054 Erlangen, Germany; karl.hilgers@uk-erlangen.de (K.F.H.); Nada.Cordasic@uk-erlangen.de (N.C.); Rainer.Wachtveitl@uk-erlangen.de (R.W.)
*   Correspondence: fabian.fahlbusch@uk-erlangen.de; Tel.: +49-9131-8533-118; Fax: +49-9131-8533-714
†   These authors contributed equally to this work.

Received: 25 October 2019; Accepted: 9 December 2019; Published: 11 December 2019

Abstract: Chemerin and its receptor, chemokine-like receptor 1 (CmklR1), are associated with chemotaxis, inflammation, and endothelial function, especially in metabolic syndrome, coronary heart disease, and hypertension. In humans, circulating chemerin levels and renal function show an inverse relation. So far, little is known about the potential role of chemerin in hypertensive nephropathy and renal inflammation. Therefore, we determined systemic and renal chemerin levels in 2-kidney-1-clip (2k1c) hypertensive and Thy1.1 nephritic rats, respectively, to explore the correlation between chemerin and markers of renal inflammation and fibrosis. Immunohistochemistry revealed a model-specific induction of chemerin expression at the corresponding site of renal damage (tubular vs. glomerular). In both models, renal expression of chemerin (RT-PCR, Western blot) was increased and correlated positively with markers of inflammation and fibrosis. In contrast, circulating chemerin levels remained unchanged. Taken together, these findings demonstrate that renal chemerin expression is associated with processes of inflammation and fibrosis-related to renal damage. However, its use as circulating biomarker of renal inflammation seems to be limited in our rat models.

Keywords: chemerin; CmklR1; 2-kidney-1-clip; 2k1c; Thy1.1 nephritis; renovascular hypertension; renal inflammation; renal injury; renal fibrosis

---

1. Introduction

The significance of end-stage renal disease (ESRD) remains clinically relevant due to its high mortality and morbidity, as well as the lack of effective preventive therapeutic interventions [1]. ESRD results from different forms of renal injury, e.g., arterial hypertension or glomerulonephritis [2,3]. Alterations in the renal microenvironment trigger pathologic immune cell responses with a subsequent acceleration of progressive renal failure, in the setting of loss of glomeruli, tubular atrophy and fibrosis, with reduced glomerular filtration rate (GFR) [2,4]. Unfortunately, the molecular pathways driving persistent renal inflammation are only partly understood to date. Therefore, further research is warranted regarding the regulatory components of inflammation-induced kidney damage in order to develop targeted therapeutics to prevent ESRD effectively. Chemokines and cytokines are both important regulatory mediators of kidney inflammation and potential therapeutic targets [5,6]. They are produced by resident kidney cells, particularly by podocytes, tubular and mesangial cells, as well as by microvascular endothelial cells [6]. Certain mediator combinations determine the recruitment of specific leukocyte subtypes to sites of renal inflammation [2].

Recently, the adipokine chemerin, also known as tazarotene-induced gene 2 protein (TIG2) or retinoic acid receptor responder protein 2 (RARRES2), was introduced as a novel chemoattractant protein [7]. It acts as a ligand for the G protein-coupled receptor CmklR1, also known as ChemR23, and was found to stimulate chemotaxis of dendritic cells and macrophages to sites of inflammation [7,8]. Beyond its classical role in adipogenesis and adipocyte metabolism [9,10], the potential involvement of chemerin in cardiovascular and renal dysfunction has recently been acknowledged [11]. Chemerin appears to form an integral link in metabolic syndrome, connecting obesity, the related dysfunctional cardiometabolic state, and the associated chronic inflammation of adipose tissue [12].

Several investigations have addressed circulating chemerin levels and their pathophysiologic relevance in cohorts with chronic kidney disease [11]. Unrelated to the method of determination [11], serum creatinine is significantly and independently associated with serum chemerin [13,14]. The level of circulating chemerin has been shown to be dependent on GFR and inversely correlated with renal function. A two-fold increase of serum chemerin has been reported in patients on hemodialysis [15]. These results were strengthened by an investigation of ESRD-patients undergoing kidney transplantation [14], whose elevated serum chemerin levels returned to baseline values observed in healthy controls three months after transplant. Furthermore, elevated chemerin levels persisted in ESRD patients on hemodialysis compared to healthy controls or kidney transplanted patients. Nonetheless, hemodialysis reduced high serum chemerin levels to some extent [16]. With adipose tissue as the main source of circulating chemerin [9], it remains to be determined whether elevated serum chemerin levels are due to the increase of fat mass in metabolic phenotypes or to the related renal damage leading to impaired renal elimination. The latter seems more likely [11], as patients with chronic kidney disease showed no difference in subcutaneous adipose tissue chemerin production at the mRNA level [16]. However, the role of visceral adipose tissue cannot be completely ruled out [11]. Also, beyond its role in chemerin elimination, the kidney itself may influence serum chemerin concentrations via its synthesis, as chemerin expression can be found in animal kidneys [9]. In order to investigate the role of renal chemerin and its potential use as a diagnostic marker of kidney disease, our current study characterized its systemic and local expression in established animal models of hypertensive nephropathy and glomerulonephritis using 2-kidney-1-clip (2k1c) hypertensive and Thy1.1 nephritic rats, respectively.

2. Results

2.1. Chemerin is Induced in Kidneys Exposed to High Blood Pressure

Five weeks after clipping of the left renal artery, the weights of the contralateral right kidneys exposed to high blood pressure were significantly higher than the right kidneys of the sham-operated controls (Table 1). Blood pressure and left ventricular weights of 2k1c rats were increased compared to controls (Table 1). Serum urea and creatinine, as markers of renal damage, were elevated in 2k1c rats compared to controls (Table 1). The expression levels of chemerin were significantly higher in the right kidneys of 2k1c hypertensive animals compared to the kidneys of controls (Figure 1A). Immunohistochemical evaluation of chemerin in kidneys revealed some discrete vascular and distal tubular staining for chemerin in control kidneys, with a prominent increase in chemerin immunoreactivity in the tubulo-interstitium of hypertensive kidneys (Figure 1B). The expression of the chemerin receptor CmklR1 was also induced in hypertensive kidneys (Figure 1C). Moreover, a Western blot analysis revealed an increase in chemerin protein in hypertensive kidneys (Figure 2).

Table 1. Physiological parameters of 2k1c experimental groups.

Physiological Parameter	Sham	2k1c	*p*-Value
Rel. right kidney weight (mg/g body weight)	3.21 ± 0.06	4.87 ± 0.25	<0.001
Serum urea (mg/dL)	37.74 ± 1.13	80.92 ± 11.26	<0.001
Serum creatinine (mg/dL)	0.195 ± 0.007	0.335 ± 0.038	<0.001
Rel. left ventricular weight (mg/g body weight)	2.05 ± 0.04	3.03 ± 0.21	0.003
Mean arterial blood pressure (mm Hg)	113.2 ± 2.6	203.7 ± 5.0	0.014

Sham, sham-operated control group; 2k1c, hypertensive group. Data are means ± standard error of the mean. $p < 0.05$ 2k1c versus sham was considered significant.

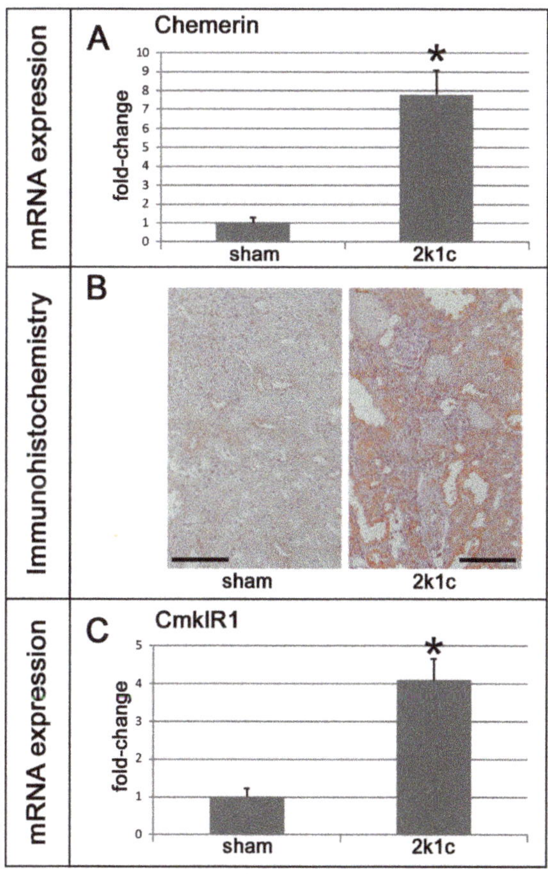

Figure 1. Chemerin and CmklR1 in 2k1c hypertensive nephropathy. (**A**) Chemerin mRNA expression levels in the kidneys of 2k1c hypertensive (2k1c) and control (sham) rats. (**B**) Exemplary photomicrographs of renal tissue from hypertensive (2k1c) and control (sham) rats stained for chemerin. Black bar represents 100 μm. (**C**) CmklR1 mRNA expression levels in the kidneys of 2k1c hypertensive (2k1c) and control (sham) rats. * $p < 0.05$ vs. sham control kidneys.

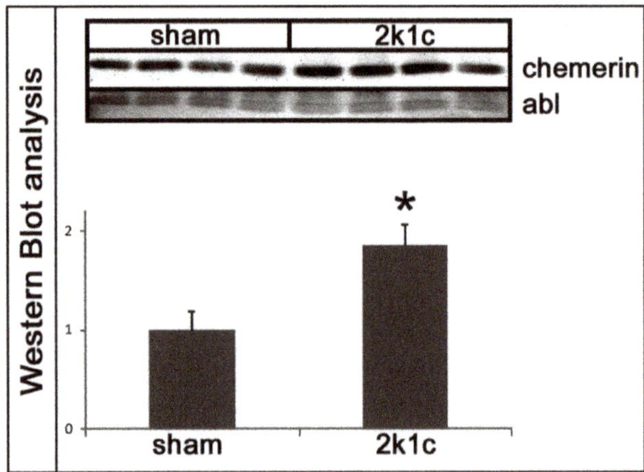

Figure 2. Western blot analysis of chemerin protein expression in the hypertensive kidneys of 2k1c rats. Amido black staining (abl) of the blot served as a loading control. Bar graph: densitometric analysis of Western Blot. * $p < 0.05$ vs. sham control kidneys.

2.2. In Kidneys Exposed to High Blood Pressure, Chemerin Expression Correlates with Markers of Renal Damage, Inflammation, and Fibrosis

Increased infiltration of M1 and M2 macrophages, neutrophil granulocytes, as well as total and helper T-cells, but not of cytotoxic T-cells into the right kidneys of 2k1c rats was observed (Table 2 and Figure 3). Exemplary photomicrographs are shown in Supplementary Figures S1–S3. The expression of TGFβ-1, a central mediator of tissue fibrosis [17], was upregulated in the kidneys of 2k1c rats (Table 3). Moreover, increased smooth muscle actin expression and the presence of more smooth muscle actin positive interstitial cells indicate pronounced fibroblast activation [18] in the right kidney of hypertensive rats (Table 3). Consequently, the expression of the matrix components fibronectin and collagens I, III, and IV was augmented in the right kidneys of these rats (Table 3). The expression of collagens I and IV in right kidney tissue was more prominent in 2k1c rats than in the right kidneys of control rats (Table 3 and Figure 3). Exemplary photomicrographs are shown in Supplementary Figure S4.

Table 2. Inflammatory cell infiltration in the kidneys of 2k1c.

Cell Type	Sham	2k1c	p-Value
M2 macrophages (CD163 pos. cells/cortical view)	0.09 ± 0.04	0.86 ± 0.20	<0.001
Neutrophil granulocytes (myeloperoxidase pos. cells/cortical view)	0.53 ± 0.15	1.49 ± 0.30	0.039
Total T-cells (CD3 pos. cells/cortical view)	1.23 ± 0.47	4.88 ± 1.81	0.046
Helper T-cells (CD4 pos. cells/cortical view)	11.56 ± 3.37	75.45 ± 14.60	0.002
Cytotoxic T-cells (CD8a pos. cells/cortical view)	3.12 ± 0.38	4.76 ± 0.35	0.456

Sham, sham-operated control group; 2k1c, hypertensive group. Data are means ± standard error of the mean. $p < 0.05$ 2k1c versus sham was considered significant.

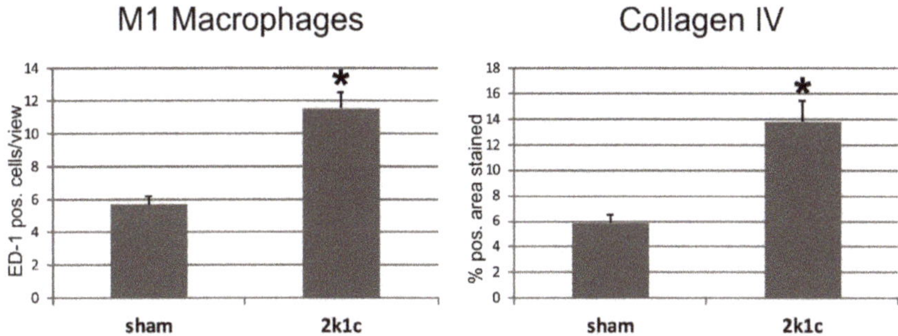

Figure 3. M1 macrophage infiltration and expansion of collagen IV in the tubulointerstitial area of rats with 2k1c hypertensive nephropathy. Sham, control sham operation; ED-1, M1 macrophage marker; * $p < 0.05$ vs. sham control kidneys, data are means ± error of the mean.

Table 3. Markers of renal fibrosis in 2k1c.

Fibrotic Marker	Sham	2k1c	*p*-Value
TGFβ-1 expression (fold change)	1.00 ± 0.25	3.69 ± 0.44	0.001
Smooth muscle actin expression (fold change)	1.00 ± 0.21	5.89 ± 0.96	0.014
Activated fibroblasts (smooth muscle actin pos. cells/cortical view)	0.26 ± 0.04	5.74 ± 1.50	0.002
Fibronectin expression (fold change)	1.00 ± 0.24	8.81 ± 1.55	0.003
Collagen I expression (fold change)	1.00 ± 0.32	4.42 ± 0.78	0.024
Collagen I stain (% pos. cells/cortical view)	4.66 ± 0.44	7.98 ± 1.14	0.001
Collagen III expression (fold change)	1.00 ± 0.49	18.25 ± 5.32	0.004
Collagen IV expression (fold change)	1.00 ± 0.22	6.03 ± 0.83	0.001

Sham, sham-operated control group; 2k1c, hypertensive group. Data are means ± standard error of the mean. $p < 0.05$ 2k1c versus sham was considered significant.

The expression of chemerin in the right kidney of hypertensive rats correlated with serum levels of urea and creatinine, but not with blood pressure levels (Table 4). There was a correlation between chemerin expression and M1 macrophage and neutrophil granulocyte infiltration into the right kidneys (Figure 4). Chemerin expression also correlated with fibroblast activation, TGFβ-1 expression and the expression of several matrix molecules (Table 4 and Figure 4). Furthermore, there was a high correlation of chemerin expression with the expression of its receptor CmklR1 (Table 4).

2.3. Chemerin is Induced in Glomeruli Afflicted with Thy1.1 Nephritis and Correlates with Markers of Renal Damage, Inflammation, and Fibrosis

Two weeks after the induction of a Thy1.1 glomerulonephritis, an increase in serum creatinine and albuminuria were observed (Table 5). Glomerular M1 macrophage infiltration and renal collagen IV expression were increased in nephritic kidneys (Figure 5 and Figure S5). Blood pressure was not altered in Thy1.1 nephritic rats (Table 5). Chemerin expression was increased in the renal tissue of Thy1.1 nephritic rats (Figure 6A). Staining for chemerin revealed prominent glomerular immunoreactivity in nephritic glomeruli, while in control glomeruli, only some podocytes stained positive (Figure 6B). The expression of the chemerin receptor CmklR1 was also somewhat increased (Figure 6C).

Table 4. Correlation of markers of renal damage, inflammation, and fibrosis with chemerin expression in 2k1c.

Chemerin (mRNA Expression)	r	*p*-Value
Serum creatinine (mg/dL)	0.62	**0.009**
Serum urea (mg/dL)	0.77	**<0.001**
Mean arterial blood pressure (mm Hg)	0.42	0.12
M1 macrophages (ED-1 pos. cells/view)	0.71	**0.001**
M2 macrophages (CD163 pos. cells/view)	0.51	0.16
Total T-cells (CD3 pos. cells/view)	0.27	0.40
Cytotoxic T-cells (CD8a pos. cells/view)	0.47	0.11
Helper T-cells (CD4 pos. cells/view)	−0.14	0.63
Neutrophil granulocytes (MPO pos. cells/view)	0.83	**<0.001**
Activated myofibroblasts (SMA-pos. cells/view)	0.74	**0.003**
Smooth muscle actin (mRNA expression)	0.65	**0.005**
Fibronectin (mRNA expression)	0.86	**<0.001**
Collagen I (% pos. area stained)	0.65	**0.043**
Collagen I (mRNA expression)	0.83	**<0.001**
Collagen III (mRNA expression)	0.84	**<0.001**
Collagen IV (% pos. area stained)	0.64	**0.014**
Collagen IV (mRNA expression)	0.90	**<0.001**
TGFβ-1 (mRNA expression)	0.73	**0.001**
CmklR1 (mRNA expression)	0.89	**<0.001**

r = Spearman–Rho correlation coefficient r, statistical significance was defined as *p*-value < 0.05.

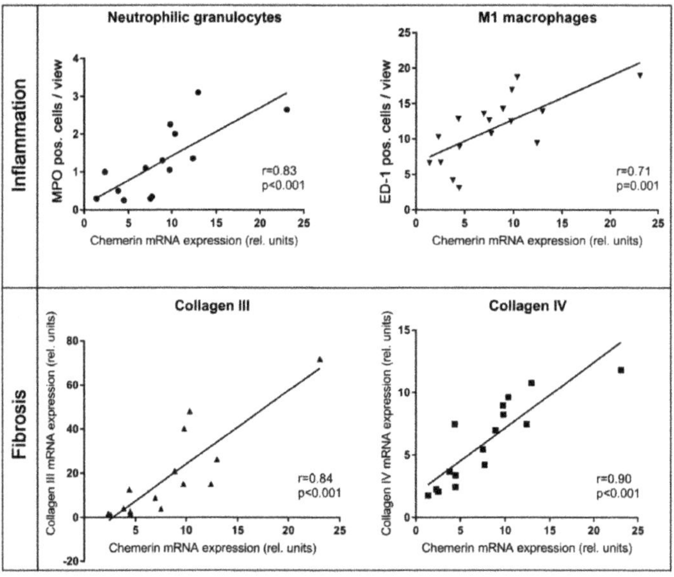

Figure 4. Correlation of chemerin expression with infiltration of neutrophilic granulocytes and M1 macrophages and the expression of collagens III and IV. MPO, myeloperoxidase (marker for neutrophil granulocytes), ED-1, marker for rat M1 macrophages.

Table 5. Markers of renal damage and blood pressure in Thy1 glomerulonephritis.

Damage Marker	NaCl	Thy1	*p*-Value
Rel. right kidney weight (mg/g body weight)	4.30 ± 0.15	8.57 ± 0.18	<0.01
Albuminuria (mg/24 h)	0.80 ± 0.19	725.79 ± 303.13	<0.01
Serum creatinine (mg/dL)	0.19 ± 0.01	0.34 ± 0.03	<0.01
Cytotoxic T-cells (CD8a pos. cells/cortical view)	3.51 ± 0.56	5.72 ± 0.41	n.s.
Helper T-cells (CD4 pos. cells/cortical view)	3.05 ± 0.61	6.23 ± 2.39	n.s.
Mean arterial blood pressure (mm Hg)	118.5 ± 1.5	123.7 ± 6.3	n.s.
Rel. left ventricular weight (mg/g body weight)	2.23 ± 0.11	2.49 ± 0.09	n.s.

NaCl, NaCl infused control group; Thy1, glomerulonephritic group. Data are means ± standard error of the mean. *p* < 0.05 2k1c versus sham was considered significant.

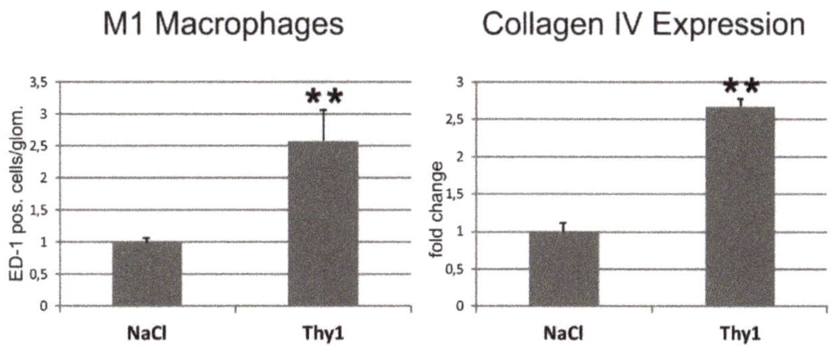

Figure 5. Glomerular M1 macrophage infiltration and collagen IV expression in the renal cortex of rats with anti-Thy1.1 mesangioproliferative glomerulonephritis. NaCl, control vehicle-injected; ED-1, M1 macrophage marker; ** *p* < 0.01; data are means ± error of the mean.

The expression of chemerin in kidneys with Thy1.1 glomerulonephritis correlated with serum creatinine levels, albuminuria, glomerular infiltration of M1 macrophages, and renal collagen IV expression (Table 6). A correlation between chemerin expression and CmklR1 expression was also detected (Table 6).

Table 6. Correlation of markers of renal damage, inflammation and fibrosis with chemerin expression in Thy1 glomerulonephritis.

Chemerin (mRNA Expression)	r	*p*-Value
CmklR1 (mRNA expression)	0.89	**0.001**
Serum creatinine (mg/dL)	0.73	**0.017**
Albuminuria (mg/24h)	0.73	**0.016**
Mean arterial blood pressure (mm Hg)	0.42	0.262
M1 macrophages (ED-1 pos. cells/view)	0.72	**0.019**
Cytotoxic T-cells (CD8a pos. cells/view)	0.58	0.082
Helper T-cells (CD4 pos. cells/view)	0.39	0.266
Collagen IV (mRNA expression)	0.83	**0.005**

r = Spearman–Rho correlation coefficient r, statistical significance was defined as *p*-value < 0.05.

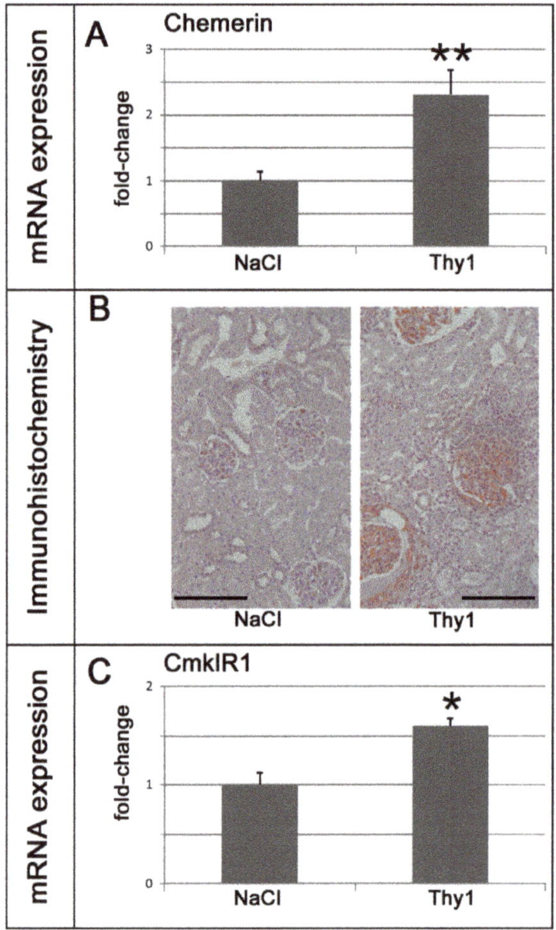

Figure 6. Chemerin and CmklR1 in anti-Thy1.1 glomerulonephritis: (**A**) mRNA expression of chemerin levels in the kidneys of Thy1.1 nephritic (Thy1) and control (NaCl) rats. (**B**) Localization of chemerin protein in renal sections of Thy1.1 nephritic and control rats. Black bar represents 100 μm. (**C**) mRNA expression of the chemerin receptor CmklR1 levels in the kidneys of Thy1.1 nephritic (Thy1) and control (NaCl) rats. NaCl, NaCl infused controls. Thy1, anti-Thy1.1 infused glomerulonephritic animals. ** $p < 0.01$, * $p < 0.05$ vs. control kidneys.

2.4. Chemerin Plasma Levels are Not Increased in Rat Models of Renal Injury

To clarify whether increases of renal tissue chemerin are also reflected by increases in plasma chemerin, ELISA assays were performed. In 2k1c hypertensive rats, plasma chemerin was not increased compared to sham-operated controls (1.15 ± 0.06 ng/mL in hypertensive rats versus 1.29 ± 0.11 ng/mL in controls). Likewise, in Thy1.1 glomerulonephritic rats, plasma chemerin levels were similar to the plasma levels of control rats (1.13 ± 0.19 ng/mL in nephritic rats versus 1.22 ± 0.10 ng/mL in controls).

3. Discussion

We have demonstrated specific induction of local expression patterns of chemerin related to the underlying model of renal injury, i.e., tubular-interstitial (2k1c, in kidneys exposed to high blood pressure) and glomerular damage (Thy1.1 nephritis). In our study, renal chemerin expression positively correlated with markers of renal damage and inflammation in 2k1c hypertensive animals and Thy1.1 nephritic rats, indicating a possible involvement of chemerin in these processes, as seen in adipose tissue [19]. Concomitantly, the expression of the chemerin receptor CmklR1 was also found to be induced in hypertensive kidneys, while somewhat increased in anti-Thy1.1 treated animals. Of the three known chemerin receptors (i.e., chemokine-like receptor 1 (CmklR1), G-protein-coupled receptor (GPR) 1, and C-C motif receptor-like (CCRL) 2, only CmklR1 sufficiently mediates intracellular signaling functions (reviewed by [12]). Besides its expression in hematopoietic tissues, CmklR1 is strongly expressed in cells of the immune system (e.g., blood monocytes, monocyte-derived human macrophages, immature dendritic cells, CD4+ T lymphocytes) [7,20]. CmklR1 directs the migration of immune cells to lymphoid organs and inflamed tissues [21]. Thus, the observed renal damage in our models might have partly resulted from chemerin-induced, CmklR1-mediated chemoattraction of immune cells to the respective sites of renal damage (i.e., tubulo-interstitium in 2k1c model and glomerulus in Thy1.1 nephritic rats).

Interestingly, CmklR1 expression was additionally observed in human microvascular endothelial cells (ECs) by Kaur et al. [22]. Thus, para-/autocrine effects of chemerin on renal vasculature in our model are also possible. Kaur et al. showed that the expression of the receptor was significantly up-regulated by pro-inflammatory cytokines in human ECs and had strong angiogenic potential via activation of PI3K/Akt and MAPK pathways in these cells [22]. The involvement of an imbalance of angiogenesis-related factors in the progression of CKD and the therapeutic potential of modulating these factors in CKD has been acknowledged (reviewed by [23]). Furthermore, Kaur et al. showed that chemerin was able to induce the activity of members of the matrix metalloproteinase (MMP) family in ECs [22], which play an important role in the degradation of the extracellular matrix (ECM) [24]. This effect is also crucial in the development and progression of CKD; however, non-proteolytic functions of MMPs might also play a role [24]. In line with these observations, we found chemerin to correlate with markers of renal fibrosis.

So far, the exact mechanisms of renal chemerin induction in our animals remain unknown. However, a potential role of angiotensin 2 (Ang II) in the regulation of chemerin expression has been proposed by others. Using a model of diabetic nephropathy, Yu et al. [25] were able to show that the expression of chemerin in the kidney of diabetic rats was significantly elevated compared to control animals, suggesting that chemerin might be relevant to the model-specific renal pathology. Treatment with irbesartan (Ang II type 1 receptor antagonist) appeared to reduce the renal chemerin expression in these diabetic animals secondary to a reduction in renin–angiotensin system (RAS) components [25].

The Goldblatt 2k1c rat hypertension model is a long-established and widely employed model in the study of renal artery stenosis and renovascular hypertension [26,27]. We have observed that the RAS, including Ang II, is closely related with the 2k1c model [28] since their levels are elevated in the development and maintenance of hypertension in these animals: Early on, hypertension in 2k1c animals is characterized by increased plasma renin levels in response to low renal arterial pressure and subsequently by an increase in circulating Ang II. Later, hypertension is maintained by a continuously activated RAS, as contralateral pressure diuresis of the unaffected kidney prevents hypervolemia [29,30]. Persistent elevation of Ang II also triggers an inflammatory response, characterized by the infiltration of macrophages (ED-1), tubular overexpression of macrophage chemotactic and adhesion molecules, such as osteopontin (OPN), MCP-1 and the expression of inflammatory cytokines, ultimately aggravating renal damage induced by hypertension [3,31,32].

A potential interaction of Ang II with chemerin in the 2k1c model remains to be determined. Ang II is a key mediator of CKD. A blockade of the Ang II type 1 receptor prevents lethal malignant hypertension [28]. It is also understood that Ang II mediates renal fibrosis by stimulating the endogenous synthesis of transforming growth factor-β (TGF-β) [33] in damaged kidney cells, thereby stimulating the synthesis of the extracellular matrix (ECM), and inhibiting the action of MMPs [34]. TGF-β induces the transformation of fibroblasts into myofibroblasts (α-smooth muscle actin-positive cells, α-SMA) and stimulates the expression of fibronectin (FN) and collagen type III (Col III).

This induces the development of renal fibrosis, leads to functional deterioration and increases kidney damage [34–36]. Notably, we have found that renal chemerin levels correlated positively with these Ang II-dependent markers of inflammation and fibrosis in both our models of renal injury. Moreover, other RAS-associated factors, such as aldosterone/mineralocorticoid receptor [37] or the activity of the angiotensin-converting enzyme (ACE) [38], might be relevant in the function of renal chemerin.

Similar to 2k1c animals, RAS activation also plays a pivotal role in the progression of glomerulonephritis (GN) in Thy1.1 nephritic rats [39]. Thus, potential cross-talk of chemerin and Ang II [25] at the glomerular level might be conceivable. The immunohistochemically observed glomerular expression of chemerin in our Thy1.1 nephritic rats closely resembled glomerular cyto/chemokine expression patterns typically found in nephritic renal damage [40], thereby underscoring the potential role of chemerin as a damage-site specific chemoattractant. The most commonly used model of selective mesangial cell damage [41–43], anti-Thy1.1-induced glomerulonephritis, resembles some human forms of GN [44], where the renal damage is characterized by the continued accumulation of ECM, related to the overproduction of glomerular TGF-β.

As a limitation, the role of Ang II in our 2k1c animals and Thy1.1. nephritic rats remains speculative due to the lack of functional data regarding RAS signaling. Future studies are needed to uncover the mechanistic insights of chemerin signaling transduction pathways in the kidney, with a special focus on the exploration of potential therapeutic targets for renal fibrosis and inflammation.

Despite the association of increased chemerin with (renal) inflammation and fibrosis, Yamamoto et al. found an association of elevated chemerin levels with a survival advantage in dialysis patients [45]. This seems controversial, as CKD induces premature vascular aging with vascular calcification and increased arterial stiffness [46]. In addition, previous studies had indicated a role of CmklR1 for the vascular smooth muscle cell (VSMC) atherosclerotic phenotype [47], characterized by vascular inflammation and intimal hyperplasia [48,49]. Surprisingly, chemerin seemed to inhibit atherogenesis through CmklR1 [48,50]. Carracedo et al. [51] were able to show that chemerin treatment of isolated wild-type mouse VSMCs significantly reduced phosphate-induced calcification and increased expression of the calcification inhibitor matrix-gla-protein (MGP). In contrast, VSMCs of CmklR1 knock-out mice were devoid of these effects. This suggests that elevated chemerin might, in fact, exert a direct protective vascular role in CKD, while negatively altering the local microenvironment via attraction of immune cells at the same time.

In contrast to findings in humans [11], we did not observe an induction of circulating chemerin. So far, the majority of existing human reports focus on elevated circulating levels of chemerin in CKD patients, while little is known about the local renal expression of the protein. Based on our finding of increased chemerin expression in ESRD, one could speculate that this may contribute to the reported increase of circulating chemerin levels in ESRD, apart from the postulated reduced chemerin renal elimination capacity associated with ESRD [14]. However, as we were unable to detect an increase of circulating chemerin levels in both animal models of our study, it remains uncertain to what extent such local changes in our rodent models might translate into a significant increase of circulating chemerin levels observed in human ESRD.

The lack of increased circulating chemerin seemed unrelated to an inoperative experimental design. Clipping of the left renal artery and anti-Thy1.1 treatment both sufficiently reduced kidney function, as determined by a ~2-fold increase in serum urea and creatinine. Also, renal weight was significantly increased in both rodent models. These results match findings previously obtained by our group in 2k1c rats [52]. It is possible that despite the detectable renal affliction of our animals and its correlation with local chemerin expression, the functional renal restriction might not have been relevant enough to fully resemble the level of kidney failure seen in human ESRD [14]. Thus, the renal capacity to eliminate increasing levels of circulating chemerin might still have been sufficient in the examined animal models.

A current methodological limitation in the field of chemerin research is the lack of analysis of the multitude of existing chemerin pre-cursors [12,19]. Chemerin is proteolytically processed (e.g., by cathepsin G, elastase, plasmin, and tryptase) into different active and inactive chemerin peptides, such as pre-prochemerin and mature prochemerin, which might exert specific functions on their own.

In summary, our findings provide novel evidence that renal chemerin expression in 2k1c and Thy1.1 nephritic rats are associated with markers of kidney inflammation and fibrosis. However, we did not find elevated levels of circulating chemerin in these animals. Thus, chemerin might not serve as a biomarker in these models.

4. Materials and Methods

4.1. Experimental Procedures

All animal experiments were performed in compliance with the DIRECTIVE 2010/63/EU of the European Parliament and were approved by the local government authorities (Regierung of Mittelfranken, AZ 54-2532.1-51/12, 22 October 2013 and AZ 55.2.2532-2-526, 18 October 2017). All efforts were made to minimize suffering in the animal cohort. Rats were housed in a room maintained at 22 ± 2 °C, exposed to a 12-h dark/light cycle. The animals had unlimited access to standard rodent nutrition and tap water.

Induction of hypertensive nephropathy: Two-kidney, one-clip renovascular hypertension (2k1c) was induced in male Sprague–Dawley rats (Charles River, Sulzfeld, Germany) weighing 150–170 g by placing a silver clip of 0.2 mm internal diameter around the left renal artery through a flank incision under isoflurane anesthesia as previously described (n = 25) [53]. Control animals underwent a sham operation without placement of the clip (n = 10). Analgesia was provided post-operatively in all animals, and as needed later on. Five weeks after the clipping of the renal artery, the experiment was terminated, and renal tissue was collected.

Induction of acute glomerulonephritis: Male Sprague-Dawley rats (150 to 200 g) were obtained from Charles River Deutschland. Anti-Thy1.1 nephritis was induced in uninephrectomized rats by a single intravenous injection of 1 mg/kg body weight anti-Thy1.1 antibody into the tail vein in light isoflurane anesthesia. Controls received solvent only (n = 5 per group). The monoclonal antibody against Thy1.1 (ER4) was from Antibody Solutions (Santa Clara, CA, USA). Anti-Thy1.1 nephritis is an acute mesangioproliferative glomerulonephritis with mesangial expansion and glomerulosclerosis peaking at days 7 to 14 of disease [42,54]. On day 13, animals were housed in metabolic cages for 24 h to collect urine. Five animals per group were sacrificed on day 14 after induction of nephritis and renal tissue was obtained for further evaluation.

4.2. Blood Pressure Measurements

At the end of the experiment, rats were weighed and instrumented with femoral artery catheters for intraarterial blood pressure measurements in anesthesia, as described previously [55]. Measurements were performed on the same day after termination of anesthesia and a recovery phase of 2 h in conscious animals via transducers connected to a polygraph (Hellige, Freiburg, Germany).

4.3. Measurement of Serum and Urine Parameters

For urine collection, anti-Thy1.1 nephritic animals were put in metabolic cages for 24 h on the day before sacrifice. Albumin excretion was assessed by enzyme-linked immunosorbent assay (Bethyl Laboratories, Biomol, Hamburg, Germany). For serum analysis, blood was collected from catheters. Thereafter, rats were euthanized by bleeding in deep anesthesia. Plasma creatinine and plasma urea were analyzed using an automatic analyzer Integra 1000 (Roche Diagnostics, Mannheim, Germany). Plasma chemerin was determined using a commercially available ELISA kit (MyBiosource, Biozol, Eching, Germany) according to the manufacturer's protocol.

4.4. Tissue Sampling

After organ weighing, kidneys were decapsulated. Both poles of each kidney and the apical tip of the left ventricle were immediately snap-frozen on liquid nitrogen for protein or RNA extraction. One 6 mm slice of the kidney was put in paraformaldehyde solution (for detection of chemerin), while another 6 mm slice of the remaining kidney was put in methyl-Carnoy solution (60% methanol, 30% chloroform and 10% glacial acetic acid) for fixation. After overnight fixation, tissues were dehydrated by bathing in increasing concentrations of alcohol and embedded in paraffin. Three μm sections were cut with a Leitz SM 2000 R microtome (Leica Instruments, Nussloch, Germany).

4.5. Immunohistochemistry

Tissue was processed as described [56]. Immunohistochemical detection of chemerin, collagen I, collagen IV, α-smooth muscle actin (SMA), ED-1, myeloperoxidase (MPO), CD3, CD4, CD8a, and CD163 was performed in methyl Carnoy-fixed tissue sections. Antibodies used are described in Supplementary Table S1. The specificity of the chemerin antibody was confirmed by staining in control tissue: rat skin, lung and testes (see Supplementary Figure S6). Interstitial collagens I and IV were quantified in 30 medium-power views (magnification x200) by means of an 11 × 11-point grid or by densitometric analysis using MetaVue software (Molecular Devices, Sunnyvale, CA, USA). The percentage of grid points corresponding with a stained area or the percentage of stained area in relation to the total area was calculated. SMA, ED-1, MPO, CD3, CD4, CD8a, and CD163 positive cells were counted in 20 medium-power cortical views. All histological evaluations were done by a single investigator blinded to the group assignment.

4.6. Western Blot Analysis

Frozen renal tissue was homogenized, protein samples were prepared as described [57] and separated on a denaturing SDS-PAGE gel [58]. After electrophoresis, the gels were electroblotted onto PVDF membranes (Hybond-P, GE Amersham, Munich, Germany), blocked with Rotiblock (Roth, Karlsruhe, Germany) for 1 h and incubated overnight with a primary antibody to chemerin. Protein bands were visualized with secondary horseradish peroxidase-conjugated IgG antibodies (Santa Cruz Biotechnology, 1:50,000), using the Pierce ECL+ system (Thermo Fisher Scientific, Waltham, MA, USA). Blots were quantified using a luminescent imager (LAS-1000, Fujifilm, Berlin, Germany) and Aida 2.1 image analysis software (Raytest, Berlin, Germany). Loading of the blot was quantified by Amido Black staining solution (Sigma, Taufkirchen, Germany).

4.7. Real-Time Polymerase Chain Reaction (PCR) Analyses

Renal tissue was homogenized in RLT buffer reagent (Qiagen, Hilden, Germany) with an ultraturrax for 30 s, total RNA was extracted from homogenates by RNeasy Mini columns (Qiagen) according to the manufacturer's protocol, and real-time RT-PCR was performed [59]. First-strand cDNA was synthesized with TaqMan reverse transcription reagents (Applied Biosystems, Darmstadt, Germany) using random hexamers as primers. Reactions without Multiscribe reverse transcriptase were used as negative controls for genomic DNA contamination. PCR was performed with a StepOnePlus™ sequence detector system (Applied Biosystems, Darmstadt, Germany) and TaqMan or SYBR Green Universal PCR master mix (Applied Biosystems), as described previously [57]. All samples were run in duplicates. Specific mRNA levels in hypertensive animals relative to sham-operated controls were calculated and normalized to a housekeeping gene (18S) with the ΔΔCt method as specified by the manufacturer (Applied Biosystems). Primer pairs used for experiments are shown in Supplementary Table S2.

4.8. Statistical Analysis

Data are expressed as mean ± standard error of the mean (SEM). After testing for normality distribution using Shapiro–Wilk's test, we performed Student's *t*-test or the Mann–Whitney U-test, where appropriate. A p-value < 0.05 was considered significant. To assess correlations between chemerin and markers of inflammation and fibrosis, Spearman's correlation coefficients (Spearman's rho) were calculated. Calculations were carried out using the SPSS 19 software (IBM, Ehningen, Germany) and GraphPad Prism 7.00 (GraphPad Software, La Jolla, CA, USA).

Supplementary Materials: Supplementary Materials can be found at http://www.mdpi.com/1422-0067/20/24/6240/s1. Figure S1: Exemplary photomicrographs of kidneys with 2k1c nephropathy and control kidneys (sham) stained for the M1 macrophage marker ED1 and the M2 macrophage marker CD163. Figure S2: Exemplary photomicrographs of kidneys with 2k1c nephropathy and control kidneys (sham) stained for the neutrophil marker myeloperoxidase and the T-cell marker CD3. Figure S3: Exemplary photomicrographs of kidneys with 2k1c nephropathy and control kidneys (sham) stained for the T-helper cell marker CD4 and the cytotoxic T-cell marker CD8a. Figure S4: Exemplary photomicrographs of kidneys with 2k1c nephropathy and control kidneys (sham) stained for collagen I and collagen IV. Figure S5: Exemplary photomicrographs of kidneys with Thy1 induced glomerulonephritis and control kidneys (NaCl) stained for the M1 macrophage marker ED1. Figure S6. Specificity testing of the chemerin antibody. The antibody stained skin (Luangsay S et al. 2009, J Immunol 183; Vermi W et al. 2005, J Exp Med 201), lung (Luangsay S et al. 2009, J Immunol 183) and testes (Li L et al. 2014, J Endocrinol 220), as described before. Black arrowheads point to the chemerin positive keratinocyte layer in a skin sample, to the chemerin positive ciliated epithelium of the lung bronchioles and to chemerin positive Leydig cells in testes. Table S1. Antibodies used for immunohistochemistry. Table S2. Primer sequences.

Author Contributions: A.M. acquired data, interpreted the results and drafted the manuscript. R.W., C.M.-C. and N.C. acquired data, interpreted the results and revised the manuscript. A.H. and F.B.F. designed the work, interpreted the data and drafted the manuscript. K.F.H. designed the work and revised the manuscript. J.W. critically revised the manuscript. All authors gave final approval of the manuscript to be published.

Funding: This research was funded by a grant from the Doktor Robert Pfleger-Stiftung to Andrea Hartner and Karl F. Hilgers and by Deutsche Forschungsgemeinschaft/Friedrich-Alexander-University Erlangen-Nürnberg (FAU) within the funding programme Open Access Publishing.

Acknowledgments: We thank Miroslava Kupraszewicz-Hutzler and Astrid Ziegler for their excellent technical assistance. A large part of the experimental procedures and respective data acquisition was performed by Alexander Mocker in fulfillment of the requirements for obtaining the degree "Dr. med." at the Friedrich-Alexander-University of Erlangen-Nürnberg, Dept. of Pediatrics and Adolescent Medicine, Germany. The authors thank J. A. Bello MD, FACR, Professor of Clinical Radiology and Neurosurgery, Director of Neuroradiology, Albert Einstein College of Medicine, Montefiore Medical Center, New York, NY, USA for language editing.

References

1. Breyer, M.D.; Susztak, K. Developing Treatments for Chronic Kidney Disease in the 21st Century. *Semin. Nephrol.* **2016**, *36*, 436–447. [CrossRef] [PubMed]

2. Ernandez, T.; Mayadas, T.N. The Changing Landscape of Renal Inflammation. *Trends Mol. Med.* **2016**, *22*, 151–163. [CrossRef] [PubMed]

3. Hilgers, K.F.; Hartner, A.; Porst, M.; Mai, M.; Wittmann, M.; Hugo, C.; Ganten, D.; Geiger, H.; Veelken, R.; Mann, J.F. Monocyte chemoattractant protein-1 and macrophage infiltration in hypertensive kidney injury. *Kidney Int.* **2000**, *58*, 2408–2419. [CrossRef] [PubMed]

4. Shafi, T.; Coresh, J. 1 - Chronic Kidney Disease: Definition, Epidemiology, Cost, and Outcomes. In *Chronic Kidney Disease, Dialysis, and Transplantation (Fourth Edition)*, Himmelfarb, J.; Ikizler, T.A., Ed.; Eds. Elsevier: Philadelphia, PA, USA, 2019.

5. Wada, T.; Matsushima, K.; Kaneko, S. The role of chemokines in glomerulonephritis. *Front. Biosci.* **2008**, *13*, 3966–3974. [CrossRef] [PubMed]

6. Chung, A.C.; Lan, H.Y. Chemokines in renal injury. *J. Am. Soc. Nephrol.* **2011**, *22*, 802–809. [CrossRef] [PubMed]

7. Wittamer, V.; Franssen, J.D.; Vulcano, M.; Mirjolet, J.F.; Le Poul, E.; Migeotte, I.; Brezillon, S.; Tyldesley, R.; Blanpain, C.; Detheux, M.; et al. Specific recruitment of antigen-presenting cells by chemerin, a novel processed ligand from human inflammatory fluids. *J. Exp. Med.* **2003**, *198*, 977–985. [CrossRef] [PubMed]

8. Xu, H.; Barnes, G.T.; Yang, Q.; Tan, G.; Yang, D.; Chou, C.J.; Sole, J.; Nichols, A.; Ross, J.S.; Tartaglia, L.A.; et al. Chronic inflammation in fat plays a crucial role in the development of obesity-related insulin resistance. *J. Clin. Investig.* **2003**, *112*, 1821–1830. [CrossRef]

9.   Bozaoglu, K.; Bolton, K.; McMillan, J.; Zimmet, P.; Jowett, J.; Collier, G.; Walder, K.; Segal, D. Chemerin is a novel adipokine associated with obesity and metabolic syndrome. *Endocrinology* **2007**, *148*, 4687–4694. [CrossRef]

10.   Goralski, K.B.; McCarthy, T.C.; Hanniman, E.A.; Zabel, B.A.; Butcher, E.C.; Parlee, S.D.; Muruganandan, S.; Sinal, C.J. Chemerin, a novel adipokine that regulates adipogenesis and adipocyte metabolism. *J. Biol. Chem.* **2007**, *282*, 28175–28188. [CrossRef]

11.   Bonomini, M.; Pandolfi, A. Chemerin in renal dysfunction and cardiovascular disease. *Vascul. Pharmacol.* **2016**, *77*, 28–34. [CrossRef]

12.   Kaur, J.; Mattu, H.S.; Chatha, K.; Randeva, H.S. Chemerin in human cardiovascular disease. *Vascul. Pharmacol.* **2018**, *110*, 1–6. [CrossRef] [PubMed]

13.   Hu, W.; Feng, P. Elevated serum chemerin concentrations are associated with renal dysfunction in type 2 diabetic patients. *Diabetes Res. Clin. Pract.* **2011**, *91*, 159–163. [CrossRef] [PubMed]

14.   Rutkowski, P.; Sledzinski, T.; Zielinska, H.; Lizakowski, S.; Goyke, E.; Szrok-Wojtkiewicz, S.; Swierczynski, J.; Rutkowski, B. Decrease of serum chemerin concentration in patients with end stage renal disease after successful kidney transplantation. *Regul. Pept.* **2012**, *173*, 55–59. [CrossRef] [PubMed]

15.   Pfau, D.; Bachmann, A.; Lossner, U.; Kratzsch, J.; Bluher, M.; Stumvoll, M.; Fasshauer, M. Serum levels of the adipokine chemerin in relation to renal function. *Diabetes Care* **2010**, *33*, 171–173. [CrossRef] [PubMed]

16.   Blaszak, J.; Szolkiewicz, M.; Sucajtys-Szulc, E.; Konarzewski, M.; Lizakowski, S.; Swierczynski, J.; Rutkowski, B. High serum chemerin level in CKD patients is related to kidney function, but not to its adipose tissue overproduction. *Ren Fail.* **2015**, *37*, 1033–1038. [CrossRef] [PubMed]

17.   Meng, X.M.; Tang, P.M.; Li, J.; Lan, H.Y. TGF-beta/Smad signaling in renal fibrosis. *Front. Physiol.* **2015**, *6*, 82. [CrossRef]

18.   Meran, S.; Steadman, R. Fibroblasts and myofibroblasts in renal fibrosis. *Int. J. Exp. Pathol.* **2011**, *92*, 158–167. [CrossRef]

19.   Ernst, M.C.; Sinal, C.J. Chemerin: At the crossroads of inflammation and obesity. *Trends Endocrinol. Metab.* **2010**, *21*, 660–667. [CrossRef]

20.   Arita, M.; Ohira, T.; Sun, Y.P.; Elangovan, S.; Chiang, N.; Serhan, C.N. Resolvin E1 selectively interacts with leukotriene B4 receptor BLT1 and ChemR23 to regulate inflammation. *J. Immunol.* **2007**, *178*, 3912–3917. [CrossRef]

21.   Vermi, W.; Riboldi, E.; Wittamer, V.; Gentili, F.; Luini, W.; Marrelli, S.; Vecchi, A.; Franssen, J.D.; Communi, D.; Massardi, L.; et al. Role of ChemR23 in directing the migration of myeloid and plasmacytoid dendritic cells to lymphoid organs and inflamed skin. *J. Exp. Med.* **2005**, *201*, 509–515. [CrossRef]

22.   Kaur, J.; Adya, R.; Tan, B.K.; Chen, J.; Randeva, H.S. Identification of chemerin receptor (ChemR23) in human endothelial cells: Chemerin-induced endothelial angiogenesis. *Biochem. Biophys. Res. Commun.* **2010**, *391*, 1762–1768. [CrossRef] [PubMed]

23.   Maeshima, Y.; Makino, H. Angiogenesis and chronic kidney disease. *Fibrogenesis Tissue Repair* **2010**, *3*, 13. [CrossRef] [PubMed]

24.   Cheng, Z.; Limbu, M.H.; Wang, Z.; Liu, J.; Liu, L.; Zhang, X.; Chen, P.; Liu, B. MMP-2 and 9 in Chronic Kidney Disease. *Int. J. Mol. Sci.* **2017**, *18*. [CrossRef] [PubMed]

25.   Yu, Q.X.; Zhang, H.; Xu, W.H.; Hao, F.; Liu, S.L.; Bai, M.M.; Mu, J.W.; Zhang, H.J. Effect of Irbesartan on Chemerin in the Renal Tissues of Diabetic Rats. *Kidney Blood Press Res.* **2015**, *40*, 467–477. [CrossRef] [PubMed]

26.   Goldblatt, H.; Lynch, J.; Hanzal, R.F.; Summerville, W.W. Studies on Experimental Hypertension : I. The Production of Persistent Elevation of Systolic Blood Pressure by Means of Renal Ischemia. *J. Exp. Med.* **1934**, *59*, 347–379. [CrossRef]

27.   Goldblatt, H.; Kahn, J.R.; Hanzal, R.F. Studies on Experimental Hypertension : Ix. The Effect on Blood Pressure of Constriction of the Abdominal Aorta above and Below the Site of Origin of Both Main Renal Arteries. *J. Exp. Med.* **1939**, *69*, 649–674. [CrossRef]

28.   Hilgers, K.F.; Hartner, A.; Porst, M.; Veelken, R.; Mann, J.F. Angiotensin II type 1 receptor blockade prevents lethal malignant hypertension: Relation to kidney inflammation. *Circulation* **2001**, *104*, 1436–1440. [CrossRef]

29.   Wiesel, P.; Mazzolai, L.; Nussberger, J.; Pedrazzini, T. Two-kidney, one clip and one-kidney, one clip hypertension in mice. *Hypertension* **1997**, *29*, 1025–1030. [CrossRef]

30. Corbier, A.; Lecaque, D.; Secchi, J.; Depouez, B.; Hamon, G. Effects of 4 weeks of treatment with trandolapril on renal hypertension and cardiac and vascular hypertrophy in the rat. *J. Cardiovasc. Pharmacol.* **1994**, *23*, S26–S29. [CrossRef]

31. Ozawa, Y.; Kobori, H.; Suzaki, Y.; Navar, L.G. Sustained renal interstitial macrophage infiltration following chronic angiotensin II infusions. *Am. J. Physiol. Renal Physiol.* **2007**, *292*, F330–F339. [CrossRef]

32. Mezzano, S.A.; Aros, C.A.; Droguett, A.; Burgos, M.E.; Ardiles, L.G.; Flores, C.A.; Carpio, D.; Vio, C.P.; Ruiz-Ortega, M.; Egido, J. Renal angiotensin II up-regulation and myofibroblast activation in human membranous nephropathy. *Kidney Int.* **2003**, *64*, S39–S45. [CrossRef] [PubMed]

33. Yang, F.; Chung, A.C.; Huang, X.R.; Lan, H.Y. Angiotensin II induces connective tissue growth factor and collagen I expression via transforming growth factor-beta-dependent and -independent Smad pathways: The role of Smad3. *Hypertension* **2009**, *54*, 877–884. [CrossRef] [PubMed]

34. Border, W.A.; Noble, N.A. Interactions of transforming growth factor-beta and angiotensin II in renal fibrosis. *Hypertension* **1998**, *31*, 181–188. [CrossRef] [PubMed]

35. Mezzano, S.A.; Ruiz-Ortega, M.; Egido, J. Angiotensin II and renal fibrosis. *Hypertension* **2001**, *38*, 635–638. [CrossRef] [PubMed]

36. Wolf, G.; Schneider, A.; Wenzel, U.; Helmchen, U.; Stahl, R.A. Regulation of glomerular TGF-beta expression in the contralateral kidney of two-kidney, one-clip hypertensive rats. *J. Am. Soc. Nephrol.* **1998**, *9*, 763–772. [PubMed]

37. Hoppmann, J.; Perwitz, N.; Meier, B.; Fasshauer, M.; Hadaschik, D.; Lehnert, H.; Klein, J. The balance between gluco- and mineralo-corticoid action critically determines inflammatory adipocyte responses. *J. Endocrinol.* **2010**, *204*, 153–164. [CrossRef] [PubMed]

38. John, H.; Hierer, J.; Haas, O.; Forssmann, W.G. Quantification of angiotensin-converting-enzyme-mediated degradation of human chemerin 145-154 in plasma by matrix-assisted laser desorption/ionization-time-of-flight mass spectrometry. *Anal. Biochem.* **2007**, *362*, 117–125. [CrossRef]

39. Urushihara, M.; Kinoshita, Y.; Kondo, S.; Kagami, S. Involvement of the intrarenal renin-angiotensin system in experimental models of glomerulonephritis. *J. Biomed. Biotechnol.* **2012**, *2012*, 601786. [CrossRef]

40. Anders, H.J.; Vielhauer, V.; Schlondorff, D. Chemokines and chemokine receptors are involved in the resolution or progression of renal disease. *Kidney Int.* **2003**, *63*, 401–415. [CrossRef]

41. Ishizaki, M.; Masuda, Y.; Fukuda, Y.; Sugisaki, Y.; Yamanaka, N.; Masugi, Y. Experimental mesangioproliferative glomerulonephritis in rats induced by intravenous administration of anti-thymocyte serum. *Acta Pathol. Jpn.* **1986**, *36*, 1191–1203. [CrossRef]

42. Hartner, A.; Schocklmann, H.; Prols, F.; Muller, U.; Sterzel, R.B. Alpha8 integrin in glomerular mesangial cells and in experimental glomerulonephritis. *Kidney Int.* **1999**, *56*, 1468–1480. [CrossRef] [PubMed]

43. Sakai, N.; Iseki, K.; Suzuki, S.; Mori, T.; Hagino, S.; Zhang, Y.; Yokoya, S.; Kawasaki, Y.; Suzuki, J.; Isome, M.; et al. Uninephrectomy induces progressive glomerulosclerosis and apoptosis in anti-Thy1 glomerulonephritis. *Pathol. Int.* **2005**, *55*, 19–26. [CrossRef] [PubMed]

44. Kawachi, H.; Iwanaga, T.; Toyabe, S.; Oite, T.; Shimizu, F. Mesangial sclerotic change with persistent proteinuria in rats after two consecutive injections of monoclonal antibody 1-22-3. *Clin. Exp. Immunol.* **1992**, *90*, 129–134. [CrossRef] [PubMed]

45. Yamamoto, T.; Qureshi, A.R.; Anderstam, B.; Heimburger, O.; Barany, P.; Lindholm, B.; Stenvinkel, P.; Axelsson, J. Clinical importance of an elevated circulating chemerin level in incident dialysis patients. *Nephrol. Dial. Transplant.* **2010**, *25*, 4017–4023. [CrossRef] [PubMed]

46. Mukai, H.; Dai, L.; Chen, Z.; Lindholm, B.; Ripsweden, J.; Brismar, T.B.; Heimburger, O.; Barany, P.; Qureshi, A.R.; Soderberg, M.; et al. Inverse J-shaped relation between coronary arterial calcium density and mortality in advanced chronic kidney disease. *Nephrol. Dial. Transplant.* **2018**. [CrossRef] [PubMed]

47. Carracedo, M.; Artiach, G.; Witasp, A.; Claria, J.; Carlstrom, M.; Laguna-Fernandez, A.; Stenvinkel, P.; Back, M. The G-protein coupled receptor ChemR23 determines smooth muscle cell phenotypic switching to enhance high phosphate-induced vascular calcification. *Cardiovasc Res.* **2019**, *115*, 1557–1566. [CrossRef] [PubMed]

48. Artiach, G.; Carracedo, M.; Claria, J.; Laguna-Fernandez, A.; Back, M. Opposing Effects on Vascular Smooth Muscle Cell Proliferation and Macrophage-induced Inflammation Reveal a Protective Role for the Proresolving Lipid Mediator Receptor ChemR23 in Intimal Hyperplasia. *Front. Pharmacol.* **2018**, *9*, 1327. [CrossRef]

49. Laguna-Fernandez, A.; Checa, A.; Carracedo, M.; Artiach, G.; Petri, M.H.; Baumgartner, R.; Forteza, M.J.; Jiang, X.; Andonova, T.; Walker, M.E.; et al. ERV1/ChemR23 Signaling Protects Against Atherosclerosis by Modifying Oxidized Low-Density Lipoprotein Uptake and Phagocytosis in Macrophages. *Circulation* **2018**, *138*, 1693–1705. [CrossRef]

50. Sato, K.; Yoshizawa, H.; Seki, T.; Shirai, R.; Yamashita, T.; Okano, T.; Shibata, K.; Wakamatsu, M.J.; Mori, Y.; Morita, T.; et al. Chemerin-9, a potent agonist of chemerin receptor (ChemR23), prevents atherogenesis. *Clin. Sci. (Lond)* **2019**, *133*, 1779–1796. [CrossRef]

51. Carracedo, M.; Witasp, A.; Qureshi, A.R.; Laguna-Fernandez, A.; Brismar, T.; Stenvinkel, P.; Back, M. Chemerin inhibits vascular calcification through ChemR23 and is associated with lower coronary calcium in chronic kidney disease. *J. Int. Med.* **2019**, *286*, 449–457. [CrossRef]

52. Hartner, A.; Jagusch, L.; Cordasic, N.; Amann, K.; Veelken, R.; Jacobi, J.; Hilgers, K.F. Impaired Neovascularization and Reduced Capillary Supply in the Malignant vs. Non-malignant Course of Experimental Renovascular Hypertension. *Front. Physiol.* **2016**, *7*, 370. [CrossRef] [PubMed]

53. Mai, M.; Hilgers, K.F.; Wagner, J.; Mann, J.F.; Geiger, H. Expression of angiotensin-converting enzyme in renovascular hypertensive rat kidney. *Hypertension* **1995**, *25*, 674–678. [CrossRef] [PubMed]

54. Baker, A.J.; Mooney, A.; Hughes, J.; Lombardi, D.; Johnson, R.J.; Savill, J. Mesangial cell apoptosis: The major mechanism for resolution of glomerular hypercellularity in experimental mesangial proliferative nephritis. *J. Clin. Investig.* **1994**, *94*, 2105–2116. [CrossRef] [PubMed]

55. Menendez-Castro, C.; Fahlbusch, F.; Cordasic, N.; Amann, K.; Munzel, K.; Plank, C.; Wachtveitl, R.; Rascher, W.; Hilgers, K.F.; Hartner, A. Early and late postnatal myocardial and vascular changes in a protein restriction rat model of intrauterine growth restriction. *PLoS ONE* **2011**, *6*, e20369. [CrossRef]

56. Menendez-Castro, C.; Hilgers, K.F.; Amann, K.; Daniel, C.; Cordasic, N.; Wachtveitl, R.; Fahlbusch, F.; Plank, C.; Dotsch, J.; Rascher, W.; et al. Intrauterine growth restriction leads to a dysregulation of Wilms' tumour supressor gene 1 (WT1) and to early podocyte alterations. *Nephrol Dial. Transplant.* **2013**, *28*, 1407–1417. [CrossRef]

57. Menendez-Castro, C.; Toka, O.; Fahlbusch, F.; Cordasic, N.; Wachtveitl, R.; Hilgers, K.F.; Rascher, W.; Hartner, A. Impaired myocardial performance in a normotensive rat model of intrauterine growth restriction. *Pediatr. Res.* **2014**, *75*, 697–706. [CrossRef]

58. Laemmli, U.K. Cleavage of structural proteins during the assembly of the head of bacteriophage T4. *Nature* **1970**, *227*, 680–685. [CrossRef]

59. Gibson, U.E.; Heid, C.A.; Williams, P.M. A novel method for real time quantitative RT-PCR. *Genome Res.* **1996**, *6*, 995–1001. [CrossRef]

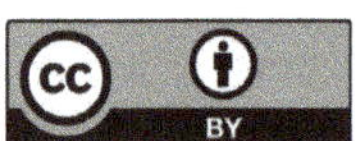

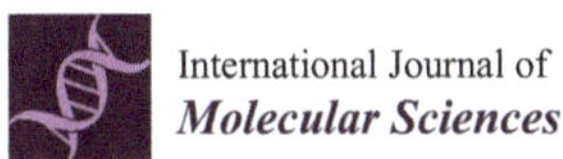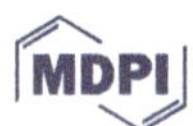

International Journal of
Molecular Sciences

Article

Xanthine Oxidase Inhibitor Febuxostat Exerts an Anti-Inflammatory Action and Protects against Diabetic Nephropathy Development in KK-Ay Obese Diabetic Mice

Yu Mizuno [1], Takeshi Yamamotoya [1], Yusuke Nakatsu [1], Koji Ueda [1], Yasuka Matsunaga [1,2], Masa-Ki Inoue [1], Hideyuki Sakoda [3], Midori Fujishiro [4], Hiraku Ono [5], Takako Kikuchi [6], Masahiro Takahashi [7], Kenichi Morii [8], Kensuke Sasaki [8], Takao Masaki [8], Tomoichiro Asano [1,*] and Akifumi Kushiyama [7,*]

[1] Department of Medical Science, Graduate School of Medicine, University of Hiroshima, 1-2-3 Kasumi, Minami-ku, Hiroshima City, Hiroshima 734-8551, Japan; d186723@hiroshima-u.ac.jp (Y.M.); ymmty@hiroshima-u.ac.jp (T.Y.); nakatsu@hiroshima-u.ac.jp (Y.N.); urouedakouji@yahoo.co.jp (K.U.); ymatsunaga@tulane.edu (Y.M.); b131831@hiroshima-u.ac.jp (M.-K.I.)

[2] Center for Translational Research in Infection & Inflammation, School of Medicine, Tulane University, 6823 St. Charles Avenue, New Orleans, LA 70118, USA

[3] Division of Neurology, Respirology, Endocrinology, and Metabolism, Department of Internal Medicine, Faculty of Medicine, University of Miyazaki, 5200 Kihara, Kiyotake, Miyazaki 889-1692, Japan; hideyuki_sakoda@med.miyazaki-u.ac.jp

[4] Division of Diabetes and Metabolic Diseases, Nihon University School of Medicine, Itabashi, Tokyo 173-8610, Japan; fujishiro.midori@nihon-u.ac.jp

[5] Department of Clinical Cell Biology, Graduate School of Medicine, Chiba University, 1-8-1 Inohana, Chuo-ku, Chiba City, Chiba 260-8670, Japan; hono@chiba-u.jp

[6] Division of Diabetes and Metabolism, The Institute for Adult Diseases, Asahi Life Foundation, 2-2-6, Nihonbashi Bakurocho, Chuo-ku, Tokyo 103-0002, Japan; kikuchi-tk@umin.ac.jp

[7] Department of Pharmacotherapy, Meiji Pharmaceutical University, 2-522-1 Noshio, Kiyose City, Tokyo 204-8588, Japan; t-masa@my-pharm.ac.jp

[8] Department of Nephrology, Hiroshima University Hospital, 1-2-3 Kasumi, Minami-ku, Hiroshima City, Hiroshima 734-8551, Japan; kenichi_morii@yahoo.co.jp (K.M.); sasakikuma@gmail.com (K.S.); masakit@hiroshima-u.ac.jp (T.M.)

* Correspondence: tasano@hiroshima-u.ac.jp (T.A.); kushiyama@my-pharm.ac.jp (A.K.); Tel./Fax: +81-42-495-8725 (A.K.)

Received: 17 August 2019; Accepted: 17 September 2019; Published: 21 September 2019

Abstract: Hyperuricemia has been recognized as a risk factor for insulin resistance as well as one of the factors leading to diabetic kidney disease (DKD). Since DKD is the most common cause of end-stage renal disease, we investigated whether febuxostat, a xanthine oxidase (XO) inhibitor, exerts a protective effect against the development of DKD. We used KK-Ay mice, an established obese diabetic rodent model. Eight-week-old KK-Ay mice were provided drinking water with or without febuxostat (15 µg/mL) for 12 weeks and then subjected to experimentation. Urine albumin secretion and degrees of glomerular injury judged by microscopic observations were markedly higher in KK-Ay than in control lean mice. These elevations were significantly normalized by febuxostat treatment. On the other hand, body weights and high serum glucose concentrations and glycated albumin levels of KK-Ay mice were not affected by febuxostat treatment, despite glucose tolerance and insulin tolerance tests having revealed febuxostat significantly improved insulin sensitivity and glucose tolerance. Interestingly, the IL-1β, IL-6, MCP-1, and ICAM-1 mRNA levels, which were increased in KK-Ay mouse kidneys as compared with normal controls, were suppressed by febuxostat administration. These data indicate a protective effect of XO inhibitors against the development of DKD, and the underlying mechanism likely involves inflammation suppression which is independent of hyperglycemia amelioration.

Keywords: diabetic kidney diseases; xanthine oxidase; glomerular damage

---

1. Introduction

Diabetic kidney disease (DKD) is currently a leading cause of end-stage renal failure [1], while treatments with renin–angiotensin–aldosterone system blockers with normalization of hyperglycemia are regarded as the gold standard [2,3]. In addition, several studies have shown hyperuricemia to be an independent factor impacting insulin resistance and also to play a significant role in the development of diabetic nephropathy [4,5]. In patients with type 1 diabetic nephropathy, usually not accompanied by insulin resistance, hyperuricemia is also shown to be an independent risk of renal dysfunction [6].

Uric acid is generated from hypoxanthine and xanthine by xanthine oxidase (XO) as the final step in the metabolism of endogenous and exogenous purines [7]. Clinical trials have proven the efficacy of XO inhibitors, including allopurinol and febuxostat, not only for lowering the serum uric acid concentration but also for protection against the progression of renal diseases [8,9]. Even for diabetic nephropathy, XO inhibition has been shown to be effective in several clinical trials [10–12]. However, whether reducing the serum uric acid level or suppression of XO activity contributes to the protective effect of XO inhibitors on renal diseases remains unclear. Therefore, elucidation of the effects and mechanisms of action of XO inhibitors is eagerly awaited.

A previous study using an insulin-deficient Type 1 diabetic model rat and XO inhibitors, including allopurinol and febuxostat, suggested the renal protective effect of febuxostat to be mediated via attenuation of oxidative and inflammatory effects [13,14]. On the other hand, a study using obese diabetic db/db mice treated with allopurinol also showed the renal protective effect of XO inhibitors to involve lowering uric acid directly [13,15]. Therefore, to date, only a few studies have focused on the mechanism, particularly that against diabetic nephropathy, underlying XO inhibitor-mediated renal protective effects.

In this study, we employed KK-Ay mice that spontaneously exhibit type 2 diabetes associated with hyperglycemia, glucose intolerance, hyperinsulinemia, obesity, and microalbuminuria [16], and investigated the effects of febuxostat on the development of diabetic nephropathy in these mice. Our observations raise the possibility that the renal protective effects of the XO inhibitor febuxostat are mediated mainly by an anti-inflammatory effect, which is independent of the effects on glycemic control.

2. Results

2.1. Effects of XO Inhibitor Febuxostat on Glycemic Control and Serum Uric Acid Levels

Diabetic KK-Ay mice were divided into two groups, with and without febuxostat in drinking water. After 12 weeks of treatment, while KK-Ay mice had higher body weights, blood glucose concentrations in the fed state, serum glycated albumin, and serum uric acid levels than the wild-type mice (Figure 1A–D), febuxostat treatment reduced the serum uric acid level of KK-Ay mice without significantly affecting other parameters. However, unexpectedly, glucose tolerance and insulin tolerance tests revealed treatment with febuxostat significantly ameliorated the impairments in KK-Ay mice (Figure 1E,F).

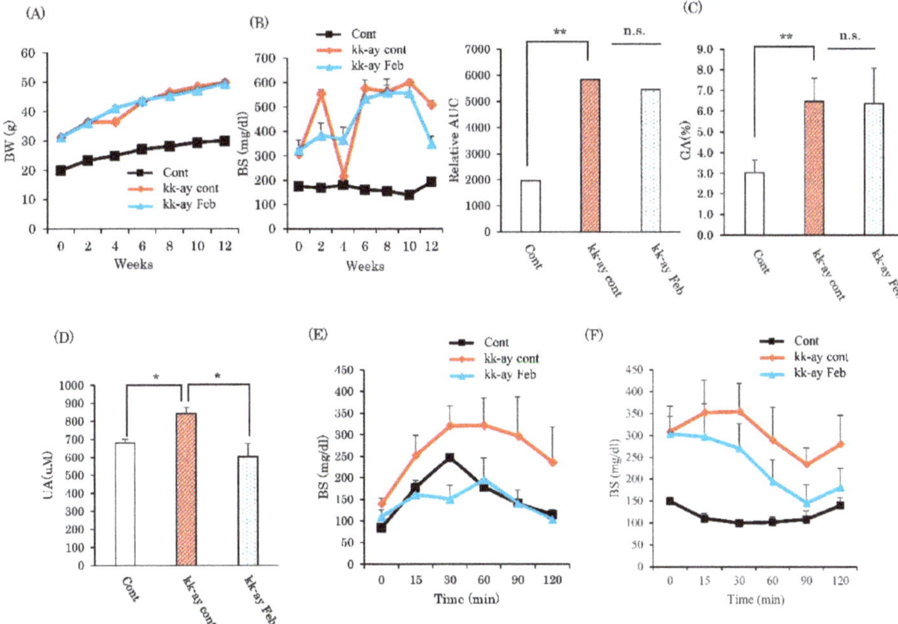

Figure 1. Inhibitory effects of xanthine oxidase inhibitor febuxostat on the progression of diabetic nephropathy. (**A**) Body weights and (**B**) blood sugar levels were measured. (**C**) Serum glycated albumin levels. (**D**) Serum uric acid levels. (**E**) Glucose tolerance test results. (**F**) Insulin tolerance test. Data are means ± SE. * $p < 0.05$, ** $p < 0.001$, n = 8 for control group, n = 10 for KK-Ay mice without febuxostat group and n = 8 for KK-Ay mice with febuxostat group.

2.2. Effects of Febuxostat Administration on Glomerular Sclerosis

Glomerular sclerosis is among the features of diabetic nephropathy. The degrees of glomerular sclerosis were estimated based on the findings of Hematoxylin–Eosin (HE) staining and positive peroxide acid-Schiff (PAS) staining (Figure 2A,B). PAS staining is reportedly useful for definitively demonstrating glomerular hypertrophy, an early feature of diabetic nephropathy [17]. Both HE and PAS staining showed glomerular sclerosis to be markedly advanced in KK-Ay mice as compared with wild-type mice, and that this progression showed significant attenuation in response to febuxostat treatment in KK-Ay mice (Figure 2B). Glomerular injury score (GIS) and glomerular areas calculated based on PAS-stained areas were markedly increased in KK-Ay mice than in wild-type controls, and these changes were partially but significantly normalized in febuxostat-treated KK-Ay mice (Figure 2C). While febuxostat treatment did not normalize the increased kidney weights of KK-Ay mice as compared with those of wild-type mice (Figure 2D), an approximately 10-fold increase in the urinary albumin-to-creatinine ratio (ACR) in KK-Ay mice was markedly ameliorated, to a level near that of control C57BL/6 mice, by febuxostat treatment (Figure 2E).

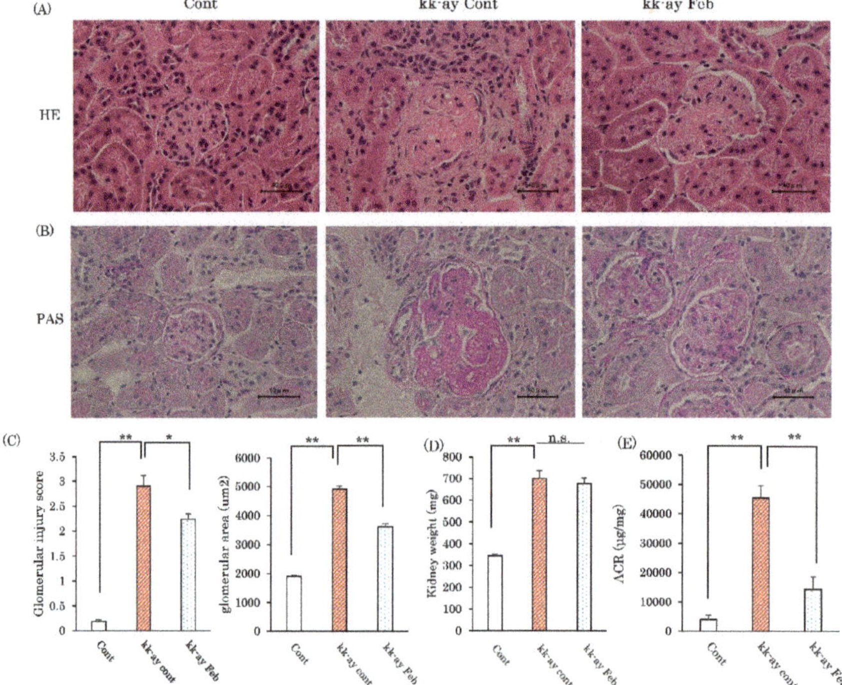

Figure 2. Febuxostat administered for prevention of glomerular sclerosis. (**A**) Hematoxylin–Eosin (HE) staining of kidney fractions. Scale bar = 40 μm. (**B**) Peroxide acid-Schiff (PAS) staining of kidney fractions. Scale bar = 40 μm. (**C**) Glomerular sclerosis score and glomerular area were calculated using image J. (**D**) Kidney weights and (**E**) the urinary albumin to creatinine ratio was measured at 20 weeks. Data are means ± SE. * $p < 0.05$, ** $p < 0.001$. n = 8 for control group, n = 10 for KK-Ay mice without febuxostat group and n = 8 for KK-Ay mice with febuxostat group.

2.3. Effects of Febuxostat on the Renal Expression Levels of Inflammatory Cytokines

Since elevated inflammation-related cytokine and chemokine expressions are reportedly involved in the pathogenesis in diabetic nephropathy, the effects of febuxostat on their mRNA levels were evaluated. In comparison with the normal mice, renal mRNA levels of IL-1β, IL-6, MCP-1, CXCL1, CXCL2, and CXCL5, but not those of the macrophage marker F4/80 and TNFα, were markedly elevated in the KK-Ay mice (Figure 3). Treatment with febuxostat essentially normalized the upregulated expressions of inflammatory cytokines (IL-1β, IL-6) without significantly affecting, though a tendency for reduction was observed, inflammatory chemokines (CKCL1, CXCL2, CXCL5) in KK-Ay mouse kidneys (Figure 3).

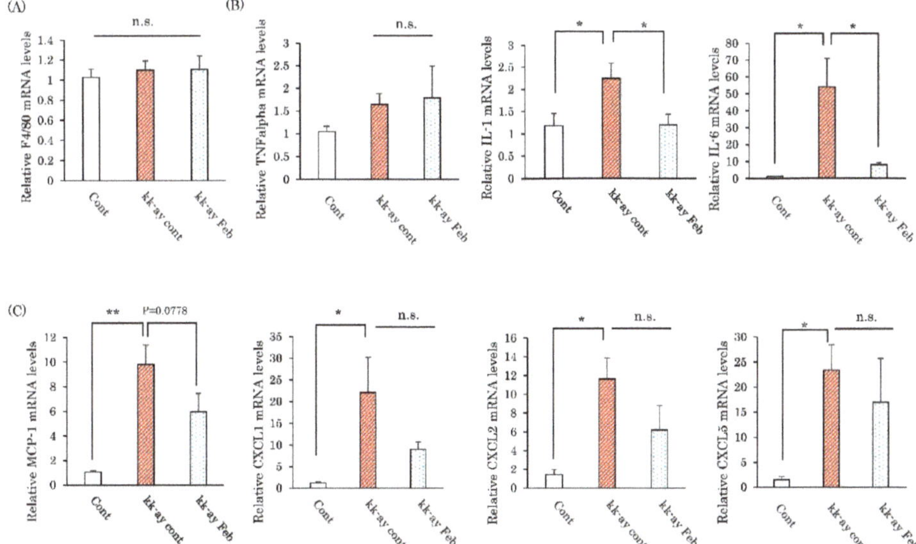

Figure 3. Febuxostat suppressed expressions of inflammatory cytokines in the kidneys of KK-Ay mice. (**A–C**) Relative mRNA levels of macrophage markers, cytokines, and chemokines in the kidneys were determined by employing real-time PCR. Data are means ± SE. * $p < 0.05$, ** $p < 0.001$. n = 8 for control group, n = 10 for KK-Ay mice without febuxostat group and n = 8 for KK-Ay mice with febuxostat group.

2.4. Effects of Febuxostat on Fibrosis-Related Collagen Gene Expressions

Azan staining was performed to evaluate the degree of fibrotic change, a change typical of the advanced stage of diabetic nephropathy. Imaging analysis of the fibrotic area based on Azan staining showed that the areas of increased fibrotic staining and fibrogenesis including glomerulosclerosis in the KK-Ay mice, as compared with control mice, were normalized by febuxostat treatment (Figure 4A). We next investigated the effects of febuxostat on the expression levels of the mRNA of genes related to the fibrotic process. The mRNA expression level of collagen 1a1 was increased in the kidneys of KK-Ay mice, but this elevation tended to be normalized by febuxostat treatment though the difference did not reach statistical significance (Figure 4B). On the other hand, mRNA expression levels of collagen 1a2, collagen 4a1, and collagen 4a2 did not show significant differences between KK-Ay and wild-type mice or between the presence and absence of febuxostat treatment (Figure 4B).

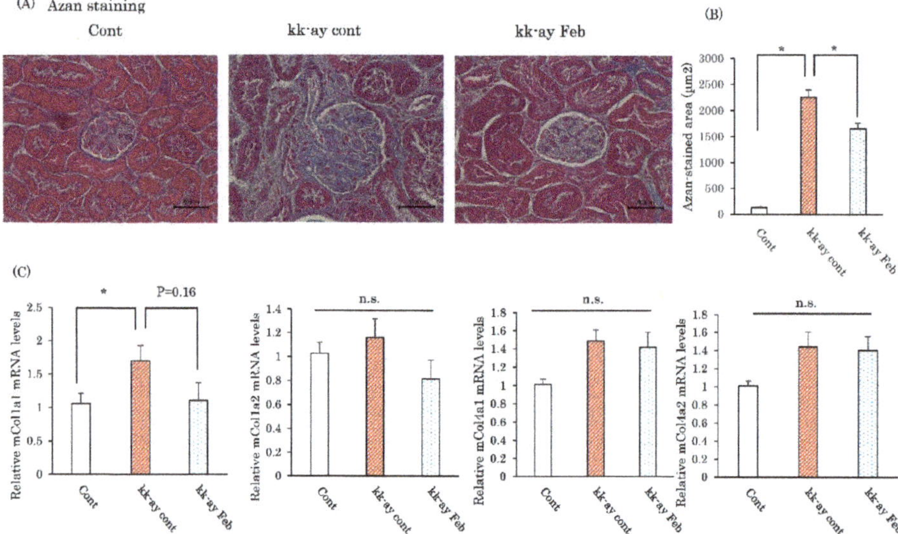

Figure 4. Febuxostat prevented progression of kidney fibrosis. (**A**) Azan staining of kidney fractions. Scale bar = 40 μm. (**B**) Relative mRNA levels of fibrotic markers in the kidneys. (**C**) The renal fibrotic area was assessed using Azan staining and then measured using image J. Data are means ± SE. * $p < 0.05$. n = 8 for control group, n = 10 for KK-Ay mice without febuxostat group and n = 8 for KK-Ay mice with febuxostat group.

2.5. Effects of Febuxostat on Markers of Oxidative Stress and the Endoplasmic Reticulum

Since febuxostat reportedly reduces the production of xanthine-induced oxidants, we measured oxidative stress in the kidneys of KK-Ay mice with and without febuxostat treatment and in wild-type mice. The amount of renal MDA, a product of lipid peroxidation, measured by the thiobarbituric acid reactive substances (TBARS) assay, showed no significant differences with wide variations among the three groups (Figure 5A). Expressions of endothelial damage markers (ICAM-1, VCAM-1) in the kidneys were elevated in KK-Ay mice as compared with wild-type mice, and febuxostat reduced these ICAM-1 elevations though not significantly (Figure 5B). Similarly, the mRNA levels of an endoplasmic reticulum stress marker (CHOP) were elevated in KK-Ay mice as compared to wild-type mice, with febuxostat reducing, though not significantly, these elevations (Figure 5C).

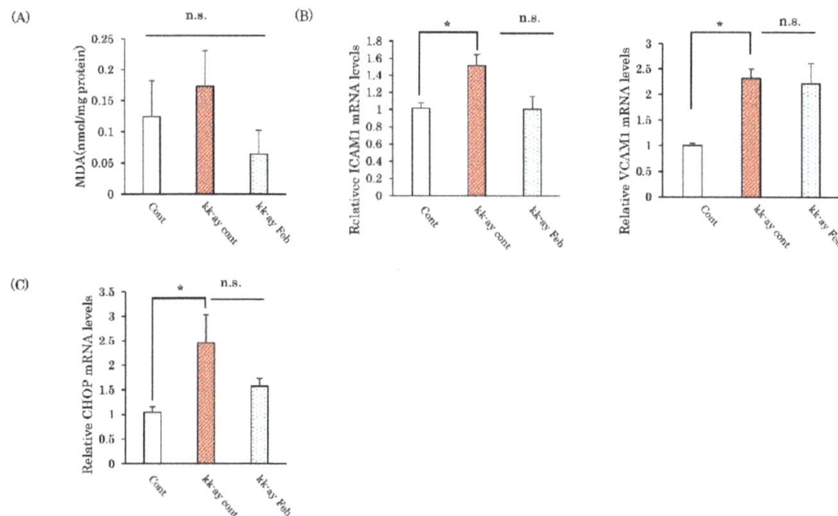

Figure 5. Febuxostat had no significant effect on either oxidative stress or endoplasmic reticulum stress. (**A**) Amounts of malondialdehyde were measured in renal tissues. (**B**) Relative mRNA levels of ICAM-1 and VCAM-1 in the kidneys. (**C**) Relative mRNA levels of CHOP in the kidney. Data are means ± SE. * $p < 0.05$, n = 8 in control group and KK-Ay mice with febuxostat, n = 10 in KK-Ay mice without febuxostat

3. Discussion

The relationship between hyperuricemia and the development of DKD is now widely recognized [18–20]. In the pathogenesis of DKD, inflammation appears to play essential roles via inflammatory mediators, adhesion molecules, and inflammatory signaling pathways directly or indirectly induced by hyperglycemia [1]. We previously demonstrated XO activity to promote inflammation in blood vessels [21] and the liver [22], while XO inhibitors suppress inflammation and oxidative stress [23] in macrophages. Thus, treatment with XO inhibitors prevented inflammatory and fibrotic changes in rodent models of atherosclerosis and non-alcoholic steatohepatitis. Another group also reported febuxostat to suppress angiotensin II-induced aortic fibrosis via XO inhibition in macrophages [24].

In this study, we showed febuxostat treatment to attenuate the development of proteinuria and to ameliorate mesangial structural changes in the kidneys of type 2 diabetic KK-Ay mice. A previous study using db/db mice also showed that allopurinol normalized hyperuricemia (to approximately 3 mg/dL) and reduced albuminuria with improvements in some of the features of diabetic nephropathy [15]. The authors insisted that high glucose accompanied by high uric acid (UA) is the causal mechanism of progressive renal function loss in db/db mice, based on a small increase in sICAM-1 detected by in vitro assay. In contrast, while KK/Ay mice showed slightly higher serum UA levels than control wild-type mice, these levels remained relatively low (around 1 mg/dL). The improved glucose tolerance and insulin tolerance test results by febuxostat obtained in this study might be consistent with the previous study using XO inhibitor [25]. However, it should be noted that the actual degree of hyperglycemia in KK/Ay mice, judging from blood sugar and glycated albumin levels, was not significantly altered by febuxostat administration. Furthermore, we recently reported treatment with febuxostat to provide significant protection from kidney failure, possibly via suppression of inflammation, in gddY mice [26], a model spontaneously developing IgA nephropathy [27] but showing no glucose metabolism defect. Taken together, these findings suggest that it would be inappropriate to interpret the mechanism underlying amelioration of renal dysfunction in KK/Ay mice as being via normalization of hyperuricemia and hyperglycemia.

The renal protective effects of febuxostat appear to be exerted through its potent anti-inflammatory actions. Despite macrophage infiltration, as indirectly evaluated by the F4/80 level, being unchanged by febuxostat treatment, renal injury was suppressed, and this was associated with reductions in inflammatory cytokines. XO inhibition was also reported to attenuate certain cellular migrations [28,29] and monocytic differentiations, such as those of foam cell formation and multinucleated giant cell formation [21,30]. Indeed, the renal protective effects of XO inhibition are consistent with previous reports showing the effects of febuxostat in mice with gddY IgA nephropathy [26] and in 5/6 nephrectomy rats, regardless of the coexisting hyperuricemia [31]. The suppressive effect on inflammation is a common feature of febuxostat treatment. Our present observations suggest febuxostat suppresses urinary albumin and glomerular injury at early stages of type 2 diabetic nephropathy, i.e., at the stage when inflammatory cytokines, such as IL-6 [32] and MCP-1, are secreted [33]. Repeated suppressions of ICAM-1 expression reportedly raised the possibility of preventing tissue injuries by administering XO inhibitors [15,34,35].

Collagenous proliferation evaluated by Azan as well as mesangial expansion, as evaluated by PAS staining, became more severe in KK/Ay mice and showed amelioration in response to febuxostat. In db/db, there are reportedly no changes in PAS staining with allopurinol treatment [15]. Febuxostat attenuated renal protein expression of TGF-β, CTGF, and collagen 4 in the kidneys of Zucker obese rats [14]. Studies using db/db mice [15] and our current experiments showed no reductions in collagen 4, though our data on collagen 1a1 and measurement of collagen 3 in db/db mice indicated both to be reduced by febuxostat administration. Despite variations in renal glomerular damage among animal models and/or species, it is reasonable to consider febuxostat to exert positive effects in terms of maintaining glomerular structure. Comparisons of the data from different sources imply that the effect of febuxostat might be more evident in KK/Ay than in db/db mice, although the mechanism underlying this difference is unclear.

Two mechanisms possibly underlying hyperuricemia-related DKD development have been suggested, elevation of the serum UA and increased superoxide free radical generation [36,37]. Oxidative stress indicators, such as the whole-kidney MDA level, and ER stress marker CHOP did not show a clearly significant difference and relatively large variance was noted. We speculate that the generation of oxidative stress would be limited to a highly localized area and that significant local changes might be difficult to detect at the whole-kidney level. Thus, we were not able to conclude that the effects of febuxostat are not due, even partially, to reduced free radical generation. Further studies are necessary to clarify this issue.

There are some limitations in this study. First, since febuxostat administration to kk-ay mice in this study showed significant changes in glomerular lesions and no obvious changes in the renal tubules or mesenchyme. Therefore, we focused on the histological glomerular change, however, the inflammation and/or fibrosis in tubulointerstitium should be evaluated in the future study. Finally, all the mRNA analysis is performed in whole kidney and not from the glomeruli, therefore the relationship between the gene expression and the effect of febuxostat on the glomerular protection might not be direct. Finally, the other xanthine oxidase inhibitors such as allopurinol, its metabolite oxypurinol, and topiroxostat should be evaluated in our model, to clarify the glomerular protective effect of febuxostat is class-effect.

In conclusion, we demonstrated that KK-Ay mice developed evident hyperglycemia and slight hyperuricemia, leading to diabetic nephropathy progression. XO inhibition by febuxostat ameliorated both proteinuria and glomerular damage, without affecting plasma glucose levels. Furthermore, the mechanism likely involves blocking intrarenal inflammation.

4. Materials and Methods

4.1. Animals

Male diabetic KK-Ay mice and age-matched C57BL/6 mice (8 weeks of age) were purchased from CLEA Japan (Tokyo, Japan). Febuxostat was obtained from Teijin Pharma Ltd., Tokyo, Japan. The mice were housed in temperature- and light-controlled rooms with free access to food (Oriental Yeast, Tokyo, Japan) and water. After the 12 weeks of treatment with or without drinking water containing febuxostat (15 μg/mL), which corresponds to approximately 1 mg/kg body weight per day, close to the clinical dose range of oral febuxostat, the mice were killed, and their kidneys and blood samples were collected. For uric acid (UA) measurement, 100 μL whole blood samples were collected with 100 μM allopurinol (Wako, Osaka, Japan). To measure the glucose concentration, blood samples were incubated on ice for 30 min and then centrifuged at 15,000 rpm for 30 min at 4 °C. All samples were preserved at −80 °C. All mice were handled in accordance with Guidelines for Care and Use of Experimental Animals published by Hiroshima University, and all protocols were approved by Hiroshima University (Approval #A17-178 Date 29 March 2018).

4.2. Metabolic Analysis

Mouse urine was collected for 24 h employing metabolic cages and preserved at −80 °C. Urine albumin and creatinine were quantified using a mouse albumin ELISA kit (FUJIFILM Wako Shibayagi, Gunma, Japan) and a mouse creatinine assay kit (Abcam, Cambridge, MA, USA), respectively. Serum UA concentrations were assayed with a UA assay kit (Cayman Chemical, Ann Arbor, UI, USA). All assays were conducted according to the manufacturers' protocols. The albumin-to-creatinine ratio (ACR) was calculated as urinary albumin/urinary creatinine.

4.3. Histological Study

Kidneys were fixed in 10% formalin, embedded in paraffin, and then cut into 2-μm sections. The sections were subjected to peroxide acid-Schiff (PAS) and Azan staining to identify glomerular sclerosis and fibrotic change, respectively [38].

Glomerular injury included mesangial matrix expansion and/or hyalinosis with focal adhesions, capillary dilation, and true glomerular tuft occlusion, and sclerosis. For the quantitative analysis of glomerular injury, the glomerular injury score (GIS) was determined on PAS-stained paraffin sections using a scale ranging from 0 to 4 for normal (0), with 1 = 25% sclerosis, 2 = 50% sclerosis, 3 = 75% sclerosis, and 4 = 100% sclerosis [39]. On average, 40 glomeruli were evaluated per mouse. GIS was calculated as [$\sum$ (each score × number of glomeruli)]/number of glomeruli. The glomerular area was measured in an average of 40 glomeruli per mouse employing image J (NIH, Bethesda, MD, USA). The renal fibrotic area was assessed using Azan staining, with an average of 10 glomeruli being measured per mouse using NIH Image J. All structural analyses were conducted in a blinded manner on unidentified sections.

4.4. Malondialdehyde (MDA) assay

Thiobarbituric acid reactive substances (TBARS) were measured using a TBARS assay kit (Cayman Chemical, Ann Arbor, UI, USA), according to the manufacturer's instructions, and absorbance was determined at 540 nm.

4.5. Quantitative Real-Time RT-PCR

Total RNA was extracted from mouse kidneys using Sepasol reagent (Nacalai Tesque, Kyoto, Japan). A 500 ng quantity of RNA was reverse transcribed using the Verso cDNA Synthesis kit (Thermo Scientific, Vilnius, Lithuania), which degrades double-stranded DNA. Quantitative real-time RT-PCR was performed using SYBR Green PCR master mix (Agilent Technologies, Santa Clara, CA, USA) on a CFX96 real-time PCR system (Bio-Rad, Hercules, CA, USA). Relative mRNA gene levels were normalized to the GAPDH mRNA level, and relative expressions were determined by the comparative Ct method. The designed primers used are shown previously [26].

4.6. Statistical Analysis

All results are expressed as means ± SE. Statistical analyses were conducted using ANOVA followed by Dunnett's test. A value of $p < 0.05$ was taken to indicate a statistically significant difference.

Author Contributions: Data curation, Y.N.; Formal analysis, T.Y., Y.N., T.K., M.T., and A.K.; Investigation, Y.M. (Yu Mizuno), T.Y., and K.U., Masa-ki Inoue, T.K., K.K., K.S., and A.K.; Methodology, K.K., K.S., T.M., and T.A.; Supervision, Y.M. (Yasuka Matsunaga), H.S., M.F., H.O., M.T., K.K., K.S., and T.M.; Validation, Y.M. (Yasuka Matsunaga); Writing—original draft, Y.M. (Yu Mizuno), T.A., and A.K.; Writing—review and editing, T.A. and A.K.

Funding: This research was funded by Grant-in-Aid for Scientific Research (C): 16K09791.

References

1. Matoba, K.; Takeda, Y.; Nagai, Y.; Kawanami, D.; Utsunomiya, K.; Nishimura, R. Unraveling the Role of Inflammation in the Pathogenesis of Diabetic Kidney Disease. *Int J. Mol. Sci.* **2019**. [CrossRef]

2. Vejakama, P.; Ingsathit, A.; McKay, G.J.; Maxwell, A.P.; McEvoy, M.; Attia, J.; Thakkinstian, A. Treatment effects of renin-angiotensin aldosterone system blockade on kidney failure and mortality in chronic kidney disease patients. *BMC Nephrol.* **2017**, *18*, 342. [CrossRef]

3. Riccio, E.; Di Nuzzi, A.; Pisani, A. Nutritional treatment in chronic kidney disease: The concept of nephroprotection. *Clin. Exp. Nephrol.* **2015**, *19*, 161–167. [CrossRef]

4. Tanaka, K.; Hara, S.; Hattori, M.; Sakai, K.; Onishi, Y.; Yoshida, Y.; Kawazu, S.; Kushiyama, A. Role of elevated serum uric acid levels at the onset of overt nephropathy in the risk for renal function decline in patients with type 2 diabetes. *J. Diabetes Investig.* **2015**, *6*, 98–104. [CrossRef]

5. Shichiri, M.; Iwamoto, H.; Marumo, F. Diabetic hypouricemia as an indicator of clinical nephropathy. *Am. J. Nephrol.* **1990**, *10*, 115–122. [CrossRef]

6. Ficociello, L.H.; Rosolowsky, E.T.; Niewczas, M.A.; Maselli, N.J.; Weinberg, J.M.; Aschengrau, A.; Eckfeldt, J.H.; Stanton, R.C.; Galecki, A.T.; Doria, A.; et al. High-normal serum uric acid increases risk of early progressive renal function loss in type 1 diabetes: Results of a 6-year follow-up. *Diabetes Care* **2010**, *33*, 1337–1343. [CrossRef]

7. Kushiyama, A.; Tanaka, K.; Hara, S.; Kawazu, S. Linking uric acid metabolism to diabetic complications. *World J. Diabetes* **2014**, *5*, 787–795. [CrossRef]

8. Pisano, A.; Cernaro, V.; Gembillo, G.; D'Arrigo, G.; Buemi, M.; Bolignano, D. Xanthine Oxidase Inhibitors for Improving Renal Function in Chronic Kidney Disease Patients: An Updated Systematic Review and Meta-Analysis. *Int. J. Mol. Sci.* **2017**. [CrossRef]

9. Siu, Y.P.; Leung, K.T.; Tong, M.K.; Kwan, T.H. Use of allopurinol in slowing the progression of renal disease through its ability to lower serum uric acid level. *Am. J. Kidney Dis.* **2006**, *47*, 51–59. [CrossRef]

10. Beddhu, S.; Filipowicz, R.; Wang, B.; Wei, G.; Chen, X.; Roy, A.C.; DuVall, S.L.; Farrukh, H.; Habib, A.N.; Bjordahl, T.; et al. A Randomized Controlled Trial of the Effects of Febuxostat Therapy on Adipokines and Markers of Kidney Fibrosis in Asymptomatic Hyperuricemic Patients With Diabetic Nephropathy. *Can. J. Kidney Health Dis.* **2016**, *3*, 2054358116675343. [CrossRef]

11. Mukri, M.N.A.; Kong, W.Y.; Mustafar, R.; Shaharir, S.S.; Shah, S.A.; Abdul Gafor, A.H.; Mohd, R.; Abdul Cader, R.; Kamaruzaman, L. Role of febuxostat in retarding progression of diabetic kidney disease with asymptomatic hyperuricemia: A 6-months open-label, randomized controlled trial. *Excli. J.* **2018**, *17*, 563–575.

12. Kojima, S.; Matsui, K.; Hiramitsu, S.; Hisatome, I.; Waki, M.; Uchiyama, K.; Yokota, N.; Tokutake, E.; Wakasa, Y.; Jinnouchi, H.; et al. Febuxostat for Cerebral and CaRdiorenovascular Events PrEvEntion StuDy. *Eur. Heart J.* **2019**, *40*, 1778–1786. [CrossRef]

13. Wang, C.; Pan, Y.; Zhang, Q.Y.; Wang, F.M.; Kong, L.D. Quercetin and allopurinol ameliorate kidney injury in STZ-treated rats with regulation of renal NLRP3 inflammasome activation and lipid accumulation. *PLoS ONE* **2012**, *7*, e38285. [CrossRef]

14. Komers, R.; Xu, B.; Schneider, J.; Oyama, T.T. Effects of xanthine oxidase inhibition with febuxostat on the development of nephropathy in experimental type 2 diabetes. *Br. J. Pharm.* **2016**, *173*, 2573–2588. [CrossRef]

15. Kosugi, T.; Nakayama, T.; Heinig, M.; Zhang, L.; Yuzawa, Y.; Sanchez-Lozada, L.G.; Roncal, C.; Johnson, R.J.; Nakagawa, T. Effect of lowering uric acid on renal disease in the type 2 diabetic db/db mice. *Am. J. Physiol. Ren. Physiol.* **2009**, *297*, F481–488. [CrossRef]

16. Iwatsuka, H.; Shino, A.; Suzuoki, Z. General survey of diabetic features of yellow KK mice. *Endocrinol Jpn.* **1970**, *17*, 23–35. [CrossRef]

17. Ruggenenti, P.; Remuzzi, G. Nephropathy of type-2 diabetes mellitus. *J. Am. Soc. Nephrol.* **1998**, *9*, 2157–2169.

18. Bo, S.; Cavallo-Perin, P.; Gentile, L.; Repetti, E.; Pagano, G. Hypouricemia and hyperuricemia in type 2 diabetes: Two different phenotypes. *Eur. J. Clin. Invest.* **2001**, *31*, 318–321. [CrossRef]

19. Rosolowsky, E.T.; Ficociello, L.H.; Maselli, N.J.; Niewczas, M.A.; Binns, A.L.; Roshan, B.; Warram, J.H.; Krolewski, A.S. High-normal serum uric acid is associated with impaired glomerular filtration rate in nonproteinuric patients with type 1 diabetes. *Clin. J. Am. Soc. Nephrol.* **2008**, *3*, 706–713. [CrossRef]

20. Tseng, C.H. Correlation of uric acid and urinary albumin excretion rate in patients with type 2 diabetes mellitus in Taiwan. *Kidney Int.* **2005**, *68*, 796–801. [CrossRef]

21. Kushiyama, A.; Okubo, H.; Sakoda, H.; Kikuchi, T.; Fujishiro, M.; Sato, H.; Kushiyama, S.; Iwashita, M.; Nishimura, F.; Fukushima, T.; et al. Xanthine oxidoreductase is involved in macrophage foam cell formation and atherosclerosis development. *Arter. Thromb. Vasc. Biol.* **2012**, *32*, 291–298. [CrossRef]

22. Nakatsu, Y.; Seno, Y.; Kushiyama, A.; Sakoda, H.; Fujishiro, M.; Katasako, A.; Mori, K.; Matsunaga, Y.; Fukushima, T.; Kanaoka, R.; et al. The xanthine oxidase inhibitor febuxostat suppresses development of nonalcoholic steatohepatitis in a rodent model. *Am. J. Physiol. Gastrointest. Liver Physiol.* **2015**, *309*, G42–51. [CrossRef]

23. Nomura, J.; Busso, N.; Ives, A.; Matsui, C.; Tsujimoto, S.; Shirakura, T.; Tamura, M.; Kobayashi, T.; So, A.; Yamanaka, Y. Xanthine oxidase inhibition by febuxostat attenuates experimental atherosclerosis in mice. *Sci. Rep.* **2014**, *4*, 4554. [CrossRef]

24. Kondo, M.; Imanishi, M.; Fukushima, K.; Ikuto, R.; Murai, Y.; Horinouchi, Y.; Izawa-Ishizawa, Y.; Goda, M.; Zamami, Y.; Takechi, K.; et al. Xanthine Oxidase Inhibition by Febuxostat in Macrophages Suppresses Angiotensin II-Induced Aortic Fibrosis. *Am. J. Hypertens* **2019**, *(3)*, 249–256. [CrossRef]

25. Yisireyili, M.; Hayashi, M.; Wu, H.; Uchida, Y.; Yamamoto, K.; Kikuchi, R.; Shoaib Hamrah, M.; Nakayama, T.; Wu Cheng, X.; Matsushita, T.; et al. Xanthine oxidase inhibition by febuxostat attenuates stress-induced hyperuricemia, glucose dysmetabolism, and prothrombotic state in mice. *Sci. Rep.* **2017**, *7*, 1266. [CrossRef]

26. Inoue, M.K.; Yamamotoya, T.; Nakatsu, Y.; Ueda, K.; Inoue, Y.; Matsunaga, Y.; Sakoda, H.; Fujishiro, M.; Ono, H.; Morii, K.; et al. The Xanthine Oxidase Inhibitor Febuxostat Suppresses the Progression of IgA Nephropathy, Possibly via Its Anti-Inflammatory and Anti-Fibrotic Effects in the gddY Mouse Model. *Int. J. Mol. Sci.* **2018**. [CrossRef]

27. Suzuki, H.; Suzuki, Y.; Novak, J.; Tomino, Y. Development of Animal Models of Human IgA Nephropathy. *Drug Discov. Today Dis. Models* **2014**, *11*, 5–11. [CrossRef]

28. Tsirmoula, S.; Lamprou, M.; Hatziapostolou, M.; Kieffer, N.; Papadimitriou, E. Pleiotrophin-induced endothelial cell migration is regulated by xanthine oxidase-mediated generation of reactive oxygen species. *Microvasc. Res.* **2015**, *98*, 74–81. [CrossRef]

29. Oh, S.H.; Choi, S.Y.; Choi, H.J.; Ryu, H.M.; Kim, Y.J.; Jung, H.Y.; Cho, J.H.; Kim, C.D.; Park, S.H.; Kwon, T.H.; et al. The emerging role of xanthine oxidase inhibition for suppression of breast cancer cell migration and metastasis associated with hypercholesterolemia. *FASEB J.* **2019**, *33*, 7301–7314. [CrossRef]

30. Mizuno, K.; Okamoto, H.; Horio, T. Inhibitory influences of xanthine oxidase inhibitor and angiotensin I-converting enzyme inhibitor on multinucleated giant cell formation from monocytes by downregulation of adhesion molecules and purinergic receptors. *Br. J. Derm.* **2004**, *150*, 205–210. [CrossRef]

31. Sanchez-Lozada, L.G.; Tapia, E.; Soto, V.; Avila-Casado, C.; Franco, M.; Wessale, J.L.; Zhao, L.; Johnson, R.J. Effect of febuxostat on the progression of renal disease in 5/6 nephrectomy rats with and without hyperuricemia. *Nephron Physiol.* **2008**, *108*, 69–78. [CrossRef]

32. Choudhary, N.; Ahlawat, R.S. Interleukin-6 and C-reactive protein in pathogenesis of diabetic nephropathy: New evidence linking inflammation, glycemic control, and microalbuminuria. *Iran. J. Kidney Dis.* **2008**, *2*, 72–79.

33. Morii, T.; Fujita, H.; Narita, T.; Shimotomai, T.; Fujishima, H.; Yoshioka, N.; Imai, H.; Kakei, M.; Ito, S. Association of monocyte chemoattractant protein-1 with renal tubular damage in diabetic nephropathy. *J. Diabetes Complicat.* **2003**, *17*, 11–15. [CrossRef]

34. Eleftheriadis, T.; Pissas, G.; Antoniadi, G.; Liakopoulos, V.; Stefanidis, I. Allopurinol protects human glomerular endothelial cells from high glucose-induced reactive oxygen species generation, p53 overexpression and endothelial dysfunction. *Int. Urol. Nephrol.* **2018**, *50*, 179–186. [CrossRef]

35. Dong, G.; Ren, M.; Wang, X.; Jiang, H.; Yin, X.; Wang, S.; Wang, X.; Feng, H. Allopurinol reduces severity of delayed neurologic sequelae in experimental carbon monoxide toxicity in rats. *Neurotoxicology* **2015**, *48*, 171–179. [CrossRef]

36. Yang, C.C.; Ma, M.C.; Chien, C.T.; Wu, M.S.; Sun, W.K.; Chen, C.F. Hypoxic preconditioning attenuates lipopolysaccharide-induced oxidative stress in rat kidneys. *J. Physiol.* **2007**, *582*, 407–419. [CrossRef]

37. Szalay, C.I.; Erdelyi, K.; Kokeny, G.; Lajtar, E.; Godo, M.; Revesz, C.; Kaucsar, T.; Kiss, N.; Sarkozy, M.; Csont, T.; et al. Oxidative/Nitrative Stress and Inflammation Drive Progression of Doxorubicin-Induced Renal Fibrosis in Rats as Revealed by Comparing a Normal and a Fibrosis-Resistant Rat Strain. *PLoS ONE* **2015**, *10*, e0127090. [CrossRef]

38. Afroz, T.; Sagar, R.; Reddy, S.; Gandhe, S.; Rajaram, K.G. Clinical and histological correlation of diabetic nephropathy. *Saudi J. Kidney Dis. Transpl.* **2017**, *28*, 836–841.

39. Lassila, M.; Seah, K.K.; Allen, T.J.; Thallas, V.; Thomas, M.C.; Candido, R.; Burns, W.C.; Forbes, J.M.; Calkin, A.C.; Cooper, M.E.; et al. Accelerated nephropathy in diabetic apolipoprotein e-knockout mouse: Role of advanced glycation end products. *J. Am. Soc. Nephrol.* **2004**, *15*, 2125–2138. [CrossRef]

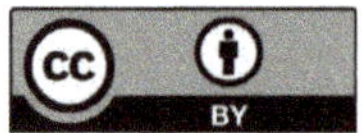

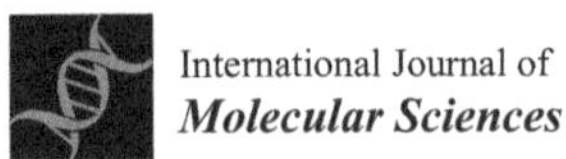
International Journal of
Molecular Sciences

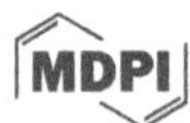

Article

Change in Renal Glomerular Collagens and Glomerular Filtration Barrier-Related Proteins in a Dextran Sulfate Sodium-Induced Colitis Mouse Model

Chia-Jung Chang [1,2], Pi-Chao Wang [3], Tzou-Chi Huang [4] and Akiyoshi Taniguchi [1,2,*]

[1] Cellular Functional Nanobiomaterials Group, Research Center for Functional Materials, National Institute for Materials Science, 1-1 Namiki, Tsukuba, Ibaraki 305-0044, Japan; CHANG.Chiajung@nims.go.jp

[2] Graduate School of Advanced Science and Engineering, Waseda University, 3-4-1 Okubo, Shinjuku-ku, Tokyo 169-8555, Japan

[3] Graduate School of Life and Environmental Sciences, University of Tsukuba, 1-1-1 Tennoudai, Tsukuba, Ibaraki 305-8572, Japan; wangpicao@gmail.com

[4] Department of Biological Science and Technology, National Pingtung University of Science and Technology, Neipu, Pingtung 912-01, Taiwan; tchuang@mail.npust.edu.tw

* Correspondence: taniguchi.akiyoshi@nims.go.jp; Tel.: +81-29-860-4505

Received: 7 March 2019; Accepted: 20 March 2019; Published: 22 March 2019

Abstract: Renal disease is not rare among patients with inflammatory bowel disease (IBD) and is gaining interest as a target of research. However, related changes in glomerular structural have rarely been investigated. This study was aimed at clarifying the changes in collagens and glomerular filtration barrier (GFB)-related proteins of glomeruli in a dextran sulfate sodium (DSS)-induced colitis mouse model. Acute colitis was induced by administering 3.5% DSS in Slc:ICR strain mice for eight days. Histological changes to glomeruli were examined by periodic acid-Schiff (PAS) and Masson's trichrome staining. Expressions of glomerular collagens and GFB-related proteins were analyzed by immunofluorescent staining and Western blot analysis. DSS-colitis mice showed an elevated disease activity index (DAI), colon shortening, massive cellular infiltration and colon damage, confirming that DSS-colitis mice can be used as an IBD animal model. DSS-colitis mice showed increased glycoprotein and collagen deposition in glomeruli. Interestingly, we observed significant changes in glomerular collagens, including a decrease in type IV collagen, and an increment in type I and type V collagens. Moreover, declined GFB-related proteins expressions were detected, including synaptopodin, podocalyxin, nephrin and VE-cadherin. These results suggest that renal disease in DSS-colitis mice might be associated with changes in glomerular collagens and GFB-related proteins. These findings are important for further elucidation of the clinical pathological mechanisms underlying IBD-associated renal disease.

Keywords: inflammatory bowel disease (IBD); DSS-colitis; glomerular filtration barrier (GFB); type IV collagen; type I collagen; type V collagen

---

1. Introduction

Inflammatory bowel disease (IBD) is a chronic, remitting and relapsing inflammatory disease of the gastrointestinal tract characterized by inflammation and mucosal tissue damage and is associated with significant morbidity. Ulcerative colitis and Crohn's disease are the two most common forms of IBD. Ulcerative colitis and Crohn's disease differ from each other in physiology, but show similar symptoms such as severe diarrhea, rectal bleeding, abdominal pain, fever, and weight loss [1,2].

Clinical and epidemiological evidence suggests that IBD is a systemic disorder that can affect almost every organ [2,3]. Renal manifestations and complications in patients with IBD are not rare, and numerous clinical studies have reported that 4–23% of IBD patients experience renal disease such as tubulointerstitial nephritis, nephrolithiasis, and glomerulonephritis [4–11], which eventually induce renal disease. The appropriate experimental animal model of IBD-associated renal disease thus has clinical importance for related studies, including pathological mechanisms, prevention and treatment strategies for IBD.

Dextran sulfate sodium (DSS) is a water-soluble sulfated polysaccharide. Oral administration of DSS to trigger acute colitis has been widely used in experimental animal models for preclinical studies of IBD, because the pathophysiology resembles human Ulcerative colitis [12–14]. Recent studies have reported that mice with colitis induced by DSS show renal tubular injury that might be associated with increased neutrophil infiltration and expressions of cytokines and chemokines in both intestines and kidneys [15,16]. However, these studies of DSS-related renal injury have not mentioned structural changes to the glomeruli. On the other hand, the renal glomerulus is included in the nephron with the tubule, and tubular necrosis has been reported to potentially lead to declines in glomerular function [17,18], suggesting that glomerular damage might be accompanied by tubular injury. The glomerulus contains a highly specialized filtration barrier structure that is essential for maintaining normal plasma ultrafiltration, and loss of glomerular filtration function can lead to poor blood filtration, resulting in renal disease [19,20]. The electively permeable glomerular filtration barrier (GFB) is a three-layered structure that separates the capillaries and Bowman's space, and comprises the interdigitating foot processes of the podocytes, the intervening glomerular basement membrane (GBM), and the fenestrated endothelium [21,22]. The GBM is constituted of specialized extracellular matrix (ECM) components, namely type IV collagen, laminin and other proteoglycans, which are essential for providing a complete structural scaffold to the glomeruli, and important for establishing and maintaining the integrity of the GFB [23,24]. Disrupted GBM has been demonstrated to lead to filtration barrier damage and eventual glomerular disease [24,25]. However, whether GFB-related proteins changes are involved in IBD associated renal disease has not yet been clarified. Herein, we hypothesized that DSS induces renal structural changes, particularly to the glomerular structure.

In this study, we investigated glomerular structural changes focusing on specific types of glomerular collagens and GFB-related proteins after DSS administration, to demonstrate the coexistence of glomerular structural changes and IBD in a DSS-induced colitis mouse model. This study should help establish an experimental animal model for further elucidation of the clinical pathological mechanisms of IBD-associated renal disease.

2. Results

2.1. Progression of DSS-Colitis

After DSS administration (Figure 1), significant body weight loss was observed on Days 4–8 as compared to those of controls (water only) ($p < 0.05$) (Figure 2A). DAI scores showed elevating values after three days of DSS administration, reaching a peak on Day 8 (Figure 2B). Colon shortening, a marker of the severity of colorectal inflammation [14], was significantly greater in DSS-colitis mice as compared to the control group by Day 8 (Figure 2C). Histological observation of the colon was subsequently performed using HE staining, which showed a normal morphology of crypts, abundant goblet cells, muscular layer, submucosa and mucosa in the control mice. However, DSS-colitis mice revealed severe epithelial damage with mucosa thickening, massive cellular infiltration into the lamina propria and colon mucosa, crypt distortion, goblet cells loss, and complete destruction of the architecture (Figure 2D). These histological changes indicated severe inflammatory colitis.

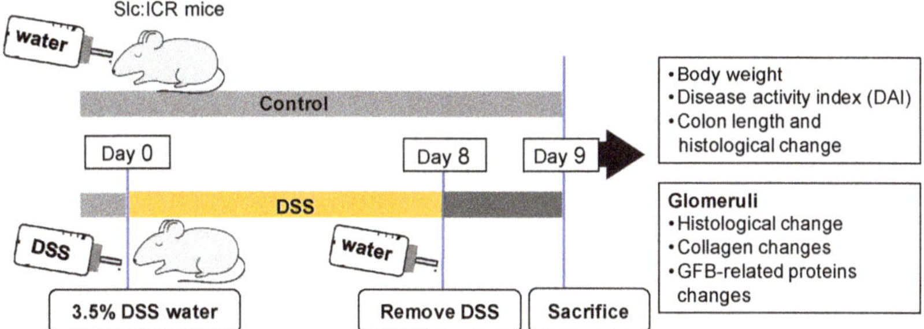

Figure 1. Investigating mouse glomerular structural changes associated with dextran sulfate sodium (DSS)-induced colitis. Slc:ICR mice were administered 3.5% DSS in drinking water for eight days, then allowed intake of filtered water on Day 8. Control mice were given filtered water. All mice were sacrificed on Day 9 and further assessments were performed. Abbreviation: GFB, glomerular filtration barrier.

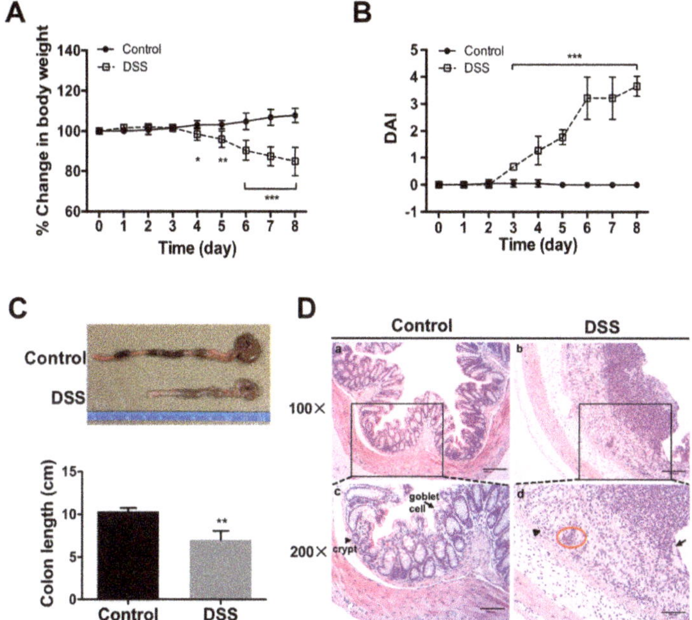

Figure 2. Macro- and microscopic changes to bowel in mice with DSS-induced colitis. Changes in body weight (**A**) and disease activity index (DAI) (**B**) were evaluated daily. Colon length was measured after sacrifice (**C**). Hematoxylin and eosin (HE) staining (**D**) showed distortion of crypts (arrowhead), loss of goblet cells (arrow), and infiltration of inflammatory cells (red circle) in colon sections from DSS-treated mice. All values are given as mean $\pm$ SEM (n = 6 mice); * $p < 0.05$, ** $p < 0.01$, and *** $p < 0.001$ vs. control. Scale bars: 200 μm (**a,b**); and 100 μm (**c,d**).

2.2. Renal Morphology and Histological Changes in DSS-Colitis Mice

Human and mouse studies have indicated the involvement of non-intestinal organs in IBD [4–9]. We therefore investigated renal changes in DSS-colitis mice. Kidney size and weight of DSS-colitis mice were decreased in mice after eight days of treatment as compared to those in controls (Figure 3A,B). To detect structural histological damage, glomerular morphology was examined in tissue sections by PAS and Masson's trichrome staining. Deep pink color (PAS-positive matrix) representing deposition of matrix glycoprotein was apparent at the GBM and mesangium, confirming increased matrix in the glomeruli of DSS-colitis mice (Figure 3C). Masson's trichrome staining was performed to detect the collagen deposition and fibrosis associated with renal disease, and blue to blue-violet staining indicated the presence of collagen in tissues. The result showed lightly stained collagen in the GBM and tubular basement membrane. On the other hand, significant collagen deposition among the glomerular capillaries and surrounding the Bowman's capsules were observed in DSS-colitis mice after eight days of DSS administration (Figure 3D) compared to control mice.

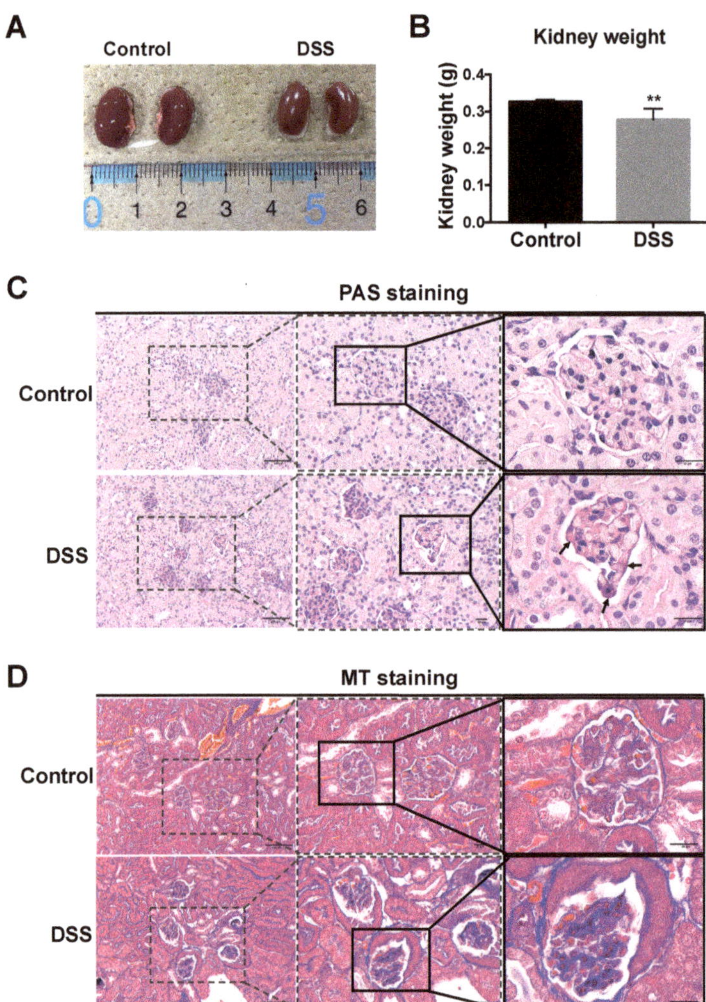

Figure 3. Macro- and microscopic changes to the kidney and glomeruli in mice after DSS administration. Mouse kidney appearance (**A**) and weight (**B**) were determined at harvest. Histological manifestations were determined by staining with periodic acid-Schiff (PAS) to assess the basement membrane of glomeruli (**C**), and Masson's trichrome (MT) staining to assess collagen deposition (**D**), respectively. Compared to control mice, glomerular accumulation of PAS-positive matrix (arrow) was prominent in DSS-treated mice (**C**). Blue staining indicates the presence of collagen fibers in tissues (**D**). All values are given as mean $\pm$ SEM (n = 6 mice); ** $p < 0.01$ vs. control. Scale bars: 100 μm and 20 μm.

2.3. Collagen Changes in Glomeruli

Glomerular collagens including type IV collagen (a typical collagen of the basement membrane matrix), type I collagen (an interstitial matrix collagen) and type V collagen (an atypical collagen that only appears at kidney development and in kidney diseases such as collagenofibrotic glomerulopathy) [26,27] were investigated by immunofluorescent microscopy and Western blot analysis. The results showed decreased type IV collagen in GBM and Bowman's capsules (Figure 4A-a′) in DSS-colitis mice as compared to controls (Figure 4A-a). In contrast to type IV collagen, type I and V collagens increased in the glomerular and renal interstitium (Figure 4A-b′,-c′) of DSS-colitis mice as compared to those in controls (Figure 4A-b,-c). Consistent with immunofluorescent microscopy results, Western blotting analysis also showed declining expressions of type IV collagen (Figure 4B-a), and increasing expressions of type I and V collagens (Figure 4B-b,-c) in the renal cortex of DSS-administered mice, indicating the influence of DSS on changes in glomerular collagens. The above results are illustrated in Figure 4C.

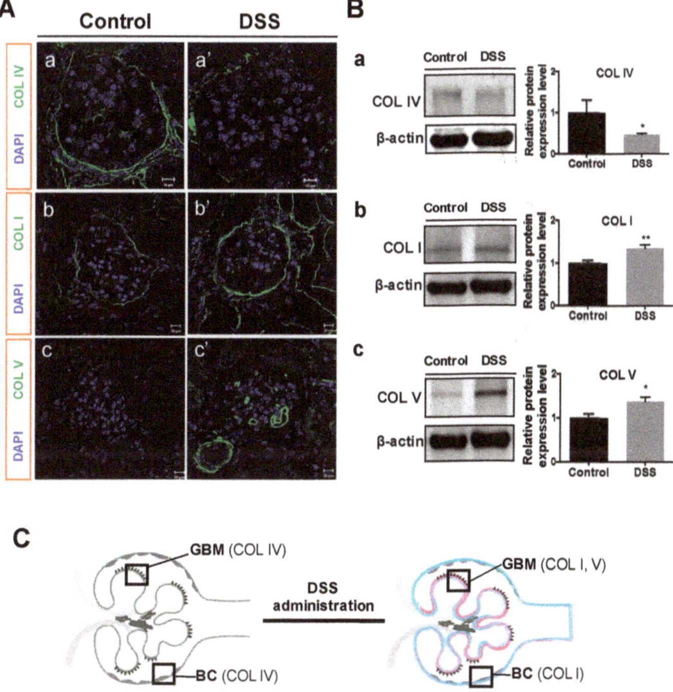

Figure 4. Changes in glomerular collagens in mice after DSS administration. Immunofluorescent microscopy (**A**) and Western blot analysis of protein expression (**B**) for type IV collagen (COL IV; A-a, A-a′; B-a; 160–190 kDa), type I collagen (COL I; A-b, A-b′; B-b; 150 kDa), and type V collagen (COL V; A-c, A-c′; B-c; 220 kDa) were conducted for control and DSS-colitis mice. Representative bands (**B**, left) and relative band intensity ratios were analyzed (**B**, right). (**C**) Illustration of glomerular collagens changes in this study. All values are means $\pm$ SEM ($n = 6$); * $p < 0.05$ and ** $p < 0.01$ vs. control. Scale bars = 10 μm. Abbreviations: GBM, glomerular basement membrane; BC, Bowman's capsule.

2.4. Changes in GFB-Related Proteins

The GFB comprises glomerular endothelial cells, the GBM and podocytes [22,23]. Podocytes and glomerular endothelial cells are located on opposite side of the GBM. Immunofluorescent investigation of podocyte-associated proteins in glomeruli (including synaptopodin, podocalyxin, and nephrin) were performed to detect changes in podocytes. The results showed that synaptopodin, podocalyxin, and nephrin were significantly expressed at capillary tufts of normal glomeruli in the control mice (Figure 5A-a, -b, -c), but declined in DSS-colitis mice after DSS administration (Figure 5A-a', -b', -c'). Similarly, the vascular-specific junctional molecule VE-cadherin in endothelial cells on the GBM, which is associated with the regulation of vascular permeability and glomerular filtration, showed lower immunofluorescence and discontinuous expression in DSS-colitis mice (Figure 5A-d') as compared to that in controls (Figure 5A-d).

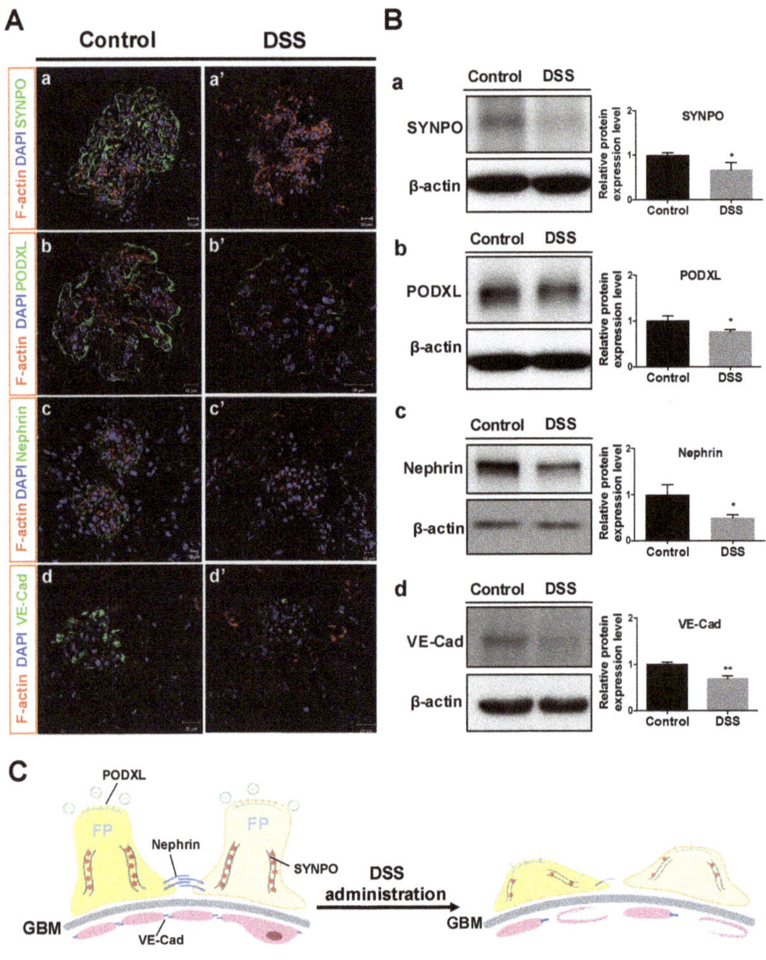

Figure 5. Changes in GFB-related proteins in mice after DSS administration. Immunofluorescent microscopy (**A**) and Western blot analysis of protein expression (**B**) against synaptopodin (A-a, A-a'; B-a; 100 kDa), podocalyxin (A-b, A-b'; B-b; 130 kDa), nephrin (A-c, A-c'; B-c; 185 kDa) and VE-cadherin (A-d, A-d'; B-d; 130 kDa) in glomeruli were conducted for control and DSS-colitis mice. (**B**) Representative bands (left), and relative band intensity ratios (right) were analyzed. (**C**) Illustration of GFB-related proteins changes in this study. All values are means ± SEM ($n = 6$), * $p < 0.05$ and ** $p < 0.01$ vs. control. Scale bars = 10 μm (A-a, A-a', A-b, A-c, A-c'); 20 μm (A-b', A-d, A-d'). Abbreviation: SYNPO, synaptopodin; PODXL, podocalyxin; VE-Cad, VE-cadherin; FP, foot processes.

Western blot analysis of these four proteins in glomeruli showed declines in all proteins (Figure 5B), consistent with the results from immunofluorescence (Figure 5A).

These findings confirmed that DSS administration caused podocyte damage (reductions in synaptopodin, podocalyxin and nephrin) and changes to endothelial adherens junctions in glomerular endothelium (reductions in VE-cadherin). These results are shown in Figure 5C.

3. Discussion

Renal manifestations and complications in patients with IBD have been reported in several clinical and experimental studies from recent years [4–11,28]. However, the coexistence of renal disease and IBD, and the related glomerular structural changes in particular, have rarely been discussed. This study provided novel data showing not only the changes in renal glomerular collagen types in a DSS-induced colitis mouse model, but also revealed the interesting fact that proteins located on both the glomerular podocyte slit diaphragm and endothelial junction declined in expression in DSS-colitis mice, reflecting GFB damage.

This study adopted the DSS-induced colitis mouse model and confirmed symptoms of DSS-induced colitis such as body weight loss, diarrhea, gross bleeding and colon architecture destruction (Figures 1 and 2), similar to IBD symptoms in humans [12,29]. Although some previous reports have mentioned that DSS might influence kidney function in mice after observing acute inflammatory responses associated with pro-inflammatory cytokine and chemokine expression in both intestines and kidneys, as well as renal tubular injury [15,16], the glomerular damage, especially the GFB damage in this DSS model still lack detailed evidence. In this study, we conducted detailed investigations into changes in the renal glomerular histology, GBM, and GFB-related protein expression, to illustrate renal damage in the DSS-induced colitis mouse model.

We noticed that kidney size and weight were decreased in DSS-colitis mice after DSS administration (Figure 3), since kidney size and weight are important indicators of renal pathology during disease development [30]. The decreased kidney size may correlate with body weight loss [30,31], and this phenomenon has been found in human patients with IBD [32]. Moreover, PAS staining revealed increasing deposition of glycoprotein matrix in GBM and mesangium, and Masson's trichome staining revealed collagen deposition was markedly increased around the glomerulus and Bowman's capsules in DSS-colitis mice. Such matrix and collagen depositions in glomeruli were also found in glomerular impairment, implicating excess ECM production as a factor in glomerular disease [27,33,34]. These observations suggest the DSS mice might show some glomerular abnormality.

To clarify the assumption that DSS induces renal structural change, we investigated the changes in specific types of collagens in the glomeruli. Our results showed that type IV collagen was decreased in the GBM, whereas type I and V collagens increased in the renal glomerular capillary loops and interstitium of DSS-colitis mice (Figure 4). Type IV collagen is well known to be the major component of the ECM in GBM, Bowman's capsule and tubular basement membranes in normal kidneys [35]. Decreased expression of type IV collagen in GBM has been reported with the increased GBM degradation associated with kidney dysfunction [35–38]. On the other hand, type I and V collagens belong to interstitial ECM and excessive deposition is known to form scar tissue in the interstitial space during fibrosis [39,40]. In fact, type I collagen seldom appears in renal vessels and glomeruli under normal conditions, but is deposited in the early stage of renal fibrosis [27,39]. Type V collagen has been reported to spread widely in glomeruli during glomerulopathy, wound healing and kidney development [26,41,42]. Our result of a decrement in type IV collagen in GBM and increments in both type I and type V collagens in renal glomerular capillary loops and interstitium suggested that DSS administration could cause these collagens changes, which may lead to glomerular structure damage.

Renal disease has been reported in human IBD patients, but GFB-related protein changes have not been closely investigated. The present study investigated four proteins (synaptopodin, podocalyxin, nephrin and VE-cadherin) to clarify GFB damage, because these proteins have not been investigated in the kidneys of DSS-colitis mice, and the relevance of GBM damage in the DSS-induced colitis mouse model has not been reported yet. Our results showed declined expression of all four proteins in glomeruli after DSS administration (Figure 5). Podocytes locating on the GBM are known to serve as the final filtration barriers of glomeruli and contain the special proteins synaptopodin, podocalyxin and nephrin. These proteins have been suggested to represent important biomarkers of podocyte deficiency [43]. Synaptopodin is known to maintain podocyte foot processes and downregulation of the podocyte actin cytoskeleton has been observed in human and rodent glomerular diseases [43]. Decreased synaptopodin expression in podocytes reflects the foot processes are associated with a loss of cytoskeletal destruction [44]. Podocalyxin is a highly electronegative sialoglycoprotein located at the apical surface of podocyte foot processes and functions to maintain the negative charge of the glomerular filtration slit diaphragm and podocyte shape by linking to the actin cytoskeleton [45]. In vivo and in vitro studies have reported that decreased podocaylxin is associated with reduced adhesiveness of cells to the GBM [43,45]. Moreover, the loss of nephrin, a structural protein located between the podocyte foot processes, causes decreased podocyte integrity of slit diaphragms, resulting in eventual damage to the GFB [19,46]. Furthermore, glomerular endothelial cells serve as the first filtration barrier through their tight adhesion to the basement membrane, and a decrease in endothelial cells can therefore worsen renal failure [20,21]. VE-cadherin is an adherens junction protein between endothelial cells that maintains vascular integrity and decreased VE-cadherin expression has been observed in the glomerular endothelium of end-stage renal disease patients [47–49].

Taken together, our results imply that DSS administration could cause the glomerular collagen changes, including decreased type IV collagen as a supporting ECM of GBM structure and deposition of type I and type V collagens in renal interstitium. These collagen changes might lead to structural damage to podocytes such as a loss of polarity and detachment from the GBM, as well as loss of endothelial cell junctions, eventually causing renal disease. Loss of the podocyte cytoskeletal proteins synaptopodin and podocalyxin and the slit diaphragms protein nephrin, as well as the defective endothelial cells adherens junction protein (VE-cadherin) which may be associated with podocyte damage.

Based on our findings, the lack or insufficiency of these GFB-related proteins in DSS-colitis mice might cause glomerular structural damage, and consequently lead to damage not only to podocytes, but also to adherens junctions in the vasculature, which might result in GFB damage.

In conclusion, this study used the DSS-induced colitis mouse model, a very common experimental model of colitis, to clarify changes in glomerular collagens and GFB-related proteins after DSS administration. These findings on glomerular structural change in experimental mice with DSS-induced colitis should lead to novel uses of the animal model for further investigations into IBD-associated renal disease.

4. Materials and Methods

4.1. Laboratory Animals

Seven-week-old male Slc:ICR strain mice weighing 28–30 g (Japan SLC, Hamamatsu, Japan) were housed in the Central Animal House at the University of Tsukuba under climate-controlled conditions (room temperature, $22 \pm 2\,°C$; 12-h light/dark cycle; relative humidity, 65%). Cages were cleaned and sterilized every week. All mice were given free access to food and water. Animal experiments were conducted in strict accordance with the recommendations of the Guide for the Care and Use of Laboratory Animals of the Science Council of Japan and Ministry of Education, Culture, Sports, Science and Technology of Japan. The protocol was approved by the Committee on the Ethics of Animal Experiments of the University of Tsukuba (Permit Number: 14-047; May 2016) based on the Institutional Animal Care and Use Committee (IACUC). All surgery was performed under sodium pentobarbital anesthesia, and all efforts were made to minimize suffering.

4.2. Induction of DSS-Colitis in Mice

As a widely used model of IBD, the DSS-induced colitis mouse model was used in this study to investigate changes to renal glomerular collagens and GFB-related proteins. This mouse model was established by inducing colitis with the administration of DSS in drinking water for eight days (Figure 1), following the previously described method [15]. Briefly, mice were administered 3.5% (*w/v*) DSS (MW 36,000–50,000 Da; MP Biomedicals, Solon, OH, USA) dissolved in drinking water for eight days. Six mice per group were used in each experiment, and were not allowed to access to any other source of water. Mouse weights were monitored daily to quantify the systemic consequences of colitis. Mice were fed with normal water in place of DSS water on Day 8 and euthanized on Day 9. Colon length and kidney weight were measured for each mouse at harvest, then fixed in 10% neutral buffered formalin (Wako, Osaka, Japan) or stored at $-80\,^{\circ}\text{C}$ for further use. Mice receiving only distilled water were used as controls.

4.3. Disease Activity Index (DAI)

Weight loss, stool consistency, and rectal bleeding were recorded daily to assess the severity of DSS-colitis. DAI was determined based on the methods described previously [50]. Briefly, DAI was scored from 0 to 4 for each parameter, and then averaged for each group. Parameters were body weight loss (0 = no weight loss; 1 = 1–5% weight loss; 2 = 6–10% weight loss; 3 = 11–15% weight loss; and 4 = $\geq$ 15% weight loss), stool consistency (0 = normal stools; 2 = loose stools; 4 = diarrhea) and gross bleeding (0 = negative, 2 = positive occult blood in stools, 4 = rectal bleeding). DAI was calculated as the sum of the weight loss, stool consistency and gross bleeding scores.

4.4. Histological Investigation

To detect injury to the colon and renal tissues, prepared tissues were cut into 2-μm thick sections using a microtome (Thermo Fisher Scientific, Waltham, MA, USA) and stained with hematoxylin and eosin (HE) for histological investigations. To assess the GBM, periodic acid-Schiff (PAS) was used to estimate the glomerular deposition of matrix glycoprotein [51]. Briefly, 3-μm-thick sections were stained using a PAS staining kit (Merck, Darmstadt, Germany) and counterstained with hematoxylin according to the instructions from the manufacturer. To detect collagen fiber deposition [52], 3-μm sections were stained with a Masson's trichrome staining kit (Muto Pure Chemicals, Tokyo, Japan) according to the manufacturer's instruction. Microscopic images were acquired using a light microscope with a charge-coupled device camera (Olympus, Tokyo, Japan).

4.5. Immunofluorescence Staining and Confocal Imaging

Immunofluorescence staining was performed by following the method described previously [53]. Briefly, kidneys were embedded in optimal cutting temperature compound (Sakura Finetek, Tokyo, Japan), and frozen in liquid nitrogen. Sections of 5-μm thickness were cut by a cryostat (CM3050; Leica, Wetzlar, Germany); then incubated with primary antibodies against type I collagen (Acris Antibodies, Germany), type IV collagen, type V collagen, synaptopodin, VE-cadherin (Santa Cruz Biotechnology, Santa Cruz, CA, USA), nephrin, and podocalyxin (R&D Systems, Minneapolis, MN, USA), respectively, at $4\,^{\circ}\text{C}$ overnight, and followed by secondary antibodies conjugated to Alexa Fluor® 488 or 568 (Invitrogen, Carlsbad, CA, USA); double-stained with rhodamine-conjugated phalloidin (Life Technologies, Gaithersburg, MD, USA) for F-actin; and finally submerged in fluoroshield mounting medium containing 4′,6-diamidino-2-phenylindole (DAPI) (Abcam, Cambridge, UK). Confocal imaging was performed according to the method described previously [26] with a confocal microscope (LSM700; Carl Zeiss, Jena, Germany). Alexa Fluor® 488, and 568 signals were detected at laser excitation wavelengths of 488 nm and 543 nm, respectively.

4.6. Renal Glomerular Isolation

Kidney cortex tissue from each mouse was removed, glomeruli were isolated using a serial sieving method described previously [54], and then washed with PBS to remove small tubular fragments. The isolated glomeruli were re-suspended by PBS for further use or dissolved in lysis buffer for protein extraction.

4.7. Protein Isolation and Western Blot Analysis

Kidney cortices (~50 mg) or isolated glomeruli from kidney cortices of each mouse were homogenized in lysis buffer (50 mM Tris pH 7.4, 250 mM NaCl, 5 mM EDTA, 2 mM Na_3VO_4, 1 mM NaF, 20 mM $Na_4P_2O_7$, 0.02% NaN_3, 1% Triton X-100, 0.1% SDS and 1 mM PMSF) with 1% protease inhibitor cocktail (Sigma-Aldrich, St. Louis, MO, USA) by sonication (Qsonica, Newtown, CT, USA), followed by incubation on ice for 10 min and centrifugation at 10,000 rpm for 10 min. Supernatant was collected and protein concentration was quantitated using the Micro BCA Protein Assay kit (Thermo Fisher Scientific, Waltham, MA, USA) according to the instructions from the manufacturer. Thirty micrograms of total protein were loaded per lane and separated by 7.5% polyacrylamide gels, followed by transferring onto methanol-activated PVDF membrane (Millipore, Billerica, MA, USA). Protein-transferred membranes were incubated with primary antibodies against type I collagen, type IV collagen, type V collagen, synaptopodin, VE-cadherin, nephrin, podocalyxin and β-actin, respectively, at 4 °C overnight, followed by incubation with horseradish peroxidase-conjugated secondary antibody for 2 h at room temperature. Blots were visualized with chemiluminescence substrate for 1 min and detected using a luminescent image analyzer (LAS-4000 mini; Fujifilm, Tokyo, Japan). Band density was quantitated densitometrically with Image J software (National Institutes of Health, MD, USA) by calculating the average optical density in each band. Relative and normalized protein expressions were calculated using the ratio of each protein density to β-actin density.

4.8. Statistical Analysis

Statistical analyses were performed using Prism software (GraphPad, San Diego, CA, USA). All data are expressed as mean $\pm$ standard error of the mean (SEM) from 6 replicates ($n = 6$ mice per group) in at least 3 independent experiments. The significance of differences between groups were analyzed using Student's *t*-test. A probability level of $p < 0.05$ was considered significant.

Author Contributions: P.-C.W. and T.-C.H. conceived the presented idea. C.-J.C. designed the study, acquired data, and drafted the manuscript. C.-J.C. and P.-C.W. analyzed and interpreted data. P.-C.W. provided critical revision. All authors discussed the results and contributed to the final manuscript. A.T. carried out final approval of the version to be published.

Funding: This study is supported by Grant-in-Aid for Scientific Research (C26450118) from the Ministry of Education, Culture, Sports, Science, and Technology of Japan.

Acknowledgments: We wish to thank Tony Hsiang-Kuang Liang for valuable medical advice, and Yusuke Murasawa, Nishimura Yusuke and Airi Akatsuka for their technical assistance.

Conflicts of Interest: The authors declare that they have no conflicts of interest, financial or otherwise, regarding this article.

Abbreviations

IBD	Inflammatory bowel disease
GFB	Glomerular filtration barrier
DSS	Dextran sulfate sodium
PAS	Periodic acid-Schiff
DAI	Disease activity index
GBM	Glomerular basement membrane
ECM	Extracellular matrix

References

1. Sartor, R.B. Current concepts of the etiology and pathogenesis of ulcerative colitis and Crohn's disease. *Gastroenterol. Clin. N. Am.* **1995**, *24*, 475–507.
2. Ricart, E.; Panaccione, R.; Loftus, E.V.; Tremaine, W.J.; Harmsen, W.S.; Zinsmeister, A.R.; Sandborn, W.J. Autoimmune disorders and Extraintestinal manifestations in First-degree familial and sporadic inflammatory bowel disease. *Inflamm. Bowel Dis.* **2004**, *10*, 207–214. [CrossRef] [PubMed]
3. Christodoulou, D.K.; Katsanos, K.H.; Kitsanou, M.; Stergiopoulou, C.; Hatzis, J.; Tsianos, E.V. Frequency of extraintestinal manifestations in patients with inflammatory bowel disease in northwest Greece and review of the literature. *Dig. Liver Dis.* **2002**, *34*, 781–786. [CrossRef]
4. Ambruzs, J.M.; Walker, P.D.; Larsen, C.P. The histopathologic spectrum of kidney biopsies in patients with inflammatory bowel disease. *Clin. J. Am. Soc. Nephrol.* **2014**, *9*, 265–270. [CrossRef] [PubMed]
5. Ambruzs, J.M.; Larsen, C.P. Renal Manifestations of Inflammatory Bowel Disease. *Rheum. Dis. Clin. N. Am.* **2018**, *44*, 699–714. [CrossRef] [PubMed]
6. Rabin, B.S.; Rogers, S. Pathologic changes in the liver and kidney produced by immunization with intestinal antigens. *Am. J. Pathol.* **1972**, *84*, 201–210.
7. Kreisel, W.; Wolf, L.M.; Grotz, W.; Grieshaber, M. Renal tubular damage: An extraintestinal manifestation of chronic inflammatory bowel disease. *Eur. J. Gastroenterol. Hepatol.* **1996**, *8*, 461–468.
8. Khosroshahi, H.T.; Shoja, M.M. Tubulointerstitial disease and ulcerative colitis. *Nephrol. Dial. Transplant.* **2006**, *21*, 2340. [CrossRef]
9. Corica, D.; Romano, C. Renal Involvement in Inflammatory Bowel Diseases. *J. Crohns Colitis* **2016**, *10*, 226–235. [CrossRef]
10. Fraser, J.S.; Muller, A.F.; Smith, D.J.; Newman, D.J.; Lamb, E.J. Renal tubular injury is present in acute inflammatory bowel disease prior to the introduction of drug therapy. *Aliment. Pharmacol. Ther.* **2001**, *15*, 1131–1137. [CrossRef]
11. Tokuyama, H.; Wakino, S.; Konishi, K.; Hashiguchi, A.; Hayashi, K.; Itoh, H. Acute interstitial nephritis associated with ulcerative colitis. *Clin. Exp. Nephrol.* **2010**, *14*, 483–486. [CrossRef] [PubMed]
12. Chassaing, B.; Aitken, J.D.; Malleshappa, M.; Vijay-Kumar, M. Dextran Sulfate sodium (DSS)-induced Colitis in mice. *Trends Pharmacol. Sci.* **2014**, *104*. [CrossRef]
13. de Lange, K.M.; Barrett, J.C. Understanding inflammatory bowel disease via immunogenetics. *J. Autoimmun.* **2015**, *64*, 91–100. [CrossRef]
14. Eichele, D.D.; Kharbanda, K.K. Dextran sodium sulfate colitis murine model: An indispensable tool for advancing our understanding of inflammatory bowel diseases pathogenesis. *World J. Gastroenterol.* **2017**, *23*, 6016–6029. [CrossRef] [PubMed]
15. Ranganathan, P.; Jayakumar, C.; Santhakumar, M.; Ramesh, G. Netrin-1 regulates colon-kidney cross talk through suppression of IL-6 function in a mouse model of DSS-colitis. *Am. J. Physiol. Renal Physiol.* **2013**, *304*, 1187–1197. [CrossRef]
16. Ranganathan, P.; Jayakumar, C.; Manicassamy, S.; Ramesh, G. CXCR2 knockout mice are protected against DSS-colitis-induced acute kidney injury and inflammation. *Am. J. Physiol. Renal Physiol.* **2013**, *305*, 1422–1427. [CrossRef]
17. Meyer, T.W. Tubular injury in glomerular disease. *Kidney Int.* **2003**, *63*, 774–787. [CrossRef] [PubMed]
18. Kriz, W.; LeHir, M. Pathways to nephron loss starting from glomerular diseases-Insights from animal models. *Kidney Int.* **2005**, *67*, 404–419. [CrossRef] [PubMed]
19. Lennon, R.; Randles, M.J.; Humphries, M.J. The Importance of Podocyte Adhesion for a Healthy Glomerulus. *Front. Endocrinol.* **2014**, *5*, 160. [CrossRef] [PubMed]
20. Arif, E.; Nihalani, D. Glomerular Filtration Barrier Assembly: An insight. *Postdoc. J.* **2013**, *1*, 33–45. [CrossRef] [PubMed]
21. Scott, R.P.; Quaggin, S.E. The cell biology of renal filtration. *J. Cell Biol.* **2015**, *209*, 199–210. [CrossRef]
22. Miner, J.H. Glomerular basement membrane composition and the filtration barrier. *Pediatr. Nephrol.* **2011**, *26*, 1413–1417. [CrossRef]
23. Byron, A.; Randles, M.J.; Humphries, J.D.; Mironov, A.; Hamidi, H.; Harris, S.; Mathieson, P.W.; Saleem, M.A.; Satchell, S.C.; Zent, R.; et al. Glomerular Cell Cross-Talk Influences Composition and Assembly of Extracellular Matrix. *J. Am. Soc. Nephrol.* **2014**, *25*, 953–966. [CrossRef]

24. Chen, Y.M.; Miner, J.H. Glomerular basement membrane and related glomerular disease. *Transl. Res.* **2012**, *160*, 291–297. [CrossRef]

25. Chew, C.; Lennon, R. Basement Membrane Defects in Genetic Kidney Diseases. *Front. Pediatr.* **2018**, *6*, 11. [CrossRef] [PubMed]

26. Hsu, H.H.; Murasawa, Y.; Qi, P.; Nishimura, Y.; Wang, P.C. Type V collagen fibrils in mouse metanephroi. *Biochem. Biophys. Res. Commun.* **2013**, *441*, 649–654. [CrossRef]

27. Genovese, F.; Manresa, A.A.; Leeming, D.; Karsdal, M.; Boor, P. The extracellular matrix in the kidney: A source of novel non-invasive biomarkers of kidney fibrosis. *Fibrogenes. Tissue Repair* **2014**, *7*, 4. [CrossRef]

28. Levine, J.S.; Burakoff, R. Extraintestinal manifestations of inflammatory bowel disease. *Gastroenterol. Hepatol.* **2011**, *7*, 235–241.

29. Da Silva, A.P.; Pollett, A.; Rittling, S.R.; Denhardt, D.T.; Sodek, J.; Zohar, R. Exacerbated tissue destruction in DSS-induced acute colitis of OPN-null mice is associated with downregulation of TNF-α expression and non-programmed cell death. *J. Cell Physiol.* **2006**, *208*, 629–639. [CrossRef] [PubMed]

30. Sandilands, E.A.; Dhaun, N.; Dear, J.W.; Webb, D.J. Measurement of renal function in patients with chronic kidney disease. *Br. J. Clin. Pharmacol.* **2013**, *76*, 504–515. [CrossRef]

31. Emamian, S.A.; Nielsen, M.B.; Pedersen, J.F.; Ytte, L. Kidney dimensions at sonography: Correlation with age, sex, and habitus in 665 adult volunteers. *Am. J. Roentgenol.* **1993**, *160*, 83–86. [CrossRef] [PubMed]

32. Lauritzen, D.; Andreassen, B.U.; Heegaard, N.H.H.; Klinge, L.G.; Walsted, A.M.; Neland, M.; Nielsen, R.G.; Wittenhagen, P. Pediatric Inflammatory Bowel Diseases: Should We Be Looking for Kidney Abnormalities? *Inflamm. Bowel Dis.* **2018**, *24*, 2599–2605. [CrossRef]

33. Kashgarian, M.; Sterze, B. The pathobiology of the mesangium. *Kidney Int.* **1992**, *41*, 524–529. [CrossRef]

34. Duffield, J.S. Cellular and molecular mechanisms in kidney fibrosis. *J. Clin. Investig.* **2014**, *124*, 2299–2306. [CrossRef] [PubMed]

35. Miner, J.H. Renal basement membrane components. *Kidney Int.* **1999**, *56*, 2016–2024. [CrossRef] [PubMed]

36. Niu, H.; Li, Y.; Li, H.; Chi, Y.; Zhuang, M.; Zhang, T.; Liu, M.; Nie, L. Matrix metalloproteinase 12 modulates high-fat-diet induced glomerular fibrogenesis and inflammation in a mouse model of obesity. *Sci. Rep.* **2016**, *6*, 20171. [CrossRef]

37. Tamsma, J.T.; van den Born, J.; Bruijn, J.A.; Assmann, K.J.; Weening, J.J.; Berden, J.H.; Wieslander, J.; Schrama, E.; Hermans, J.; Veerkamp, J.H. Expression of glomerular extracellular matrix components in human diabetic nephropathy: Decrease of heparan sulphate in the glomerular basement membrane. *Diabetologia* **1994**, *37*, 313–320. [CrossRef]

38. Morita, M.; Uchigata, Y.; Hanai, K.; Ogawa, Y.; Iwamoto, Y. Association of urinary type IV collagen with GFR decline in young patients with type 1 diabetes. *Am. J. Kidney Dis.* **2011**, *58*, 915–920. [CrossRef] [PubMed]

39. Yoshioka, K.; Tohda, M.; Takemura, T.; Akano, N.; Matsubara, K.; Ooshima, A.; Maki, S. Distribution of type I collagen in human kidney diseases in comparison with type III collagen. *J. Pathol.* **1990**, *162*, 141–148. [CrossRef] [PubMed]

40. Sumiyoshi, H.; Kitamura, H.; Matsuo, N.; Tatsukawa, S.; Ishikawa, K.; Okamoto, O.; Fujikura, Y.; Fujiwara, S.; Yoshioka, H. Transient expression of mouse Pro-α3(V) collagen gene (Col5a3) in wound healing. *Connect. Tissue Res.* **2012**, *5*, 313–317. [CrossRef] [PubMed]

41. Morita, H.; Hasegawa, T.; Minamoto, T.; Oda, Y.; Inui, K.; Tayama, H.; Nakao, N.; Nakamoto, Y.; Ideura, T.; Yoshimura, A. Collagenofibrotic glomerulopathy with a widespread expression of type-v collagen. *Virchows Arch.* **2003**, *442*, 163–168. [PubMed]

42. Murasawa, Y.; Hayashi, T.; Wang, P.C. The role of type V collagen fibril as an ECM that induces the motility of glomerular endothelial cells. *Exp. Cell Res.* **2008**, *314*, 3638–3653. [CrossRef] [PubMed]

43. Sekulic, M.; Pichler, S. A compendium of urinary biomarkers indicative of glomerular podocytopathy. *Pathol. Res. Int.* **2013**, *2013*, 782395. [CrossRef] [PubMed]

44. Kwon, S.K.; Kim, S.J.; Kim, H.Y. Urine synaptopodin excretion is an important marker of glomerular disease progression. *Korean J. Intern Med.* **2016**, *31*, 938–943. [CrossRef] [PubMed]

45. Nielsen, J.S.; McNagny, K.M. The role of podocalyxin in health and disease. *J. Am. Soc. Nephrol.* **2009**, *20*, 1669–1676. [CrossRef] [PubMed]

46. Greka, A.; Mundel, P. Cell biology and pathology of podocytes. *Annu. Rev. Physiol.* **2012**, *74*, 299–323. [CrossRef]

47. Spagnuolo, R.; Corada, M.; Orsenigo, F.; Zanetta, L.; Deuschle, U.; Sandy, P.; Schneider, C.; Drake, C.J.; Breviario, F.; Dejana, E. Gas1 is induced by VE-cadherin and vascular endothelial growth factor and inhibits endothelial cell apoptosis. *Blood* **2004**, *103*, 3005–3012. [CrossRef] [PubMed]

48. Giannotta, M.; Trani, M.; Dejana, E. VE-Cadherin and endothelial Adherens Junctions: Active guardians of vascular integrity. *Dev. Cell* **2013**, *26*, 441–454. [CrossRef]

49. Hernandez, N.M.; Casselbrant, A.; Joshi, M.; Johansson, B.R.; Sumitran-Holgersson, S. Antibodies to kidney endothelial cells contribute to a "leaky" glomerular barrier in patients with chronic kidney diseases. *Am. J. Physiol. Renal Physiol.* **2012**, *302*, F884–F894. [CrossRef]

50. Murthy, S.N.; Cooper, H.S.; Shim, H.; Shah, R.S.; Ibrahim, S.A.; Sedergran, D.J. Treatment of dextran sulfate sodium-induced murine colitis by intracolonic cyclosporine. *Dig. Dis. Sci.* **1993**, *38*, 1722–1734. [CrossRef]

51. McManus, J.F. The Periodic Acid Routine Applied to the Kidney. *Am. J. Pathol.* **1948**, *24*, 643–653. [PubMed]

52. Cohen, A.H. Masson's trichrome stain in the evaluation of renal biopsies. An appraisal. *Am. J. Clin. Pathol.* **1976**, *65*, 631–643. [CrossRef] [PubMed]

53. Nishimura, Y.; Hsu, H.H.; Wang, P.C. Detection of initial angiogenesis from dorsal aorta into metanephroi and elucidation of its role in kidney development. *Regener. Ther.* **2016**, *4*, 27–35. [CrossRef]

54. Nagao, T.; Suzuki, K.; Utsunomiya, K.; Matsumura, M.; Saiga, K.; Wang, P.C.; Minamitani, H.; Aratani, Y.; Nakayama, T.; Suzuki, K. Direct activation of glomerular endothelial cells by anti-moesin activity of anti-myeloperoxidase antibody. *Nephrol. Dial. Transplant.* **2011**, *26*, 2752–2760. [CrossRef] [PubMed]

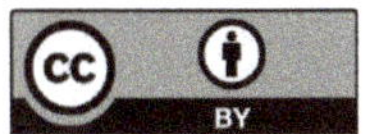

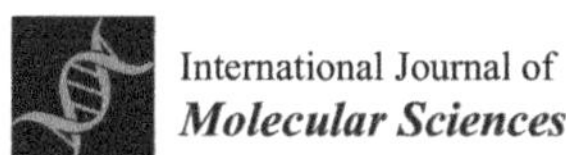
International Journal of
Molecular Sciences

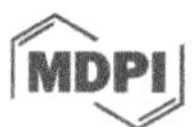

Article

Kidney Injury by Variants in the *COL4A5* Gene Aggravated by Polymorphisms in Slit Diaphragm Genes Causes Focal Segmental Glomerulosclerosis

Jenny Frese [1,†], Matthias Kettwig [2,†], Hildegard Zappel [2], Johannes Hofer [3], Hermann-Josef Gröne [4], Mato Nagel [5], Gere Sunder-Plassmann [6], Renate Kain [7], Jörg Neuweiler [8] and Oliver Gross [1,*]

1   Clinic of Nephrology and Rheumatology, University Medical Center Goettingen, 37075 Goettingen, Germany; jenny.frese@dpdhl.com
2   Clinic of Pediatrics and Adolescent Medicine, University Medical Center Goettingen, 37075 Goettingen, Germany; matthias.kettwig@med.uni-goettingen.de (M.K.); hzappel@med.uni-goettingen.de (H.Z.)
3   Department of Pediatrics, Pediatrics I, Innsbruck Medical University, 6020 Innsbruck, Austria; Johannes.Hofer@i-med.ac.at
4   Department of Cellular and Molecular Pathology, German Cancer Research Center, 69120 Heidelberg, Germany; h.-j.groene@dkfz-heidelberg.de
5   Center for Nephrology and Metabolic Disorders, Molecular Diagnostics, 02943 Weißwasser, Germany; nagel@moldiag.de
6   Division of Nephrology and Dialysis, Department of Medicine III, Medical University of Vienna, 1090 Vienna, Austria; Gere.Sunder-Plassmann@meduniwien.ac.at
7   Department of Pathology, Medical University of Vienna, 1090 Vienna, Austria; renate.kain@meduniwien.ac.at
8   Institute of Pathology, Kantonsspital, 9007 St. Gallen, Switzerland; joerg.neuweiler@kssg.ch
*   Correspondence: gross.oliver@med.uni-goettingen.de; Tel.: +49-551-396331; Fax: +49-551-398906
†   These authors contributed equally to this work.

Received: 14 December 2018; Accepted: 21 January 2019; Published: 26 January 2019

Abstract: Kidney injury due to focal segmental glomerulosclerosis (FSGS) is the most common primary glomerular disorder causing end-stage renal disease. Homozygous mutations in either glomerular basement membrane or slit diaphragm genes cause early renal failure. Heterozygous carriers develop renal symptoms late, if at all. In contrast to mutations in slit diaphragm genes, hetero- or hemizygous mutations in the X-chromosomal *COL4A5* Alport gene have not yet been recognized as a major cause of kidney injury by FSGS. We identified cases of FSGS that were unexpectedly diagnosed: In addition to mutations in the X-chromosomal *COL4A5* type IV collagen gene, nephrin and podocin polymorphisms aggravated kidney damage, leading to FSGS with ruptures of the basement membrane in a toddler and early renal failure in heterozygous girls. The results of our case series study suggest a synergistic role for genes encoding basement membrane and slit diaphragm proteins as a cause of kidney injury due to FSGS. Our results demonstrate that the molecular genetics of different players in the glomerular filtration barrier can be used to evaluate causes of kidney injury. Given the high frequency of X-chromosomal carriers of Alport genes, the analysis of genes involved in the organization of podocyte architecture, the glomerular basement membrane, and the slit diaphragm will further improve our understanding of the pathogenesis of FSGS and guide prognosis of and therapy for hereditary glomerular kidney diseases.

Keywords: kidney injury; alport syndrome; modifier gene; nephrin; podocin; glomerular basement membrane; slit diaphragm; focal segmental glomerulosclerosis

1. Introduction

Focal segmental glomerulosclerosis (FSGS) is the most common primary glomerular disorder causing end-stage renal disease (ESRD) in the United States [1]. Podocyte injury plays a critical role in the pathogenesis of proteinuric kidney diseases, as podocytes are important for maintaining the glomerular filtration barrier [2]. They restore crucial components of the glomerular basement membrane (GBM), such as $\alpha3/\alpha4/\alpha5$ type IV collagen chains (*COL4A3/4/5*), and of the slit diaphragm, such as nephrin (*NPHS1*) and podocin (*NPHS2*). Homozygous or hemizygous mutations in glomerular filtration barrier genes, such as the *COL4A3/4/5* genes, result in Alport syndrome (AS) [3–5], while homozygous mutations in the *NPHS1* and *NPHS2* genes result in congenital nephrotic syndrome [6,7]. The development of these syndromes leads to early ESRD. Few heterozygous carriers develop late changes, and they rarely (or never, in the case of *NPHS1/2* heterozygotes) develop ESRD. Polymorphisms in these genes are thought to result in an even milder phenotype or no phenotype.

The typical clinical signs of FSGS are marked proteinuria and podocyte injury. FSGS often manifests as nephrotic syndrome and frequently leads to renal failure. As FSGS is much less responsive to steroid therapy than minimal change disease, its prognosis for preserving renal function is (much) worse, with a high recurrence rate after renal transplantation [8].

The initial injuries leading to FSGS vary widely from monogenetic forms to secondary forms, which can be triggered by maladaptation of the podocyte to hyperfiltration, virus infections, drug use, or (unknown) circulating factors [8]. Primary (monogenetic) FSGS is caused by variants in the structural genes of the podocyte or the extracellular matrix (GBM). Primary FSGS typically results in in early onset of disease during childhood or adolescence.

Approximately 80% of adult cases of FSGS are primary (idiopathic) [1]. Up to 10% of familial FSGS can be explained by autosomal *COL4A3/4* mutations [9]; however, *COL4A5* mutations leading to X-linked Alport syndrome (XLAS) are much more common. Here, we describe three families with FSGS, which was unexpectedly diagnosed in toddlers with XLAS and in adolescent XLAS carriers with renal failure. In addition to mutations in the XLAS-related *COL4A5* gene, nephrin and podocin polymorphisms seem to have aggravated kidney damage, including severe FSGS with GBM ruptures in a toddler and unusually early renal failure in heterozygous girls.

2. Results

Patient 1 (case 1) was the index patient, in whom a severe kidney phenotype and GBM ruptures led to the discovery that in FSGS due to genetic GBM diseases, such as AS, polymorphisms in slit diaphragm genes can aggravate kidney damage. Subsequently, two other families with X-chromosomal AS were found to have FSGS, which was aggravated by slit diaphragm gene polymorphisms (Table 1).

Table 1. Summary of patient phenotypes and genotypes.

Patient	Sex	First Clinical Presentation > Symptoms	Genotype COL4A5	Genotype Nphs-1/-2	Ear/Eye	Dialysis/Tx	Medication	Affected Family Members
Case 1 A.N. II-1	♂	27 months macrohematuria acanthocytes proteinuria urinary tract infection	COL4A5 p.W1538X (TGG>TGA) hemizygous	Nphs1: p.R408Q (CGG>CAG) polymorphism heterozygous Nphs1:p.S1105S(TCG>TCA) polymorphism homozygous Nphs2: p.G34G (GGA>GGG) polymorphism homozygous	no pathological findings	none	2012–today ACEi	no kidney diseases known mother without symptoms: Nphs1: p.R408Q (CGG>CAG) polymorphism heterozygous
Case 2 C.V. II-4	♀	11 years macrohematuria proteinuria urinary tract infection	COL4A5 Exon 49, Codon 1510, IVS49+3A>G heterozygous	Nphs2: p.R229Q (CGA>CAA) polymorphism heterozygous	no pathological findings	Tx age: 15	/refused treatment	no other family members affected
S.V. III-1	♀	1 year macrohematuria Proteinuria	COL4A5 Exon 49, Codon 1510, IVS49+3A>G heterozygous	Nphs2: p.R229Q (CGA>CAA) polymorphism heterozygous	no pathological findings	none	/refused treatment	
M.V. III-2	♂	4 months macrohematuria proteinuria	COL4A5 Exon 49, Codon 1510, IVS49+3A>G hemizygous	none	no pathological findings	none	/refuse treatment	
Case 3 L.U. II-3	♀	27 years hematuria proteinuria	COL4A5 p.G624D (GGT>GAT) heterozygous	Nphs2: p.R229Q (CGA>CAA) polymorphism heterozygous Nphs2: p.G34G(GGA>GGG) polymorphism homozygous	minimal high-frequency hearing loss (2013)	Tx age: 51	<u>Before Tx</u>: ACEi from 33 years	see pedigree of family (Figure 3)
W.T. II-7	♀	40 years: microhematuria 42 years: proteinuria	COL4A5 p.G624D (GGT>GAT) heterozygous	none	retinal detachment	none	02/2013: ACEi (discontinued due to angioedema)	
T.O. II.4	♀	microhematuria	COL4A5 p.G624D (GGT>GAT) heterozygous	none	high-frequency hearing loss (2013)	none	none	
S.O. III-7	♂	microhematuria	COL4A5 p.G624D (GGT>GAT) heterozygous	none	no pathological findings (2013)	none	none	
O.T. III-12	♀	no symptoms	COL4A5 p.G624D (GGT>GAT) heterozygous	not investigated	not investigated	none	none	

2.1. Clinical Presentation

Patient 1 was a 27-month-old boy with persistent macrohematuria, proteinuria (1300 mg/L), active sediment, and normal renal function. His older sister and his non-consanguineous Lithuanian parents were healthy, with no family history of kidney diseases (Figure 1a). Post-infectious glomerulonephritis was excluded. Due to the initial suspicion of an infection and normal renal morphology on ultrasound examination, a cystoscopy was performed, which revealed hemorrhagic cystitis. However, common causes of hemorrhagic cystitis in childhood [10,11], such as cytomegalovirus or BK-polyomavirus infection, were ruled out. Consequently, a renal biopsy was performed. Light microscopy and immunohistochemistry (Figure 1b,c) revealed profound FSGS, IgM-positive deposits, and slight mesangial expansion. Ultrastructurally, the GBM presented with diffuse splitting, thinning, and ruptures (Figure 1d–f). The podocytes showed foot process effacement, with partial loss of the slit diaphragm (Figure 1d). These structural changes led to the diagnosis of AS. Hearing and eye evaluations did not reveal any abnormalities. Nephroprotective angiotensin-converting enzyme (ACE)-inhibitor therapy with ramipril was started [12,13], and the proteinuria slowly decreased from 1300 mg/L to less than 400 mg/L (Figure 1g). No further macrohematuria was reported.

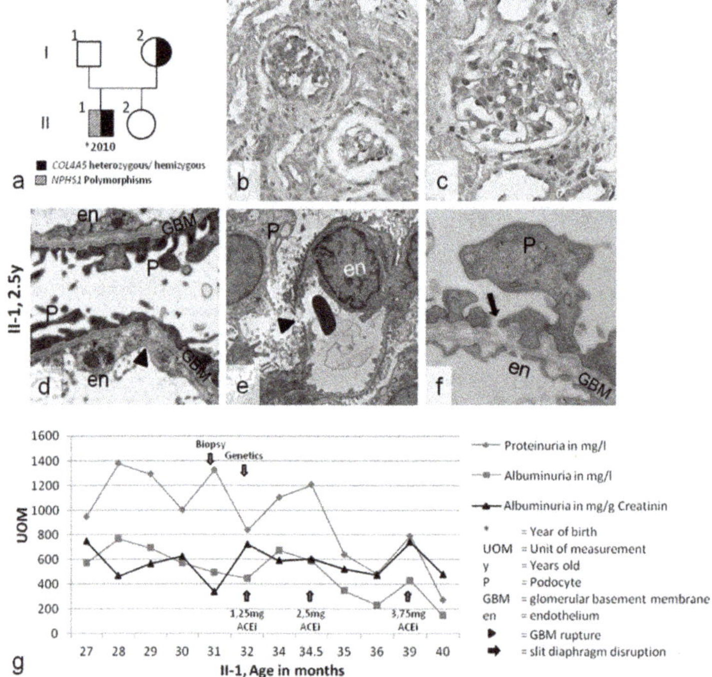

Figure 1. (**a**) Pedigree of case 1. (**b–f**) Nephropathological evaluation of the kidney biopsy of patient II-1. (**b,c**) Light microscopy showing focal segmental glomerulosclerosis (FSGS) and slight mesangial matrix expansion. (**d–f**) Ultrastructural analysis showing gross broadening of the podocyte foot processes; partial loss of the slit diaphragm (black arrow); and splitting, thinning, and ruptures of the glomerular basement membrane (GBM) (arrowhead). (**g**) The course of disease during ACE-inhibitor therapy: proteinuria constantly decreased (arrow). The diagnostic timescale is indicated by the blue arrows. Magnification: (**b,c**) 400×, (**d**) 20,000×, (**e**) 8000×, (**f**) 25,000×.

Case 2 was an Austrian family with severe kidney disease in the mother, daughter, and son (Figure 2). The mother presented with hematuria and proteinuria in childhood. She soon developed ESRD and received a kidney transplant from her father at the age of 15. Her kidney biopsy at 11 years of age revealed advanced FSGS, hyalinosis, tubulointerstitial foam cells, podocyte effacement, splitting, lamellations, and partial thinning of the GBM. AS was considered; however, due to the unusual nature of a severe manifestation in a girl with healthy parents, she was diagnosed as having FSGS and nephrotic syndrome, with secondary structural changes in the GBM (Figure 2b,c).

Her daughter and son both presented with hematuria and progressive proteinuria during the first year of life. A kidney biopsy performed when the daughter was two years old appeared relatively normal under light microscopy, although ultrastructural analysis showed advanced pathology, with podocyte effacement and splitting and thinning of the GBM, similar to the mother's biopsy (Figure 2d–g). Hearing and eye evaluations did not reveal any pathological abnormalities in any family member. The family refused therapeutic intervention, leading to progressive proteinuria in both siblings (Figure 2h). Currently, the daughter and son have reached stage 3 of chronic kidney disease.

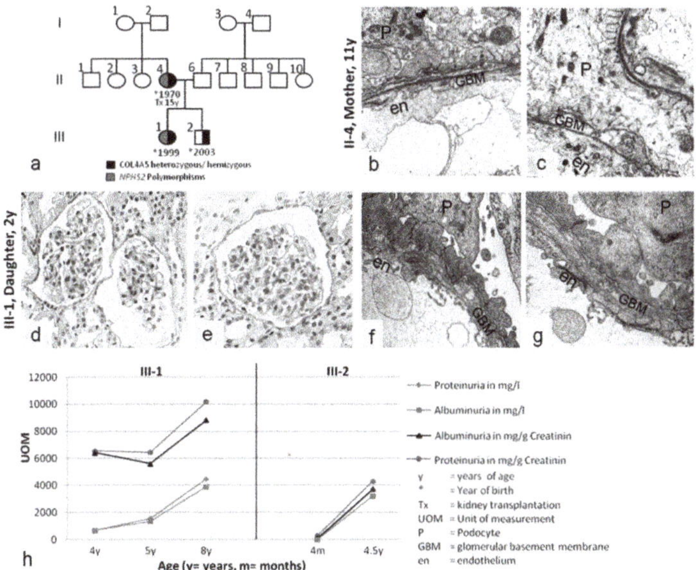

Figure 2. (**a**) Pedigree of case 2. (**b,c**) Kidney biopsy of the mother (11 y) revealing partial GBM thinning, splitting, and laminations in the lamina densa, with plump podocyte (P) foot processes. (**d–g**) Kidney biopsy of the daughter (3 y). (**d,e**) Light microscopy showing relatively normal glomerular and tubulointerstitial structures. Electron microscopy uncovered GBM pathology with splitting and thinning, similar to the mother's nephropathology. (**h**) The course of disease without therapy in this X-chromosomal *COL4A5* genotype was unexpectedly very similar in the heterozygous girl (III-1) and her hemizygous brother (III-2): proteinuria constantly increased into the nephrotic range. Magnification: (**b,c**) 10,000×, (**d,e**) 400×, (**f,g**) 12,500×.

Case 3 was a family originating from Austria and Poland (Figure 3a). A kidney biopsy performed in a 27-year-old female (II-3) with hematuria and proteinuria showed advanced FSGS (Figure 3b,c). The biopsied material was not sufficient for ultrastructural analysis. A definite diagnosis was not possible; however, FSGS was suspected. The patient developed ESRD at approximately 40 years of age and received a kidney transplant at 51 years of age. Kidney disease progressed more slowly in her sister (II-7), who first presented with microhematuria at the age of 40. Further evaluation of several other affected family members (Figure 3a) revealed moderate hearing loss in patients II-3 and II-4 and eye involvement in patient II-7. Therefore, a complex hereditary kidney disease was considered.

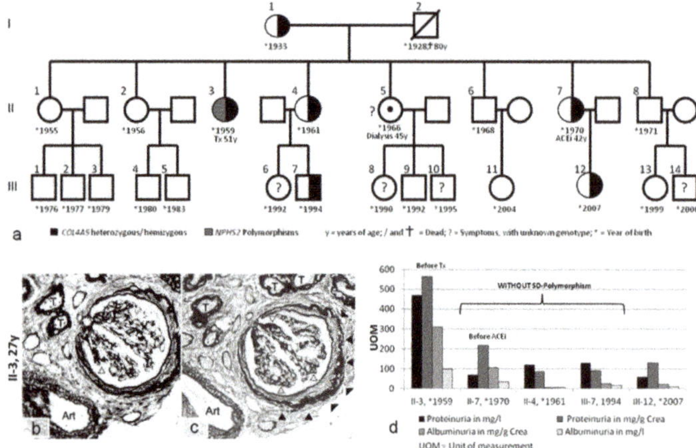

Figure 3. (**a**) Pedigree of case 3, with I-1 and family members (II-1, II-2, II-5, II-6, and II-8) living in Poland. Further evaluation was performed on family members living in Vienna (II-3, II-4, II-7, III-7, and III-12). Tx = kidney transplant. (**b,c**) Kidney biopsy in case II-3. Only a small core of renal tissue could be obtained for light microscopy. This tissue contained only one relatively intact glomerulus and three glomerular scars. The pathology was described as nonspecific and dominated by sclerosis. The glomerulus showed segmental scarring of the capillary loops (open arrowheads) and pronounced periglomerular fibrosis (solid arrowheads). The tubules (T) were dissociated by interstitial fibrosis, and thickening of the tubular basement membranes confirmed advanced atrophy. One small artery (Art) exhibited minimal intimal fibrosis. (**d**) Proteinuria and albuminuria in family members with and without additional slit diaphragm (SD) polymorphisms. Methenamine silver (**b**) and PAS staining (**c**); magnification: 400×.

2.2. Genetic Analyses of COL4A3/4/5 GBM Genes and NPHS1/2 Slit Diaphragm Genes

In case 1, the suspected diagnosis of AS was confirmed by genetic testing. A hemizygous X-chromosomal *COL4A5* de novo mutation was discovered in the boy but not in his parents: p.W1538X (TGG>TGA), c.4614 G>A. *COL4A5* mutations are typically associated with microhematuria in the first few years of life, slowly progressing to microalbuminuria below 300 mg [14], but not with high levels of proteinuria such as the 1300 mg/L observed in the two-year-old boy. Therefore, the severe phenotype of the two-year-old boy, an origin close to Scandinavia, and unusually severe FSGS led to the exploration of the slit diaphragm genes *NPHS1* and *NPHS2*. A polymorphism (p.R408Q (CGG>CAG), c.1223G>A) in *NPHS1* (nephrin) was identified in the boy and in his mother, who was not affected by the *COL4A5* mutation. Furthermore, homozygous silent polymorphisms in *NPHS1* (p.S1105S (TCG>TCA), c.102A>G) and *NPHS2* (p.G34G (GGA>GGG) c.3315G>A) were discovered in the boy (Table 1).

In case 2, a *COL4A5* splice mutation (exon 49, codon 1510, IVS49+3A>G) was hemizygous in the boy and heterozygous in the girl and the mother. No other family members were affected, suggesting that this was a de novo mutation in the mother (Figure 2 and Table 1). The heterozygous mother and daughter were both severely affected; however, proteinuria is usually mild or absent in young heterozygous *COL4A5* females, and early progression to ESRD before the third decade of life has never been described [14,15]. As in case 1, the severe phenotype of the heterozygous carriers led to an exploration of the slit diaphragm genes. Both heterozygous females, but not the hemizygous son, had a heterozygous *NPHS2* polymorphism (p.R229Q (CGA>CAA), c.686G>A; Table 1) that has been described as a modifier gene in thin basement membrane disease [16,17]. The clinical course of the son, who lacked the *NPHS2* polymorphism, was consistent with X-chromosomal AS in males. In contrast, the clinical courses of his heterozygous sister and mother, who had the *NPHS2* polymorphism, were very unusual.

In case 3, patient II-3 had a heterozygous *COL4A5* mutation (p.G624D (GGT>GAT), c.1871 G>A) that generally results in benign hematuria in females and late-onset ESRD in hemizygous males (in the 4th decade of life) [16]. Again, the severe phenotype resulted in further evaluation, and a polymorphism in *NPHS2* (p.R229Q (CGA>CAA), c.686G>A) in addition to a silent single-nucleotide polymorphism (SNP) in *NPHS2* (p.G34G (GGA>GGG), c.102A>G) were identified. Importantly, the G34G variant was found independently in case 1 and case 3, but represents a polymorphism of unknown relevance. All other family members presented only the *COL4A5* mutation (Figure 3a), and their clinical courses were consistent with benign hematuria (in females) and slowly progressing renal disease (in males) (Table 1). The heterozygous female with the *NPHS2* polymorphism (II-3) had higher proteinuria compared with her heterozygous sisters (II-7 and II-4) at the same age, who did not have the *NPHS2* polymorphism (Figure 3d).

2.3. Slit Diaphragm Gene Polymorphisms Aggravate Glomerular Architecture towards FSGS in Patients with GBM Mutations

Morphological analysis of case 1 further underscored the evidence that a *COL4A5* mutation in a basement membrane component can be aggravated by polymorphisms in slit diaphragm genes: (1) pronounced FSGS has not been previously described in toddlers with AS (Figure 1b,c); however, (2) initial thinning (and splitting) of the GBM is a common feature in children with AS (Figure 1d). GBM ruptures have not been previously described in patients with AS (Figure 1e). (3) Gross broadening of the podocyte foot processes, with partial loss of the slit diaphragm (Figure 1d), is a very notable and unusual finding in toddlers with AS, and (4) a high level of proteinuria (1300 mg/l with persistent macrohematuria) is unusual for a toddler with AS. The last feature and the FSGS were judged as being indicative of additional podocyte pathology. The structural changes led to the presumptive diagnosis of AS, though with the differential diagnosis of mutations in podocyte genes, as the atypically progressive structural changes could not be attributed to the patient's age and his primary diagnosis of AS.

In case 2, the mother was diagnosed in childhood as having nephrotic-range FSGS with secondary GBM changes (Figure 2b,c). Kidney pathology in the 3-year-old daughter, with gross broadening of the podocyte foot processes (Figure 2f,g), was similar to that of her mother. In both individuals, despite their "merely" heterozygous AS status, the *NPHS2* polymorphism aggravated GBM pathology toward FSGS and early ESRD. Despite X-inactivation, ESRD has not been previously described in heterozygous AS carriers during adolescence. Notably, the hemizygous son, who had full-pattern AS but lacked the *NPHS2* polymorphism, had a clinical course that was identical to that of his "merely" heterozygous sister with the *NPHS2* polymorphism.

In case 3, the kidney pathology of the *COL4A5* carrier (II-3) was dominated by sclerosis (Figure 3b,c). This finding is a clear contradiction to the thin GBM that one would have expected in a young female with a heterozygous p.G624D mutation. This glomerulosclerosis may be due to the *NPHS2* polymorphism, as proteinuria was much lower in all other p.G624D-affected family members without the *NPHS2* polymorphism (e.g., the sister (II-4) at the same age). Even the *COL4A5* hemizygous adult male presented with less than 20% of the proteinuria of his aunt (II-3).

3. Discussion

It has been predicted that next-generation sequencing will identify most of the monogenic disease-causing genes by the year 2020 [18]. Next-generation sequencing has recently been shown to improve mutation screening in familial hematuric nephropathies [19]. However, the increasing knowledge of human genetic pathology will be associated with major challenges. Here, we show that for personalized medical care, physicians need all (1) a careful clinical evaluation of their patients,

(2) close cooperation with the pathologist interpreting (kidney) specimens, and (3) genetic information about mutations and polymorphisms that might influence disease. Remarkably, thorough clinical exploration and its correlation with the kidney histology by the pathologist were essential tools guiding disease-focused genetic evaluation in the three families that we described. Without clinical and histological assessment preceding mutation analysis, physicians would not be able to understand and interpret the pathology of the glomerular filtration barrier [20].

As a limitation of our study, phenotyping of all family members and the extension of genetic correlation to other slit diaphragm genes was restricted by regional barriers, as family members originated from four different countries. The use of Sanger sequencing limited our search for possible disease-causing mutations to only five genes, whereas mutations in other podocyte genes could be contributory [21]. Additional regional legal barriers hindered us from extending the genetic analysis beyond the *COL4A3/4/5* and *NPHS1/2* genes. Still, our study was able to correlate the phenotype to the genetic changes in most members of a large three-generation pedigree, with a less severe phenotype in patients II-4, II-7, and III-7 without polymorphisms in slit diaphragm genes (Figure 3).

Podocytes evolve into crucial cells that maintain the glomerular filtration barrier in renal diseases. Because of their need to withstand permanent filtration pressure, these cells adhere tightly to the underlying GBM [22]. The dynamic control of their cytoskeleton is affected by the slit diaphragm [22]. As a consequence, podocyte dedifferentiation, effacement, and FSGS are very common features in renal diseases [23]. Reducing the filtration pressure and thus protecting podocytes is a crucial therapeutic goal, even in children with congenital renal diseases [24].

Malone and coworkers demonstrated that up to 10% of familial FSGS can be explained by autosomal *COL4A3/4* mutations [9]. Our investigations expand previous findings that FSGS can also be caused by *COL4A5* mutations, the most common cause of AS, aggravated by polymorphisms in slit diaphragm genes [20,25]. $\alpha3/\alpha4/\alpha5$ type IV collagen chains stabilize the GBM against filtration pressure [26]. Loss of any of the $\alpha3/\alpha4/\alpha5$ type IV collagen chains results in a weaker GBM and increased podocyte cytoskeleton vulnerability [27]. As the cell–cell adhesions of the slit diaphragm are closely linked to the podocyte cytoskeleton, any polymorphism in slit diaphragm genes [28–31], as demonstrated in our study, might result in further damage in the histological picture of FSGS. This hypothesis should be tested in animal models using heterozygous $NPHS2^{+/R140Q}$ mice, which correspond to the most common p.R138Q mutation found in humans and $COL4A3^{+/-}$ mice [32–35]. $NPHS2^{+/R140Q}$ mice develop no phenotype [32], while $COL4A3^{+/-}$ mice develop benign familial hematuria [33,34]. The mature GBM with the $\alpha3/4/5$ (IV) collagen chains can solely be built by podocytes, which sense the integrity of the GBM via their type IV collagen receptors, such as discoidin receptor 1 (DDR1) and integrins [4]. On the other hand, the crosstalk between the collagen receptor and the podocyte actin cytoskeleton, which also interacts with the slit diaphragm, might be the crucial link between the GBM and slit diaphragm that causes FSGS in our patients [4].

In conclusion, our findings demonstrate that after thorough clinical evaluation, the molecular genetics of different players in the glomerular filtration barrier can be used to evaluate FSGS. The analysis of genes involved in the organization of podocyte architecture, the GBM, and the slit diaphragm will further our understanding of the histological picture of FSGS. Our increasing knowledge of genes, arising from next-generation sequencing, will help to personalize the diagnosis and prognosis of and therapy for glomerular kidney diseases. Experienced physicians and pathologists are still needed to classify genetic results for the benefit of the patient.

4. Methods

4.1. Ethical Considerations

Written informed consent was given by the families for the publication of their cases. ICH-GCP data acquisition and storage of the European Alport registry was approved by the IRB of the University Medicine Goettingen, Germany (AZ 10/11/06; updated version from 2014).

The European Alport registry has been registered at ClinicalTrials.gov (NCT 02378805) and as EudraCT number 2014-003533-25.

4.2. Genetic Analyses

EDTA-treated blood was obtained after written informed consent was provided. Genomic DNA was extracted from peripheral blood leukocytes. The coding regions of *COL4A3*, *COL4A4*, *COL4A5*, *NPHS1*, and *NPHS2* were analyzed: The entire coding regions and splice sites of the *NPHS1* (transcript NM_004646.3; 29 exons), *NPHS2* (transcript NM_014625.2; 8 exons), *COL4A3* (transcript NM_000091.4; 52 exons), *COL4A4* (transcript NM_000092.4; 48 exons), and *COL4A5* (transcript NM_033380.2; 53 exons) genes were sequenced using unidirectional tagged primer Sanger sequencing in a 96-well format. Polymerase chain reaction (PCR) primers were designed using Primer-BLAST® from the NCBI (National Center for Biotechnology Information, Bethesda, MD, USA). PCR products were generated using Buffer HOT Fire Polymerase® (Solis Biodyne Solis, Tartu, Estonia) at an annealing temperature of 60 °C and were cleaned up using an Illustra ExoProStar One-Step® kit (GE Healthcare, Freiburg, Germany). Sequencing was performed using a BigDye® Terminator v1.1 cycle kit (Applied Biosystems®, Life Technologies GmbH, Darmstadt, Germany), and products were cleaned up using a CentriSep ABI® kit (Applied Biosystems®, Life Technologies GmbH, Darmstadt, Germany). The sequences were read with an ABI Prism® 3130XL DNA analyzer (Applied Biosystems®, Life Technologies GmbH, Darmstadt, Germany) and were analyzed using our in-house sequence analysis software (SeqEdit).

4.3. Morphological Analyses

Kidney biopsies were analyzed by light microscopy, immunohistochemistry, and electron microscopy.

Author Contributions: H.-J.G., R.K. and J.N. analyzed and interpreted the kidney biopsies, including the interpretation of the clinical and genetic data, and co-wrote the manuscript. M.N. analyzed and interpreted all mutations and polymorphisms, including the interpretation of the clinical and histological data, and co-wrote the manuscript. M.K., H.Z., J.H. and G.S.-P. took care of the patients, analyzed and interpreted the clinical data, including the interpretation of the genetic and histological data, and co-wrote the manuscript. J.F. collected all data, was involved in all data analysis and interpretation, and wrote the primary version of the manuscript. O.G. conceived the study design and concept, was involved in all data analysis and interpretation, and wrote the final version of the manuscript. All authors read and approved the manuscript.

Funding: Parts of the work has been supported by German research foundation DFG (to OG, GR 1852/6-1).

Acknowledgments: We thank all families for their contribution and consent for the publication of their cases.

Conflicts of Interest: The authors declare no conflict of interest.

References

1. D'Agati, V.D.; Kaskel, F.J.; Falk, R.J. Focal segmental glomerulosclerosis. *N. Engl. J. Med.* **2011**, *365*, 2398–2411. [CrossRef] [PubMed]
2. Brinkkoetter, P.T.; Ising, C.; Benzing, T. The role of the podocyte in albumin filtration. *Nat. Rev. Nephrol.* **2013**, *9*, 328–336. [CrossRef] [PubMed]
3. Hudson, B.G.; Tryggvason, K.; Sundaramoorthy, M.; Neilson, E.G. Alport's syndrome, Goodpasture's syndrome, and type IV collagen. *N. Engl. J. Med.* **2003**, *348*, 2543–2556. [CrossRef] [PubMed]
4. Kruegel, J.; Rubel, D.; Gross, O. Alport syndrome—Insights from basic and clinical research. *Nat. Rev. Nephrol.* **2013**, *9*, 170–178. [CrossRef] [PubMed]
5. Storey, H.; Savige, J.; Sivakumar, V.; Abbs, S.; Flinter, F.A. COL4A3/COL4A4 mutations and features in individuals with autosomal recessive Alport syndrome. *J. Am. Soc. Nephrol.* **2013**, *24*, 1945–1954. [CrossRef] [PubMed]
6. Gubler, M.C. Podocyte differentiation and hereditary proteinuria/nephrotic syndromes. *J. Am. Soc. Nephrol.* **2003**, *14* (Suppl. 1), S22–S26. [CrossRef] [PubMed]
7. Niaudet, P. Genetic forms of nephrotic syndrome. *Pediatr. Nephrol.* **2004**, *19*, 1313–1318. [CrossRef]

8. Fogo, A.B. Causes and pathogenesis of focal segmental glomerulosclerosis. *Nat. Rev. Nephrol.* **2015**, *11*, 76–87. [CrossRef]

9. Malone, A.F.; Phelan, P.J.; Hall, G.; Cetincelik, U.; Homstad, A.; Alonso, A.S.; Jiang, R.; Lindsey, T.B.; Wu, G.; Sparks, M.A.; et al. Rare hereditary COL4A3/COL4A4 variants may be mistaken for familial focal segmental glomerulosclerosis. *Kidney Int.* **2014**, *86*, 1253–1259. [CrossRef]

10. Megged, O.; Stein, J.; Ben-Meir, D.; Shulman, L.M.; Yaniv, I.; Shalit, I.; Levy, I. BK-virus-associated hemorrhagic cystitis in children after hematopoietic stem cell transplantation. *J. Pediatr. Hematol. Oncol.* **2011**, *33*, 190–193. [CrossRef]

11. Kloos, R.Q.; Boelens, J.J.; de Jong, T.P.; Versluys, B.; Bierings, M. Hemorrhagic cystitis in a cohort of pediatric transplantations: Incidence, treatment, outcome, and risk factors. *Biol. Blood Marrow Transplant.* **2013**, *19*, 1263–1266. [CrossRef] [PubMed]

12. Gross, O.; Licht, C.; Anders, H.J.; Hoppe, B.; Beck, B.; Tönshoff, B.; Höcker, B.; Wygoda, S.; Ehrich, J.H.; Pape, L.; et al. Early angiotensin-converting enzyme inhibition in Alport syndrome delays renal failure and improves life expectancy. *Kidney Int.* **2012**, *81*, 494–501. [CrossRef] [PubMed]

13. Gross, O.; Friede, T.; Hilgers, R.; Görlitz, A.; Gavénis, K.; Ahmed, R.; Dürr, U. Safety and Efficacy of the ACE-Inhibitor Ramipril in Alport Syndrome: The Double-Blind, Randomized, Placebo-Controlled, Multicenter Phase III EARLY PRO-TECT Alport Trial in Pediatric Patients. *ISRN Pediatr.* **2012**, *2012*, 436046. [CrossRef] [PubMed]

14. Gross, O.; Netzer, K.O.; Lambrecht, R.; Seibold, S.; Weber, M. Meta-analysis of genotype-phenotype correlation in X-linked Alport syndrome: Impact on clinical counselling. *Nephrol. Dial. Transplant.* **2002**, *17*, 1218–1227. [CrossRef] [PubMed]

15. Jais, J.P.; Knebelmann, B.; Giatras, I.; De Marchi, M.; Rizzoni, G.; Renieri, A.; Weber, M.; Gross, O.; Netzer, K.O.; Flinter, F.; et al. X-linked Alport syndrome: Natural history and genotype-phenotype correlations in girls and women belonging to 195 families: A "European Community Alport Syndrome Concerted Action" study. *J. Am. Soc. Nephrol.* **2003**, *14*, 2603–2610. [CrossRef] [PubMed]

16. Knebelmann, B.; Breillat, C.; Forestier, L.; Arrondel, C.; Jacassier, D.; Giatras, I.; Drouot, L.; Deschênes, G.; Grünfeld, J.P.; Broyer, M.; et al. Spectrum of mutations in the COL4A5 collagen gene in X-linked Alport syndrome. *Am. J. Hum. Genet.* **1996**, *59*, 1221–1232. [PubMed]

17. Voskarides, K.; Arsali, M.; Athanasiou, Y.; Elia, A.; Pierides, A.; Deltas, C. Evidence that NPHS2-R229Q predisposes to proteinuria and renal failure in familial hematuria. *Pediatr. Nephrol.* **2012**, *27*, 675–679. [CrossRef]

18. Boycott, K.M.; Vanstone, M.R.; Bulman, D.E.; MacKenzie, A.E. Rare-disease genetics in the era of next-generation sequencing: Discovery to translation. *Nat. Rev. Genet.* **2013**, *14*, 681–691. [CrossRef]

19. Morinière, V.; Dahan, K.; Hilbert, P.; Lison, M.; Lebbah, S.; Topa, A.; Bole-Feysot, C.; Pruvost, S.; Nitschke, P.; Plaisier, E.; et al. Improving Mutation Screening in Familial Hematuric Nephropathies through Next Generation Sequencing. *J. Am. Soc. Nephrol.* **2014**, *25*, 2740–2751. [CrossRef]

20. Gibson, J.; Gilbert, R.D.; Bunyan, D.J.; Angus, E.M.; Fowler, D.J.; Ennis, S. Exome analysis resolves differential diagnosis of familial kidney disease and uncovers a potential confounding variant. *Genet. Res.* **2014**, *28*, 1–9. [CrossRef]

21. Bullich, G.; Trujillano, D.; Santín, S.; Ballarín, J.; Torra, R.; Estivill, X.; Ars, E. Targeted next-generation sequencing in steroid-resistant nephrotic syndrome: Mutations in multiple glomerular genes may influence disease severity. *Eur. J. Hum. Genet.* **2014**, *23*, 1192. [CrossRef] [PubMed]

22. Cravedi, P.; Kopp, J.B.; Remuzzi, G. Recent progress in the pathophysiology and treatment of FSGS recurrence. *Am. J. Transplant.* **2013**, *13*, 266–274. [CrossRef] [PubMed]

23. Sachs, N.; Sonnenberg, A. Cell-matrix adhesion of podocytes in physiology and disease. *Nat. Rev. Nephrol.* **2013**, *9*, 200–210. [CrossRef] [PubMed]

24. Ingelfinger, J.R. Blood-pressure control and delay in progression of kidney disease in children. *N. Engl. J. Med.* **2009**, *361*, 1701–1703. [CrossRef] [PubMed]

25. Adam, J.; Connor, T.M.; Wood, K.; Lewis, D.; Naik, R.; Gale, D.P.; Sayer, J.A. Genetic testing can resolve diagnostic confusion in Alport syndrome. *Clin. Kidney J.* **2014**, *7*, 197–200. [CrossRef] [PubMed]

26. Fidler, A.L.; Vanacore, R.M.; Chetyrkin, S.V.; Pedchenko, V.K.; Bhave, G.; Yin, V.P.; Stothers, C.L.; Rose, K.L.; McDonald, W.H.; Clark, T.A.; et al. A unique covalent bond in basement membrane is a primordial innovation for tissue evolution. *Proc. Natl. Acad. Sci. USA* **2014**, *111*, 331–336. [CrossRef] [PubMed]

27. Welsh, G.I.; Saleem, M.A. The podocyte cytoskeleto—Key to a functioning glomerulus in health and disease. *Nat. Rev. Nephrol.* **2011**, *8*, 14–21. [CrossRef]

28. Tsukaguchi, H.; Sudhakar, A.; Le, T.C.; Nguyen, T.; Yao, J.; Schwimmer, J.A.; Schachter, A.D.; Poch, E.; Abreu, P.F.; Appel, G.B.; et al. NPHS2 mutations in late-onset focal segmental glomerulosclerosis: R229Q is a common disease-associated allele. *J. Clin. Invest.* **2002**, *110*, 1659–1666. [CrossRef]

29. Ozaltin, F.; Ibsirlioglu, T.; Taskiran, E.Z.; Baydar, D.E.; Kaymaz, F.; Buyukcelik, M.; Kilic, B.D.; Balat, A.; Iatropoulos, P.; Asan, E.; et al. Disruption of PTPRO causes childhood-onset nephrotic syndrome. *Am. J. Hum. Genet.* **2011**, *89*, 139–147. [CrossRef]

30. Tory, K.; Menyhárd, D.K.; Woerner, S.; Nevo, F.; Gribouval, O.; Kerti, A.; Stráner, P.; Arrondel, C.; Huynh Cong, E.; Tulassay, T.; et al. Mutation-dependent recessive inheritance of NPHS2-associated steroid-resistant nephrotic syndrome. *Nat. Genet.* **2014**, *46*, 299–304. [CrossRef]

31. Kerti, A.; Csohány, R.; Wagner, L.; Jávorszky, E.; Maka, E.; Tory, K. NPHS2 homozygous p.R229Q variant: Potential modifier instead of causal effect in focal segmental glomerulosclerosis. *Pediatr. Nephrol.* **2013**, *28*, 2061–2429. [CrossRef] [PubMed]

32. Philippe, A.; Weber, S.; Esquivel, E.L.; Houbron, C.; Hamard, G.; Ratelade, J.; Kriz, W.; Schaefer, F.; Gubler, M.C.; Antignac, C. A missense mutation in podocin leads to early and severe renal disease in mice. *Kidney Int.* **2008**, *73*, 1038–1047. [CrossRef] [PubMed]

33. Tonna, S.; Wang, Y.Y.; Wilson, D.; Rigby, L.; Tabone, T.; Cotton, R.; Savige, J. The R229Q mutation in NPHS2 may predispose to proteinuria in thin-basement-membrane nephropathy. *Pediatr. Nephrol.* **2008**, *23*, 2201–2207. [CrossRef] [PubMed]

34. Beirowski, B.; Weber, M.; Gross, O. Chronic renal failure and shortened lifespan in COL4A3$^{+/-}$ mice: An animal model for thin basement membrane nephropathy. *J. Am. Soc. Nephrol.* **2006**, *17*, 1986–1994. [CrossRef] [PubMed]

35. Cosgrove, D.; Meehan, D.T.; Grunkemeyer, J.A.; Kornak, J.M.; Sayers, R.; Hunter, W.J.; Samuelson, G.C. Collagen COL4A3 knockout: A mouse model for autosomal Alport syndrome. *Genes Dev.* **1996**, *10*, 2981–2992. [CrossRef] [PubMed]

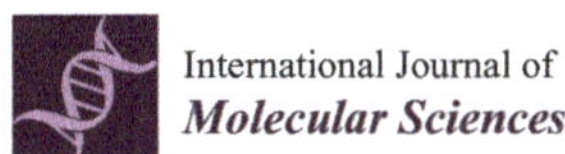
International Journal of
Molecular Sciences

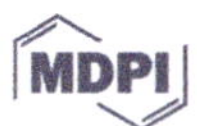

Article

Renal Regenerative Potential of Extracellular Vesicles Derived from miRNA-Engineered Mesenchymal Stromal Cells

Marta Tapparo [1,†], Stefania Bruno [1,†], Federica Collino [2], Gabriele Togliatto [1], Maria Chiara Deregibus [3], Paolo Provero [4], Sicheng Wen [5], Peter J. Quesenberry [5] and Giovanni Camussi [1,*]

[1] Department of Medical Sciences and Molecular Biotechnology Center, University of Torino, 10126 Torino, Italy; marta.tapparo@unito.it (M.T.); stefania.bruno@unito.it (S.B.); gabriele.togliatto@unito.it (G.T.)

[2] Department of Biomedical Sciences and Paediatric Research Institute "Citta della Speranza", University of Padova, 35129 Padova, Italy; federica.collino@unipd.it

[3] 2i3T Società per la gestione dell'incubatore di imprese e per il trasferimento tecnologico Scarl, University of Torino, 10126 Torino, Italy; mariachiara.deregibus@unito.it

[4] Department of Molecular Biotechnology and Health Sciences and Molecular Biotechnology Center, University of Torino, 10126 Torino, Italy; paolo.provero@unito.it

[5] Division of Hematology/Oncology, Brown University, Rhode Island Hospital, Providence, Rhode Island, RI 02912, USA; swen@lifespan.org (S.W.); PQuesenberry@lifespan.org (P.J.Q.)

* Correspondence: giovanni.camussi@unito.it; Tel.: +39-011-670-9588

† These authors contributed equally to this work.

Received: 1 April 2019; Accepted: 10 May 2019; Published: 14 May 2019

Abstract: Extracellular vesicles (EVs) derived from mesenchymal stromal cells (MSCs) possess pro-regenerative potential in different animal models with renal injury. EVs contain different molecules, including proteins, lipids and nucleic acids. Among the shuttled molecules, miRNAs have a relevant role in the pro-regenerative effects of EVs and are a promising target for therapeutic interventions. The aim of this study was to increase the content of specific miRNAs in EVs that are known to be involved in the pro-regenerative effect of EVs, and to assess the capacity of modified EVs to contribute to renal regeneration in in vivo models with acute kidney injuries. To this purpose, MSCs were transiently transfected with specific miRNA mimics by electroporation. Molecular analyses showed that, after transfection, MSCs and derived EVs were efficiently enriched in the selected miRNAs. In vitro and in vivo experiments indicated that EVs engineered with miRNAs maintained their pro-regenerative effects. Of relevance, engineered EVs were more effective than EVs derived from naïve MSCs when used at suboptimal doses. This suggests the potential use of a low amount of EVs (82.5×10^6) to obtain the renal regenerative effect.

Keywords: mesenchymal stromal cells; extracellular vesicles; acute kidney injury; modified-MSCs; microRNA

---

1. Introduction

Mesenchymal stromal cells (MSCs) are one of the most studied adult stem cells and have been extensively applied in the field of regenerative medicine. In the last years, many studies have demonstrated that their therapeutic effects are mainly mediated by the secretion of bioactive molecules (such as RNAs, proteins, and lipids) that can be directly released in the local microenvironment or packaged in extracellular vesicles (EVs) [1]. Paracrine factors released by MSCs, including EVs, induce the recovery of injured tissue and modulate the immune response and inflammation [2,3]. Many reports have demonstrated the application of MSCs and of their derived EVs in the recovery of renal dysfunction [4]. Different preclinical models of acute and chronic kidney injuries have been used to demonstrate the efficacy of EVs from MSCs in the amelioration of acute kidney injury (AKI) and in preventing progression at the chronic stage [5]. Recently, we tested different subpopulations of MSC-derived EVs in renal regeneration. Most of the effects observed in the recovery from AKI were ascribed to the exosomal fraction, which carried mRNA, miRNAs and proteins that induced the proliferation of tubular cells. Despite the inefficiency of the non-exosomal fraction, we observed that the effect of the exosomal fraction and the total-EVs was not significantly different in terms of pro-regenerative potential, suggesting that the ineffective fraction did not interfere with the exosomal fraction activity [6]. Moreover, MSCs may be manipulated in culture by transferring specific miRNA to EV-producing cells to obtain modified-EVs with potentiated pro-regenerative or reparative effects [7–11]. In this work, we set up a method to increase—in MSCs and in their total-EVs—the content of specific miRNAs involved in renal regeneration. To assess the capacities of modified-EVs to contribute to AKI recovery, we tested them in vitro on murine renal tubular epithelial cells and in vivo in a model of AKI induced by glycerol injection.

2. Results

2.1. Identification of Pro-Regenerative miRNAs Carried by EVs

In our previous study, we performed RNA sequencing (RNA-Seq) analysis to detect the molecular changes that occurred in the kidneys of AKI mice treated with MSC-derived EVs (EV-CTRL) vs. untreated AKI mice (AKI) (Gene Expression Omnibus accession number GSE59958) [12]. In this study, the potential healing miRNAs were selected from among known human miRNAs that were predicted to significantly down-regulate RNAs modulated in our treatments with a bio-informatic approach, as described in the Methods section. The obtained miRNA families (Table 1) were posteriorly cross-matched with a list of 50 miRNAs with increased expression in the MSC-derived EVs [6]. The following miRNAs were identified: miR-10a-5p, miR-127-3p, miR-29a-3p, let-7a and miR-30a-5p. miR-486-5p was also selected because it was the most enriched miRNA in the exosomal fraction, which was the more effective fraction in promoting AKI recovery [6].

Table 1. List of miRNA families for which targets were significantly modulated by extracellular vesicle (EV) administration in acute kidney injury (AKI) mice.

	FC Non-Targets	FC Targets	p	Rank
miR-10abc/10a-5p	0.03	0.06	0.0313	1
let-7/98/4458/4500	0.03	0.06	0.0476	2
miR-127/127-3p	0.03	0.25	0.0431	12
miR-30abcdef/30abe-5p/384-5p	0.03	0.07	0.0003	13
miR-29abcd	0.03	0.07	0.0047	24
miR-192/215	0.03	0.14	0.0035	50
miR-140/140-5p/876-3p/1244	0.03	0.10	0.0177	72
miR-377	0.03	0.08	0.0203	96
miR-202-3p	0.03	0.08	0.0060	124

miRNAs with targets that showed significant down-regulation in EV treated-vs. untreated-AKI mice were listed and correlated with their enrichment in EVs isolated at 100,000 g (p value < 0.05). Non-targets: Median fold change (FC, logarithmic treated vs. untreated) of the genes that are not miRNA targets. Targets: Median FC of the genes that are miRNA targets. p: p-value generated by Mann–Whitney test, comparing the FC of targets vs. non-target miRNAs. Rank: List of the expressed miRNAs based on their abundance inside EVs.

To evaluate the potential of selected miRNAs to promote tubular cell proliferation, murine tubular epithelial cells (mTECs) were treated with miRNA mimics and submitted to hypoxia/reoxygenation conditions. mTECs treated with miR-10a-5p (miR10a), miR-127-3p (miR127), miR-29a-3p (miR29a) and miR-486-5p (miR486) were able to proliferate to some degree in the hypoxia/reoxygenation culture, even if the obtained results did not reach statistical significance, unlike let-7b- and miR-30a-5p-

(miR30a-)treated tubular cells (Figure 1), which only supported the beneficial effects of selected EV-miRNAs in AKI.

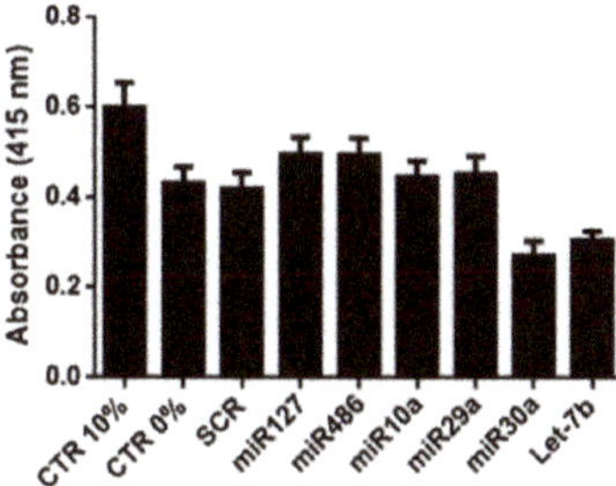

Figure 1. In vitro effect of selected miRNA mimics. Different miRNA mimics (miR127, miR486, miR10a, miR29a, miR30a and let-7b-100 nM) were added to murine tubular epithelial cells (mTECs) maintained in hypoxia for 48 h, after which proliferation was evaluated following 24 h of re-oxygenation. mTECs were maintained in medium supplemented with 10% fetal calf serum (FCS) or 0% FCS, used respectively as the positive (CTR 10%) and negative (CTR 0%) controls. Data are reported as mean ± SEM for three different experiments performed in quadruplicate.

2.2. Generation of MSCs and Derived EVs Engineered with miRNAs

MSCs were subjected to electroporation (MSC-EP) in order to enrich their content of the selected miRNAs. Different electroporation protocols were tested (EP1-3, Table 2, Materials and Methods section) and transfection efficiency was evaluated by qRT-PCR. The EP1 protocol (990 V, 40 msec, 1 pulse) was selected because of the enhanced expression of the control miRNA mimic observed in the MSCs and the maintained cell viability (Figure 2A). We also set up the optimal dose of miRNA mimic to transfect MSCs. As seen in Figure 2B, 25 pmol/4 × 10^4 cells was the lowest dose tested that increased the expression of the control miRNA. Expression of the selected miRNAs was then assessed using the transfection condition identified during setting. We detected an increased expression of the selected miRNAs in MSC-EP after 24 h (Figure 2C) that remained stable until day 7. Of notice, we observed a higher expression for miR-127 and miR-486 with respect to the other two miRNAs, suggesting a different efficiency of transfection.

EVs from MSC-EP (EV-EP), enriched with different miRNA mimics (Figure 3), were isolated 24 h after transfection and subsequently characterized for size distribution and particle number by NanoSight. EVs derived from MSC-EP showed similar size profiles to naïve MSC EVs. No differences were observed among EV-EP that were simply electroporated or transfected with scramble (SCR) mimic (EV-SCR) or with different miRNAs mimics (EV-miR127, EV-miR486, EV-miR10a, EV-miR29a) (Figure 4A). Moreover, evaluation of particle number did not show any variation between the different mimic-enriched EV-EP.

Additionally, typical MSC marker expression on EV-EP was maintained, suggesting that electroporation did not affect surface molecule expression. As described in Reference [6], EVs derived from naïve MSCs or MSC-EP in the presence of different miRNA mimics expressed the typical exosomal marker (CD63) and MSC markers (CD73, CD44 and CD29) (Figure 4B). Electron microscopy confirmed that EV-EP maintained the same morphology as EV-CTRL (Figure 4C).

miRNA enrichment was then evaluated by real-time PCR for the different EV-EP. The expression of miR-127, miR-10a, miR-29a and miR-486 was increased in MSC-EP-derived EVs with respect to MSC-EVs derived from cells that were only electroporated or from SCR-transfected MSC-EP (Figure 2D). As seen in the MSC-EP and their respective EVs, the efficiency of enrichment was slightly different according to the mimic used. For instance, miR-29a was less enriched in EVs with respect to the other mimics. Instead, we observed a higher increase in the expression for miR-127 and miR-486.

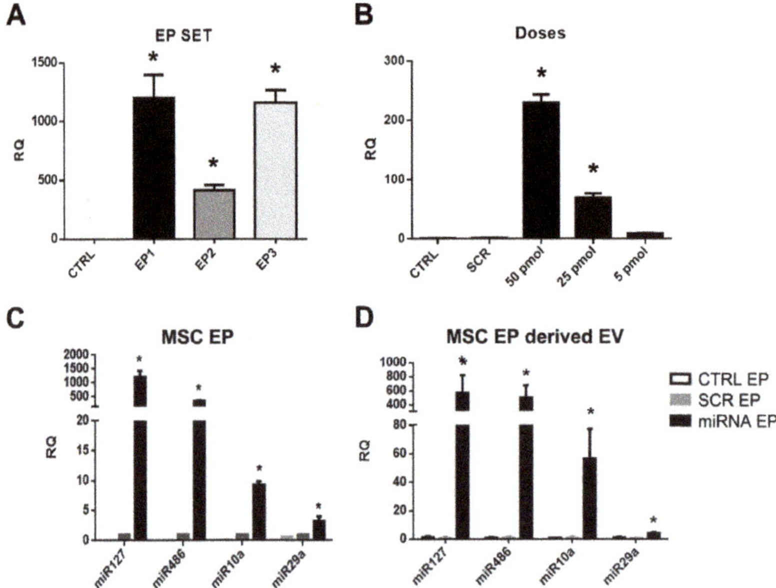

Figure 2. miRNA enrichment evaluation in mesenchymal stromal cells subjected to electroporation (MSC-EP) and derived EVs. (**A**) Representative real-time PCR showing the efficiency of transfection for different electroporation protocols (EP1-3). ANOVA with Dunnett's multiple comparison test was performed. * $p < 0.05$ EP protocol vs. CTRL (non elecroporated cells); (**B**) representative real-time PCR showing the efficiency of transfection for different doses of control miRNA mimic obtained with EP1 electroporation conditions. ANOVA with Dunnett's multiple comparison test was performed. $p < 0.05$ different control miRNA doses vs. scramble (SCR); (**C**) representative real-time PCR showing the increased expression of the selected miRNAs (miR10a, miR29a, miR127, miR486) 24 h after transfection in MSC-EP and (**D**) in derived EVs collected 24 h after transfection. Data were normalized in respect to MSC transfected with the SCR. Data are represented as relative quantification (RQ) $\pm$ SEM. * $p < 0.05$ MSC-EP SCR vs. MSC-EP transfected with mimics and * $p < 0.05$ EV-SCR vs. EV transfected with mimics. Multiple *t* test with Holm–Sidak method correction was performed.

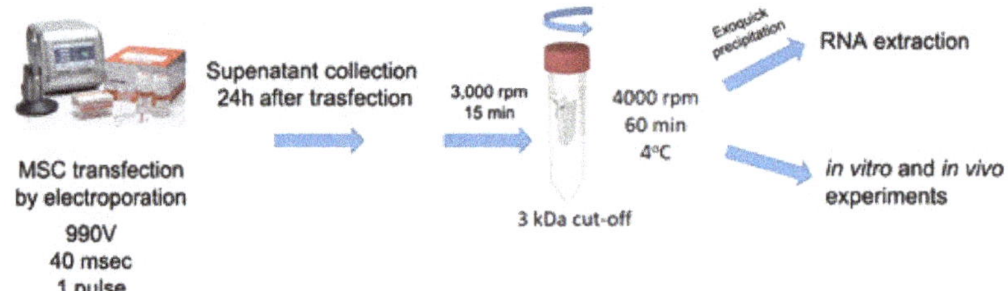

Figure 3. Schematic illustration of the engineering method used to transiently transfect MSCs. MSCs were transfected via a neon electroporation system with different miRNA mimics. EVs were collected after 24 h and supernatant, previously centrifuged at 2000 *g* to eliminate cell debris, was concentrated by 3 kDa filter tube. EVs were then used for in vitro and in vivo experiments or precipitated by Exoquick and used for RNA extraction.

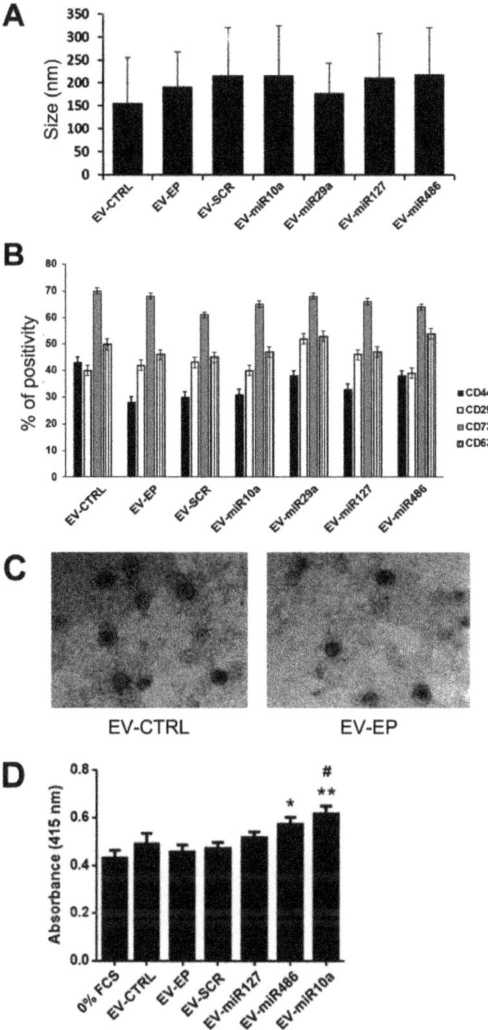

Figure 4. Characterization of EVs derived from naïve MSCs and from EP MSCs. (**A**) Size of EVs obtained from naïve MSC (EV-CTRL), from electroporated MSC (EV-EP) and transfected with scramble (EV-SCR) or with different miRNA mimics (EV-mir10a, EV-miR29a, EV-miR127, EV-miR486), evaluated by nanoparticle tracking analysis (NTA). Data reported are mean ± SD for three different experiments. No statistically significant differences were observed among the different types of EVs; (**B**) cytofluorimetric analysis of the expression of MSC (CD44, CD29 and CD73) and exosomal (CD63) markers, in different EV populations. Data reported are the mean ± SD for three different experiments. No statistically significant differences were observed in marker expression among the different types of EVs; (**C**) representative micrographs of transmission electron microscopy of EV-CTRL (left) and EV-EP (right). EVs negatively stained with NanoVan (magnification ×100,000); and (**D**) different types of EVs (1000/cells) were added to mTECs maintained for 48 h in hypoxia, after which proliferation was evaluated following 24 h of reoxygenation. Data are reported as mean ± SEM for three different experiments in quadruplicate. ANOVA with Dunnett's multiple comparison test was performed. ** $p < 0.01$ and * $p < 0.05$ mTEC stimulated with EV-mimic vs. mTEC maintained in 0% FCS, # $p < 0.05$ EV-miR10a vs. mTEC stimulated with EV-EP.

2.3. In Vitro and In Vivo Effects of EVs

EVs obtained from naïve MSCs and from MSC-EP transfected with SCR or with 10a, 127 and 486 miRNA mimics were tested in vitro on mTECs cultured in hypoxia. EV-miR29a was not further tested since the miR-29a in EVs after transfection was less enriched in comparison with the other miRNAs considered. EVs from MSC-EP transfected with 10a and 486 miRNA mimics induced significant proliferation of mTECs with respect to the negative controls (mTECs maintained with 0% fetal calf serum [FCS]). Only EVs enriched with miR10a induced a significant increase in proliferation with respect to EVs obtained by MSC-EP (Figure 4D).

MSC electroporation did not interfere with the renal pro-regenerative capacity of EVs; EV-EP significantly improved renal function and morphology similarly to naïve MSC-EVs (Figure 5).

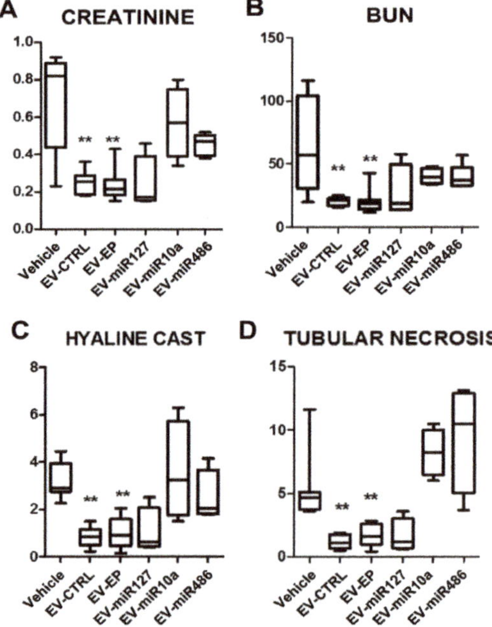

Figure 5. Effect of EVs derived from naïve or electroporated MSC in AKI mice: Functional and morphological evaluation. (**A**) Creatinine and (**B**) blood urea nitrogen (BUN) values in AKI mice injected with vehicle alone (Vehicle) or with 165×10^6 EVs derived from naïve MSCs (EV-CTRL) or from electroporated MSCs (EV-EP) transfected with different miRNA mimics (EV-miR127, EV-miR10a, EV-miR486). EVs were injected at day 3 and mice were sacrificed at day 5 after glycerol administration. Results are expressed as mean ± SD; ANOVA with Dunnett's multiple comparison test was performed. ** $p < 0.01$ EV-CTRL and EV-EP vs. Vehicle. Morphometric evaluaïon of (**C**) hyaline casts and (**D**) tubular necrosis in AKI mice treated with vehicle alone (Vehicle) or injected with 165×10^6 EVs derived from naïve MSCs (EV-CTRL) or from electroporated MSCs (EV-EP) transfected with different miRNA mimics (EV-miR127, EV-miR10a, EV-miR486). Results are expressed as mean ± SD; ANOVA with Dunnett's multiple comparison test was performed. ** $p < 0.01$ EV-CTRL and EV-EP vs. Vehicle.

Treatment of AKI mice with a dose of miRNA-enriched EVs comparable to the effective dose of EV-CTRL (165×10^6 EV/mouse) did not show any significant improvement. In fact, in some experimental conditions (EV-miR10a and EV-miR486), a worsening was even observed, suggesting that changing the composition of miRNAs content in MSC-EVs altered their pro-regenerative properties

(Figure 5). The administration of EV-miR127 did not show a worsening of kidney function and morphology, nor an amelioration of kidney function (Figure 5).

To better understand whether miRNA-enriched EVs could improve the biological activities of EVs, we treated AKI mice with an ineffective dose of unmodified EVs. A half-dose of these EVs (82.5×10^6 EV/mouse) did not induce significant functional or morphological improvements (Figure 6). In contrast, half-doses of EVs obtained from MSC-EP transfected with miRNA mimic-486 or -10a induced a significant amelioration of renal function and morphology (Figure 6). These findings suggest that the regenerative effect of MSC-derived EVs is related to a balanced composition of miRNAs and, therefore, modification in miRNA content may increase the effectiveness of EVs at lower doses, but not improve the effective dose of naïve EVs.

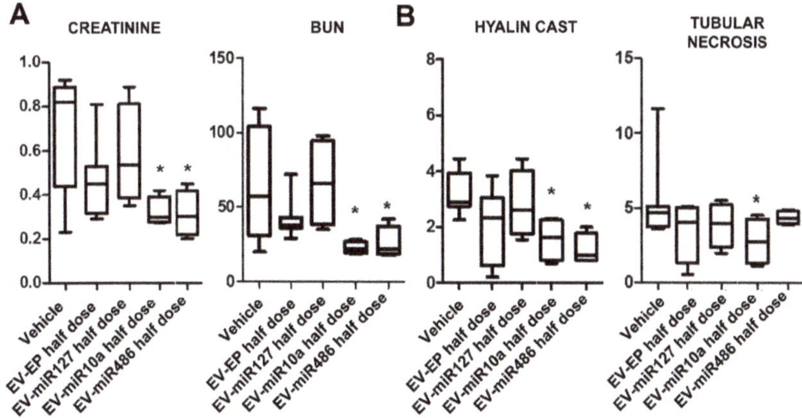

Figure 6. Effect of EVs derived from naïve or miRNA-enriched MSC in AKI mice: Functional and morphological evaluation. (**A**) Creatinine and BUN values in AKI mice injected with vehicle alone (Vehicle) or with 82.5×10^6 EVs derived from electroporated MSCs (EV-EP) and transfected with different miRNA mimics (EV-miR127, EV-miR10a, EV-miR486). EVs were injected at day 3 and mice were sacrificed at day 5 after glycerol administration. Results are expressed as mean ± SD; ANOVA with Dunnett's multiple comparison test was performed. * $p < 0.05$ EV-miR10a half-dose and EV-miR486 half-dose vs. Vehicle. (**B**) Morphometric evaluation of hyaline casts and tubular necrosis in AKI mice treated with vehicle alone (Vehicle) or with 82.5×10^6 EVs derived from electroporated MSCs (EV-EP) and transfected with different miRNA mimics (EV-miR127, EV-miR10a, EV-miR486). Results are expressed as mean ± SD; ANOVA with Dunnett's multiple comparison test was performed. * $p < 0.05$ EV-miR10a half-dose and EV-miR486 half-dose vs. Vehicle for hyaline cast; * $p < 0.05$ EV-miR10a half-dose vs. Vehicle, for tubular necrosis.

3. Discussion

Recent studies have shown that paracrine mechanisms, including EVs, are responsible for stem/progenitor cell-mediated renal regenerative effect [5]. EVs derived from MSCs shuttle different molecules (proteins, lipids, and nucleic acids) that may contribute to their pro-regenerative potential. Among the different shuttled molecules, miRNAs have been reported to be one of the factors involved in the pro-regenerative effects of MSC-EVs. Indeed, miRNA deregulation by Drosha-knockdown in MSCs has been reported to inhibit the regenerative potential of MSCs and of their derived EVs in a murine model of AKI [12]. This suggests a critical role of miRNA content in MSCs and MSC-EVs in the recovery following an AKI.

The idea of using EVs as carriers for selected miRNA cargo became very attractive in the last decades. EVs overcome many problems related to stability and preservation of their cargo from degradation in circulation. Different approaches were developed in order to modify EV content to enhance their homing capacity (proteins) or their effect (miRNAs, mRNAs and drugs) [13]. Direct manipulation of EVs implies the temporary disruption of EV membranes by different techniques, such as electroporation, sonication or chemical transfection [14]. Another technique used to enhance miRNA content in EVs is engineering of the parental cells. Some recent works demonstrated that is possible to load miRNA mimic or antimiR into MSCs by transfection, as well as to increase the pro-regenerative properties of EVs in different tissue injuries [7–11,15] or to potentiate their anti-tumor effect [16,17].

In this study, we set up a method to increase the content of specific miRNAs involved in renal regeneration in MSCs and their respective EVs. Potentially regenerative miRNAs were selected using a bio-informatic approach based on predicted interactions between the miRNAs present inside the MSC-EVs with genes modulated during AKI treatment with MSC-EVs. Moreover, this list was implemented with miR-486-5p, which was highly expressed in the exosomal fraction of MSC-EVs [6]. Of relevance, miR-486-5p and some of the miRNAs selected by bio-informatic analyses (miR-10a-5p, miR-29a-3p) were found to be down-regulated in EVs obtained by Drosha knock-down MSCs, which were ineffective in glycerol induced AKI [12].

In this work, we demonstrated that the miRNA mimics transfected in MSCs were also up-regulated in their EVs. Among the different miRNA mimics transfected, miR-127 and miR-486 were more enriched than miR-29a in cells and, consequently, in their EVs, suggesting differences in efficiency of transfection for different miRNAs.

The EVs obtained from transfected cells with miR-10a, -127 and -486 were tested in vivo. Treatment with a dose of miRNA-enriched EVs known to be effective in the AKI model [6] did not provide any significant improvement, while a worsening was observed for miR-10a- and miR-486-enriched EVs. These data suggest that changing the miRNA composition of MSC-EVs can alter their renal regenerative capacities. When we used an ineffective dose of naïve-EVs as the control, and a similar dose miR-10a- and miR-486-enriched EVs, a significant improvement of renal function and morphology was invariably observed. These findings indicate that in order to detect biological activity of miRNA-enriched EVs, low doses of EV should be studied. Moreover, these data highlight the important role of miR-10a and of miR-486 in the pro-regenerative effect exerted by MSC-EVs in AKI. Interestingly, miR-486 is also in exosomes derived from human endothelial progenitor cells, which have been shown to possess renal regenerative capacity in ischemia-reperfusion injury models [18].

In conclusion, our study has demonstrated that it is possible to modify the miRNA content of MSCs and their EVs. Changing the amount of pro-regenerative miRNAs in EVs was found to modify the window of biological activity of these EVs. Therefore, this may be a strategy to reduce the amount of EVs used in therapy. We previously showed that EVs derived from MSCs accumulated specifically in the kidneys of mice with AKI compared to healthy controls [19]. Since in the present study the bio-distribution of miRNA-enriched EVs was not evaluated, we cannot rule out the possibility that miRNA-enriched EVs have a different bio-distribution.

4. Materials and Methods

4.1. Cell Cultures and EV-CTRL Isolation

Bone marrow MSCs were purchased from Lonza (Basel, Switzerland) and cultured in a mesenchymal stem cells basal medium bullet kit (Lonza). MSCs were used for the different experiments until passage 6 and expressed the typical MSC markers (CD105, CD29, CD73, CD44 and CD90).

MSC-EVs, used as control (EV-CTRL), were obtained by ultracentrifugation, as described in Reference [6]. Briefly, EVs were obtained from supernatants of MSCs cultured overnight in (Roswell Park Memorial Institute (RPMI) medium. After removal of cell debris and apoptotic bodies by centrifugation at 3000× g for 20 min, EVs were purified by 2 h ultracentrifugation at 100,000× g at 4 °C. EVs from control MSCs or from modified MSCs were used freshly or stored at −80 °C after resuspension in RPMI supplemented with 1% dimethyl sulfoxide (DMSO, Sigma, St. Louis, MO, USA).

Murine renal tubular epithelial cells (mTECs) were obtained as previously described [20] and cultured in Dulbecco's Modified Eagle Medium (DMEM) low glucose (Euroclone, Pero, Italy) supplemented with 10% fetal calf serum (FCS, Euroclone), penicillin (50 IU/mL), and streptomycin (50 µg/mL) (Sigma). Murine TECs were characterized for positive staining to cytokeratin, alkaline phosphatase and aminopeptidase A, and for negative staining for endothelial (von Willebrand factor), hematopoietic (CD45) and glomerular (nephrin) markers.

4.2. MSC Transfection and Collection of Engineered MSC-EVs

To obtain miRNA-enriched MSCs, cells were transiently transfected by electroporation (MSC-EP) (neon transfection system) using a 100 µl tip (Thermo Fisher Scientific, Waltham, MA, USA), according to the manufacturer's protocol. Different electroporation conditions with a control miRNA mimic (100 nM) were tested in order to find the optimal protocol (Table 2 and Figure 2A). The electroporation conditions were set to 990 V, 40 msec and 1 pulse (EP1 protocol).

Table 2. Electroporation protocols tested to transfect MSCs.

	EP1	EP2	EP3
Voltage	990	1100	990
msec	40	30	30
Pulse	1	1	2

Three different doses (5, 25 and 50 nmol $/4 \times 10^4$ cells) of a control miRNA mimic were evaluated to find the optimal dose to transfect MSCs (Figure 2B). The dose 25 nmol/4×10^4 cells was selected for subsequent experiments. The transfection efficiency was evaluated by qRT-PCR with the miScript PCR system (Qiagen, Venlo, The Netherlands), following the manufacturer's protocol.

These electroporation conditions did not affect cell viability.

Selected miRNA mimics (hsa-miR-10a-5p, hsa-miR-29a-3p, hsa-miR-127-3p, hsa-miR-486-5p) (Qiagen) were used to enrich MSCs (600 pmol/10^6 cells). As a control, MSCs were transfected with AllStars Negative Control siRNA (SCR-Qiagen) and used for normalization of transfection with different mimics. For modified MSCs, EV collection was carried out starting from a four sub-confluent flask (T75, Euroclone S.p.A) 24 h after the electroporation, starving MSCs over-night in RPMI (Euroclone). The collected medium was centrifuged at 2000 *g* for 20 min to eliminate cell debris. Supernatant was then micro-filtrated and concentrated by an Amicon® Ultra 15 mL 3 kDa cut off filter (Merck-Millipore, Darnstadt, Germany) at 4000 rpm 60 min at 4 °C. EV samples were stored at −80 °C, with addition of 1% DMSO (Sigma).

4.3. EV Characterization

Analysis of size distribution and enumeration of EVs from naïve MSCs and from MSC-EP (enriched or not with specific miRNA mimics) were performed using NanoSight NS300 (NanoSight Ltd., Amesbury, UK) equipped with a 405 nm laser and nanoparticle tracking analysis (NTA) 3.2 software, as described in Reference [6]. Using a laser light source, particles in the sample are illuminated and the scattered light is captured by the camera and displayed on a connected computer running NTA. Using NTA, the particles are automatically tracked and sized based on Brownian motion and the diffusion coefficient. Three videos of 30 s were recorded to perform the analyses.

EV-surface expression markers were analyzed by Guava easyCyte™ Flow Cytometer (Millipore), as previously described [21]. FITC-, PE- or APC-conjugated antibodies against CD44, CD29, CD73 and CD63 (all from Miltenyi Biotec GmbH, Bergisch Gladbach, Germany) were employed. Isotopic IgG was used as the negative control. Briefly, EVs were incubated at 4 °C for 15 min with the antibodies, then diluted 1:3 and acquired immediately. Samples were acquired using a Guava easyCyte Flow Cytometer (Millipore) and analyzed with InCyte software.

Transmission electron microscopy was performed on CTRL-EVs and EV-EP placed on 200 mesh nickel formvar carbon-coated grids (Electron Microscopy Science, Hatfield, PA, USA) and left to adhere for 20 min, as described in Reference [22]. The grids were then incubated with 2.5% glutaraldehyde containing 2% sucrose and, after washings in distilled water, the EVs were negatively stained with NanoVan (Nanoprobes, Yaphank, NK, USA) and observed using a Jeol JEM 1010 electron microscope (Jeol, Tokyo, Japan).

4.4. RNA Analysis

RNA from MSC-EP was extracted by TRIzol™ (Ambion, Thermo Fisher Scientific, Waltham, MA, USA) according to the manufacturer's protocol.

Only for RNA analysis, Exoquick (System Biosciences, LLC, Palo Alto, CA, USA) was used to precipitate EVs obtained from MSC-EP (EV-EP), MSC transfected with scrambled siRNA (EV-SCR) or with the selected mimics (EV-miR127, EV-miR10a, EV-miR486, EV-miR29a). RNA was extracted with RNA/DNA/Protein Purification Plus Kit (Norgen Biotek Corp, Thorold, ON, Canada), following the manufacturer's protocol.

RNA concentration was spectroscopically determined by NanoDrop2000 (Thermo Fisher Scientific). cDNA was synthetized and RT-PCR was performed by using miRCURY™ LNA™ Universal RT microRNA PCR (Exiqon-Qiagen, Vedbaek, Denmark). Specific primers set for hsa-miR-127-3p, hsa-miR-10a-5p, hsa-miR-29a-3p, hsa-miR-486-5 were used. U6 spike-in was used for housekeeping (Exiqon-Qiagen). Data were normalized with respect to MSC transfected with the SCR and were represented as relative quantification (RQ) ± SEM.

4.5. Integrating miRNA Expression in MSC EVs and RNA Analysis in AKI Animals

To identify potentially relevant miRNAs carried by MSC EVs and involved in the positive readout associated with EVs treatment, we proceeded as follows: For each miRNA family listed in TargetScan we generated a list of predicted targets. We then compared the fold-change in expression of these targets with the fold-change in expression of all the genes that were predicted targets of miRNAs but not of the miRNA families under analysis. The miRNA families selected were those for which the targets showed significant down-regulation in the kidneys of AKI mice treated with MSC-derived EVs vs. untreated AKI mice (AKI), as detected in Reference [12]. The obtained miRNA families were then matched with the list of miRNAs detected inside the total extracellular vesicle population (100K TOT) in Reference [6].

4.6. mTEC Proliferation Assay

mTEC were seeded in 96-well plates at a density of 1000 cells/well and maintained in a hypoxia chamber (Stem Cell Technology, Vancouver)) for 48 h with 1% O_2 in DMEM + 10% FCS (positive control), DMEM + 0% FCS (negative control). During the reoxygenation step, mTEC were treated for 24 h with mimics of selected miRNAs (100 nM) or 500 EV/mTEC. Cell proliferation was assessed by a 5-bromo-2′-deoxy-uridine (BrdU) incorporation assay (Roche Applied Science, Mannheim, Germany).

4.7. SCID Mouse Model of AKI

Animal studies were conducted in accordance with the National Institutes of Health Guide for the Care and Use of Laboratory Animals. All procedures were approved by the Italian Health Ministry (authorization number: 211/2016-PR).

AKI was induced by an intramuscular injection (IM) of glycerol (Sigma) in SCID mice, as described previously [6,20]. Male SCID mice were anesthetized with an IM injection of zolazepam (80 mg/kg) and xilazina (16 mg/kg) and then injected with 8 mL/kg of 50% glycerol in water. Half the dose was injected into each muscle of the inferior hind limbs. Three days after the glycerol injection, the mice were treated intravenously with either 120 µL of the vehicle alone ($n = 7$) or containing 165×10^6 or 82.5×10^6 particles of EVs derived from control MSCs (EV-CTRL, $n = 8$), from MSC-EP

(EV-EP, *n* = 8/doses), or from EP-MSC enriched with specific miRNA mimics (EV-miR127, EV-miR486, EV-miR10a, *n* = 6/group/doses). The mice were sacrificed 5 days after the glycerol injection (2 days after EV treatment).

Blood samples were collected 5 days after glycerol-induced AKI for the measurement of blood urea nitrogen (BUN) and creatinine. BUN was measured by direct quantification of serum urea with a colorimetric assay kit according to the manufacturer's protocol (Arbor Assays, Ann Arbor, MI, USA). Serum creatinine was measured using a colorimetric microplate assay based on the kinetic Jaffe reaction as per the manufacturer's protocol (Quantichrom Creatinine Assay; BioAssay Systems, Hayward, CA, USA).

Renal morphology was evaluated through formalin-fixed paraffin-embedded tissue staining, as previously described [6,20]. Briefly, 5-μm-thick paraffin kidney sections were routinely stained with hematoxylin and eosin (Merck-Millipore) for microscopic evaluation. Luminal hyaline casts and cell necrosis (denudation of the tubular basement membrane) were assessed in non-overlapping fields (10 for each section) using a 40× objective (high-power field [HPF]). The number of casts and tubular profiles showing necrosis were recorded in a single-blind manner.

4.8. Statistical Analyses

Data were analyzed using the GraphPad Prism 6.0 program. Statistical analysis was performed by employing Student's *t*-tests, analysis of variance (ANOVA) with Dunnett's multi-comparison tests or Multiple t test with Helm–Sidak method correction as deemed appropriate. A *p*-value of <0.05 was considered significant. For the bioinformatic analyses, *p* values were generated by Mann–Whitney statistical test comparing the median fold change of genes down-regulated in EV treated animals (Log EV treated vs. AKI untreated) that were target of miRNAs with the non-target genes. Nine miRNA families (Table 1) achieved nominal significance ($p < 0.05$).

Author Contributions: S.B. and G.T. performed in vivo studies and tissues analysis; M.T. performed transfection experiments and in vitro assay; F.C. performed in vitro experiments; P.P. performed bioinformatics analyses; S.W. and P.J.Q. data interpretation and revised the manuscript; M.C.D. performed electron microscopy analyses of the vesicle preparations; S.B., M.T., F.C. and G.C. performed study design, data interpretation and manuscript writing. All authors approved the submitted version of the manuscript. M.T. and S.B. equally contributed to this work.

Funding: This work was supported by the NIH grants UH2-TR000880, UH3TR000880-03S1. The content is solely the responsibility of the authors and does not necessarily represent the official views of the National Institutes of Health.

Acknowledgments: The technical assistance of Federica Antico and Massimo Cedrino are gratefully acknowledged.

Conflicts of Interest: G.C. is component of the Scientific Advisory Board of Unicyte. Other authors declare no conflict of interest.

References

1.	Heldring, N.; Mager, I.; Wood, M.J.A.; Le Blanc, K.; Andaloussi, S.E. Therapeutic potential of multipotent mesenchymal stromal cells and their extracellular vesicles. *Hum. Gene Ther.* **2015**, *26*, 506–517. [CrossRef]

2.	Lamichhane, T.N.; Sokic, S.; Schardt, J.S.; Raiker, R.S.; Lin, J.W.; Jay, S.M. Emerging roles for extracellular vesicles in tissue engineering and regenerative medicine. *Tissue Eng. Part B Rev.* **2015**, *21*, 45–54. [CrossRef]

3.	Robbins, P.D.; Morelli, A.E. Regulation of immune responses by extracellular vesicles. *Nat. Rev. Immunol.* **2014**, *14*, 195–208. [CrossRef]

4.	Wang, Y.; He, J.; Pei, X.; Zhao, W. Systematic review and meta-analysis of mesenchymal stem/stromal cells therapy for impaired renal function in small animal models. *Nephrology* **2013**, *8*, 201–218. [CrossRef] [PubMed]

5.	Grange, C.; Iampietro, C.; Bussolati, B. Stem cell extracellular vesicles and kidney injury. *Stem Cell Investig.* **2017**, *4*, 90. [CrossRef]

6.	Bruno, S.; Tapparo, M.; Collino, F.; Chiabotto, G.; Deregibus, M.C.; Soares Lindoso, R.; Neri, F.; Kholia, S.; Giunti, S.; Wen, S.; et al. Renal Regenerative Potential of Different Extracellular Vesicle Populations Derived from Bone Marrow Mesenchymal Stromal Cells. *Tissue Eng. Part A* **2017**, *23*, 1262–1273. [CrossRef]

7. Tao, S.C.; Yuan, T.; Zhang, Y.L.; Yin, W.J.; Guo, S.C.; Zhang, C.Q. Exosomes derived from miR-140-5p-overexpressing human synovial mesenchymal stem cells enhance cartilage tissue regeneration and prevent osteoarthritis of the knee in a rat model. *Theranostics* **2017**, *7*, 180–195.

8. Lou, G.; Yang, Y.; Liu, F.; Ye, B.; Chen, Z.; Zheng, M.; Liu, Y. MiR-122 modification enhances the therapeutic efficacy of adipose tissue-derived mesenchymal stem cells against liver fibrosis. *J. Cell Mol. Med.* **2017**, *21*, 2963–2973. [CrossRef] [PubMed]

9. Song, J.L.; Zheng, W.; Chen, W.; Qian, Y.; Ouyang, Y.M.; Fan, C.Y. Lentivirus-mediated microRNA-124 gene-modified bone marrow mesenchymal stem cell transplantation promotes the repair of spinal cord injury in rats. *Exp. Mol. Med.* **2017**, *49*, e332. [CrossRef] [PubMed]

10. Li, D.; Zhang, P.; Yao, X.; Li, H.; Shen, H.; Li, X.; Wu, J.; Lu, X. Exosomes Derived From miR-133b-Modified Mesenchymal Stem Cells Promote Recovery After Spinal Cord Injury. *Front. Neurosci.* **2018**, *22*, 845. [CrossRef] [PubMed]

11. Shen, H.; Yao, X.; Li, H.; Li, X.; Zhang, T.; Sun, Q.; Ji, C.; Chen, G. Role of Exosomes Derived from miR-133b Modified MSCs in an Experimental Rat Model of Intracerebral Hemorrhage. *J. Mol. Neurosci.* **2018**, *64*, 421–430. [CrossRef]

12. Collino, F.; Bruno, S.; Incarnato, D.; Dettori, D.; Neri, F.; Provero, P.; Pomatto, M.; Oliviero, S.; Tetta, C.; Quesenberry, P.J.; et al. AKI Recovery Induced by Mesenchymal Stromal Cell-Derived Extracellular Vesicles Carrying MicroRNAs. *J. Am. Soc. Nephrol.* **2015**, *26*, 2349–2360. [CrossRef]

13. Mentkowski, K.I.; Snitzer, J.D.; Rusnak, S.; Lang, J.K. Therapeutic Potential of Engineered Extracellular Vesicles. *AAPS J.* **2018**, *20*, 50. [CrossRef]

14. Janas, T.; Janas, M.M.; Sapoñ, K.; Janas, T. Mechanisms of RNA loading into exosomes. *FEBS Lett.* **2015**, *589*, 1391–1398. [CrossRef] [PubMed]

15. Wang, B.; Yao, K.; Huuskes, B.M.; Shen, H.H.; Zhuang, J.; Godson, C.; Brennan, E.P.; Wilkinson-Berka, J.L.; Wise, A.F.; Ricardo, S.D. Mesenchymal Stem Cells Deliver Exogenous MicroRNA-let7c via Exosomes to Attenuate Renal Fibrosis. *Mol. Ther.* **2016**, *24*, 1290–1301. [CrossRef]

16. Sutaria, D.S.; Badawi, M.; Phelps, M.A.; Schmittgen, T.D. Achieving the promise of therapeutic extracellular vesicles: The devil is in details of therapeutic loading. *Pharm. Res.* **2017**, *34*, 1053–1066. [CrossRef] [PubMed]

17. Lou, G.; Song, X.; Yang, F.; Wu, S.; Wang, J.; Chen, Z.; Liu, Y. Exosomes derived from miR-122-modified adipose tissue derived MSCs increase chemosensitivity of hepatocellular carcinoma. *J. Hematol. Oncol.* **2015**, *8*, 122. [CrossRef] [PubMed]

18. Viñas, J.L.; Burger, D.; Zimpelmann, J.; Haneef, R.; Knoll, W.; Campbell, P.; Gutsol, A.; Carter, A.; Allan, D.S.; Burns, K.D. Transfer of microRNA-486-5p from human endothelial colony forming cell-derived exosomes reduces ischemic kidney injury. *Kidney Int.* **2016**, *90*, 1238–1250. [CrossRef] [PubMed]

19. Bruno, S.; Grange, C.; Deregibus, M.C.; Calogero, R.A.; Saviozzi, S.; Collino, F.; Morando, L.; Busca, A.; Falda, M.; Bussolati, B.; et al. Mesenchymal stem cell-derived microvesicles protect against acute tubular injury. *J. Am. Soc. Nephrol.* **2009**, *20*, 1053–1067. [CrossRef]

20. Grange, C.; Tapparo, M.; Bruno, S.; Chatterjee, D.; Quesenberry, P.J.; Tetta, C.; Camussi, G. Biodistribution of mesenchymal stem cell-derived extracellular vesicles in a model of acute kidney injury monitored by optical imaging. *Int. J. Mol. Med.* **2014**, *33*, 1055–1063. [CrossRef]

21. Lindoso, R.S.; Collino, F.; Bruno, S.; Araujo, D.S.; Sant'Anna, J.F.; Tetta, C.; Provero, P.; Quesenberry, P.J.; Vieyra, A.; Einicker-Lamas, M.; et al. Extracellular vesicles released from mesenchymal stromal cells modulate miRNA in renal tubular cells and inhibit ATP depletion injury. *Stem Cells Dev.* **2014**, *23*, 1809–1819. [CrossRef] [PubMed]

22. Deregibus, M.C.; Figliolini, F.; D'Antico, S.; Manzini, P.M.; Pasquino, C.; De Lena, M.; Tetta, C.; Brizzi, M.F.; Camussi, G. Charge-based precipitation of extracellular vesicles. *Int. J. Mol. Med.* **2016**, *38*, 1359–1366. [CrossRef] [PubMed]

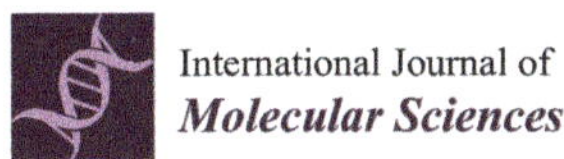 International Journal of
Molecular Sciences

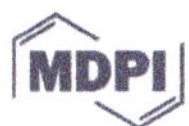

Article

Contribution of Inflammatory Cytokine Interleukin-18 Genotypes to Renal Cell Carcinoma

Wen-Shin Chang [1,†], Te-Chun Shen [1,†], Wei-Lan Yeh [2,†], Chien-Chih Yu [3], Hui-Yi Lin [3], Hsi-Chin Wu [1,4], Chia-Wen Tsai [1,*] and Da-Tian Bau [1,5,6,*]

[1] Terry Fox Cancer Research Laboratory, Translational Medicine Research Center, China Medical University Hospital, Taichung 40447, Taiwan; halittlemelon@hotmail.com (W.-S.C.); chestshen@gmail.com (T.-C.S.); wuhc@mail.cmuh.org.tw (H.-C.W.)
[2] Institute of New Drug Development, China Medical University, Taichung 40402, Taiwan; wlyeh@mail.cmu.edu.tw
[3] School of Pharmacy, China Medical University, Taichung 40402, Taiwan; ccyu@mail.cmu.edu.tw (C.-C.Y.); hylin@mail.cmu.edu.tw (H.-Y.L.)
[4] School of Medicine, China Medical University, Taichung 40402, Taiwan
[5] Graduate Institute of Biomedical Sciences, China Medical University, Taichung 40402, Taiwan
[6] Department of Bioinformatics and Medical Engineering, Asia University, Taichung 41354, Taiwan
*   Correspondence: wenwen816@gmail.com (C.-W.T.); artbau2@gmail.com (D.-T.B.)
†   These authors contributed equally to this work.

Received: 14 January 2019; Accepted: 26 March 2019; Published: 28 March 2019

Abstract: Interleukin-18 (*IL-18*) is a multi-functional immuno-mediator in the development and progression of many types of infectious and inflammatory diseases. In this study, we evaluated the contribution of *IL-18* genotypes to renal cell carcinoma (RCC) in Taiwan via the genotyping of *IL-18* -656 (A/C), -607 (A/C), and -137 (G/C). Moreover, we analyzed their interactions with smoking, alcohol drinking, hypertension, and diabetes status. The results showed an association of the AC and CC genotypes of *IL-18* -607 with a significant decrease in the risk of RCC compared with the AA genotype (odds ratio (OR) = 0.44 and 0.35, 95% confidence interval (CI) = 0.27–0.72 and 0.18–0.66, p = 0.0008 and 0.0010, respectively). Furthermore, a significantly lower frequency of the C allele at -607 was observed in the RCC group (35.3% vs. 49.8%; OR = 0.53; 95% CI = 0.35–0.71, p = 0.0003). However, *IL-18* -656 and -137 did not exhibit a likewise differential distribution of these genotypes between the control and case groups. Stratifying the population according to smoking, alcohol drinking, hypertension, and diabetes status revealed a different distribution of *IL-18* -607 genotypes among non-smokers, non-drinkers, and patients without diabetes, but not among smokers, drinkers, or patients with diabetes. These findings suggest that *IL-18* -607 genotypes may play a role in the etiology and progression of RCC in Taiwan and may serve as a useful biomarker for early detection.

Keywords: genotype; *IL-18*; polymorphism; renal cell carcinoma; Taiwan

---

1. Introduction

Renal cell carcinoma (RCC) is the sixth most frequently diagnosed cancer in men (5%) and the tenth in women (3%) worldwide, thus posing a serious disease burden [1]. From an epidemiological viewpoint, RCC is the most common renal cancer and includes several subtypes that may be distinguished from each other by their histology, genetic background, clinical course, and response to treatment [2,3]. Moreover, there are several potential risk factors for RCC, including physical activity level, obesity, fruit and vegetable intake, cigarette smoking, and alcohol consumption. In addition, there are some common medical comorbidities for RCC, such as hypertension, diabetes, urinary stones, and other forms of chronic kidney diseases [3]. However, to date, no clinically practical genomic biomarker is available for RCC risk prediction. Unfortunately, many RCC patients, even those with advanced-stage tumors, remain asymptomatic [2,4], and the disease proceeds undetected. To make matters worse, up to 30% of RCC patients treated by radical nephrectomy suffer from many adverse effects and will relapse soon after their surgery [5]. Current personal prognostication of RCC is mainly based on histological validation, which may be labor intensive and time consuming, but frequently not useful for establishing a suitable course of treatment. Therefore, genomic molecular markers for early detection of RCC are urgently needed.

Interleukin-18 (IL-18), initially named IFN-γ inducing factor, is a proinflammatory cytokine encoded by the human *IL-18* gene and produced by activated macrophages, epithelial cells, osteoblasts, keratinocytes, and most importantly, cancer cells [6,7]. In syngeneic mice models, supplementary IL-18 administration suppressed the growth of Meth A sarcoma and mouse glioma cells [7–9], suggesting that IL-18 plays an essential role in host mechanisms of defense against tumors. On a molecular level, IL-18 homeostasis is under the control of highly complex machinery involved in chronic inflammation and carcinogenesis, which is of great interest to both immunologists and oncologists. However, the promotive or suppressive effects of IL-18 on carcinogenesis are not yet fully understood. First, IL-18 may exert its tumor-suppressive influences by stimulating IFN-γ production, promoting Th1 differentiation, enhancing the cytotoxic capacities of CD8+ lymphocytes and natural killer cells [7], inducing cancer cells to undergo programmed cell death [10], and suppressing the angiogenesis [7,11]. Second, IL-18 can inhibit the recognition of cancer cells by immune cells, enhancing cancer cell adherence to the vascular wall, increasing the production of angiogenic and growth factors, and providing a pro-metastatic microenvironment [12,13]. Third, the serum levels of IL-18 were found to be higher in cancer patients than in healthy subjects, including bladder cancer [14], ovarian cancer [15], gastrointestinal cancer [16], and non-small cell lung cancer [17]. Fourth, the serum levels of IL-18 were much higher in those from breast cancer patients with metastasis than in those from patients without metastasis and non-cancer healthy subjects, supporting the hypothesis that elevated serum IL-18 levels can be used as non-invasive markers for suspected metastatic potential [18]. All the above findings support the hypothesis that the pleiotropic cytokine IL-18 can biphasically exert both anti-cancerous and pro-cancerous activities [13]. To summarize, the molecular interactions of IL-18 and other molecules are very complex and deeply involved in tumorigenesis.

From a genomic perspective, the expression level of IL-18 appears to be determined by at least two single nucleotide polymorphisms (SNPs) in the promoter at positions -607 (A/C) and -137 (G/C) of the human *IL-18* gene. The former involves an A to C shift that disrupts a potential binding site for the cAMP responsive element binding protein, and the latter involves a G to C shift that abolishes the human histone H4 gene-specific transcription factor-1 (H4TF-1) nuclear factor binding site [19]. The alterations in transcription factor binding capacities determined by these two promoter polymorphisms may affect the overall activity of *IL-18*. Another SNP located in the *IL-18* promoter is -656 (A/C); however, the effects of different genotypes at *IL-18* -656 on cancer risk have not yet been well elucidated. That is to say, the contribution of -656 genotypes in human *IL-18* to autoimmune diseases has started to be examined [15], but their involvement in any type of cancer has not.

As mentioned above, most of the previous genomic studies on human *IL-18* were devoted to examining the association of *IL-18* -607 and -137 polymorphisms with various types of cancer. Some of them revealed positive associations with cancer risk [20–24], while others identified negative ones [25,26]. However, only one such study investigated the association of the -137 and -607 genotypes of *IL-18* with RCC [27]. In that paper, although the authors reported a negative association, they found that the -137 and -607 genotypes of *IL-18* were correlated with more advanced stages of RCC, and the genotype related to a higher production of IL-18 was associated with a larger size and T stage of the tumor [27]. In the present study, the promoter SNPs at positions -656 (A/C, rs1946519), -607 (A/C, rs1946518), and -137 (G/C, rs187238) of the *IL-18* gene were first examined and their genotype distributions analyzed in patients with RCC in Taiwan. In addition, we investigated the interaction of these *IL-18* promoter genotypes with personal behavioral and clinical factors that contribute to RCC susceptibility.

2. Results

2.1. Comparison of Characteristics Among Patients with Renal Cell Carcinoma (RCC) and Controls

The frequency distributions in terms of age, gender, and personal behavioral habits for the 92 patients with RCC and the 580 cancer-free controls are summarized and compared in Table 1. Because the control subjects were already matched with patients with RCC for these factors, no difference was observed in terms of age and gender between these groups ($p > 0.05$). Moreover, there was no significant difference between the two groups in the frequency distributions in terms of personal behavioral habits, smoking, alcohol consumption, diabetes status, and family history ($p > 0.05$) (Table 1). An interesting finding was that there was a higher proportion of subjects with hypertension in the RCC group (66.3%) than in the cancer-free group (52.1%) ($p = 0.0130$). The percentage histologically identified as clear cell RCC patients is 77.2%. The percentages of "low" grade and "middle and high grade" are 52.2 and 47.8%, respectively (Table 1).

Table 1. Distributions of the frequencies of selected characteristics among the renal cell carcinoma (RCC) cases and healthy controls.

Characteristics	Cases ($n = 92$)		Controls ($n = 580$)		*p*-Value
	N	%	N	%	
Age (year) (mean ± SD)	58.8 ± 11.7		58.3 ± 11.5		0.8971
≤60	47	51.1%	307	52.9%	0.8223
>60	45	48.9%	273	47.1%	
Gender					
Male	59	64.1%	371	64.0%	1.0000
Female	33	35.9%	209	36.0%	
Smoking status					
Smokers	41	44.6%	220	37.9%	0.2499
Non-smokers	51	55.4%	360	62.1%	
Alcohol drinking status					
Drinkers	37	40.2%	209	36.0%	0.4848
Non-drinkers	55	59.8%	371	64.0%	
Hypertension					
Yes	61	66.3%	302	52.1%	0.0130 *
No	31	33.7%	278	47.9%	
Diabetes					
Yes	21	22.8%	104	17.9%	0.2523
No	71	77.2%	476	82.1%	
Family cancer history					
Yes	6	6.5%	17	2.9%	0.1125
No	86	93.5%	563	97.1%	
Histological types					
Clear cell	71	77.2%			
Non-clear cell	21	22.8%			
Histological grades					
Low	48	52.2%			
Middle and high	44	47.8%			

* Statistically identified as significant based on Chi-square test without Yates' correction.

2.2. Analysis of the Association of IL-18 Promoter Genotypes and RCC Risk in Taiwan

The genotype frequencies of *IL-18* -656 (A/C, rs1946519), -607 (A/C, rs1946518), and -137 (G/C, rs187238) for the 92 patients with RCC and the 580 age- and gender-matched healthy control subjects were determined, and the comparative results of codominant, dominant, and recessive models are presented in Table 2. The frequencies of *IL-18* -656 and -137 genotypes in the control group, but not those of *IL-18* -656 ($p = 0.0206$), were in agreement with the Hardy–Weinberg equilibrium.

Table 2. Distribution of *interleukin-18 (IL-18)* genotypes among the renal cell carcinoma patients and non-cancer healthy control subjects.

Genotypes	Controls		Patients		OR (95% CI) [a]	aOR (95% CI) [a]	p-Value
	n	%	n	%			
IL-18 -656							
AA	221	38.1%	32	34.8%	1.00 (Reference)	1.00 (Reference)	
AC	252	43.5%	44	47.8%	1.21 (0.74–1.97)	1.20 (0.69–1.84)	0.4535
CC	107	18.4%	16	17.4%	1.03 (0.54–1.96)	1.04 (0.52–1.93)	0.9218
P_{trend}							0.7311
Carrier comparison							
AA + AC	473	81.6%	76	82.6%	1.00 (Reference)	1.00 (Reference)	
CC	107	18.4%	16	17.4%	0.93 (0.52–1.66)	0.96 (0.56–1.46)	0.8076
AA	221	38.1%	32	34.8%	1.00 (Reference)	1.00 (Reference)	
AC + CC	359	61.9%	60	65.2%	1.15 (0.73–1.83)	1.12 (0.70–1.79)	0.5414
IL-18 -607							
AA	144	24.8%	41	44.6%	1.00 (Reference)	1.00 (Reference)	
AC	294	50.7%	37	40.2%	0.44 (0.27–0.72)	0.41 (0.22–0.64)	0.0008 *
CC	142	24.5%	14	15.2%	0.35 (0.18–0.66)	0.33 (0.15–0.58)	0.0010 *
P_{trend}							0.0004 *
Carrier comparison							
AA + AC	438	75.5%	78	84.8%	1.00 (Reference)	1.00 (Reference)	
CC	142	24.5%	14	15.2%	0.55 (0.30-1.00)	0.51 (0.32–0.96)	0.0505
AA	144	24.8%	41	44.6%	1.00 (Reference)	1.00 (Reference)	
AC + CC	436	75.2%	51	55.4%	0.41 (0.26–0.65)	0.39 (0.25–0.66)	0.0001 *
IL-18 -137							
GG	463	79.8%	72	78.3%	1.00 (Reference)	1.00 (Reference)	
GC	108	18.6%	18	19.5%	1.07 (0.61-1.87)	1.06 (0.60-1.66)	0.8074
CC	9	1.6%	2	2.2%	1.42 (0.30-6.75)	1.37 (0.35-6.23)	0.6505
P_{trend}							0.8825
Carrier comparison							
GG + GC	571	98.4%	90	97.8%	1.00 (Reference)	1.00 (Reference)	
CC	9	1.6%	2	2.2%	1.41 (0.30-6.63)	1.38 (0.32-5.98)	0.6622
GG	463	79.8%	72	78.3%	1.00 (Reference)	1.00 (Reference)	
GC + CC	117	20.2%	20	21.7%	1.10 (0.64-1.88)	1.10 (0.65-1.85)	0.7289

OR: odds ratio; [a] The ORs were estimated with multivariate logistic regression analysis after being adjusted with age, gender, smoking, alcohol drinking, hypertension, diabetes, and family history status; * Statistically identified as significant based on Chi-square test without Yates' correction.

For the first time, the genotypes at the *IL-18* promoter -607 (A/C) polymorphic site were found to be differentially distributed between RCC cases and control groups (*p* for trend = 0.0004) (Table 2, middle panel). To explain in detail, the *IL-18* -607 heterozygous AC and homozygous CC genotypes were associated with decreased risks for RCC (OR = 0.44 and 0.35, 95% CI = 0.27–0.72 and 0.18–0.66, *p* = 0.0008 and 0.0010, respectively) (Table 2, middle panel). After adjusting for the potential confounders, including age, gender, smoking, alcohol consumption, hypertension, diabetes status, and family history status, the significances still existed (Table 2, middle panel). In the dominant and recessive analyzing models, a significant association with the risk for RCC still persisted, as observed for the homozygous CC genotype (Table 2, middle panel). In contrast, none of the genotypes or alleles for *IL-18*, -656, and -137 demonstrated any correlation with RCC risk in any of the subgroups (Table 2).

We further performed allelic frequency analysis for these three *IL-18* genotypes; the results are shown in Table 3. These results demonstrated that the variant allele C comprised only 35.3% in the RCC group, which was significantly less than that (49.8%) in the control group (adjusted OR = 0.53, 95% CI = 0.35–0.71, *p* = 0.0003), and these results fully confirmed the conclusion derived in Table 2. Consistently, the other two genotypes, *IL-18* -656 and -137, showed no significant association with the risk for RCC (Table 3).

Table 3. Allelic frequency analysis for *interleukin-18 (IL-18)* polymorphisms and renal cell carcinoma.

Allele	Controls *n* (%)	Patients *n* (%)	aOR (95% CI) [a]	*p*-Value
IL-18 -656				
G	694 (59.8%)	108 (58.7%)	1.00 (Reference)	
T	466 (40.2%)	76 (41.3%)	1.06 (0.73-1.31)	0.7712
IL-18 -607				
A	582 (50.2%)	119 (64.7%)	1.00 (Reference)	
C	578 (49.8%)	65 (35.3%)	0.53 (0.35-0.71)	0.0003 *
IL-18 -137				
G	1034 (89.1%)	162 (88.0%)	1.00 (Reference)	
C	126 (10.9%)	22 (12.0%)	1.11 (0.69-1.83)	0.6595

[a] The ORs were estimated with multivariate logistic regression analysis after being adjusted with age, gender, smoking, alcohol drinking, hypertension, diabetes, and family history status. * Statistically identified as significant based on chi-square test without Yates' correction.

2.3. Stratified Analysis of IL-18 Genotypes According to Personal Behavioral and Clinical Factors

We further conducted stratification analysis of the association between *IL-18* -607 genotypes and the risk for RCC based on potential personal behavioral and clinical risk factors among Taiwanese people, including cigarette smoking, alcohol consumption, hypertension, and diabetes status. First, the distributions of the genotype frequencies between the case and control groups among nonsmokers were significantly different, but showed similar proportions for cases and controls among smokers (Figure 1). The adjusted ORs for carriers with genotypes AC and CC at *IL-18* -607 were 0.36 and 0.22 for nonsmokers (95% CI = 0.21–0.63 and 0.11–0.56, respectively) and 0.61 and 0.58 for smokers (95% CI = 0.33–1.31 and 0.24–1.35, respectively), respectively (Figure 1). It appeared that the protective effects of *IL-18* -607 genotypes on the risk for RCC were obvious among nonsmokers, but not among smokers (Figure 1). Second, the distributions of the genotype frequencies between the case and control groups among nondrinkers were significantly different, but showed similar proportions for cases and controls among alcohol drinkers (Figure 2). The adjusted ORs for carriers with genotypes AC and CC at *IL-18* -607 were 0.38 and 0.21 among nondrinkers (95% CI = 0.22–0.70 and 0.09–0.51, respectively) and 0.56 and 0.62 among alcohol drinkers (95% CI = 0.31–1.23 and 0.28–1.41, respectively), respectively (Figure 2). The protective effects of *IL-18* -607 genotypes on the risk for RCC appeared to be obvious among nondrinkers, but not among alcohol drinkers (Figure 2). Third, the distributions of the genotype frequencies between case and control groups among non-hypertensive and hypertensive subjects were both significantly different (Figure 3). The adjusted ORs for carriers with genotypes AC and CC at *IL-18* -607 were 0.39 and 0.24 among subjects without hypertension (95% CI = 0.18–0.81 and 0.11–0.69, respectively) and 0.41 and 0.39 among those with hypertension (95% CI = 0.26–0.84 and 0.18–0.94, respectively), respectively (Figure 3). The protective effects of *IL-18* -607 genotypes on the risk for RCC appeared to be obvious among people with or without hypertension (Figure 3). Finally, the distributions of the genotype frequencies between the case and control groups among subjects without diabetes were significantly different, but presented similar proportions for cases and controls among subjects with diabetes (Figure 4). The adjusted ORs for carriers with genotypes AC and CC at *IL-18* -607 were 0.44 and 0.35 among subjects without diabetes (95% CI = 0.28–0.81 and 0.21–0.68, respectively) and 0.38 and 0.36 among those with diabetes (95% CI = 0.18–1.02 and 0.13–1.58, respectively), respectively (Figure 4). The effects of *IL-18* -607 genotypes on the risk for RCC appeared to be protective among subjects without diabetes, but not among those with diabetes (Figure 4). The sample size of those with a family history of cancer was too small for stratification analysis.

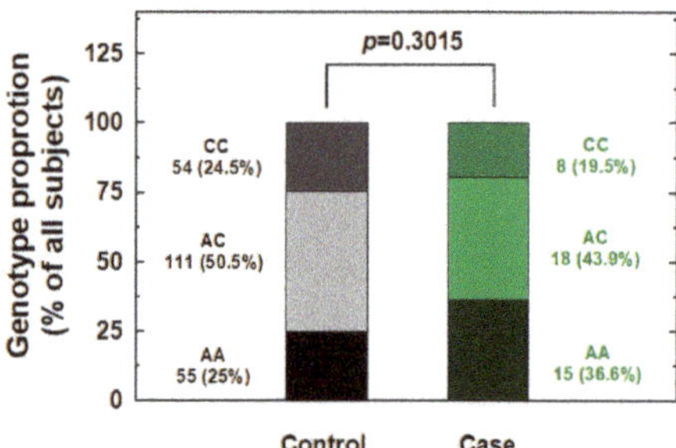

Figure 1. Contribution of *interleukin-18 (IL-18)* promoter -607 genotype to the risk of renal cell carcinoma after stratification by smoking status. The distributions of AA, AC, and CC genotypes at *IL-18* promoter -607 among nonsmokers (**A**) and smokers (**B**). *** Statistically significant between case and control groups.

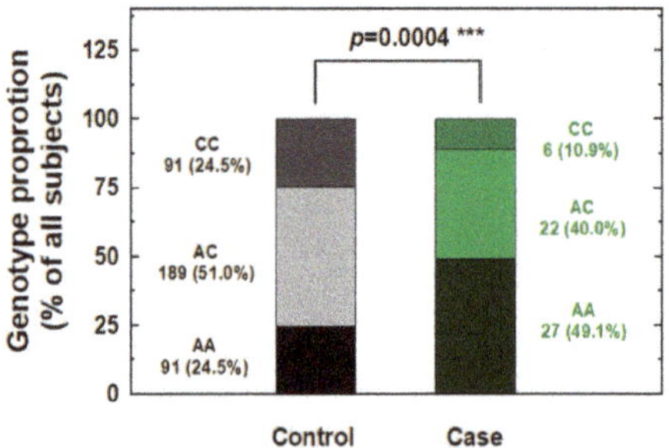

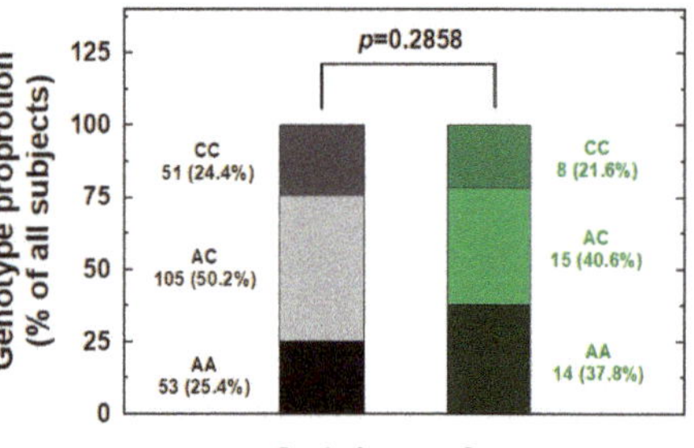

Figure 2. Contribution of *interleukin-18 (IL-18)* promoter -607 genotype to the risk of renal cell carcinoma after stratification by alcohol consumption status. The distributions of AA, AC, and CC genotypes at *IL-18* promoter -607 among nondrinkers (**A**) and drinkers (**B**). *** Statistically significant between case and control groups.

A. Non-hypertension
B. Hypertension

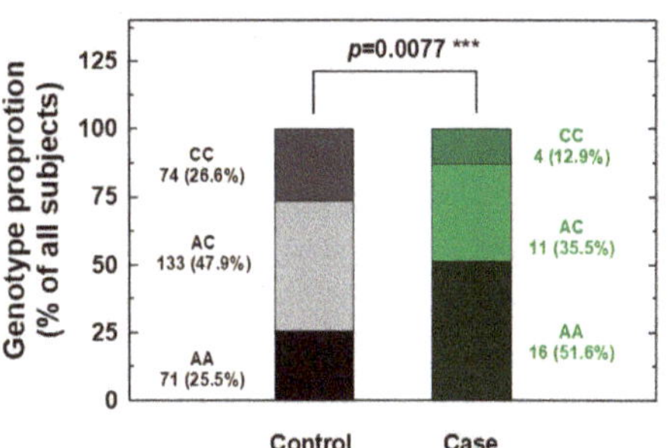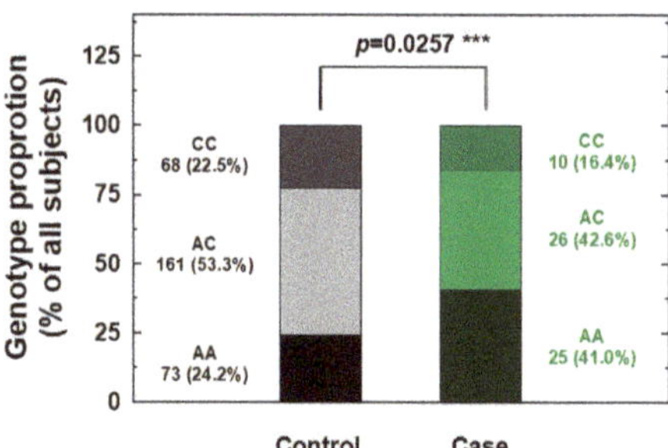

Figure 3. Contribution of *interleukin-18 (IL-18)* promoter -607 genotype to the risk of renal cell carcinoma after stratification by hypertension status. The distributions of AA, AC, and CC genotypes at *IL-18* promoter -607 among non-hypertensive (**A**) and hypertensive subjects (**B**). *** Statistically significant between case and control groups.

A. Non-diabetes
B. Diabetes

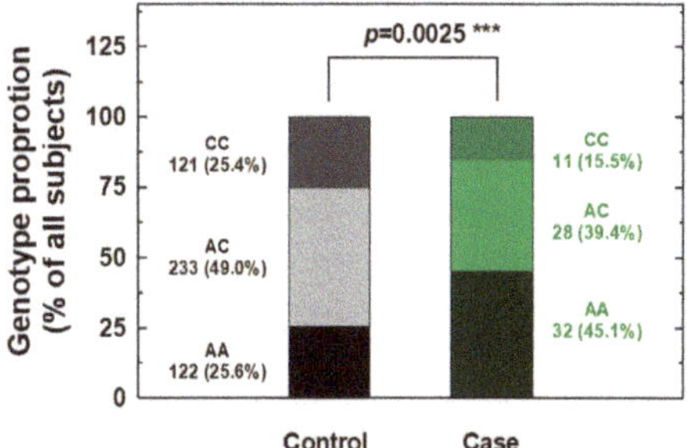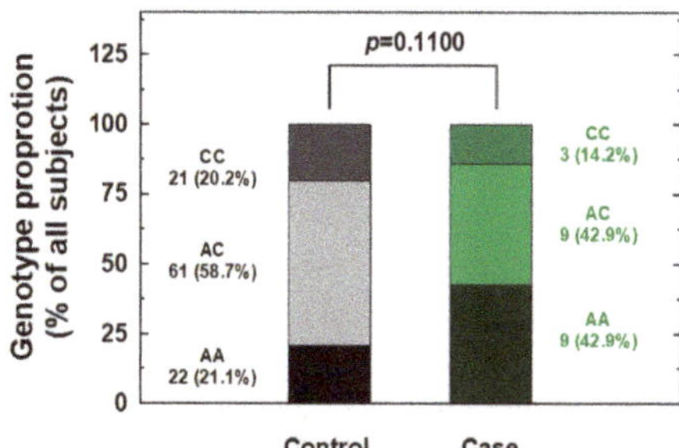

Figure 4. Contribution of *interleukin-18 (IL-18)* promoter -607 genotype to the risk of renal cell carcinoma after stratification by diabetes status. The distributions of AA, AC, and CC genotypes at *IL-18* promoter -607 among subjects without (**A**) and with (**B**) diabetes. *** Statistically significant between case and control groups.

The levels of IL-18 in the serum of 10 RCC patients and 10 healthy controls were determined using ELISA. The results demonstrated that the basal IL-18 levels were significantly higher in RCC patients (212.80 ± 21.39 pg/mL) than those of control subjects (113.70 ± 9.94 pg/mL) ($p = 0.0001$) (Figure 5). According to their *IL-18* -607 genotype distribution, the 10 RCC patients were divided into three subgroups: four patients with the AA genotype (216.25 ± 12.79 pg/mL), four with AC (206.25 ± 31.31 pg/mL), and two with CC (219.00 ± 19.80 pg/mL). There were no significant differences in serum IL-18 levels between different *IL-18* -607 genotypes (AC versus AA: $p = 0.5759$; CC versus AA: $p = 0.8412$; and CC versus AC: $p = 0.6369$).

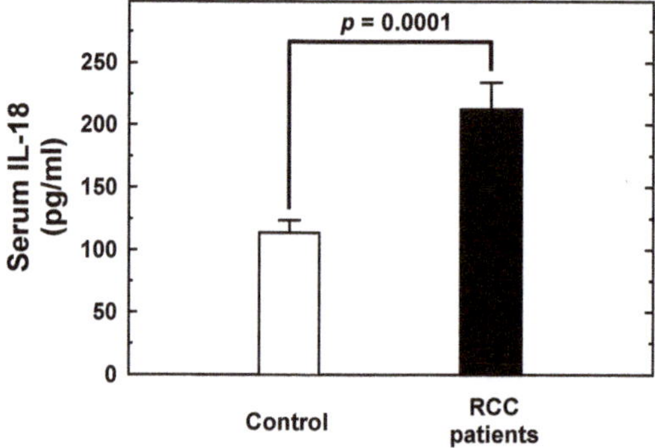

Figure 5. Serum IL-18 levels in 10 RCC patients and 10 healthy control subjects. The serum IL-18 levels were measured by ELISA methodology. The basal levels of serum IL-18 were higher in RCC patients (212.80 ± 21.39 pg/mL) than those of control subjects (113.70 ± 9.94 pg/mL) (p = 0.0001). However, no association was found between serum IL-18 levels and specific genotypes. The values are shown as mean ± standard deviation. IL-18, interleukin-18; RCC, renal cell carcinoma; ELISA, enzyme-linked immunosorbent assay.

3. Discussion

The prevalence and death rates of RCC are not ranked as high as those of other cancers in Taiwan. Clinically, surgery is the major course of RCC treatment. However, the symptoms of early-stage RCC are not obvious, and early detection of RCC is not available. Thus, the findings of genomic biomarker(s), which are very useful in rapid and convenient screening, may contribute to early detection and prediction of RCC susceptibility and outcome. For many years, members of the Terry Fox Cancer Fox Cancer Research foundation, including translational scientists and surgeons, have devoted themselves to elucidating specific and practical genomic biomarkers for early detection and prediction in Taiwan, where RCC is a prevalent condition and the cause of many cancer deaths [28–32]. Cytokines play an essential but complex role in the initiation and progression of inflammation and tumorigenesis [33], which is currently still under investigation. The proinflammatory cytokine IL-18 confers protective effects against cancer proliferation, such as that of lung cancer, in several murine models [13,34], and the benefits of recombinant human IL-18 have been shown in preclinical trials for cancer treatment [35]. However, despite the conventional view of IL-18 as an anticancer agent, some studies have also proposed a procancerous behavior for IL-18 under specific conditions [13]. Recently, mounting studies have reported that various cytokine genotypes may influence the serum levels of their counterpart cytokines, which may be closely associated with susceptibility to certain human diseases [19–23,25,26]. Among the numerous SNPs in *IL-18*, three polymorphisms are present in the promoter region of this gene: -656 (G/T), -607 (C/A), and -137 (G/C), and they were reported to cause differences in the transcription factor binding capacity and expression level of IL-18 in serum [19]. The polymorphic genotypes of *IL-18* promoter -607 and -137 were previously found to be associated with the risk of esophageal squamous cell carcinoma [20] and prostate cancer [21] in China, colorectal cancer in Greece [22], ovarian cancer in the USA (Hawaii) [23], and breast cancer in Iran [24]. On the contrary, there were also some negative associations reported between *IL-18* polymorphisms and the risk of head and neck cancers in Iran [26], as well as oral cancer in Greece [25]. Reasonable explanations for these discrepant and diverse findings may involve three possibilities: the dual impact of IL-18 on tumor-immune responses [13], the different types of cancer investigated, and variation among the populations under study [26].

In the current study, the genotypes at polymorphic locations -656 (G/T), -607 (C/A), and -137 (G/C) of the *IL-18* promoter region among RCC patients and healthy individuals in a Taiwan population were first determined and evaluated for their contribution to RCC risk. The results indicated a significantly lower risk for the heterozygous AC and homozygous CC variant genotypes and for the C allele at position -607 of the *IL-18* gene than their counterparts about RCC susceptibility (Tables 2 and 3), even after statistical adjustment for personal behavioral and clinical risk factors. In contrast, no significant association between any genotype or allelic type with RCC risk was found for -656 or -137 of *IL-18* (Tables 2 and 3). The positive findings indicating that genotypes of *IL-18* -607 may be determinants for personal RCC susceptibility were inconsistent with previous findings from the only paper investigating the contribution of *IL-18* genotypes to RCC [27], which returned negative findings. Once again, the inconsistency may be due to the location of Taiwan located in East Asia and the fact that it is an island with a conserved genetic, cultural, and environmental background, much different from the investigated Spanish population [27]. Although the sample size of the current study was similar to theirs (case:control = 92:580 vs. 158:506), we brought forward two novel findings: *IL-18* -607 was a determinant of RCC susceptibility (Tables 2 and 3), and there were positive interactions of this polymorphic site with personal behavioral and clinical factors (Figures 1–4). In the near future, the significant contribution of *IL-18* genotypes to RCC risk evaluation, especially those at *IL-18* -607, should be validated in larger samples and other populations worldwide.

In detail, the stratification of RCC patients and non-cancer subjects according to personal behavior revealed that *IL-18* -607 genotypes may play a significant role in the determination of susceptibility to RCC in non-smokers (Figure 1), non-alcohol drinkers (Figure 2), those with and without hypertension (Figure 3), and those without diabetes (Figure 4), but not in smokers, alcohol drinkers, or those with diabetes (Figures 1, 3 and 4). However, the undermined subtle mechanisms and signaling networks that are responsible for the interaction of IL-18 and other molecules related to the etiology of RCC require further investigation.

The genotype-phenotype association was performed after the measurement of serum levels of IL-18 in 10 RCC patients and 10 healthy controls. The results showed that: (a) the AA genotype at *IL-18* -607 was higher in the RCC patients than the healthy controls (Table 2); (b) the IL-18 levels were higher in the RCC patients than the healthy controls (Figure 5), which is consistent with the previous findings [36]; and (c) there was no difference in the IL-18 levels among RC patients of different *IL-18* -607 genotypes. This finding is consistent with the previous finding in lung cancer [37], but inconsistent with another [38]. The difference and similarity may due to the fact that different populations were investigated. Ours and the former were investigating Taiwanese and Chinese people, respectively, while the latter one was investigating people from Iran.

As for the perspective molecular mechanism, there is literature mentioning that the A to C shift at IL-18 -607 may disrupt the potential binding site for the cAMP responsive element binding protein, thus lowering the expression level of IL-18 [19]. That is to say, the differential genotype at *IL-18* -607 may associate with elevated expression levels of IL-18, as the early detector for RCC, like we showed in Figure 5. The current study does not provide supporting evidence for the hypothesis that any genotype at *IL-18* -607 may associate with elevated expression levels of IL-18, due to the limited samples examined, and confirmation in larger samples is an urgent need. We also have to notice that the alteration of IL-18 may not be the only indicator during RCC carcinogenesis. In 2015, Xu et al. reported that elevated IL-18 together with IL-1b were significantly associated with advanced RCC stages, an elevated recurrence rate, and a shortened survival period among patients with localized RCC [35].

To summarize, this pilot study indicated a significant association between the *IL-18* -607 polymorphism and RCC in Taiwan. Furthermore, to the best of our knowledge, it is also the first to investigate the interaction of *IL-18* genotypes and behavioral and clinical factors in RCC risk. Our results showed a significant association between the *IL-18* -607 polymorphism and RCC, particularly in people without smoking or alcohol drinking behavior, and those without diabetes. However, it should be pointed out that the samples sizes of affected subjects (i.e., smokers, drinkers, and particularly patients with diabetes) were much smaller than those of un-affected subjects, which might be the main reason for the lack of statistically significant associations in the affected subjects. Future larger studies in various populations are needed to validate *IL-18* genotypes as early detective and predictive determinants of RCC.

4. Materials and Methods

4.1. Selected Subjects

This case-control study was performed in the China Medical University Hospital and involved the collection of data from 92 patients with RCC and 580 cancer-free controls matched by age and gender; none of the participants were related to each other by any biological relationship. The diagnosis of RCC, and the grades and types of each patient were histopathologically confirmed by the surgeons and pathologists led by Hsi-Chin Wu. In addition, the age- and gender-matched cancer-free controls were genetically unrelated to any of the recruited participants and had no prior history of any cancer. Originally, we frequency matched seven controls, which were collected in the Health Examination Center of the China Medical University Hospital, for each RCC patient with the same gender and age at ±2 years. After the first-term matching, those with incomplete demographic data about smoking, alcohol drinking status, hypertension, diabetes, or family cancer history, were excluded. A further exclusion criterion for the control subjects was any symptom suggestive of RCC, such as hematuria. Finally, only 580 controls were collected in the study. After obtaining written informed consent, 3–5 mL of venous blood was collected from each participant for genotyping. The study was approved by the Institutional Review Board of China Medical University, and expert members of the Tissue Bank of China Medical University Hospital (DMR98-IRB-209 in 2009) provided their kind assistance. The overall agreement rate among the participants was >85%. Select characteristics of all the participants are summarized and compared in Table 1.

4.2. DNA Preparation and Storage

Genomic DNA from the leukocytes of each study subject was extracted using the QIAamp Blood Mini Kit (Qiagen, Valencia, CA, USA), stored for the long term at $-80\,^{\circ}\mathrm{C}$, simultaneously diluted, and aliquoted and stored for genotyping as a working stock at $-20\,^{\circ}\mathrm{C}$, as we have frequently performed previously [32,39,40].

4.3. IL-18 Genotype Discrimination Methodology

The genotype discrimination methodology for *IL-18* -137, -607, and -656 genotypes was performed as we described in 2018 [41]. Briefly, -137 (G/C, rs187238) and -607 (A/C, rs1946518) genotyping was performed using the ABI StepOne™ Real-Time PCR System (Applied Biosystems, Foster City, CA, USA) and analyzed using the typical TaqMan assay. Regarding the genotyping of *IL-18* -656 (A/C, rs1946519), the polymerase chain reaction-restriction fragment length polymorphism (PCR-RFLP) methodology was carried out using the primers originally reported in 2005 by Flowaczny et al. [42], with the forward primer being 5′-AGGTCAGTCTTTGCTATCATTCCAGG-3′ and the reverse primer being 5′-CTGCAACAGAAAGTAAGCTTGCGGAGAGG-3′, and a 120-bp fragment nearby the *IL-18* -656 polymorphism was amplified. In detail, approximately 100 ng of genomic DNA of each sample was subjected to PCR, in which the reaction mixture of 25-µL contained 300 mM dNTP, 2 U of Taq DNA polymerase, 1× PCR buffer, 1.5 mM MgCl$_2$, and 0.8 mM of each primer. After mixing up and briefly spinning down, the reaction mixture was heated to 94 $^{\circ}$C for 4 min and amplified by 30 cycles using the My Cycler (Biorad, Hercules, CA, USA) with the following steps: denaturation at 94 $^{\circ}$C for 60 s, annealing at 60 $^{\circ}$C for 60 s, extension at 72 $^{\circ}$C for 60 s for each cycle, and a final extension step at 72 $^{\circ}$C for 5 min. The volume of the restriction assay was set at 12.5 µL, containing 8 µL of PCR products, 2 U *Mwo* I restriction enzyme, and 1× buffer. The reaction mixture was then incubated for 16 h or overnight at 60 $^{\circ}$C. The resultant DNA fragments were subject to electrophoresis in 3.0% agarose gel at 100 V for 30 min. After electrophoresis, ethidium bromide staining was done to observe the DNA fragments under UV (260 nm) light. For the A allele of *IL-18* -656, there was no digestion of the 120-bp PCR fragment, whereas for the C allele of *IL-18* -656, two (96- and 24-bp) fragments were identified.

4.4. Enzyme-linked Immunosorbent Assay (ELISA) for Serum IL-18 Levels

Ten milliliters of blood samples were collected from 10 healthy controls and 10 RCC patients. The blood samples were collected in serum tubes with an accelerating agent for serum separation and kept at a room temperature for 30 min before their further centrifugation for 20 min at $1500\times$ g. Serum was then isolated and stored at -80 °C until IL-18 measurement. The individual level of IL-18 in serum was measured by enzyme-linked immunosorbent assay (ELISA, Newwark, DE, USA) kits.

4.5. Statistical Analysis Methodology

The data of 580 cancer-free healthy controls and 92 patients with RCC who had complete genotypic and clinical details were finally included for statistical analysis, whose results are presented in the form of tables and figures. To ensure that the control subjects in this study were representative of the Taiwanese general population and to exclude the possibility of genotyping error, the deviation of the genotype frequencies of *IL-18* SNPs in the control subjects from those expected under the Hardy–Weinberg equilibrium was assessed using the goodness-of-fit test. Pearson's Chi-square test was used to compare the distribution of *IL-18* genotypes between cases and control groups and in the stratification analysis. The comparison of the continuous factor age was performed and evaluated by the Student's *t*-test. The contribution of *IL-18* genotypes to the risk of developing RCC was estimated by the odds ratios (ORs) and their counterpart 95% confidence intervals (CIs) obtained through logistic regression analysis with adjustment for possible confounders. Any *p* value < 0.05 was considered to be statistically significant.

Author Contributions: Conceived and designed the experiments: W.-S.C., T.-C.S., and W.-L.Y. Performed the experiments: W.-S.C. and C.-W.T. Analyzed the data: C.-C.Y. and H.-Y.L. Contributed reagents/materials/analysis tools: W.-L.Y. and H.-C.W. Wrote the paper: C.-W.T. and D.-T.B.

Funding: This research was mainly funded by China Medical University Hospital (DMR107-175) to Shen.

Acknowledgments: We thank the Tissuebank and colleagues of the Urinary Department in the China Medical University Hospital for their excellent technical assistance. The genotyping and analyzing work was partially helped by Yun-Chi Wang, Hsin-Ting Li, and Huai-Mei Hsu. The statistical analyses were kindly double checked by Cheng-Li Lin (manpower under MOHW108-TDU-B-212-133004).

Conflicts of Interest: The authors declare no conflict of interest.

References

1. Siegel, R.L.; Miller, K.D.; Jemal, A. Cancer statistics, 2018. *CA Cancer J. Clin.* **2018**, *68*, 7–30. [CrossRef] [PubMed]
2. Ferlay, J.; Shin, H.R.; Bray, F.; Forman, D.; Mathers, C.; Parkin, D.M. Estimates of worldwide burden of cancer in 2008: GLOBOCAN 2008. *Int. J. Cancer* **2010**, *127*, 2893–2917. [CrossRef] [PubMed]
3. Klaassen, Z.; Sayyid, R.K.; Wallis, C.J.D. Lessons learned from the global epidemiology of kidney cancer: A refresher in epidemiology 101. *Eur. Urol.* **2019**, *75*, 85–87. [CrossRef]
4. Niedworok, C.; Dorrenhaus, B.; Vom Dorp, F.; Piotrowski, J.A.; Tschirdewahn, S.; Szarvas, T.; Rubben, H.; Schenck, M. Renal cell carcinoma and tumour thrombus in the inferior vena cava: Clinical outcome of 98 consecutive patients and the prognostic value of preoperative parameters. *World J. Urol.* **2015**, *33*, 1541–1552. [CrossRef]
5. Cohen, H.T.; McGovern, F.J. Renal-cell carcinoma. *N. Engl. J. Med.* **2005**, *353*, 2477–2490. [CrossRef]
6. Okamura, H.; Tsutsi, H.; Komatsu, T.; Yutsudo, M.; Hakura, A.; Tanimoto, T.; Torigoe, K.; Okura, T.; Nukada, Y.; Hattori, K.; et al. Cloning of a new cytokine that induces IFN-gamma production by T cells. *Nature* **1995**, *378*, 88–91. [CrossRef] [PubMed]
7. Nakanishi, K.; Yoshimoto, T.; Tsutsui, H.; Okamura, H. Interleukin-18 is a unique cytokine that stimulates both Th1 and Th2 responses depending on its cytokine milieu. *Cytokine Growth Factor Rev.* **2001**, *12*, 53–72. [CrossRef]
8. Golab, J. Interleukin 18–interferon gamma inducing factor–a novel player in tumour immunotherapy? *Cytokine* **2000**, *12*, 332–338. [CrossRef] [PubMed]

9. Kikuchi, T.; Akasaki, Y.; Joki, T.; Abe, T.; Kurimoto, M.; Ohno, T. Antitumor activity of interleukin-18 on mouse glioma cells. *J. Immunother.* **2000**, *23*, 184–189. [CrossRef] [PubMed]

10. Okano, F.; Yamada, K. Canine interleukin-18 induces apoptosis and enhances Fas ligand mRNA expression in a canine carcinoma cell line. *Anticancer Res.* **2000**, *20*, 3411–3415.

11. Cao, R.; Farnebo, J.; Kurimoto, M.; Cao, Y. Interleukin-18 acts as an angiogenesis and tumor suppressor. *FASEB J.* **1999**, *13*, 2195–2202. [CrossRef] [PubMed]

12. Park, C.C.; Morel, J.C.; Amin, M.A.; Connors, M.A.; Harlow, L.A.; Koch, A.E. Evidence of IL-18 as a novel angiogenic mediator. *J. Immunol.* **2001**, *167*, 1644–1653. [CrossRef] [PubMed]

13. Vidal-Vanaclocha, F.; Mendoza, L.; Telleria, N.; Salado, C.; Valcarcel, M.; Gallot, N.; Carrascal, T.; Egilegor, E.; Beaskoetxea, J.; Dinarello, C.A. Clinical and experimental approaches to the pathophysiology of interleukin-18 in cancer progression. *Cancer Metastasis Rev.* **2006**, *25*, 417–434. [CrossRef] [PubMed]

14. Jaiswal, P.K.; Singh, V.; Srivastava, P.; Mittal, R.D. Association of IL-12, IL-18 variants and serum IL-18 with bladder cancer susceptibility in North Indian population. *Gene* **2013**, *519*, 128–134. [CrossRef]

15. Samsami Dehaghani, A.; Shahriary, K.; Kashef, M.A.; Naeimi, S.; Fattahi, M.J.; Mojtahedi, Z.; Ghaderi, A. Interleukin-18 gene promoter and serum level in women with ovarian cancer. *Mol. Biol. Rep.* **2009**, *36*, 2393–2397. [CrossRef]

16. Haghshenas, M.R.; Hosseini, S.V.; Mahmoudi, M.; Saberi-Firozi, M.; Farjadian, S.; Ghaderi, A. IL-18 serum level and IL-18 promoter gene polymorphism in Iranian patients with gastrointestinal cancers. *J. Gastroenterol. Hepatol.* **2009**, *24*, 1119–1122. [CrossRef]

17. Okamoto, M.; Azuma, K.; Hoshino, T.; Imaoka, H.; Ikeda, J.; Kinoshita, T.; Takamori, S.; Ohshima, K.; Edakuni, N.; Kato, S.; et al. Correlation of decreased survival and IL-18 in bone metastasis. *Intern. Med.* **2009**, *48*, 763–773. [CrossRef]

18. Gunel, N.; Coskun, U.; Sancak, B.; Gunel, U.; Hasdemir, O.; Bozkurt, S. Clinical importance of serum interleukin-18 and nitric oxide activities in breast carcinoma patients. *Cancer* **2002**, *95*, 663–667. [CrossRef]

19. Giedraitis, V.; He, B.; Huang, W.X.; Hillert, J. Cloning and mutation analysis of the human IL-18 promoter: A possible role of polymorphisms in expression regulation. *J. Neuroimmunol.* **2001**, *112*, 146–152. [CrossRef]

20. Wei, Y.S.; Lan, Y.; Liu, Y.G.; Tang, H.; Tang, R.G.; Wang, J.C. Interleukin-18 gene promoter polymorphisms and the risk of esophageal squamous cell carcinoma. *Acta. Oncol.* **2007**, *46*, 1090–1096. [CrossRef]

21. Liu, Y.; Lin, N.; Huang, L.; Xu, Q.; Pang, G. Genetic polymorphisms of the interleukin-18 gene and risk of prostate cancer. *DNA Cell. Biol.* **2007**, *26*, 613–618. [CrossRef] [PubMed]

22. Nikiteas, N.; Yannopoulos, A.; Chatzitheofylaktou, A.; Tsigris, C. Heterozygosity for interleukin-18 -607 A/C polymorphism is associated with risk for colorectal cancer. *Anticancer Res.* **2007**, *27*, 3849–3853. [PubMed]

23. Bushley, A.W.; Ferrell, R.; McDuffie, K.; Terada, K.Y.; Carney, M.E.; Thompson, P.J.; Wilkens, L.R.; Tung, K.H.; Ness, R.B.; Goodman, M.T. Polymorphisms of interleukin (IL)-1alpha, IL-1beta, IL-6, IL-10, and IL-18 and the risk of ovarian cancer. *Gynecol. Oncol.* **2004**, *95*, 672–679. [CrossRef] [PubMed]

24. Khalili-Azad, T.; Razmkhah, M.; Ghiam, A.F.; Doroudchi, M.; Talei, A.R.; Mojtahedi, Z.; Ghaderi, A. Association of interleukin-18 gene promoter polymorphisms with breast cancer. *Neoplasma* **2009**, *56*, 22–25. [CrossRef]

25. Vairaktaris, E.; Serefoglou, Z.C.; Yapijakis, C.; Agapi, C.; Vassiliou, S.; Nkenke, E.; Antonis, V.; Sofia, S.; Neukam, F.W.; Patsouris, E. The interleukin-18 -607A/C polymorphism is not associated with risk for oral cancer. *Anticancer Res.* **2007**, *27*, 4011–4014. [PubMed]

26. Asefi, V.; Mojtahedi, Z.; Khademi, B.; Naeimi, S.; Ghaderi, A. Head and neck squamous cell carcinoma is not associated with interleukin-18 promoter gene polymorphisms: A case-control study. *J. Laryngol. Otol.* **2009**, *123*, 444–448. [CrossRef]

27. Saenz-Lopez, P.; Carretero, R.; Vazquez, F.; Martin, J.; Sanchez, E.; Tallada, M.; Garrido, F.; Cozar, J.M.; Ruiz-Cabello, F. Impact of interleukin-18 polymorphisms-607 and -137 on clinical characteristics of renal cell carcinoma patients. *Hum. Immunol.* **2010**, *71*, 309–313. [CrossRef]

28. Chang, W.S.; Ke, H.L.; Tsai, C.W.; Lien, C.S.; Liao, W.L.; Lin, H.H.; Lee, M.H.; Wu, H.C.; Chang, C.H.; Chen, C.C.; et al. The role of XRCC6 T-991C functional polymorphism in renal cell carcinoma. *Anticancer Res.* **2012**, *32*, 3855–3860.

29. Chang, W.S.; Tsai, C.W.; Wang, S.M.; Wang, S.W.; Wu, H.C.; Ji, H.X.; Lin, C.H.; Wang, Z.H.; Chou, J.C.; Bau, D.T.; et al. Association of caveolin-1 genotypes with renal cell carcinoma risk in Taiwan. *Chin. J. Physiol.* **2014**, *57*, 220–226. [CrossRef]

30. Chang, W.S.; Liao, C.H.; Miao, C.E.; Wu, H.C.; Hou, L.L.; Hsiao, C.L.; Ji, H.X.; Tsai, C.W.; Bau, D.T. The role of functional polymorphisms of cyclooxygenase 2 in renal cell carcinoma. *Anticancer Res.* **2014**, *34*, 5481–5486.

31. Chang, W.S.; Liao, C.H.; Tsai, C.W.; Hu, P.S.; Wu, H.C.; Hsu, S.W.; Ji, H.X.; Hsiao, C.L.; Bau, D.T. The Role of IL-10 Promoter Polymorphisms in Renal Cell Carcinoma. *Anticancer Res.* **2016**, *36*, 2205–2209.

32. Liao, C.H.; Chang, W.S.; Hu, P.S.; Wu, H.C.; Hsu, S.W.; Liu, Y.F.; Liu, S.P.; Hung, H.S.; Bau, D.T.; Tsai, C.W. The Contribution of MMP-7 Promoter Polymorphisms in Renal Cell Carcinoma. *In Vivo* **2017**, *31*, 631–635. [PubMed]

33. Aggarwal, B.B.; Shishodia, S.; Sandur, S.K.; Pandey, M.K.; Sethi, G. Inflammation and cancer: How hot is the link? *Biochem. Pharmacol.* **2006**, *72*, 1605–1621. [CrossRef] [PubMed]

34. Lian, H.; Jin, N.; Li, X.; Mi, Z.; Zhang, J.; Sun, L.; Li, X.; Zheng, H.; Li, P. Induction of an effective anti-tumor immune response and tumor regression by combined administration of IL-18 and Apoptin. *Cancer Immunol. Immunother.* **2007**, *56*, 181–192. [CrossRef] [PubMed]

35. Herzyk, D.J.; Bugelski, P.J.; Hart, T.K.; Wier, P.J. Preclinical safety of recombinant human interleukin-18. *Toxicol. Pathol.* **2003**, *31*, 554–561. [CrossRef] [PubMed]

36. Sozen, S.; Coskun, U.; Sancak, B.; Bukan, N.; Gunel, N.; Tunc, L.; Bozkirli, I. Serum levels of interleukin-18 and nitrite+nitrate in renal cell carcinoma patients with different tumor stage and grade. *Neoplasma* **2004**, *51*, 25–29. [PubMed]

37. Jia, Y.; Zang, A.; Jiao, S.; Chen, S.; Yan, F. The interleukin-18 gene promoter -607 A/C polymorphism contributes to non-small-cell lung cancer risk in a Chinese population. *Onco. Targets. Ther.* **2016**, *9*, 1715–1719. [CrossRef]

38. Xu, L.; Zhu, Y.; An, H.; Liu, Y.; Lin, Z.; Wang, G.; Xu, J. Clinical significance of tumor-derived IL-1β and IL-18 in localized renal cell carcinoma: Associations with recurrence and survival. *Urol. Oncol.* **2015**, *33*, 68.e9–68.e16. [CrossRef]

39. Yueh, T.C.; Wu, C.N.; Hung, Y.W.; Chang, W.S.; Fu, C.K.; Pei, J.S.; Wu, M.H.; Lai, Y.L.; Lee, Y.M.; Yen, S.T.; et al. The Contribution of MMP-7 Genotypes to Colorectal Cancer Susceptibility in Taiwan. *Cancer Genomics Proteomics* **2018**, *15*, 207–212. [CrossRef]

40. Shen, T.C.; Chang, W.S.; Tsai, C.W.; Chao, C.Y.; Lin, Y.T.; Hsiao, C.L.; Hsu, C.L.; Chen, W.C.; Hsia, T.C.; Bau, D.T. The Contribution of Matrix Metalloproteinase-1 Promoter Genotypes in Taiwan Lung Cancer Risk. *Anticancer Res.* **2018**, *38*, 253–257.

41. Huang, C.Y.; Chang, W.S.; Tsai, C.W.; Hsia, T.C.; Shen, T.C.; Bau, D.T.; Shui, H.A. Interleukin-18 promoter genotype is associated with the risk of nasopharyngeal carcinoma in Taiwan. *Cancer Manag. Res.* **2018**, *10*, 5199–5207. [CrossRef] [PubMed]

42. Folwaczny, M.; Glas, J.; Torok, H.P.; Tonenchi, L.; Paschos, E.; Bauer, B.; Limbersky, O.; Folwaczny, C. Polymorphisms of the interleukin-18 gene in periodontitis patients. *J. Clin. Periodontol.* **2005**, *32*, 530–534. [CrossRef] [PubMed]

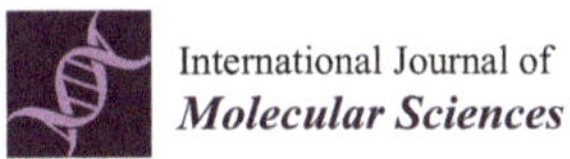

International Journal of
Molecular Sciences

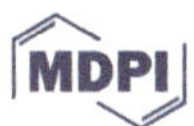

Article

Chemokine CXCL13 as a New Systemic Biomarker for B-Cell Involvement in Acute T Cell-Mediated Kidney Allograft Rejection

Lena Schiffer [1,2,†], Flavia Wiehler [1,†], Jan Hinrich Bräsen [3], Wilfried Gwinner [1], Robert Greite [1], Kirill Kreimann [1], Anja Thorenz [1], Katja Derlin [4], Beina Teng [1], Song Rong [1], Sibylle von Vietinghoff [1], Hermann Haller [1], Michael Mengel [5], Lars Pape [2], Christian Lerch [2], Mario Schiffer [1,6,†] and Faikah Gueler [1,*,†]

[1] Nephrology, Hannover Medical School, 30625 Hannover, Germany; Schiffer.Lena@mh-hannover.de (L.S.); Wiehler.Flavia@mh-hannover.de (F.W.); Gwinner.Wilfried@mh-hannover.de (W.G.); Greite.Robert@mh-hannover.de (R.G.); Kirill.Kreimann@stud.mh-hannover.de (K.K.); athorenz@gmx.de (A.T.); teng.beina@mh-hannover.de (B.T.); rong.song@mh-hannover.de (S.R.); vonvietinghoff.sibylle@mh-hannover.de (S.v.V.); haller.hermann@mh-hannover.de (H.H.); Mario.Schiffer@uk-erlangen.de (M.S.)

[2] Pediatric Nephrology, Hannover Medical School, 30625 Hannover, Germany; pape.lars@mh-hannover.de (L.P.); Lerch.christian@mh-hannover.de (C.L.)

[3] Pathology, Hannover Medical School, 30625 Hannover, Germany; Braesen.Jan@mh-hannover.de

[4] Radiology, Hannover Medical School, 30625 Hannover, Germany; derlin.katja@mh-hannover.de

[5] Laboratory Medicine & Pathology, University of Alberta, Edmonton, AB T6G 2R3, Canada; mmengel@ualberta.ca

[6] Nephrology and Hypertension, University Hospital Erlangen, 91054 Erlangen, Gerrmany

[*] Correspondence: gueler.faikah@mh-hannover.de; Tel.: +49-511-5323722; Fax: +49-511-552366

[†] These authors contributed equally to this work.

Received: 26 March 2019; Accepted: 19 May 2019; Published: 24 May 2019

Abstract: The presence of B-cell clusters in allogenic T cell-mediated rejection (TCMR) of kidney allografts is linked to more severe disease entities. In this study we characterized B-cell infiltrates in patients with TCMR and examined the role of serum CXCL-13 in these patients and experimentally. CXCL-13 serum levels were analyzed in 73 kidney allograft recipients at the time of allograft biopsy. In addition, four patients were evaluated for CXCL13 levels during the first week after transplantation. ELISA was done to measure CXCL-13 serum levels. For further mechanistic understanding, a translational allogenic kidney transplant (ktx) mouse model for TCMR was studied in BalbC recipients of fully mismatched transplants with C57BL/6 donor kidneys. CXCL-13 serum levels were measured longitudinally, CD20 and CD3 composition and CXCL13 mRNA in tissue were examined by flow cytometry and kidneys were examined by histology and immunohistochemistry. We found significantly higher serum levels of the B-cell chemoattractant CXCL13 in patients with TCMR compared to controls and patients with borderline TCMR. Moreover, in patients with acute rejection within the first week after ktx, a >5-fold CXCL13 increase was measured and correlated with B-cell infiltrates in the biopsies. In line with the clinical findings, TCMR in mice correlated with increased systemic serum-CXCL13 levels. Moreover, renal allografts had significantly higher CXCL13 mRNA expression than isogenic controls and showed interstitial CD20+ B-cell clusters and CD3+ cell infiltrates accumulating in the vicinity of renal vessels. CXCL13 blood levels correlate with B-cell involvement in TCMR and might help to identify patients at risk of a more severe clinical course of rejection.

Keywords: B-cell attracting chemokine; CXCL13; kidney transplantation; allograft rejection; T cell-mediated rejection

---

1. Introduction

Kidney allograft rejection is the major cause for loss of graft function and may have a negative impact on long-term allograft survival. Currently, besides donor specific antibodies or non-HLA antibodies, which are linked to humoral rejection, no reliable serum markers for ktx rejection exist [1,2]. Impaired allograft function with elevated serum creatinine drives the decision to perform a biopsy. The majority (about 90%) of acute rejections, especially in the first year after ktx, are T cell-mediated [3]. However, emerging evidence has revealed that intra-graft B-cell accumulation plays an important role in T cell-mediated rejection as well and correlates with a worse outcome [4–6]. However, the mechanistic details are not completely resolved. The chemokine CXC ligand 13 (CXCL13), also known as B-cell-attracting chemokine-1 (BAC-1) or B-lymphocyte-chemoattractant (BLC), is a CXC subtype member of the chemokine superfamily. CXCL13 is particularly important in the context of leukocyte recruitment and is sufficient to induce secondary lymphoid nodes [7,8]. Besides B-cell attraction CXCL13 activates different intracellular pathways that are involved in cell survival, invasion and growth and is able to stimulate resident kidney cells to produce pro-inflammatory cytokines and chemokines [7,9–11]. In sum, these biological functions of CXCL13 have led us to hypothesize that CXCL13 may also be linked to B-cell accumulation in kidney allografts in the presence of TCMR.

Here, we were able to show that CXCL13 can be monitored systemically and is elevated in TCMR compared to borderline rejection and controls. In addition, increasing CXCL13 values in the first week after ktx were indicators for acute rejection with B-cell rich infiltrates in two more patients. Furthermore, in a murine model for TCMR after ktx with similar histological TCMR patterns as in patients, we verified systemic upregulation of CXCL13 in blood as well as on an mRNA-level in the allografts. Taken together, our data indicate that CXCL13 blood levels can function as a readily available biomarker for B-cell involvement in T cell-mediated rejection and possibly as a therapeutic target.

2. Results

2.1. B-cell Involvement in Kidney Allograft Rejection in Patients

Different morphologies have been described for renal allograft rejection. We characterized different B-cell expression patterns (Figure 1A–E) in 67 randomly selected human biopsies with TCMR and graded them as B-cell rich infiltrates if more than 30 CD20+ cells were detected per high power field (HPF) (Figure 1E).

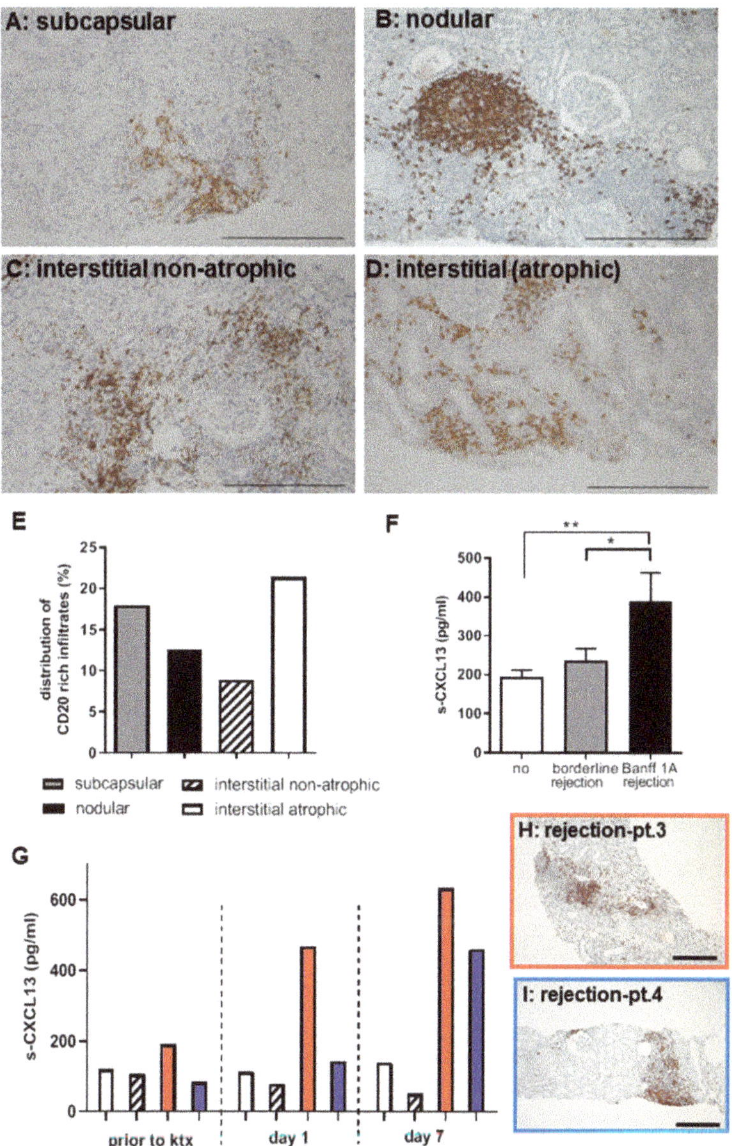

Figure 1. CD20+ cells were detected as part of inflammatory infiltrates in patient biopsies with TCMR (**A–D**, bar: 100 μm)) in subcapsular, tubular-interstitial (atrophic and non-atrophic) areas as well as in nodular infiltrates. In the non-rejection state, no CD20 positivity is detectable (data not shown). CD20+ cells were quantified in 67 randomly selected human biopsies with TCMR and graded as B-cell rich (>30 CD20-positive cells/hpf). In subcapsular infiltrates, 17.9%, in interstitial-nodular infiltrates, 12.5%, and in interstitial/atrophic areas, 21.4% were B-cell rich. The Banff-relevant interstitial non-atrophic areas contained 8.9% B-cell rich infiltrates (**E**). Serum CXCL13 levels are increased in patients with TCMR (Banff1a) compared to patients with borderline or no rejection (** $p = 0.01$; * $p = 0.05$) (**F**). Four patients had CXCL13 measurements during the first week after ktx (**G**). All had low levels of CXCL13 prior to ktx and two patients developed a relevant increase of CXCL13 levels up to day 7. Biopsy revealed a rejection with B-cell rich infiltrates (**H,I**, bar: 200 μm).

We found CD20+ rich infiltrates in 83.6% ($n = 56$) of the biopsies while only 16.4% were negative for CD20. The B-cell infiltrates were localized in the subcapsular region in 28.6% of renal biopsies, of these 17.9% contained more than 30 CD20+ cells per HPF. In 19.6% of the biopsies, interstitial-nodular infiltrates occurred, and 12.5% contained more than 30 CD20+ cells per HPF. The majority of CD20+ infiltrates was detected in interstitial/atrophic areas of biopsies (60.7%), more than 30 CD20+ cells per HPF were detected in 21.4% of the biopsies. Interestingly, the nodular infiltrates showed starry sky macrophages and signs of tertiary lymphoid organ formation (TLO) as depicted by CD3 and CD68-stains (Figure S1).

2.2. CXCL13 as a Systemic Biomarker of TCMR Rejection in Patients

Serum samples of 73 patients undergoing kidney transplant biopsies with an interval of 39–214 days after surgery ($n = 28$ with allograft rejection and $n = 45$ without rejection) were analyzed by ELISA for systemic CXCL13 expression (Figure 1F). Patient characteristics are summarized in Table 1. Serum CXCL13 was significantly higher in patients with TCMR than in the control group (rejection ($n = 10$ samples); mean 357.6 ±73.2 pg/mL versus controls ($n = 65$ samples; 211.4 ± 19 pg/mL, $p = 0.006$) and also higher compared to patients with borderline rejection ($n = 24$ samples; CXCL13: 214.2 ± 33.7 pg/mL, $p = 0.06$). No significant difference was observed between patients without rejection compared to borderline rejection. In four patients CXCL13 levels were measured longitudinally prior to ktx, at day 1 and 7 after surgery (Figure 1G). All patients had low initial CXCL13 levels and only the two patients with allograft rejection with B-cell rich infiltrates (Figure 1H,J) had >5-fold CXCL13 elevation. Allograft biopsy was indicated when serum-creatinine levels stayed high. Serum-creatinine decreased after anti-rejection therapy (serum-creatinine levels are shown in Figure S2).

Table 1. Patient characteristics (study 2001–2006).

Type of Rejection	Banff 1A or Higher	Borderline	No Rejection
Number of patients	9	19	45
Number of serum samples	10	24	65
Time between transplantation and biopsy (days; ±SD)	108.9 (±56.2)	110.4 (±59.0)	117.0 (±53.6)
Age at transplantation (years; ±SD)	54.1 (±19.6)	48.3 (±10.2)	54.5 (±12.6)
HLA-Mismatch (mean ± SD)	1.5 (±2.3)	1.9 (±1.6)	2.1 (±1.7)
Data available for the following number of patients	8 (9)	15 (19)	41 (45)
Creatinine level at time of biopsy (μmol/l; ±SD)	160.1 (±72.9)	194.0 (±91.8)	154.1 (±72.4)
Creatinine level after 1 year (μmol/l; ±SD)	156.4 (±41.1)	188.1 (±73.7)	142.2 (±63.9)
Creatinine level after 5 year (μmol/l; ±SD)	146.2 (±41.9)	196.9 (±91.5)	162.9 (±99.9)
Immunosuppression at time of biopsy			
Number of immunosuppressants (±SD)	2.2 (±0.6)	2.2 (±0.4)	2.6 (±0.6)
Data available for the following number of samples	10 (10)	23 (24)	62 (65)
Prednisolon dose (mg; ±SD)	10.5 (±5.7)	12.2 (±5.3)	9.6 (±5.4)
Cyclosporine A	50%	91.7%	88.7%
Mycophenolat mofetil	20%	25%	59.7%
Sirolimus	0%	8.3%	16.1%
Tacrolimus	30%	4.2%	3.2%
Belatacept	20%	0%	4.8%
Number of rejections (mean ± SD)	1.2 (±0.4)	0.2 (±0.4)	0 (±0)
DSA-Status	n.d.	n.d.	n.d.

2.3. Allograft Rejection in a Translational Mouse Model for TCMR

To study CXCL13 up-regulation in more detail, we investigated a well described translational mouse model of kidney transplantation. The fully mismatched B6 to BALB/c ktx resulted in TCMR and was compared to isogenic ktx (Figure 2).

Histology at three weeks after transplantation revealed Banff 1A or higher rejection in the allografts which had severe interstitial inflammation (Figure 2A–C). The majority of infiltrating cells were CD3+ (Figure 2D–F). In addition, dense, nodular CD22+ B-cell clusters around the vessels could be identified (Figure 2G–I). By flow cytometry, significantly more CD3+ T-cells and also to a lesser extent CD19+ B-cells were observed in the allografts compared to isografts (Figure 2J). In the spleen no differences between T- and B-lymphocytes from allo- or isografts were observed. When measuring systemic CXCL13 expression, a significant increase at day 6 and 14 after ktx in allograft recipients was detected (Figure 3A).

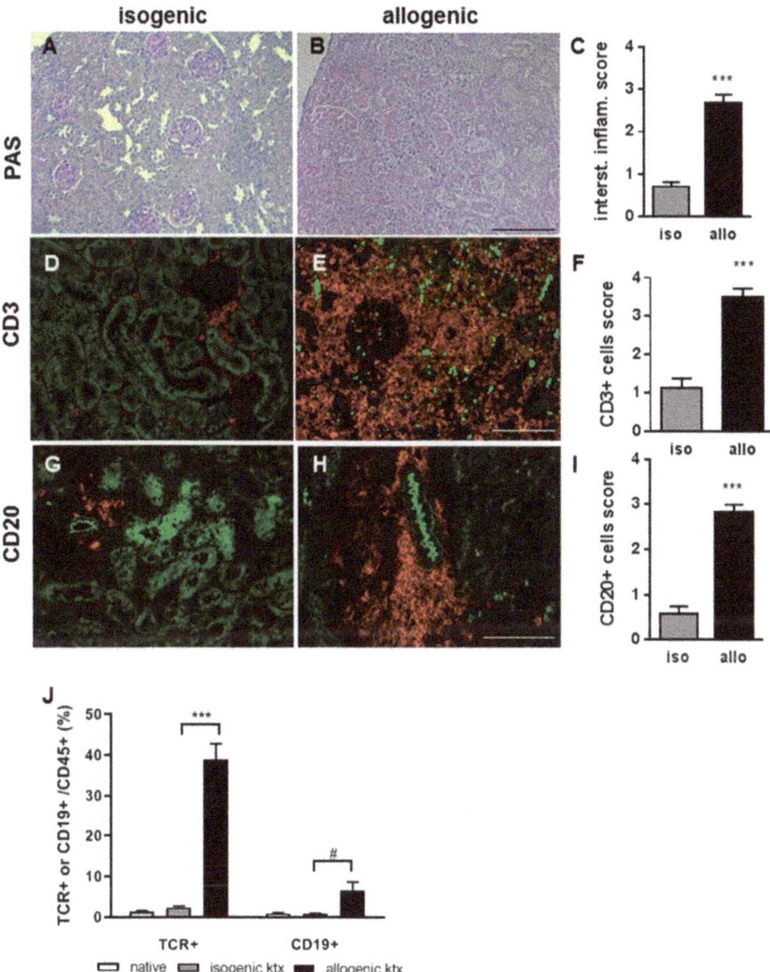

Figure 2. At three weeks after ktx, renal allograft rejection was characterized by severe inflammation and Banff 1A, and higher rejection grades in comparison to isogenic grafts without inflammation (**A–C**, representative PAS stains, bar: 200 μm). The majority of infiltration cells were CD3+ T-lymphocytes, which formed interstitial dense infiltrates and clustered around vessels and glomeruli (**D–F**, bar: 200 μm). CD20+ nodular B-cell clusters were identified with much higher cell count in allografts compared to isografts (**G–I**, bar: 100 μm). Flow cytometry of the infiltrating leukocytes of the grafts showed significantly enhanced proportion of CD3+ T-lymphocytes in allografts and also enhanced CD20+ B-lymphocytes (**J**, *** $p < 0.001$, # $p < 0.05$).

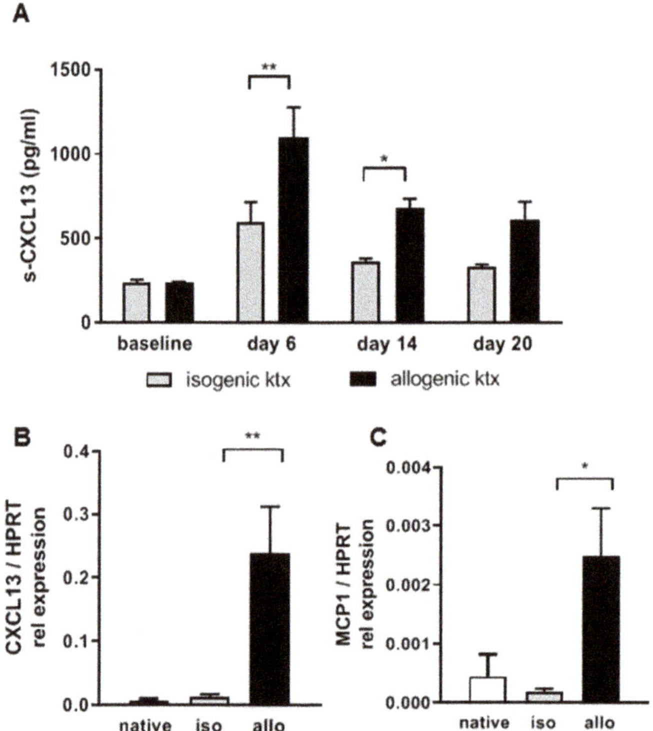

Figure 3. In the mouse ktx model, allograft recipients showed significantly increased serum CXCL13 levels towards day 6 and 14 (**A**). Rejecting kidney allografts showed significantly enhanced CXCL13 mRNA expression compared to isografts and native controls (**B**). MCP-1 mRNA was significantly up-regulated in rejecting kidneys (**C**, $n = 6$ in each group, HPRT served as house keeper, * $p < 0.05$, ** $p < 0.01$).

This was in line with the increased systemic CXCL13 levels in patients. Furthermore, in the renal tissue, significantly enhanced CXCL13 mRNA expression was detected in allografts compared to isografts (Figure 3B). As expected, the pro-inflammatory cytokine monocyte chemoattractant protein (MCP-1) was also significantly upregulated in allografts compared to isografts (Figure 3C).

3. Discussion

Kidney allograft rejection remains a major complication after transplantation along with the risk of graft loss or limited long term graft survival. The majority of rejection types in the early phase after ktx are TCMR [12]. In this context it is known that a significant proportion of TCMR cases additionally contain relevant number of B-cells in the infiltrates [13]. B-cell involvement has been linked to more severe clinical courses of allograft rejection, which were more difficult to control [13,14]. It is generally accepted that B-cells act as positive mediators of inflammation through their production of immunoglobulins and of cytokines such as IL-4 and IL-6. B-cells also support T cell activation by acting as antigen presenting cells and exacerbate renal damage through this interaction [15]. Even though the pathophysiological role is not completely resolved, the association of B-cell infiltrates and an inferior ktx outcome is beyond controversy: different clinical studies have confirmed an association of B-cell infiltrates and a worse transplant survival rate [16,17].

Previously, Steinmetz et al. described an association between CXCL13 expression and CXCR5+ and CD 20+ B-cells in acute renal transplant rejection in patients [18]. Interestingly, in the current study we were able to show that B-cells can be detected in the majority of cases with TCMR in patients. We demonstrated that B-cells were, besides localizations in the subcapsular region and the interstitium, mainly located in interstitial non-atrophic areas. Of note, the revised Banff-classification newly introduced the inflammation-interstitial fibrosis and tubular atrophy (i-IFTA) score, which recognizes inflammation within areas of fibrosis and atrophy as relevant [19].

Previously, we found that the expression of the B-cell attracting chemokine CXCL13 plays a pivotal role in patients with different B-cell mediated diseases [20]. Besides its role in B-cell homeostasis, the CXCL13/CXCR5 interaction also leads to an activation of different important intracellular pathways such as PI3K/AKT, Raf/MEK/ERK, Integrin-beta3/Scr/FAK and DOCK/Rac/JNK [7,9,10]. These pathways are involved in cell survival, invasion and growth, underlining a more complex function of CXCL13 than initially suspected. In addition, we were able to show that the chemokine CXCL13 was able to stimulate resident kidney cells to produce pro-inflammatory cytokines and chemokines [21]. These mediators lead to a neutrophil respiratory burst, indicating that CXCL13 aggravated the course of disease [21].

In the current study, we demonstrated that CXCL13 was significantly increased in the serum of patients with an acute transplant rejection. Of clinical interest, a statistically significant increase was only detected in patients with a clinically relevant rejection, but not in patients with borderline rejection [22]. In a pilot study with four patients we showed that prior to ktx, serum CXCL13 levels were low and increased due to rejection in two patients. A clinical trial is ongoing to validate CXCL13 as a biomarker for early B-cell activation and to study its relevance in the context with allograft rejection shortly after transplantation. Especially in times of organ shortage, this is of clinical interest since allograft rejections are one of the main reasons for transplant loss and early identification of patients at risk allows for early medical intervention.

The sources of CXCL13 production are not completely understood. So far, a variety of transient and non-transient cells have been shown to express CXCL13 [21,23]. Steinmetz et al. showed that CXCL13 expression is exclusively present in areas of B-cell clusters [18].

To further investigate the role of CXCL13 and B-cells in acute allograft rejection we used a well-established translational ktx mouse model of TCMR [22]. By using a non-life supporting model where one native kidney remained in situ, we were able to perform longitudinal follow up for three weeks despite ongoing TCMR. In this model, TCMR onset starts at 4–5 days after ktx and is triggered by a prolonged cold ischemia time of 60 min. Flow cytometry and immunohistochemistry showed that the main infiltrating cell type was CD3+ T-lymphocytes. However, similar to the findings in human biopsies, nodular B-cell clusters were also identified in rejecting renal allograft specimens in mice. Accordingly, enhanced CD19+ B-cell population were also identified by flow cytometry in the allografts. Interestingly, the circulating CD19+ B-cell population was reduced in allograft recipients compared to the isogenic controls. This might be explained by the fact that the B-cells were recruited into the lymphoid organs and the rejecting allograft where they form tertiary lymphoid organs [24].

Taken together, our data show that CXCL13 could serve as a relevant circulating biomarker to identify B-cell involvement in ktx recipients with TCMR and relevant B-cell involvement. CXCL13 serum levels may be a readily available surrogate marker for ktx rejection and it is tempting to speculate that CXCL13 could function as a potential therapeutic target.

4. Materials and Methods

4.1. Patient Samples

The first clinical study (2001 and 2006) was approved by the Institutional Review Board of Hannover Medical School (approval number 2765). Following informed consent, serum samples from 73 patients were collected at the time of a kidney graft biopsy. Samples for 28 patients with allograft rejection (9 patients with Bannf1A or higher and 19 with Borderline rejection) and 45 patients without rejection were collected. Some patients had repeated biopsies over time so that total sample number was (*n* = 99) (see Table 1). In addition, in an ongoing clinical study (approval number 6895) with longitudinal blood sampling prior to ktx, at day 1 and 7 after ktx we identified two patients with early rejection and two with initial function, and tested for CXCL13 levels in correlation to ktx biopsy (*n* = 4, patient characteristics are shown in Table 2). All patients had standard triple therapy with prednisolone, MMF and tacrolimus and induction therapy with basiliximab. Patient 2 had high panel reactive antibodies (77%) and received plasmapheresis at the day of ktx and afterwards. All serum samples were stored at −80°C.

Table 2. Pilot study in the early phase after ktx.

Patient Characteristics	Patient 1	Patient 2	Patient 3	Patient 4
Recipient age (years)	22	48	51	50
Hemodialysis (years)	None	6	12	12
Type of ktx	living donation	postmortal, AM-Program	postmortal	postmortal
Plasmapheresis	no	2× day 0 + 1	day 15, 16, 17	no
Delayed graft function	no	no	no	yes
Allograft biopsy (day)	n/a	n/a	10	14
In hospital stay (days)	8	8	21	14
Steroid boli for rejection treatment	n.a.	n.a.	3× 500 mg prednisolone	3× 500 mg prednisolone
Creatinine at 4 weeks after ktx (μmol/L)	145	178	162	169

4.2. CXCL13 ELISA

CXCL13 serum levels in human and mice samples were analyzed by ELISA (Quantikine Human CXCL13/BLC/BCA-1 Immunoassay Catalog Number DCX130, Quantikine Mouse CXCL13/BLC/BCA-1, Immunoassay Catalog Number MCX130), respectively, as described previously [10,20]. Color development was measured by using an ELISA reader (Tecan spectra mini, Crailsheim, Germany). The color intensity was correlated with the amounts of bound CXCL13 by comparison with internal standards.

4.3. Renal Morphology and Immunohistochemistry of Patient Allograft Biopsies

Human kidney transplant biopsies were fixed in 4% neutral buffered formaldehyde and embedded in paraffin. Two μm sections were stained for routine histochemical diagnostics (H&E, PAS, Jones Methenamine) according to standard protocols, immunohistochemical stains were performed for CD20 (Dako, clone L26, 1:500 after heat pretreatment with EDTA at pH8.4 for 16 minutes) on an automated platform (Ventana Benchmark Ultra). Normal biopsies can contain single B-cell infiltrates without any clinical relevance. Therefore, we developed a cutoff of >30 CD20+ cells per hpf for definition of relevant "B-cell rich" infiltrates. For the evaluation we used a visual analog scale that we have developed ourselves for standardized evaluation of the samples Figure S3).

4.4. Mice

Male C57Bl/6N (B6, H2b) and BALB/cAnCrl (H2d) mice (Charles River, Sulzfeld Germany) weighing 25–28 g at 10–12 weeks of age were used for all experiments. B6 mice served as donors, BALB/c mice as recipients.

4.5. Kidney Transplantation

For allogenic kidney transplantation (ktx), B6 mice served as donors and BALB/c as recipients and for isogenic controls, B6 mice served as donors and recipients. Surgeries were done in general anesthesia with isoflurane (induction 3–5% and maintenance 1.5%) by a vascular surgeon with >15 years' experience in small animal surgery. For analgesia, butorphanol (2.5 mg/kg bodyweight ip) was given prior to surgery [25]. Briefly, the kidney graft was retrieved en bloc with the renal vessels and the ureter. After left recipient nephrectomy, the kidney graft was transplanted. Vessel anastomosis with the abdominal aorta and the caval vene was done. Afterwards, the ureter was directly anastomosed into the bladder dome. Cold ischemia time was standardized to 60 min and warm ischemia time to 30 min. The prolonged cold ischemia time is needed to induce 100% allograft rejection. To overcome mortality in the allograft model, a non-live supporting model was chosen and the right native kidney remained in situ to ensure normal renal function throughout the three weeks observation time. The model has been described previously in detail by functional MRI studies [26,27]. After surgery, animals were monitored until fully awake and had free access to a standard diet (Altromin, Lippe) and tap water. Daily monitoring of physical well-being and behavior was done throughout the follow up of three weeks. Criteria for study termination were impaired food uptake, passive behavior and scrubby appearance. Animals were cared for in accordance to the national and international guidelines of animal welfare and animal protection. Ethical approval was given by the local authority (Lower Saxony Ministry for Food and Drug Safety number: 33.9-42502-04-11/0492).

4.6. Renal Morphology and Immunohistochemistry of Mouse Kidney Grafts

For mouse kidney graft histology and immunohistochemistry two µm paraffin sections were analyzed by PAS stain to define the type and degree of rejection according to the Banff classification [28]. The analysis was done without knowledge of animal group assignment by a nephropathologist with >20 years of experience. Immunohistochemistry for CD3+ T-cell (Acris Antibodies GmbH, Herford, Germany) infiltrates was done on paraffin sections. CD22+ B cells (Southern Biotech, Birmingham, AL, USA) were stained on four µm cryosections. Semi-quantitative assessment of the density of CD3+ cell infiltration was done as follows: 0 < 5 cells per view field (VF40x), 1 mild infiltration: 5–10 cells/VF, 2 moderate infiltration: 11–25 cells/VF, 3 severe: 26–50 cells/VF, 4 very severe >50 cells/VF. B-cell clusters were quantified with 0.5: single CD22+ cell, 1: B-cell cluster with 2–9 CD22+ cells, 2: B-cell cluster with 10–20 CD22+ cells, 3: B-cell cluster with >21 CD22+ cells.

4.7. Flow Cytometry

Flow cytometry of the kidney grafts, whole blood and spleen was done to characterize leukocyte subsets as described previously [27]. FACS Canto-I (BD Biosciences, San Jose, CA, USA) was used for all experiments with FACSDiva software version 6·0. Data were analyzed using WinList™ software (Verity Software House, Topsham, ME, USA). After collagen digest of the renal tissue, live death stain was done. Living leukocytes were stained by CD45+ and CD19+ B-lymphocytes and TCR+ T lymphocytes were gated from CD11b+ cells. Quantification is given in % from CD45+ cell counts.

4.8. CXCL13 Expression in Kidney Graft Tissue

After organ retrieval, tissue was immediately fixed in RNAlater. Total mRNA was extracted using the RNeasy mini kit system (Qiagen, Hilden, Germany) and transcribed with Quiagen mini kits. For quantitative PCR (qPCR), 1 µg of DNase-treated total RNA was reverse transcribed using Superscript II Reverse transcriptase (Invitrogen, Carlsbad, CA, USA) and qPCR was performed on a Lightcycler 420 II (Roche Diagnostics, Penzberg, Germany) using FastStart Sybr-Green. Gene-specific primers for CXCL13 (Primer-sequence: fwd-TCT GGA CCA AGA rev-TGA AGA AAG TT) and monocyte chemoattractant protein-1 (MCP-1; Mm_Ccl2_1_SG QuantiTect Primer Assay QT00167832) were used. Quantification was carried out using QGene software.

4.9. Statistical Analysis

For human data we used R (Version 3.3.3) for analysis [29]. As some patients were investigated more than once, we had to account for the correlated nature of the data. We used the multgee package, which applies a generalized estimating equations (GEE) approach for correlated multinomial responses using a local odds ratios parameterization [30]. Besides, statistical analysis was performed with GraphPad Prism 6.0 (GraphPad Software, Inc., La Jolla, CA, USA). One-way ANOVA for multiple comparison was used with post-hoc Tukey correction. For comparison of two groups, T-test was done. Values are expressed as mean with standard error of mean (SEM). Significance was assumed at * $p < 0.05$, ** $p < 0.01$, *** $p < 0.001$.

Supplementary Materials: Supplementary materials can be found at http://www.mdpi.com/1422-0067/20/10/2552/s1.

Author Contributions: L.S.: Research design, result evaluation, manuscript writing; F.W.: Performed experimental work-up, result evaluation, manuscript writing, approval of the manuscript; J.H.B.: Performed histology work-up and evaluation of patient ktx biopsies, approval of the manuscript; W.G.: Participated in manuscript writing; A.T.: Participated in mouse ktx analysis, discussed and approved the manuscript; R.G.: enrolled patients for the clinical study, retrieved blood samples and discussed and approved the manuscript; K.K.: measured CXCL13 ELISA, did data analysis and approved the manuscript; K.D.: discussed and approved the manuscript; B.T.: discussed and approved the manuscript; S.R.: performed ktx in mice, approved the manuscript; S.v.V.: participated in analysis of flow cytometry data, approved the manuscript; H.H.: discussed and approved the manuscript; M.M.: Analyzed mouse kidney transplants, approved the manuscript; L.P.: Participated in statistical evaluation, approved the manuscript; C.L.: Participated in statistical evaluation, approved the manuscript; M.S.: Research design, participated in result evaluation, discussed and approved the manuscript; F.G.: designed kidney transplant mouse study, result evaluation, manuscript writing.

Funding: This work was supported by the BMBF grants 01EO1302 to LS, 03INT502AB to FG and 01GM1518A and 01GM1901D to MS and the German Science Foundation grant: GU 613/1-1 to FG.

Acknowledgments: We thank Heike Lührs, Herle Chlebusch and Barbara Hertel for excellent technical support. We thank Patricia Schroder for critical reading of the manuscript.

Conflicts of Interest: The authors declare no conflict of interest.

Abbreviations

BCA	B-cell attracting chemokine
CXCL13	CXC ligand 13 protein
ktx	Kidney transplantation
allograft rejection	T cell-mediated rejection

References

1. Cardinal, H.; Dieude, M.; Hebert, M.J. The Emerging Importance of Non-HLA Autoantibodies in Kidney Transplant Complications. *J. Am. Soc. Nephrol.* **2017**, *28*, 400–406. [CrossRef] [PubMed]
2. Lefaucheur, C.; Viglietti, D.; Bouatou, Y.; Philippe, A.; Pievani, D.; Aubert, O.; Duong Van Huyen, J.P.; Taupin, J.L.; Glotz, D.; Legendre, C.; et al. Non-HLA agonistic anti-angiotensin II type 1 receptor antibodies induce a distinctive phenotype of antibody-mediated rejection in kidney transplant recipients. *Kidney Int.* **2019**. (Epub ahead of print). [CrossRef] [PubMed]
3. Sellares, J.; de Freitas, D.G.; Mengel, M.; Reeve, J.; Einecke, G.; Sis, B.; Hidalgo, L.G.; Famulski, K.; Matas, A.; Halloran, P.F. Understanding the causes of kidney transplant failure: The dominant role of antibody-mediated rejection and nonadherence. *Am. J. Transpl.* **2012**, *12*, 388–399. [CrossRef]
4. Mengel, M.; Gwinner, W.; Schwarz, A.; Bajeski, R.; Franz, I.; Brocker, V.; Becker, T.; Neipp, M.; Klempnauer, J.; Haller, H.; et al. Infiltrates in protocol biopsies from renal allografts. *Am. J. Transpl.* **2007**, *7*, 356–365. [CrossRef]
5. Hasegawa, J.; Honda, K.; Omoto, K.; Wakai, S.; Shirakawa, H.; Okumi, M.; Ishida, H.; Fuchinoue, S.; Hattori, M.; Tanabe, K. Clinical and Pathological Features of Plasma Cell-Rich Acute Rejection After Kidney Transplantation. *Transplantation* **2018**, *102*, 853–859. [CrossRef]

6. Kwun, J.; Manook, M.; Page, E.; Burghuber, C.; Hong, J.; Knechtle, S.J. Crosstalk Between T and B Cells in the Germinal Center After Transplantation. *Transplantation* **2017**, *101*, 704–712. [CrossRef]

7. Ansel, K.M.; Ngo, V.N.; Hyman, P.L.; Luther, S.A.; Forster, R.; Sedgwick, J.D.; Browning, J.L.; Lipp, M.; Cyster, J.G. A chemokine-driven positive feedback loop organizes lymphoid follicles. *Nature* **2000**, *406*, 309–314. [CrossRef]

8. Luther, S.A.; Ansel, K.M.; Cyster, J.G. Overlapping roles of CXCL13, interleukin 7 receptor alpha, and CCR7 ligands in lymph node development. *J. Exp. Med.* **2003**, *197*, 1191–1198. [CrossRef]

9. Gunn, M.D.; Ngo, V.N.; Ansel, K.M.; Ekland, E.H.; Cyster, J.G.; Williams, L.T. A B-cell-homing chemokine made in lymphoid follicles activates Burkitt's lymphoma receptor-1. *Nature* **1998**, *391*, 799–803. [CrossRef] [PubMed]

10. El-Haibi, C.P.; Singh, R.; Gupta, P.; Sharma, P.K.; Greenleaf, K.N.; Singh, S.; Lillard, J.W., Jr. Antibody Microarray Analysis of Signaling Networks Regulated by Cxcl13 and Cxcr5 in Prostate Cancer. *J. Proteom. Bioinform.* **2012**, *5*, 177–184. [CrossRef]

11. Chen, D.; Zhang, J.; Peng, W.; Weng, C.; Chen, J. Urinary CXC motif chemokine 13 is a noninvasive biomarker of antibodymediated renal allograft rejection. *Mol. Med. Rep.* **2018**, *18*, 2399–2406. [CrossRef]

12. Halloran, P.F.; Famulski, K.; Reeve, J. The molecular phenotypes of rejection in kidney transplant biopsies. *Curr. Opin. Organ Transpl.* **2015**, *20*, 359–367. [CrossRef]

13. Einecke, G.; Reeve, J.; Mengel, M.; Sis, B.; Bunnag, S.; Mueller, T.F.; Halloran, P.F. Expression of B cell and immunoglobulin transcripts is a feature of inflammation in late allografts. *Am. J. Transpl.* **2008**, *8*, 1434–1443. [CrossRef] [PubMed]

14. Carpio, V.N.; Noronha Ide, L.; Martins, H.L.; Jobim, L.F.; Gil, B.C.; Kulzer, A.S.; Loreto Mda, S.; Goncalves, L.F.; Manfro, R.C.; Veronese, F.V. Expression patterns of B cells in acute kidney transplant rejection. *Exp. Clin. Transpl.* **2014**, *12*, 405–414.

15. Firl, D.J.; Benichou, G.; Kim, J.I.; Yeh, H. A Paradigm Shift on the Question of B Cells in Transplantation? Recent Insights on Regulating the Alloresponse. *Front Immunol.* **2017**, *8*, 80. [CrossRef] [PubMed]

16. Hippen, B.E.; DeMattos, A.; Cook, W.J.; Kew, C.E., 2nd; Gaston, R.S. Association of CD20+ infiltrates with poorer clinical outcomes in acute cellular rejection of renal allografts. *Am. J. Transpl.* **2005**, *5*, 2248–2252. [CrossRef]

17. Tsai, E.W.; Rianthavorn, P.; Gjertson, D.W.; Wallace, W.D.; Reed, E.F.; Ettenger, R.B. CD20+ lymphocytes in renal allografts are associated with poor graft survival in pediatric patients. *Transplantation* **2006**, *82*, 1769–1773. [CrossRef]

18. Steinmetz, O.M.; Panzer, U.; Kneissler, U.; Harendza, S.; Lipp, M.; Helmchen, U.; Stahl, R.A. BCA-1/CXCL13 expression is associated with CXCR5-positive B-cell cluster formation in acute renal transplant rejection. *Kidney Int.* **2005**, *67*, 1616–1621. [CrossRef] [PubMed]

19. Loupy, A.; Haas, M.; Solez, K.; Racusen, L.; Glotz, D.; Seron, D.; Nankivell, B.J.; Colvin, R.B.; Afrouzian, M.; Akalin, E.; et al. The Banff 2015 Kidney Meeting Report: Current Challenges in Rejection Classification and Prospects for Adopting Molecular Pathology. *Am. J. Transpl.* **2017**, *17*, 28–41. [CrossRef]

20. Schiffer, L.; Henke-Gendo, C.; Wilsdorf, N.; Hussein, K.; Pape, L.; Schmitt, C.; Haller, H.; Schiffer, M.; Klein, C.; Kreipe, H.; et al. CXCL13 as a novel marker for diagnosis and disease monitoring in pediatric PTLD. *Am. J. Transpl.* **2012**, *12*, 1610–1617. [CrossRef]

21. Worthmann, K.; Gueler, F.; von Vietinghoff, S.; Davalos-Misslitz, A.; Wiehler, F.; Davidson, A.; Witte, T.; Haller, H.; Schiffer, M.; Falk, C.S.; et al. Pathogenetic role of glomerular CXCL13 expression in lupus nephritis. *Clin. Exp. Immunol.* **2014**, *178*, 20–27. [CrossRef] [PubMed]

22. Gueler, F.; Rong, S.; Gwinner, W.; Mengel, M.; Brocker, V.; Schon, S.; Greten, T.F.; Hawlisch, H.; Polakowski, T.; Schnatbaum, K.; et al. Complement 5a receptor inhibition improves renal allograft survival. *J. Am. Soc. Nephrol.* **2008**, *19*, 2302–2312. [CrossRef] [PubMed]

23. Ishikawa, S.; Nagai, S.; Sato, T.; Akadegawa, K.; Yoneyama, H.; Zhang, Y.Y.; Onai, N.; Matsushima, K. Increased circulating CD11b+CD11c+ dendritic cells (DC) in aged BWF1 mice which can be matured by TNF-alpha into BLC/CXCL13-producing DC. *Eur. J. Immunol.* **2002**, *32*, 1881–1887. [CrossRef]

24. Xu, X.; Han, Y.; Wang, Q.; Cai, M.; Qian, Y.; Wang, X.; Huang, H.; Xu, L.; Xiao, L.; Shi, B. Characterisation of Tertiary Lymphoid Organs in Explanted Rejected Donor Kidneys. *Immunol. Invest.* **2016**, *45*, 38–51. [CrossRef]

25. Rong, S.; Lewis, A.G.; Kunter, U.; Haller, H.; Gueler, F. A knotless technique for kidney transplantation in the mouse. *J. Transpl.* **2012**, *2012*, 127215. [CrossRef]

26. Gueler, F.; Shushakova, N.; Mengel, M.; Hueper, K.; Chen, R.; Liu, X.; Park, J.K.; Haller, H.; Wensvoort, G.; Rong, S. A novel therapy to attenuate acute kidney injury and ischemic allograft damage after allogenic kidney transplantation in mice. *PLoS ONE* **2015**, *10*, e0115709. [CrossRef]

27. Hueper, K.; Gutberlet, M.; Brasen, J.H.; Jang, M.S.; Thorenz, A.; Chen, R.; Hertel, B.; Barrmeyer, A.; Schmidbauer, M.; Meier, M.; et al. Multiparametric Functional MRI: Non-Invasive Imaging of Inflammation and Edema Formation after Kidney Transplantation in Mice. *PLoS ONE* **2016**, *11*, e0162705. [CrossRef] [PubMed]

28. Haas, M.; Sis, B.; Racusen, L.C.; Solez, K.; Glotz, D.; Colvin, R.B.; Castro, M.C.; David, D.S.; David-Neto, E.; Bagnasco, S.M.; et al. Banff 2013 meeting report: Inclusion of c4d-negative antibody-mediated rejection and antibody-associated arterial lesions. *Am. J. Transpl.* **2014**, *14*, 272–283. [CrossRef] [PubMed]

29. Team, R.C. *A Language and Environment for Statistical Computing*; R Foundation for Statistical Computing: Vienna, Austria; Available online: https://www.R-project.org (accessed on 1 May 2018).

30. Touloumis, A. R Package multgee: A Generalized Estimating Equations Solver for Multinomial Responses. *J. Stat. Softw.* **2015**, *64*, 1–14. [CrossRef]

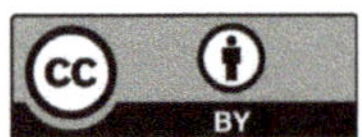

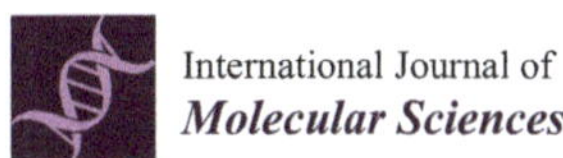
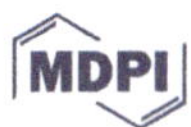

Communication

Noninvasive Urinary Monitoring of Progression in IgA Nephropathy

Joshua Y. C. Yang [1,2], Reuben D. Sarwal [1], Fernando C. Fervenza [3], Minnie M. Sarwal [1,2,*] and Richard A. Lafayette [4,*]

1   Department of Surgery, University of California San Francisco, San Francisco, CA 94143, USA
2   KIT Bio, 665 3rd St, Suite 280, San Francisco, CA 94107, USA
3   Division of Nephrology and Hypertension, Mayo Clinic, Rochester, MN 55905, USA
4   Division of Nephrology and Hypertension, Stanford University, Stanford, CA 94305, USA
*   Correspondence: minnie.sarwal@ucsf.edu (M.M.S.); czar@stanford.edu (R.A.L.)

Received: 26 July 2019; Accepted: 7 September 2019; Published: 10 September 2019

Abstract: Standard methods for detecting and monitoring of IgA nephropathy (IgAN) have conventionally required kidney biopsies or suffer from poor sensitivity and specificity. The Kidney Injury Test (KIT) Assay of urinary biomarkers has previously been shown to distinguish between various kidney pathologies, including chronic kidney disease, nephrolithiasis, and transplant rejection. This validation study uses the KIT Assay to investigate the clinical utility of the non-invasive detection of IgAN and predicting the progression of renal damage over time. The study design benefits from longitudinally collected urine samples from an investigator-initiated, multicenter, prospective study, evaluating the efficacy of corticosteroids versus Rituximab for preventing progressive IgAN. A total of 131 urine samples were processed for this study; 64 urine samples were collected from 34 IgAN patients, and urine samples from 64 demographically matched healthy controls were also collected; multiple urinary biomarkers consisting of cell-free DNA, methylated cell-free DNA, DMAIMO, MAMIMO, total protein, clusterin, creatinine, and CXCL10 were measured by the microwell-based KIT Assay. An IgA risk score (KIT-IgA) was significantly higher in IgAN patients as compared to healthy control (87.76 vs. 14.03, $p < 0.0001$) and performed better than proteinuria in discriminating between the two groups. The KIT Assay biomarkers, measured on a spot random urine sample at study entry could distinguish patients likely to have progressive renal dysfunction a year later. These data support the pursuit of larger prospective studies to evaluate the predictive performance of the KIT-IgA score in both screening for non-invasive diagnosis of IgAN, and for predicting risk of progressive renal disease from IgA and utilizing the KIT score for potentially evaluating the efficacy of IgAN-targeted therapies.

Keywords: IgA nephropathy; KIT assay; KIT-IgA score; noninvasive; diagnostics; prediction

---

1. Introduction

IgA nephropathy (IgAN) remains the most common type of primary chronic glomerulonephritis worldwide [1]. Its prevalence varies among different groups of people, where IgAN makes up about 20–40% of primary glomerular disease in Asia, and about 15–20% in Northern Europe [2]. The onset of IgAN may occur at any age, but the condition most frequently develops in patients in their second and third decades of life [3]. Many patients who present with mild symptoms will not require treatment, though they will be monitored for disease progression, but up to 40% of patients with IgAN will eventually develop end-stage renal disease [1]. Trials have established the benefit of agents that antagonize the renin-angiotensin-aldosterone system (RAAS) in reducing or delaying progression, but even patients treated with RAAS blockade still face deterioration of their kidney function over time [4]. One major issue in the treatment of IgAN is that there are few biomarkers that can predict progression of disease and monitor the efficacy of treatment [5].

Currently, IgAN is diagnosed by renal biopsy which is often performed to confirm causes of mild urinary abnormalities, particularly hematuria; however, biopsies are invasive procedures [6] that carry the risk for complications such as bleeding, and the majority of cases of microscopic hematuria are not associated with any kidney pathology. Recent advances in the analysis of the urinary proteome suggest that the excreted polypeptides include disease-specific patterns [7] and as such, much of the current research has investigated urinary biomarkers of IgA-associated glomerulonephritides. Biomarkers such as urinary neutrophil gelatinase-associated lipocalin or cystatin C [8] and protein/polypeptide patterns [9] have been studied in IgAN; however, their discriminative abilities appear modest and many studies exclude patients undergoing treatment, thus limiting any determination of the monitoring utility of such biomarkers. As a result, there exists a need for a reliable and non-invasive method to diagnose and monitor IgAN, especially in the context of treatment.

Recently, the Kidney Injury Test (KIT) Assay was developed by our group as a noninvasive test to measure kidney injury and function in the context of chronic kidney disease [10], nephrolithiasis [11], and transplant rejection [12]. The KIT Assay measures a panel of urinary biomarkers in a microwell-based format that were identified through a combination of proteomics, genomics, and metabolomics approaches [13–15] to be the most sensitive indicators of various etiologies of kidney injury and functional changes. In this investigator-initiated, multicenter, prospective study, we investigated the utility of the KIT Assay, a urine-based, microwell format assay for the detection of patients with IgAN who were treated with standard of care or with Rituximab. We additionally investigated the utility of the KIT-IgA score to predict progression of renal functional decline longitudinally on a subset of these patients who had longitudinally collected samples.

2. Results

2.1. Study Design and Patient Disposition

Sixty-nine spot urine samples were collected from 34 enrolled patients in the IgAN clinical trial over the study follow-up of 1 year (Figure 1). Patients were randomized at study entry 1:1, to receive either standard of care (corticosteroids) or Rituximab. Patients had biopsy-confirmed IgAN at study entry and serial urine samples were collected at study entry, 6 and 12 months. Two or more samples were available from 25 patients, and a complete set of three time-points were available from 14 patients. The baseline characteristics and disposition of the 34 patients are listed in Table 1.

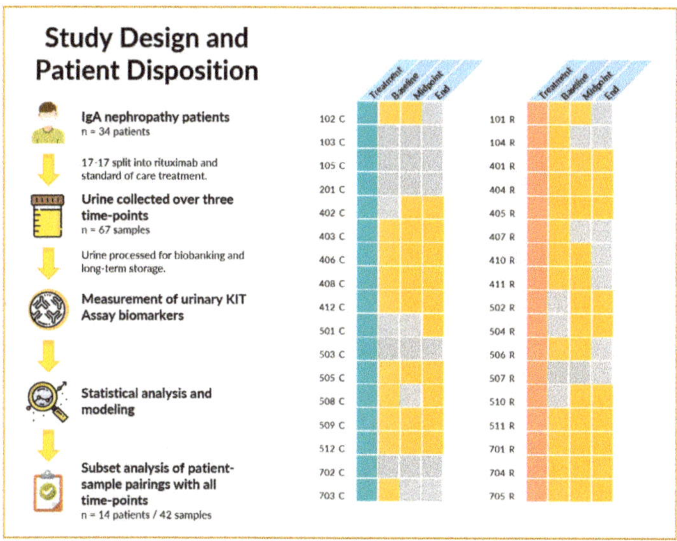

Figure 1. Study design and patient disposition. (Left) In the original trial, 34 patients met inclusion criteria and were randomized into Rituximab and standard of care treatment groups. At least one urine sample was available from 28 of the 34 patients, with 14 having urine samples at all three designated time-points. (Right) Pictorial depiction of patients, treatment, and sample availability. Patients were segregated based on treatment, either with standard of care (turquoise) or Rituximab (coral), with individual patients as rows. A yellow square indicates a urine sample was available at the indicated time-point, while gray indicates that no urine sample was available for analysis due to failure to collect or insufficient sample volume.

Table 1. Baseline characteristics of IgA nephropathy (IgAN) patients.

Baseline Characteristics	IgA Cohort (n = 34) [1]
Age, years	40 (21–63)
Sex	
• Female	9
• Male	25
Race	
• Caucasian	24
• Asian/Pacific Islander	6
• Hispanic/Latino	3
• African American	1
Weight, kg	89.7 (57–120)
eGFR, mL/min per 1.73 m^2	49 (30–122)
Treatment	
• Rituximab	17
• Standard of Care	17

[1] Data are reported as median (range) or count. n indicates the number of patients in the cohort.

As concluded by the original study, and as shown in Figure 2, there was no statistically significant difference between the change in eGFR over the course of the study by treatment with Rituximab (coral) over standard of care (teal). However, while some patients maintained or even recovered kidney function as seen in an increase in eGFR, some patients had IgAN progression with functional decline. This finding motivated us to investigate whether the KIT Assay biomarkers could be used to not only detect IgA nephropathy through urine alone, but also predict and monitor kidney function changes longitudinally.

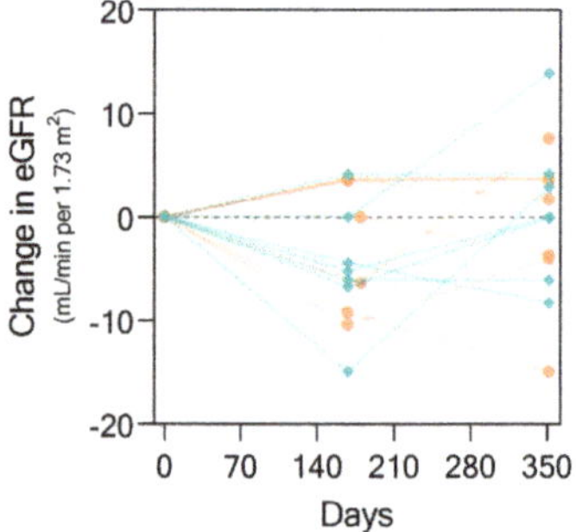

Figure 2. Changes in eGFR (by Modification of Diet in Renal Disease (MDRD) [16]) from baseline. Data shown here for the change in eGFR values over the time-course of the study for a subset of 14 patients who had complete urine samples collected at all three study time-points. Each line represents an individual patient trajectory. Trajectories in teal represent patients who received standard of care while those in salmon represent those who received Rituximab.

2.2. The KIT Assay Biomarkers Can Discriminate Healthy Controls from Patients with IgA Nephropathy

Urine samples from 64 healthy control patients were assessed and compared to those collected from the IgA nephropathy patients for the KIT biomarkers. A KIT-IgA risk score, ranging from 0 to 100, was developed on these biomarkers using a Bootstrap Forest ensemble model. The KIT-IgA scores for each of the patients in the two groups are depicted in Figure 3A. The KIT-IgA score could distinguish between healthy controls (median 14.03, 95% CI 8.94–18.52) and IgA patients (median 87.76, 95% CI 83.39–90.32) ($p < 0.0001$). Receiver–operator characteristic curves (Figure 3B) comparing the discrimination abilities of the IgA risk score and proteinuria identifies the IgA risk score (AUC 0.9935, 95% CI 0.985–1.000) as performing better than proteinuria (AUC 0.9100, 95% CI 0.855–0.965), suggesting that the KIT-IgA risk score is more sensitive and may detect IgAN earlier than proteinuria. For the KIT-IgA risk score, the sensitivity and specificity were 95.5% and 98.4% respectively.

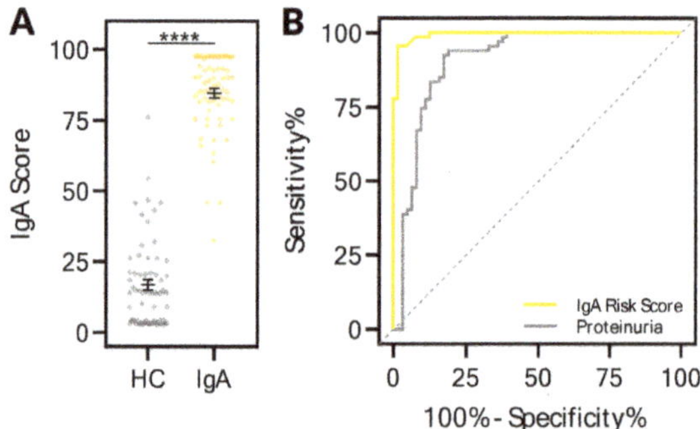

Figure 3. The urinary KIT biomarkers could segregate healthy controls from those with IgA nephropathy. (**A**) An IgA risk score ranging from 0 to 100 segregated healthy control patients from those with IgA nephropathy. Urine samples were collected from healthy controls ($n = 64$) who had no evidence of kidney disease or injury as assessed by both absence of proteinuria and eGFR greater than 120. All urine samples from IgA patients ($n = 67$) were used, as none of these patients had remission of IgA during the treatment duration. (**B**) Receiver–operator characteristic (ROC) curves of the IgA risk score with AUC of 0.994 ($p < 0.0001$) and proteinuria. For the IgA risk score, the sensitivity and specificity were 95.5% and 98.4% respectively. **** $p < 0.0001$.

2.3. The KIT Assay Biomarkers Can Discriminate Progressors from Non-Progressors and Predict Progression

We further investigated whether the KIT Assay biomarkers and the KIT-IgA score could distinguish progressors versus non-progressors. Progression was assessed based on a composite clinical evaluation of changes in proteinuria and eGFR from baseline (>50% increase in proteinuria and/or a 25% reduction in eGFR) and, as such, was dependent on both urine and serum biomarker values. We first sought to investigate whether urinary biomarkers alone could be used to classify progressor status. Looking at the 1-year endpoint biomarkers (Figure 4A), progressor status could be classified using nominal logistic regression with 100% accuracy based on urinary measurements alone ($p = 0.0154$). We then investigated whether midpoint (0.5 year prior to progression determination) and baseline (1 year prior) urinary biomarkers could predict progression status. We found that the KIT-IgA score could predict progressor status with 100% accuracy at both time-points (midpoint $p = 0.0269$, baseline $p = 0.0383$). For both the baseline and midpoint predictions, the cfDNA values were the most important predictors, with chi square likelihood ratios of 25.92 and 141.98, respectively, and with $p < 0.0001$ for both. However, neither baseline nor midpoint proteinuria alone could predict progression (Figure 4B). As the progressor definition was based on a composite of proteinuria and eGFR changes, there was no expectation that endpoint proteinuria alone could predict progressor status, as reflected in the probabilities. We further assessed the ability of the baseline urinary biomarkers to predict progression status on the entire set of patients who had baseline urine samples, regardless of the presence of additional longitudinal samples. For these 23 urine-patient pairs, the results were similar to the original analysis in that the KIT biomarkers could segregate progressors from non-progressors with 100% accuracy ($p < 0.0001$) (ROC AUC = 1.00).

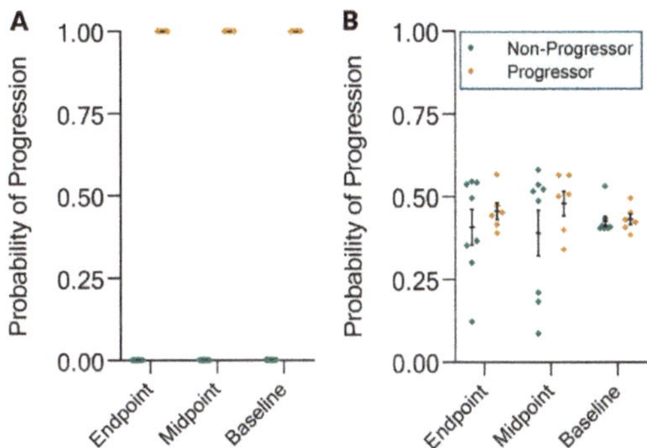

Figure 4. KIT Assay biomarker modeling of progression status after one year of treatment. Modeling was performed on endpoint, midpoint, and baseline biomarker data on either (**A**) the set of KIT Assay biomarkers or (**B**) proteinuria alone. The y-axis shows the probability of progression as determined by a nominal logistic regression model.

3. Materials and Methods

3.1. Patients and Study Characteristics

Samples were those from a study done in 2017 (NCT00498368) and the study was registered with clinicaltrials.gov [17]. Patient inclusion and exclusion criteria were as described in the previous study. Subjects included adults, ages 18–70 years old, with biopsy-proven IgAN within 2 years of enrollment were included. Patients were excluded if their biopsy showed >50% glomerular sclerosis or interstitial fibrosis or >10% glomerular crescents. Subjects were then randomly assigned to receive Rituximab or continue standard care. Baseline Oxford classification score [18] was recorded in blinded fashion by an expert renal pathologist. eGFR (by Modification of Diet in Renal Disease (MDRD) [16]) or measured creatinine clearance had to be <90 and >30 mL/min per 1.73 m^2. To establish continued risk, baseline proteinuria needed to be >1000 mg/day while on stable doses of angiotensin-converting enzyme inhibitor, angiotensin receptor blocker, or renin inhibitor therapy for at least 2 months. However, patients who were on dual therapy with agents that inhibit angiotensin II required a lower proteinuria threshold of >500 mg/day. Baseline BP was controlled to <130/80 mmHg. Patients with secondary forms of IgAN, such as cirrhosis, were excluded, although subjects with Henoch–Schönlein purpura nephritis (HSPN) could be included. Patients were excluded if they had previously received Rituximab, were receiving other immunosuppressive therapy, or had ever received >6 months of prednisone or other systemic corticosteroid therapy in the past. There was no corticosteroid exposure within 3 months of study initiation. Randomization was done centrally by a random assignment by prefilled envelopes. The protocol was approved by the institutional review board of each participating center. The study was registered with clinicaltrials.gov, protocol NCT00498368. Informed consent was obtained before all study procedures, and the study adhered to the Declaration of Helsinki.

The primary outcome measures were the change in proteinuria and the change in eGFR from baseline to 12 months. The secondary outcome was safety related, comparing overall adverse events and monitoring for potential intervention-specific complications, such as infusion-related reactions, hypogammaglobulinemia, and infections. Progression was defined as a >50% increase in proteinuria and/or a 25% reduction in eGFR at the one-year time-point. Results showed that treatment with Rituximab resulted in statistically insignificant changes in proteinuria or partial remissions that could not be distinguished from the response to supportive therapy alone.

For the healthy control cohort, urine samples were collected from healthy controls ($n = 64$) who had no evidence of kidney disease or injury as assessed by both absence of proteinuria and eGFR greater than 120. Demographics of this cohort include a median age of 24 (range 2 to 64), median weight of 57.5 kg (range 13.7 to 120.2), 53.1% female, 9.4% African American, and median eGFR of 132 (range 120 to 213).

3.2. Urine Sample Processing

Voided urine samples were collected in sterile containers. Urine samples were centrifuged at $2000\times g$ for 30 min at 4 °C. The supernatant was separated from the urine pellet containing cells and cell debris. The pH of the supernatant was adjusted to 7.0 using Tris-HCl and stored at −80 °C in the UCSF Biorepository until further analysis.

3.3. KIT Assay Biomarkers

Measurement of the KIT Assay biomarkers was performed as previously described [10]. Total protein was measured using the Pierce™ Coomassie Plus Assay Kit (Thermo Fisher Scientific, Waltham, MA, USA). Urinary creatinine was measured using the Creatinine Assay Kit (BioAssay Systems, Hayward, CA, USA) as a method for urinary concentration and hydration status normalization. Briefly, cell-free DNA (cfDNA), methylated cell-free DNA (m-cfDNA), CXCL10, Clusterin, (Dimethylamino)iminomethyl-ornithine (DMAIMO), and (Methylamino)(methylimino)methyl-ornithine (MAMIMO), were measured using the KIT Assay (KIT Bio, San Francisco, CA, USA), a set of in-house developed ELISA assays. Microwell plate readings were measured using a SpectraMax iD3 Multi-Mode Microplate Reader (Molecular Devices, San Jose, CA, USA). All assays were run in duplicates.

3.4. Statistical Analysis

Comparisons involving two groups were performed using the nonparametric Mann–Whitney U test. Comparisons involving three groups were performed using the nonparametric Kruskal–Wallis test with Dunn's post-hoc multiple comparisons correction. The IgA risk score was determined using a Bootstrap Forest ensemble model by averaging numerous decision trees each fit to a bootstrap sample of the training data. The final prediction is the average of the predicted values over all the decision trees. Specifically, six trees were used in the forest, with a minimum of ten splits per tree and a minimum size split of five. The number of splits for trees 1–6 were 9, 17, 15, 7, 13, and 11 respectively. The top contributing biomarkers as based on G^2 were total protein, MAMIMO, creatinine, and DMAIMO, with G^2 values of 36.02, 21.12, 9.72, and 6.74 respectively. The overall statistics for the Entropy R^2 was 0.7422, Generalized R^2 was 0.8568, and Root Mean Square Error (RMSE) was 0.1996.

Modeling of progressor status was done using nominal logistic regression. All analyses were performed using either GraphPad Prism 8.0.2 (GraphPad Software, Carlsbad, CA, USA) or JMP 14.3 (SAS Institute, Cary, NC, USA).

4. Discussion

In this study, we used urine samples from IgA nephropathy (IgAN) patients to evaluate the predictive capacity of the KIT Assay biomarkers to discriminate IgAN from healthy controls as well as predict progression of renal functional decline. Our results show that these urinary biomarkers could distinguish between healthy control patients and those with IgAN better than urinary protein alone. Furthermore, the biomarkers could predict progressor status up to one year in advance of status determination while urinary protein could not.

Such findings are important because IgAN is the most prevalent chronic glomerular disease worldwide [19], with diagnosis historically requiring kidney biopsy. While recent studies have identified serum and urinary biomarkers that can diagnose IgAN with high accuracy [7,8,20], the clinical utility of individual biomarkers is limited by the high overlap between the healthy and diseased ranges of these biomarkers in an individual and temporal manner. Such biomarkers, while indicative of IgAN, have shown less utility in predicting progression of disease. While some studies have suggested the use of GC–MS and similar technologies to identify a panel of biomarkers, these proteomic studies are not easily transferrable to the clinical setting. Identifying biomarkers that not only can identify IgAN but can also predict progression is important for the future development and evaluation of therapies that seek to treat and prevent functional decline in IgAN.

The multi-hit hypothesis for the pathogenesis of IgA nephropathy is the leading theory behind the mechanism of progression [20]. In this hypothesis, deposition of IgA1-containing circulating immune complexes in the glomeruli induce renal injury by subsequent induction of local cytokine, growth factor, and complement system production and activation [21–24]. While currently approved therapies for IgAN are largely non-IgAN specific and consist of supportive therapy with corticosteroids and blood pressure control [25], future directed therapies targeting the specific "hits" in IgAN will address these acute causes of glomerular injury. Monitoring the efficacy of such therapies will require biomarkers that not only reflect kidney function, but also convey the acute status of kidney injury and resolution of that injury.

We had previously validated the utility of the biomarkers comprising the KIT Assay in chronic kidney disease [10], chronic lung transplant rejection [26,27], nephrolithiasis [11], and kidney transplant rejection [12,28], suggesting its utility across a range of diseases and chronicity states. The KIT Assay biomarkers are measured in a microwell format, contributing to their ease of use and deployment. Additionally, urine is a completely noninvasive biofluid that is available in virtually unlimited quantities, enabling a frequency of monitoring that can be adjusted to the functional status of the patient. Due to the acute and chronic injury mechanism present in IgAN [29], we investigated whether the KIT Assay biomarkers could also be applied to detection of IgAN as well as prediction of progression status.

We have discussed the rationale of the KIT Assay biomarkers previously [10], with selection of these biomarkers due to the various temporal and regional differences in levels as dependent upon renal injury and function. While proteinuria has been shown to be a predictor of outcome in IgAN [30] and is a commonly used endpoint, proteinuria did not perform as well as the composite IgA risk score in discriminating patients with IgAN from healthy controls, likely because many patients with IgAN present with low levels of proteinuria despite disease progression [31]. That the KIT-IgA risk score could identify IgAN more accurately is likely due to the composite integration of functional, injury, and renal-specific markers that may reflect IgAN across a spectrum of disease states.

Further, proteinuria alone was not a significant predictor for progression at one-year of treatment duration measured at either the baseline or midpoint time-points. It is notable that the cfDNA values at baseline and midpoint were the strongest predictors of progression at the one-year timepoint. Urinary cfDNA has been previously reported to be a sensitive indicator of kidney injury and reflects ongoing damage to the kidney prior to functional changes or decline [15,32,33]. This finding is in concordance with these reports, suggesting that while progression may be defined by functional measures such as eGFR and proteinuria, the underlying cause of such progression may be acute injury such as that measured by cfDNA burden. As such, measurement of cfDNA, as done in the KIT Assay, may be beneficial for measuring the efficacy of treatment in IgAN.

In summary, our data indicate that the non-invasive KIT Assay panel of urinary biomarkers can distinguish between healthy controls and patients with IgAN. Furthermore, this panel could monitor progression of disease and changes in kidney function. We believe that the KIT-IgA score would have great utility in (1) screening for IgAN in patients with hematuria, as a replacement for biopsy as done in many Asian countries; (2) diagnosis; (3) monitoring efficacy of treatment; and (4) predicting progression and monitoring disease activity. While our sample size is limited by the small size of the parent study, these results add to a growing body of evidence of the generalizability and utility of the KIT Assay biomarkers in renal disease and beyond. Additionally, while all comparisons in this study were between healthy control and IgAN patients, we have planned additional studies where we will include samples from patients with other types of renal diseases so that we can assess the performance of these and other biomarkers in discriminating IgAN from other nephropathies. Future studies using additional kidney disease cohorts will clarify whether there is a specific pattern among these biomarkers to discriminate one disease from another. Future multi-center, prospective studies are planned to further build on the clinical utility of these observations to assess serial performance of the KIT assay in IgAN patients as a non-invasive tool to monitor disease progression and evaluate the efficacy of new reno-protective therapies for IgA disease.

Author Contributions: M.M.S. and R.A.L. designed the study and experiments; J.Y.C.Y. and R.D.S. carried out experiments; J.Y.C.Y., M.M.S., and R.A.L. analyzed the data; J.Y.C.Y. made the figures; J.Y.C.Y., R.D.S., F.C.F., M.M.S., and R.A.L. drafted and revised the paper; all authors revised the manuscript critically for important intellectual content and approved the final version of the manuscript. R.A.L. had full access to all the data in the study and takes responsibility for the integrity of the data and the accuracy of the data analysis.

Funding: This research and the APC was funded by Genentech, grant number 249 (ML 01579), via an Investigator initiated study award to Minnie Sarwal linked to the parent IgA clinical IST trial. This research was funded by the Sarwal Laboratory of the University of California, San Francisco (UCSF), via startup funding.

Acknowledgments: We are grateful for the help from physicians, clinical coordinators, research personnel, patients, and patient families.

Conflicts of Interest: The samples from the patient cohort in this study came from an investigator-initiated study sponsored by Genentech/Roche, Inc. and the Fulk Family Foundation. The sponsors had no role in study design, protocol development, data analysis, or preparation of the manuscript. M.M.S. and J.Y.C.Y. are founders of KIT Bio, Inc. (San Francisco, CA), now operating under NephroSant, IP for which is exclusively owned by the Regents, University of California San Francisco and licensed to KIT Bio. R.L. is a scientific advisor of KIT Bio. All other authors declare no conflict of interest.

Abbreviations

AUC	area-under-curve
BMI	body mass index
cfDNA	cell-free deoxyribonucleic acid
DMAIMO	(dimethylamino)iminomethyl-ornithine
eGFR	estimated glomerular filtration rate
GC–MS	gas chromatography–mass spectrometry
HSPN	Henoch–Schönlein purpura nephritis
IgAN	immunoglobulin alpha nephropathy
KIT	Kidney Injury Test

m-cfDNA	methylated cfDNA
MAMIMO	(methylamino)(methylimino)methyl-ornithine
MDRD	Modification of Diet in Renal Disease
RAAS	renin–angiotensin–aldosterone system
ROC	Receiver-operator characteristic

References

1. Wyatt, R.J.; Julian, B.A. IgA Nephropathy. *N. Engl. J. Med.* **2013**, *368*, 2402–2414. [CrossRef]
2. D'Amico, G. Clinical features and natural history in adults with IgA nephropathy. *Am. J. Kidney Dis.* **1988**, *12*, 353–357. [CrossRef]
3. Yap, H.K.; Quek, C.M.; Shen, Q.; Joshi, V.; Chia, K.S. Role of urinary screening programmes in children in the prevention of chronic kidney disease. *Ann. Acad. Med. Singap.* **2005**, *34*, 3–7. [PubMed]
4. Boyd, J.K.; Cheung, C.K.; Molyneux, K.; Feehally, J.; Barratt, J. An update on the pathogenesis and treatment of IgA nephropathy. *Kidney Int.* **2012**, *81*, 833–843. [CrossRef] [PubMed]
5. Maixnerova, D.; Reily, C.; Bian, Q.; Neprasova, M.; Novak, J.; Tesar, V. Markers for the progression of IgA nephropathy. *J. Nephrol.* **2016**, *29*, 535–541. [CrossRef]
6. Donadio, J.V.; Joseph, P. Grande IgA Nephropathy. *N. Engl. J. Med.* **2002**, *347*, 738–748. [CrossRef] [PubMed]
7. Julian, B.A.; Wittke, S.; Haubitz, M.; Zürbig, P.; Schiffer, E.; McGuire, B.M.; Wyatt, R.J.; Novak, J. Urinary biomarkers of IgA nephropathy and other IgA-associated renal diseases. *World J. Urol.* **2007**, *25*, 467–476. [CrossRef] [PubMed]
8. Ding, H.; He, Y.; Li, K.; Yang, J.; Li, X.; Lu, R.; Gao, W. Urinary neutrophil gelatinase-associated lipocalin (NGAL) is an early biomarker for renal tubulointerstitial injury in IgA nephropathy. *Clin. Immunol.* **2007**, *123*, 227–234. [CrossRef] [PubMed]
9. Haubitz, M.; Wittke, S.; Weissinger, E.M.; Walden, M.; Rupprecht, H.D.; Floege, J.; Haller, H.; Mischak, H. Urine protein patterns can serve as diagnostic tools in patients with IgA nephropathy. *Kidney Int.* **2005**, *67*, 2313–2320. [CrossRef]
10. Watson, D.; Yang, J.Y.C.; Sarwal, R.D.; Sigdel, T.K.; Liberto, J.M.; Damm, I.; Louie, V.; Sigdel, S.; Livingstone, D.; Soh, K.; et al. A Novel Multi-Biomarker Assay for Non-Invasive Detection and Quantitative Monitoring of Kidney Injury. *J. Clin. Med.* **2019**, *8*, 499. [CrossRef]
11. Yang, J.Y.C.; Sarwal, R.D.; Ky, K.; Dong, V.; Stoller, M.; Watson, D.; Sarwal, M.M.; Chi, T. Non-Radiologic Assessment of Kidney Stones by KIT, a Spot Urine Assay. *Br. J. of Urol. Int.* **2019**. under review.
12. Yang, J.Y.C.; Sarwal, R.D.; Sigdel, T.K.; Sarwal, M.M. Predicting Transplant Rejection by a Composite Urinary Injury Score. *Am. J. Transpl.* **2019**, *17*, 519.
13. Sigdel, T.K.; Gao, Y.; He, J.; Wang, A.; Nicora, C.D.; Fillmore, T.L.; Shi, T.; Webb-Robertson, B.-J.; Smith, R.D.; Qian, W.-J.; et al. Mining the human urine proteome for monitoring renal transplant injury. *Kidney Int.* **2016**, *89*, 1244–1252. [CrossRef] [PubMed]
14. Yang, J.Y.C.; Sigdel, T.K.; Sarwal, M.M. Self-antigens and rejection: A proteomic analysis. *Curr. Opin. Organ Transpl.* **2016**, *21*, 362–367. [CrossRef] [PubMed]
15. Yang, J.Y.C.; Sarwal, M.M. Transplant genetics and genomics. *Nat. Rev. Genet.* **2017**, *18*, 309–326. [CrossRef] [PubMed]
16. Levey, A.S.; Bosch, J.P.; Lewis, J.B.; Greene, T.; Rogers, N.; Roth, D. A more accurate method to estimate glomerular filtration rate from serum creatinine: A new prediction equation. Modification of Diet in Renal Disease Study Group. *Ann. Intern. Med.* **1999**, *130*, 461–470. [CrossRef]
17. Lafayette, R.A.; Canetta, P.A.; Rovin, B.H.; Appel, G.B.; Novak, J.; Nath, K.A.; Sethi, S.; Tumlin, J.A.; Mehta, K.; Hogan, M.; et al. A Randomized, Controlled Trial of Rituximab in IgA Nephropathy with Proteinuria and Renal Dysfunction. *J. Am. Soc. Nephrol.* **2017**, *28*, 1306–1313. [CrossRef]
18. Cattran, D.C.; Coppo, R.; Cook, H.T.; Feehally, J.; Roberts, I.S.D.; Troyanov, S.; Alpers, C.E.; Amore, A.; Barratt, J.; Berthoux, F.; et al. The Oxford classification of IgA nephropathy: Rationale, clinicopathological correlations, and classification. *Kidney Int.* **2009**, *76*, 534–545. [CrossRef]
19. Schena, F.P.; Nistor, I. Epidemiology of IgA Nephropathy: A Global Perspective. *Semin. Nephrol.* **2018**, *38*, 435–442. [CrossRef]

20. Suzuki, H. Biomarkers for IgA nephropathy on the basis of multi-hit pathogenesis. *Clin. Exp. Nephrol.* **2019**, *23*, 26–31. [CrossRef]

21. Lai, K.N. Pathogenesis of IgA nephropathy. *Nat. Rev. Nephrol.* **2012**, *8*, 275–283. [CrossRef] [PubMed]

22. Sigdel, T.K.; Woo, S.H.; Dai, H.; Khatri, P.; Li, L.; Myers, B.; Sarwal, M.M.; Lafayette, R.A. Profiling of Autoantibodies in IgA Nephropathy, an Integrative Antibiomics Approach. *J. Am Soc. Nephrol.* **2011**, *6*, 2775–2784. [CrossRef] [PubMed]

23. Woo, S.H.; Sigdel, T.K.; Dinh, V.T.; Vu, M.T.; Sarwal, M.M.; Lafayette, R.A. Mapping novel immunogenic epitopes in IgA nephropathy. *Clin. J. Am. Soc. Nephrol.* **2015**, *10*, 372–381. [CrossRef] [PubMed]

24. Rizk, D.V.; Saha, M.K.; Hall, S.; Novak, L.; Brown, R.; Huang, Z.-Q.; Fatima, H.; Julian, B.A.; Novak, J. Glomerular Immunodeposits of Patients with IgA Nephropathy Are Enriched for IgG Autoantibodies Specific for Galactose-Deficient IgA1. *J. Am. Soc. Nephrol.* **2019**, *30*, 9. [CrossRef] [PubMed]

25. Floege, J.; Eitner, F. Current Therapy for IgA Nephropathy. *J. Am. Soc. Nephrol.* **2011**, *22*, 1785–1794. [CrossRef] [PubMed]

26. Yang, J.Y.C.; Verleden, S.E.; Zarinsefat, A.; Vanaudenaerde, B.M.; Vos, R.; Verleden, G.M.; Sarwal, R.D.; Sigdel, T.K.; Liberto, J.M.; Damm, I.; et al. Cell-Free DNA and CXCL10 Derived from Bronchoalveolar Lavage Predict Lung Transplant Survival. *J. Clin. Med.* **2019**, *8*, 9. [CrossRef] [PubMed]

27. Sacreas, A.; Yang, J.Y.C.; Vanaudenaerde, B.M.; Sigdel, T.K.; Liberto, J.M.; Damm, I.; Verleden, G.M.; Vos, R.; Verleden, E.; Sarwal, M.M. The common rejection module in chronic rejection post lung transplantation. *PLoS ONE* **2018**, *13*, 1–16. [CrossRef]

28. Sigdel, T.K.; Yang, J.Y.C.; Bestard, O.; Schroeder, A.; Hsieh, S.-C.; Liberto, J.M.; Damm, I.; Geraedts, A.C.M.; Sarwal, M.M. A urinary Common Rejection Module (uCRM) score for non-invasive kidney transplant monitoring. *PLoS ONE* **2019**, *7*, 1–15. [CrossRef] [PubMed]

29. Kusano, T.; Takano, H.; Kang, D.; Nagahama, K.; Aoki, M.; Morita, M.; Kaneko, T.; Tsuruoka, S.; Shimizu, A. Endothelial cell injury in acute and chronic glomerular lesions in patients with IgA nephropathy. *Hum. Pathol.* **2016**, *49*, 135–144. [CrossRef]

30. Reich, H.N.; Troyanov, S.; Scholey, J.W.; Cattran, D.C. Remission of Proteinuria Improves Prognosis in IgA Nephropathy. *J. Am. Soc. Nephrol.* **2007**, *18*, 3177–3183. [CrossRef]

31. Gutiérrez, E. IgA nephropathy: Is a new approach beyond proteinuria necessary? *Pediatr. Nephrol.* **2019**, 921–924. [CrossRef] [PubMed]

32. Burnham, P.; Dadhania, D.; Heyang, M.; Chen, F.; Westblade, L.F.; Suthanthiran, M.; Lee, J.R.; De Vlaminck, I. Urinary cell-free DNA is a versatile analyte for monitoring infections of the urinary tract. *Nat. Commun.* **2018**, *9*, 1–10. [CrossRef] [PubMed]

33. Celec, P.; Vlková, B.; Lauková, L.; Bábíčková, J.; Boor, P. Cell-free DNA: The role in pathophysiology and as a biomarker in kidney diseases. *Expert Rev. Mol. Med.* **2018**, *20*, 1–14. [CrossRef] [PubMed]

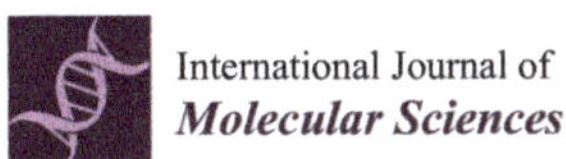

International Journal of
Molecular Sciences

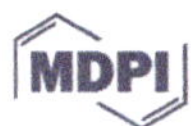

Article

No Cytotoxic and Inflammatory Effects of Empagliflozin and Dapagliflozin on Primary Renal Proximal Tubular Epithelial Cells under Diabetic Conditions In Vitro

Patrick C. Baer [1,*], **Benjamin Koch** [1], **Janina Freitag** [1], **Ralf Schubert** [2] and **Helmut Geiger** [1]

[1] Division of Nephrology, Department of Internal Medicine III, University Hospital, Goethe-University, 60596 Frankfurt/M., Germany; b.koch@med.uni-frankfurt.de (B.K.); janinafreitag@gmx.net (J.F.); h.geiger@em.uni-frankfurt.de (H.G.)

[2] Division of Allergology, Pneumology and Cystic Fibrosis, Department for Children and Adolescents, University Hospital, Goethe-University, 60596 Frankfurt/M., Germany; ralf.schubert@kgu.de

* Correspondence: patrick.baer@kgu.de or p.baer@em.uni-frankfurt.de; Tel.: +49-69-6301-5554; Fax: +49-69-6301-4749

Received: 12 December 2019; Accepted: 7 January 2020; Published: 8 January 2020

Abstract: Gliflozins are inhibitors of the renal proximal tubular sodium-glucose co-transporter-2 (SGLT-2), that inhibit reabsorption of urinary glucose and they are able to reduce hyperglycemia in patients with type 2 diabetes. A renoprotective function of gliflozins has been proven in diabetic nephropathy, but harmful side effects on the kidney have also been described. In the current project, primary highly purified human renal proximal tubular epithelial cells (PTCs) have been shown to express functional SGLT-2, and were used as an in vitro model to study possible cellular damage induced by two therapeutically used gliflozins: empagliflozin and dapagliflozin. Cell viability, proliferation, and cytotoxicity assays revealed that neither empagliflozin nor dapagliflozin induce effects in PTCs cultured in a hyperglycemic environment, or in co-medication with ramipril or hydro-chloro-thiazide. Oxidative stress was significantly lowered by dapagliflozin but not by empagliflozin. No effect of either inhibitor could be detected on mRNA and protein expression of the pro-inflammatory cytokine interleukin-6 and the renal injury markers KIM-1 and NGAL. In conclusion, empa- and dapagliflozin in therapeutic concentrations were shown to induce no direct cell injury in cultured primary renal PTCs in hyperglycemic conditions.

Keywords: renal tubular cells; epithelial cells; proximal tubule; cytotoxicity; injury; inflammation; empagliflozin; dapagliflozin; kidney

---

1. Introduction

Over 90% of the filtered glucose in the kidney is reabsorbed by the sodium-glucose co-transporter 2 (SGLT-2) expressed in the apical brush border membrane of tubular epithelial cells [1,2]. Inhibition of SGLT-2 blocks the reabsorption of glomerularly filtered glucose (and sodium) in the ensuing proximal S1/S2 segment, a mechanism that has been exploited to reduce hyperglycemia in patients with type 2 diabetes mellitus [1]. Based on the selective inhibition of SGLT-2, gliflozins increase urinary glucose excretion by reducing the reabsorption into the bloodstream. Gliflozins are a class of antidiabetic drugs used to lower glucose in type 2 diabetes mellitus [3,4]. The mechanism of action is independent of endogenous insulin and shows a very low risk of hypoglycemia. In the last few years, the renoprotective function of gliflozins has been described in diabetic nephropathy, which affects approximately 40% of patients with diabetes and is a leading cause of chronic kidney disease worldwide. SGLT2 inhibition has been described as reducing inflammation and attenuating the progression of diabetic nephropathy [4].

As the first active substance, the European Medicines Agency granted marketing authorization for dapagliflozin in 2012. Empagliflozin and ertugliflozin have also been approved; in the meantime, canagliflozin has been taken off the market in Germany. Other substances are in advanced clinical trials or are approved in the United States. The pleiotropic effects of SGLT2 inhibitors have the potential to generate benefits beyond the inhibition of glucose reuptake, and there is increasing evidence that gliflozins may reduce the risk of progression of renal impairment in diabetic patients [5]. It has been shown that in patients with type 2 diabetes and kidney disease, the risk of kidney failure and cardiovascular events was lower in the canagliflozin group than in the placebo group [6]. A post-hoc analysis from recent published trial revealed the risk of AKI may be lower under SGLT2 inhibition [7]. In another study of patients with diabetes, initiation of SGLT2 inhibitor therapy has been shown to be associated with a slower rate of kidney function decline and lower risk of major kidney events compared with initiation of other glucose-lowering drugs [8]. Although current evidence supports their safety, additional efforts are needed to elucidate the long-term impact of these compounds on chronic kidney disease, mineral metabolism, and bone health. Indeed, the limited study follow-up precludes a definitive answer on the impact of gliflozins (e.g., on electrolyte and mineral metabolism changes), especially in high-risk subgroups of patients [9]. The findings of ongoing and future clinical trials will help shed further light on the role of gliflozins in the long-term protection of renal function.

Nevertheless, despite overall good clinical tolerability [10], harmful effects also can occur during daily gliflozin intake. Reported adverse events are especially acute kidney injury (AKI) [11,12], acute tubular necrosis [13], genital infections, and bone fractures [3]. Although current evidence supports their safety, additional efforts are needed to elucidate the long-term impact of these compounds on chronic kidney disease, mineral metabolism, and bone health. Indeed, the limited follow-up studies and the heterogeneity of the case-mix of different randomized controlled trials preclude a definitive answer on the impact of these compounds on long-term outcomes such as the risk of bone fracture.

The US Food and Drug Administration (FDA) issued a warning in June 2016 covering the increased risk of AKI following the use of gliflozins [14]. A total of 101 cases were reported between March 2013 and October 2015, but a much higher number is expected worldwide. The FDA warning was based on data suggesting a link between the development of AKI and two approved gliflozins [3]. In this alert, patients with diabetes and heart failure, chronic renal insufficiency, and/or decreased circulating blood volume were included in the risk group. The risk is potentiated by the additional intake of ACE inhibitors, diuretics, and/or nonsteroidal anti-inflammatory drugs, warned the FDA. In November 2019, the German Drug Commission concluded that treatment with gliflozins should be stopped if patients are hospitalized due to major surgery or acute serious illness [15]. However, despite these relevant safety issues, the points are still under investigation and no firm conclusion can be currently drawn.

Possible pathophysiologic mechanisms of AKI induced by SGLT-2 inhibitors have been highlighted recently [16]. Osmotic diuresis can lead to volume depletion, while uricosuria as a consequence of increased glucose–uric acid exchange in the proximal tubule, has the potential of direct tubular damage through crystal formation. High glucose concentrations in renal tubules may lead to altered fructose metabolism in proximal tubular cells and, thus, to local cytotoxicity and tubular injury from increased oxidative stress and the release of inflammatory molecules [16]. Summing up all current data, it can be concluded that a very detailed study of why some patients on gliflozin therapy develop acute renal failure, but not others, and details about the underlying cellular pathomechanisms in the kidney are needed urgently. To date, there is only speculation about the exact pathomechanisms of the renal side effect of gliflozins. No clear investigations have been published to elucidate these mechanisms.

In this project, highly purified and cultured human renal proximal tubular epithelial cells (PTCs) were used as an in vitro model to study the cellular damage of gliflozins. This is the first study using primary highly differentiated PTCs to investigate possible effects of two gliflozins: empa- and dapagliflozin. As PTCs are the direct site of action for SGLT2 inhibitors, a simulation of different environmental variables, such as high glucose, or combinations with other drugs were used to investigate the influence on the renal tubule system in the in vitro model and possibly to simulate the conditions in the human nephron.

2. Results

2.1. Characterization of SGLT-2 Expression and Function in PTCs

Immunofluorescence staining clearly showed the expression of SGLT-2 in the apical membrane of cells of the proximal tubule in situ (Figure 1A) and PTCS in vitro (Figure 1C). The staining of human renal sections showed that SGLT-2 is exclusively expressed in the apical brush border membrane of tubular epithelial cells.

Cultured PTCs displayed an epithelial morphology with a highly compact cell monolayer (Figure 1B). The expression of SGLT2 mRNA and protein in cultured PTCs was also proven by standard PCR analysis (Figure 1D) and western blotting (Figure 1E). The RNA and protein isolated from human kidneys (renal extracts) were used as positive controls in both verifications (Figure 1D,E).

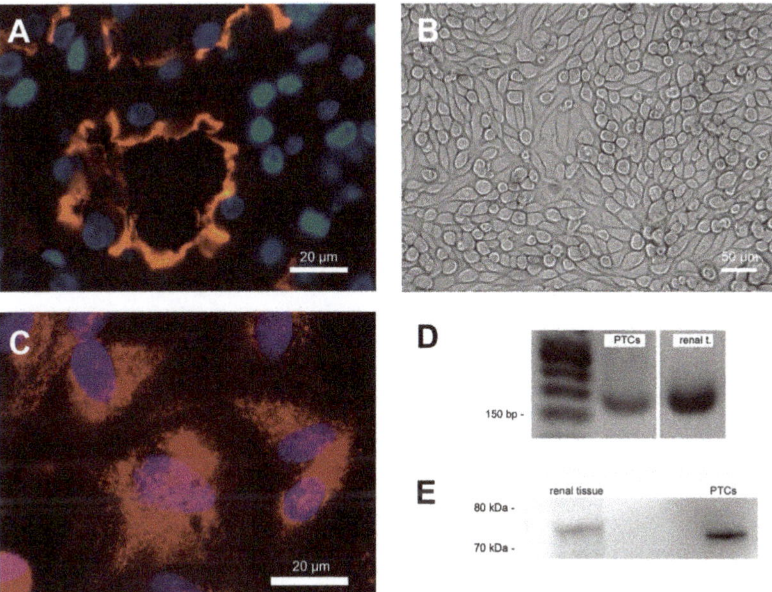

Figure 1. Cell characterization. (**A**) Immunofluorescence staining of human renal paraffin-embedded tissue sections showing sodium-glucose co-transporter 2 (SGLT-2) expression on the apical cell membrane in the proximal tubular nephron. Nuclei were counterstained with 4,6-diamino-2-phenylindole (DAPI; blue). (**B**) Characteristic phase contrast microscopy of confluent PTCs cultured in standard cell culture. (**C**) Immunofluorescence staining of SGLT-2 expression in cultured PTCs. Nuclei were counterstained with DAPI (blue). (**D**) Proof of SGLT-2 mRNA expression in cultured PTCs and RNA from human renal tissue extracts using PCR. (**E**) Proof of SGLT-2 protein expression in cultured PTCs and protein from human renal tissue extracts using western blotting.

As a functional assay, the glucose uptake was evaluated using the fluorescent glucose analog NBDG-2. Loading of NBDG-2 into PTCs was shown by the measurement of unloaded cells as a negative control. The SGLT2-mediated NBDG-2 influx from the cell culture medium into the cells was sensitive to inhibition by the SGLT inhibitors in a dose-dependent manner (Figure 2). Incubation of PTC with 10 nM empa- or dapagliflozin had no inhibitory effect on the glucose uptake of PTCs. The

NBDG-2 assay confirms the activity of the sodium-glucose co-transporter in cultured PTCs and the inhibitory effect of the gliflozins.

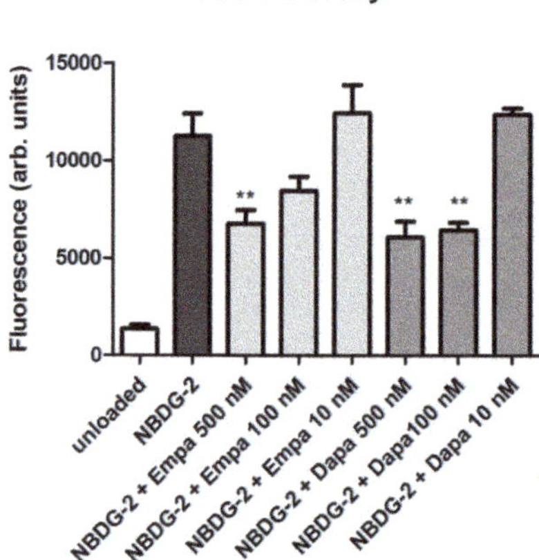

Figure 2. Functional assay. NBDG-2, a fluorescent glucose analog, was used to monitor glucose uptake in cultured PTCs. NBDG-2 was added either alone or with decreasing concentrations of gliflozins (500, 100, 10 nM) for 60 min at 37 °C. Cells incubated in buffer without NBDG-2 were used as background controls (unloaded). Fluorescence was measured using a fluorescence reader with excitation and emission wavelengths of 485 and 538 nm (arbitrary units, mean ± standard deviation (SD), $n = 4$, ** $p<0.01$ versus NBDG-2).

2.2. Cell Viability, Proliferation, and Cytotoxicity Assays

We used two viability assays using calcein-acetoxymthyl (calcein-AM) and XTT to investigate the effects of empa- and dapagliflozin on PTCs viability. Calcein-AM is a cell-permeant non-fluorescent dye, which is exclusively in viable cells converted into calcein, a dye with intense green fluorescence. The XTT assay is a colorimetric assay used to estimate the metabolic activity of viable cells.

Both assays demonstrated that empa- and dapagliflozin induce no cytotoxic effects on cultured PTCs. Depending on the experiment, media were additionally supplemented by a combination of empa- or dapagliflozin with ramipril or hydro-chloro-thiazide (HCT). Nevertheless, no statistically significant difference could be detected compared to the control (high glucose medium: HG) either with the calcein assay (Figure 3A) or the XTT assay (Figure 3B). In addition, we used different internal negative controls within the two assays. In the calcein assay, we used a mixture of cytokines which significantly reduced the viability of PTCs over the incubation period (43.5 ± 8.4% versus HG (=100%)) (Figure 3A). For the XTT, we used a low glucose medium 199 (LG) as a control. Incubation in LG resulted in a reduced metabolic activity, due to reduced cell proliferation (72.2 ± 5.5% versus HG (=100%)) (Figure 3B).

In addition, both a proliferation and a cytotoxicity assay were used to detect further effects of empa- and dapagliflozin on PTCs. The fluorometric assay with 4,6-diamino-2-phenylindole (DAPI), measuring the DNA content as an indirect determination of cell number and proliferation, verified that both gliflozins had no influence on cell proliferation. Furthermore, the combinations with ramipril or HCT also showed no effects on cell proliferation, whereas the negative control (LG) reduced proliferation of PTCs significantly (77.8 ± 2.5% versus HG (=100%)) (Figure 4A). Cytotoxic effects, measured by quantification of lactate dehydrogenase (LDH) in the supernatant of PTCs after incubation in gliflozin-containing media or co-medications, were also not detectable (Figure 4B). Only the incubation with the cytomix induced a significant increase in LDH activity in the supernatant (148.3 ± 16.7% versus HG (=100%)) (Figure 4B).

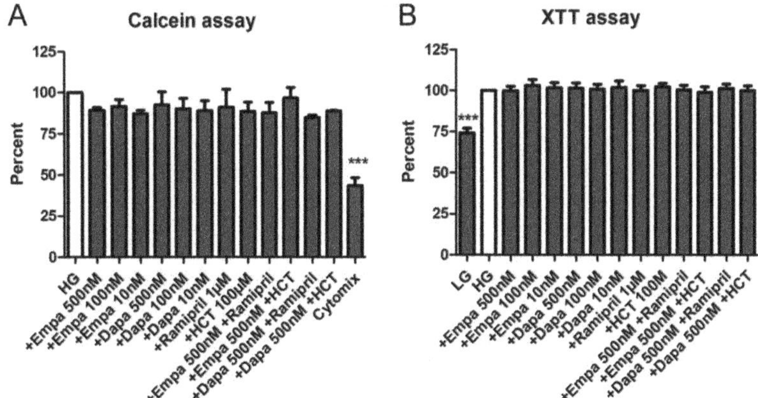

Figure 3. Cell viability assays. The PTCs cultured in 96-well plates were incubated for 6 d in media containing empa- or dapagliflozin and co-medications. No significant effects of the different pretreatments on the cell viability were detected. (**A**) Calcein assay. After loading with calcein-AM for 1h, fluorescence was measured immediately using a fluorescence reader (ex 485 nm, em 538 nm, arbitrary units, calculated as percent in relation to the control (high glucose medium: HG), mean ± SD, n = 5). Cells incubated with a mixture of cytokines (Cytomix) were used as a negative control (*** p < 0.001). (**B**) XTT assay. The XTT assay was performed and optical density (OD) was measured in a microplate reader at 490 vs. 650 nm (arbitrary units, calculated as percent in relation to the control (HG), mean ± SD, n = 4). Cells cultured in low glucose medium 199 (LG) were used as a negative control (*** p < 0.001).

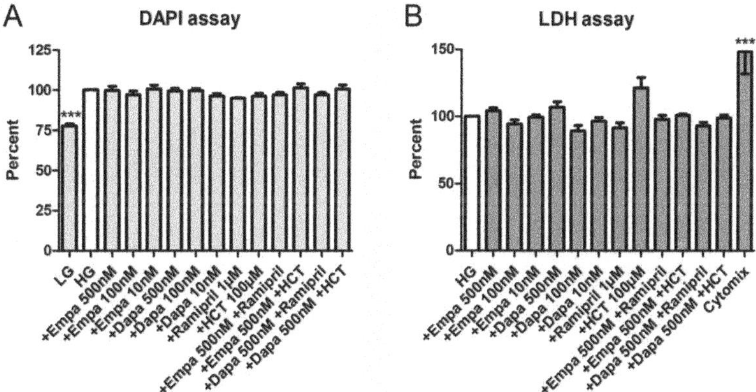

Figure 4. Cell proliferation and cytotoxicity assays. (**A**) DAPI assay. The assay was used to measure the DNA content as an indirect determination of cell number and proliferation [17]. Fluorescence was measured using a fluorescence reader (ex 355 nm, em 460 nm, arbitrary units, calculated as percent in relation to the control (HG), mean ± SD, n = 4). Cells cultured in LG were used as a negative control. (**B**) Lactate dehydrogenase (LDH) assay. The measurement of LDH activity released from the cytosol of damaged cells into the supernatant was used for the quantification of cell death and cell lysis. Absorbance was measured in a microplate reader (490 vs. 650 nm, arbitrary units, calculated as percent in relation to the control (HG), mean ± SD, n = 4–6). A mixture of pro-inflammatory cytokines was used as a positive control (*** p < 0.001).

2.3. Measurement of Oxidative Stress and Tubular Injury Markers

Formation of intracellular oxidative stress was proven using fluorescence measurements of intracellular 2′,7′-dichlorofluorescein (DCF). Incubation of PTCs in HG increased oxidative stress levels in a significant manner. Addition of empagliflozin (500 nM) to HG could not reduce the oxidative stress level (Figure 5). By contrast, oxidative stress generation evoked by high glucose exposure was significantly suppressed by the treatment with dapagliflozin (500 nM). We further checked the effect of H_2O_2 (250 µM) after loading for establishment of the DCF measurements, resulting in a maximum signal (positive control, data not shown). Unloaded cells were used as negative controls and compared with cells after DCF loading (data not shown).

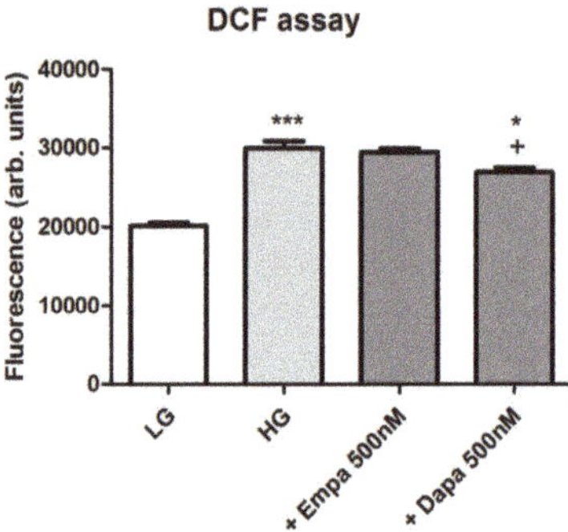

Figure 5. Formation of oxidative stress under diabetic culture conditions. Confluent PTCs in 96-well plates were cultured in LG, HG or with gliflozins (500 nM) for 6 d. Then, 2′,7′-dichlorodihydrofluorescein diacetate (20 µM in Hank's buffered saline solution) was added for 30 min at 37 °C. Fluorescence of intracellular DCF was measured using a fluorescence reader with excitation and emission wavelengths of 485 and 538 nm (arbitrary units, mean ± SD, $n = 6$, *** $p < 0.001$ vs. LG, + $p < 0.05$ vs. HG, * $p < 0.05$ vs. Empa 500 nM).

We further studied the role of SGLT2 inhibition in the induction and release of pro-inflammatory and injury markers. Firstly, we checked the mRNA levels of the pro-inflammatory cytokine interleukin-6 (IL-6) and two renal tubular injury markers (kidney injury molecule-1 (KIM-1), and neutrophil gelatinase-associated lipocalin (NGAL)) after 24 h incubation in HG with gliflozins. As shown in Figure 6, neither empagliflozin nor dapagliflozin influenced the mRNA expression of all three readouts. Comparison between LG and HG showed an induction of IL-6 and NGAL mRNA after incubation for 24 h, but not of KIM-1 (data not shown). Stimulation with a mixture of cytokines was used as a positive control. The cytomix induced a significant induction of IL-6 and NGAL mRNA but not KIM-1 mRNA expression (Figure 6).

We then checked the release of all three molecules in the supernatant of PTCs (Figure 7). At the protein level, IL-6 is constitutively released by PTCs cultured in HG (11.9 ± 1.7 ng/mL; mean ± SD, $n = 6$). When the cells were incubated with gliflozins, no significant effect on the release of IL-6 protein was detected. Incubation in the presence of the cytomix increased the release of IL-6 protein significantly (417 ± 117 %, calculated as percent in relation to the control (HG), $n = 6$). In addition, we also found no effect of empa- or dapagliflozin on the release of KIM-1 and NGAL. The cytomix induced the release of NGAL protein in a significant manner (269 ± 57 %, $n = 4$), whereas release of KIM-1 was not increased. At the protein level, KIM-1 and NGAL are also constitutively released by PTCs cultured in HG (11.6 ± 2.1 ng/mL and 115.7 ± 26.2 ng/mL, respectively; mean ± SD, $n = 4$).

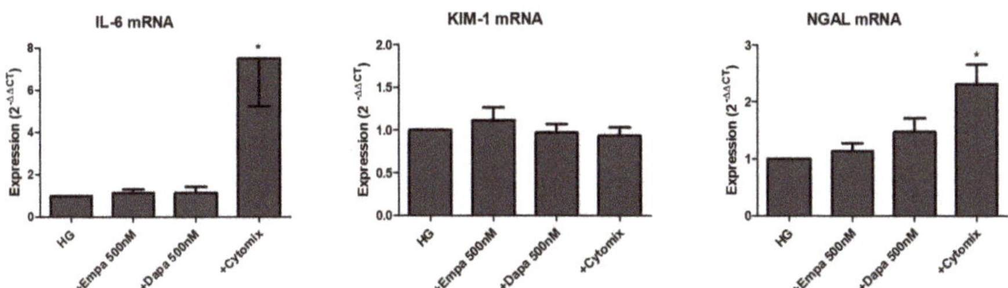

Figure 6. Effect of empagliflozin and dapagliflozin on mRNA expression of selected factors. Cells were grown in small culture flasks until confluence, serum depleted for 2 h and stimulated in HG for 24 h. The expression levels in each experiment were normalized to a housekeeping gene (β-actin) and are expressed relative to the control using the ΔΔCT method. A mixture of pro-inflammatory cytokines (cytomix) was used as a control, whereas only IL-6 mRNA was significantly increased after incubation with the cytomix (* $p < 0.05$ versus HG; IL-6 and NGAL $n = 6$; KIM-1 $n = 7$).

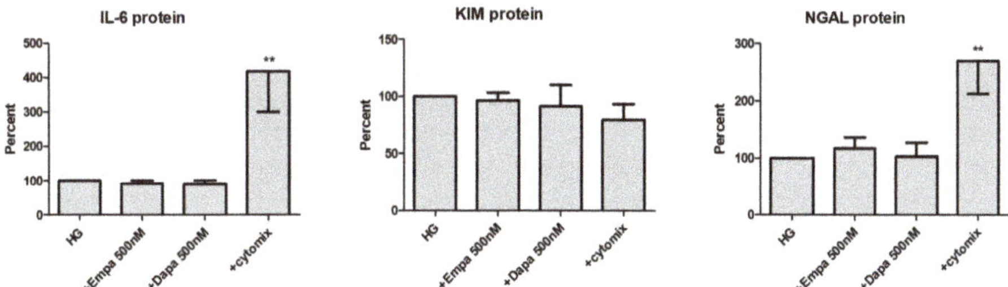

Figure 7. Effect of empagliflozin and dapagliflozin on the release of pro-inflammatory and injury proteins. Cells were grown in a 24-well plate until confluence, serum depleted for 2 h and stimulated in HG for 48 h. Supernatants were then harvested and quantified using commercially available immunoassays (optical density 450/620 nm, calculated as percent in relation to the control (HG), mean ± SD). A mixture of pro-inflammatory cytokines (cytomix) was used as a positive control. (** $p < 0.01$ versus HG, IL-6 $n = 6$, KIM-1 and NGAL $n = 4$).

3. Discussion

Gliflozins are the latest class of hypoglycemic agents for the treatment of diabetes mellitus type 2 and have a unique mechanism of lowering glucose by the inhibition of renal proximal tubular sodium-glucose co-transporter-2. SGLT-2 inhibitors have been shown to increase urinary glucose excretion and decrease serum glucose and HbA1c. In addition, compared to other topical antidiabetic medications, gliflozin intake can also reduce body weight. The drug group is further attributed to an improvement in hypertension, a reduction in cardiovascular mortality risk, and multiple effects on the kidney. Nevertheless, despite good overall clinical tolerability, several harmful effects have been published related to daily intake. Caution is still advised regarding possible adverse events described such as AKI and acute tubular necrosis [3,13]. Under certain circumstances—possibly dehydration of the patient, low blood pressure, or certain co-medications—gliflozin may damage the organ. Currently, however, there is only speculation about the exact pathomechanisms of the renal side effects [16]. No clear investigations have been published to elucidate these mechanisms. The influence of osmotic pressure and the development of excess uric acid on the function of tubular epithelial cells in the nephron might be involved in this context [18]. Increased osmotic pressure (hyperosmolarity) in the tubular system may activate the polyol pathway in epithelial cells [19], leading to osmotic damage via the accumulation of sorbitol and the formation of oxidative stress with cellular damage, inflammation, and pathological tissue change [20,21]. The main site of action of SGLT-2 inhibition raises the question whether inhibition of the transporter induces direct cytotoxic or inflammatory effects on renal proximal tubular epithelial cells.

In the current study, we focus on the effects of two currently available gliflozins on renal proximal tubular epithelial cells. For the first time, we examined the cytotoxic and inflammatory effects of empa- and dapagliflozin on primary and highly differentiated PTCs under diabetic conditions in vitro. High levels of circulating glucose and inflammation are the main causes of tissue damage in diabetes mellitus by inducing cell injury and high levels of oxidative stress in the kidney [22]. In this case, it should also be mentioned that diabetes itself is a systemic pro-inflammatory condition, involving not only the kidney, but also the cardiovascular system and bone [23,24].

Several in vitro studies using immortalized human tubular epithelial cells (e.g., HK2 cell line) [25–28], murine tubular epithelial cells [29] or non-renal cells [30,31] investigated either the effects of empa- or of dapagliflozin. Some of them have shown that SGLT2 inhibition reduced the release of inflammatory or fibrotic factors induced by high glucose levels [25–27], others found effects on oxidative stress responses [26,30,31]. Our current study looked at whether high glucose induced changes were influenced by either of the two gliflozins. Whereas we found no effect on cell viability, proliferation, and cytotoxicity, a significant reduction in the oxidative stress was found after incubation with dapagliflozin. Chen and co-workers also demonstrated decreased reactive oxidative species after incubation with dapagliflozin in a fructose-induced diabetic milieu [31]. Others investigated the subcellular mechanisms underlying the protective effects of empagliflozin from high glucose-mediated injuries on HK-2 cells [26]. As oxidative stress plays pathologic roles in diabetic kidneys [32] and empagliflozin may reduce this effect [33], the authors analyzed the effects of empagliflozin and described the protection of HK-2 cells from high glucose-mediated injuries through a mitochondrial mechanism.

In addition, a series of in vitro cytotoxicological investigations were conducted to evaluate a mode of action for gliflozin-associated effects. In addition to the in vitro studies, the effects of gliflozins on the kidney were also assessed in several in vivo studies and in clinical trials (currently reviewed by Ninčević and co-workers [34]), which should not be discussed here. Cytotoxicity and inflammation mediated by high glucose is directly responsible for pathological changes in diabetic nephropathy [35]. The in vitro data presented by Smith and co-workers demonstrated no genotoxic, cytotoxic, or mitogenic role for empagliflozin. However, the data indicate that an oxidative metabolite of empagliflozin is cytotoxic to renal tubular cells, but is not genotoxic [29]. Others described a canagliflozin-induced cytotoxicity at particularly low concentrations in proliferating immortalized tubular epithelial cells in vitro [36]. We also checked the influence of often used co-medications, such as ramipril or HCT, on the cytotoxicity and viability of PTCs. Co-incubation of gliflozins with either ramipril, clinically used to lower hypertension via inhibition of the renal angiotensin-converting enzyme, or HCT, clinically used as diuretic medication, did not induce significant effects on PTCs. We did not check the co-medications by PCR and enzyme-linked immunosorbent assay (EIA) due the negative results of the cytotoxicity and viability assays (and also to the low availability of primary isolated PTCs). Measurement of the inflammatory marker (IL-6) and two injury markers (KIM-1 and NGAL) showed that the gliflozins did not influence their expression in vitro. In contrast to our study, other have shown that SGLT-2 inhibition with empagliflozin reduces high glucose-induced IL-6 release in HK-2 cells [27]. Dekkers and co-workers further described in a post-hoc analysis of a clinical trial that dapagliflozin decreased urinary KIM-1 and IL-6 excretion, suggesting that dapagliflozin may beneficially affect renal inflammation and reduces tubular cell injury [37].

In summary, our current study describes the expression and function of SGLT-2 on primary, highly differentiated PTCs and investigated the effects of SGLT-2 inhibition using two gliflozins: empa- and dapagliflozin. Cell viability, proliferation and cytotoxicity assays revealed that neither empagliflozin nor dapagliflozin induces effects in PTCs cultured in diabetic medium, or co-medication with ramipril or HCT. Oxidative stress was significantly lowered by dapagliflozin but not empagliflozin. No effect of either inhibitor could be detected on the mRNA and protein expression of inflammatory or injury markers. In conclusion, empa- and dapagliflozin in therapeutic concentrations (C_{max} 500 nM) induce no direct cell injury in cultured primary renal proximal tubular cells. Nevertheless, further future studies are needed to investigate potential specific factors leading to tubular injury. First, the effects of incubation in high concentrations of fructose and in hyperosmotic media, both in the presence of gliflozins and high glucose media, should be investigated. High fructose, in vivo generated due to consumption of high fructose dietary products, may also affect tubular epithelial cells [38]. Dietary fructose has been shown to cause tubular injury in vitro and in vivo [21,39]. In addition, an increment in osmotic pressure, generated in vivo by dehydration, may cause activation of the polyol pathway also leading in the accumulation of fructose [16,20]. On the other hand, high concentrations of uric acid could be another factor involved [18], whereas it has been shown that canagliflozin therapy decreased serum uric acid in patients with type 2 diabetes [40]. Finally, the in vitro effects of supratherapeutic gliflozin concentrations that may mimic the accumulation of the drug in conditions of renal failure in vivo should also be investigated in future studies.

4. Materials and Methods

4.1. Isolation and Culture of Primary Human Renal Proximal Tubular Epithelial Cells

Human renal tissue was obtained from patients undergoing tumor nephrectomies. The donors gave written informed consent. The study was approved by the ethics committee of the clinic of the Goethe University, Frankfurt (05 Dec 2014, UGO 03/10, Amendment). The ethical standards defined by the World Medical Association Declaration of Helsinki were complied with.

Primary human renal proximal tubular epithelial cells (PTC) were separated as described previously [41]. In brief, cells were isolated after tumor nephrectomies from renal tissue not involved in renal cell carcinoma. The tissue was disintegrated using crossed blades, digested with collagenase/dispase, and passed through a 106 µm mesh. Remaining cohered cells were then incubated with collagenase IV, DNase, and $MgCl_2$ and further purified by a Percoll density gradient centrifugation. The cells were then isolated by a mAb against aminopeptidase M (CD13) and the Mini-MACS system (Miltenyi, Bergisch Gladbach, Germany) to enrich highly purified PTC. Primary isolated PTC were strongly positive for aminopeptidase M (98.6 %). Ultrastructural analysis revealed highly preserved brush border microvilli, a well-developed endocytosis apparatus, and numerous mitochondria [41,42]. Isolated cells were seeded in 6-well plates. Medium 199 (M4530, Sigma-Aldrich, Taufkirchen, Germany) with a physiologic glucose concentration (100 mg/dl) was supplemented with 10% fetal bovine serum (FBS; Biochrom, Berlin, Germany), used as standard culture medium and replaced every three to four days. Confluent cells were passaged by trypsinization. Cells between passages 2 and 5 were used for the experiments.

4.2. Characterization of SGLT-2 Expression

Regarding histological staining, a small portion of human renal tissue normally used for PTC isolation was fixed with 10% formalin at room temperature for 4–6 h. Subsequently, paraffin-embedded tissue sections (4 µm) were dewaxed and rehydrated in xylol, 100, 96, and 70 % ethanol, boiled in TRIS-buffer (10 mM Tris Base, 1 mM EDTA, 0.05 % Tween 20, pH 9.0) for 20 min for antigen retrieval and washed with phosphate-buffered saline (PBS). Samples were blocked with normal goat serum at 37 °C for 30 min and incubated with anti-SGLT-2 (Santa Cruz Biotechnology, Heidelberg, Germany, no. sc-393350, 1:50) overnight at 4 °C. After washing with PBS, a Cy3-conjugated goat-anti-mouse IgG (Jackson Immuno Research, Cambridgeshire, UK, no. 115-165-062; 1:300) was applied for 1 h at 37 °C. Sections were subsequently, mounted in mounting medium and examined using Zeiss fluorescence microscope equipment.

Regarding fluorescence microscopy, PTC cultured on chamber slides was rinsed three times with PBS, and fixed with paraformaldehyde (4%) for 10 min. The fixed cells were washed twice. Unspecific binding sites were blocked by PBS containing 5% normal goat serum for 20 min. Primary antibody anti-SGLT-2 (Santa Cruz Biotechnology, no. sc-393350; 1:50) was applied without washing and incubated for 30 min at 37 °C with gentle shaking. After washing with PBS, cells were incubated with a Cy3-conjugated goat-anti-mouse IgG (1:300) for 30 min at 37 °C. Controls of autofluorescence or non-specific fluorescence were performed on fixed cells processed without the primary antibody. Monolayers were mounted in mounting medium and examined using Zeiss fluorescence microscope equipment.

Proof of SGLT-2 mRNA expression in cultured PTCs was done by PCR analysis (described in Section 4.7). The expression of SGLT-2 protein on PTC was examined using western blotting, as described previously [43]. In brief, the cells were lysed using 10 mM Tris pH 7.4, 0.1% sodium dodecyl sulphate (SDS), 0.1% Tween20, 0.5 % TritonX100, 150 mM NaCl, 10 mM EDTA, 1 M urea, 10 mM NEM, 4 mM benzamidine, and 1 mM PMSF and collected by scraping. After centrifugation, the pellet was suspended in Laemmli's buffer and heated at 95 °C for 5 min prior to electrophoresis on a 10 % SDS polyacrylamide gel. The protein content was determined by a standard assay and an equal volume of protein was loaded into each lane. The separated proteins were transferred electrophoretically to Immobilon transfer membrane (Millipore). Membranes were blocked for 2 h. Immunoblotting was performed by incubating with antibodies against SGLT-2 (resulting in a 73 kDa band; Santa Cruz Biotechnology, no. sc-393350; 1:200), followed by a secondary antibody (horseradish peroxidase-conjugated anti-mouse IgG; DAKO P0447, 1:1000). Protein bands were made visible using the Peqlab Fusion FX system (VWR, Darmstadt, Germany).

4.3. Stimulations

Cells were grown in 24- or 96-well culture plates, or small culture flasks (25cm^2) in standard cell culture medium (described in Section 4.1) until confluence. PTCs in selected experiments were grown to subconfluence and used for the assays (as indicated). The cells were then washed and kept in serum-free medium 199 for 2 h and stimulated as indicated in the particular assay. In most assays, LG with 10 % FBS (glucose content 100 mg/dl (5.5 mM)) was used as a negative control. Stimulations were done in HG with 10% FBS (glucose content 450 mg/dl (25 mM)) which induced a diabetic milieu in the cultures. In case of protein measurements in the supernatants (EIA, Section 4.8), stimulations were done in high glucose medium 199 without 10% FBS. For stimulations, empagliflozin (Adipogen, San Diego, CA, USA; no. AG-CR1-3619) was dissolved in dimethylsulfoxide and diluted in medium (500, 100, 10 nM). Dapaglifozin (Cayman Chemical, Ann Arbor, MI, USA; no. 11574) was dissolved in dimethyl sulfoxid and diluted in medium (500, 100, 10 nM). Maximal concentration of both gliflozins (500 nM) is matched to the published maximal therapeutic concentration observed (C$_{max}$) [44,45]. The interactions of gliflozin with ramipril (Cayman Chemicals, no. 15558; stock solution 1mM in dimethyl sulfoxide) or HCT (Sigma-Aldrich, Taufkirchen, Germany, no. H-4759; stock solution 100mM in dH$_2$O) were investigated in selected experiments (viability, cytotoxicity, and proliferation assays).

4.4. Functional Assay

We used 2-Deoxy-2-[(7-nitro-2,1,3-benzoxadiazol-7-yl)amino]-D-glucose (NBDG-2; Hoelzel Diagnostika, Köln, Germany, no. M6327), a fluorescent glucose analogon for usage in fluorescence measurements [46], to monitor glucose uptake in cultured PTCs. Confluent PTCs in 96-well plates were washed with pre-warmed HBSS. The HBSS containing NBDG-2 (100 µg/mL) either alone or with decreasing concentrations of gliflozins (500, 100, 10 nM) was added for 60 min at 37 °C (in quadruplicate for each biological replicate). Cells incubated in buffer without NBDG-2 were used as background controls. The cells were then washed with HBSS and fluorescence was measured directly using a fluorescence reader (BMG Fluostar, Ortenberg, Germany) with excitation and emission wavelengths of 485 nm and 538 nm, respectively. Data are expressed as arbitrary fluorescence units.

4.5. Cell Viability, Proliferation, and Cytotoxicity Assays

The cell viability of PTC was determined by two viability assays, a photometric assay using 2,3-Bis-(2-Methoxy-4-Nitro-5-Sulfophenyl)-2*H*-Tetrazolium-5-Carboxanilide (XTT) and a fluorescence-based assay using calcein-AM (Biolegend, San Diego, CA, USA) to investigate any possible cytotoxic effects, as described previously [43]. In brief, confluent PTCs in 96-well plates were incubated for 6 d in media containing empa- or dapagliflozin and co-medications (in quintuplicate for each biological replicate). The XTT reagent was then added to the wells, as described by the manufacturer (AppliChem, Darmstadt, Germany), and incubated at 37 °C for 4 h. Absorbance was measured in an Apollo LB911 microplate reader (Berthold, Bad Wildbad, Germany) at 492 nm vs. 650 nm. For the fluorescence assay, cells were washed and calcein-AM (1 µM) was added incubated at 37 °C for 30 min. Fluorescence was then measured immediately using a fluorescence reader (BMG Fluostar, Ortenberg, Germany) with excitation and emission wavelengths of 485 nm and 515 nm, respectively. Cells incubated in buffer without calcein-AM were used as background controls. Data are calculated as a percent in relation to the control (HG). Cells cultured in LG were used as a negative control.

Epithelial cell proliferation was determined by a fluorometric assay using DAPI, measuring the DNA content as an indirect determination of cell number and proliferation [17]. In brief, subconfluent PTCs in 96-well plates were incubated for 6 d in media containing empa- or dapagliflozin and co-medications (in quintuplicate for each biological replicate). Then, cells were permeabilized using 0.02% SDS, 150 mM NaCl, and 15 mM sodium citrate. Finally, DAPI (2 µg/mL) was added to each well. Fluorescence was measured in a fluorescence reader (FluoStar, BMG Labtech, Offenburg, Germany) with excitation and emission wavelengths of 355 nm and 460 nm, respectively. Data are calculated as a percent in relation to the control (HG). Cells cultured in LG were used as a negative control.

The measurement of LDH activity released from the cytosol of damaged cells into the supernatant was used for the quantification of cell death and cell lysis to determine cytotoxic effects. Supernatants were harvested after incubation in gliflozin-containing media for 6 d and processed as described by the manufacturer (Sigma-Aldrich, Taufkirchen, Germany, no. 11644793001). Absorbance was measured in a microplate reader at 490 nm vs. 650 nm. Data are calculated as a percent in relation to the control (HG). Cells cultured in medium 199 containing a mixture of cytokines (Cytomix: γ-interferon, 200 U/mL; IL-1β, 25 U/mL; and tumor necrosis factor-α, 10 ng/mL) were used as a positive control.

4.6. Measurement of Oxidative Stress

The cell-permeant 2′,7′-dichlorodihydrofluorescein diacetate (H_2DCFDA) was used to detect reactive oxygen species in PTCs. Upon cleavage of the acetate groups by intracellular esterases and oxidation, nonfluorescent H_2DCFDA is converted to highly fluorescent DCF. Confluent PTCs in 96-well plates were cultured in LG, HG or with gliflozins (500 nM) for 6 d. The cells were then washed with pre-warmed HBSS and H_2DCFDA (20 µM in HBSS) was added for 30 min at 37 °C (in quintuplicate for each biological replicate). Cells incubated in buffer without DCF were used as background controls. The cells were then washed with HBSS and fluorescence was measured immediately using a fluorescence reader (BMG Fluostar, Ortenberg, Germany) with excitation and emission wavelengths of 485 nm and 538 nm, respectively. Data are expressed as arbitrary fluorescence units.

4.7. PCR

The RNA extraction was performed using single-step RNA isolation from cultured PTC by a standard protocol. After the RNA extraction, cDNAs were synthesized for 30 min at 37 °C using 1 µg RNA, 50 µM random hexamers, 1 mM deoxynucleotide-triphosphate-mix, 50 units of reverse transcriptase (Fermentas, St. Leon-Rot, Germany) in 10× PCR buffer, 1 mM β-mercaptoethanol and 5 mM $MgCl_2$. A Hot FIREPol EvaGreen Mix Plus was used (Solis Biodyne, Tartu, Estonia) for the master mix; the primer mix and RNAse-free water were added. Quantitative PCR was carried out in 96-well plates using the following conditions: 12 min at 95 °C for enzyme activation, 15 s at 95 °C for denaturation, 20 s at 63 °C for annealing, and 30 s at 72 °C for elongation (40 cycles). Finally, a melting curve analysis was conducted. Products were checked by agarose gel electrophoresis in selected experiments. The PCR fragment quantification was realized using the ABI Prism ® 7900HT Fast Real-Time PCR System with a Sequence Detection System SDS 2.4.1 (Thermo Fisher Scientific,

Waltham, MA, USA). Relative quantification was estimated by the $\Delta\Delta$CT method [47] with β-actin as a housekeeper. The level of target gene expression was calculated using $2^{-\Delta\Delta Ct}$. The PCR products in selected experiments were separated by agarose electrophoresis (2 %) and observed under ultraviolet illumination. Primer pairs were synthesized by Invitrogen (Karlsruhe, Germany) and are listed in Table 1.

Table 1. Primer used for PCR analyses

Gene	Primer Forward	Primer Reverse	Product Length (bp)	NCBI Reference Sequence
SGLT-2	TGG GCT GGA ACA TCT ATG CC	GTG GAA GGC GTA ACC CAT GA	155	NM_003041.3
IL-6	AAA GAT GGC TGA AAA AGA TGG ATG C	ACA GCT CTG GCT TGT TCC TCA CTA C	150	NM_000600.4
KIM-1	CAG TGG CGT ATA TTG TTG CCG	CAG TCG TGA CGG TTG GAA CA	134	NM_001173393.2
NGAL	GAC CCG CAA AAG ATG TAT GCC	CTC ACC ACT CGG ACG AGG TA	197	NM_005564.4
β-Actin	ACT GGA ACG GTG AAG GGT GAC	AGA GAA GTG GGG TGG CTT TT	169	NM_001101

4.8. Immunoassays

After stimulation for 48 h (described in Section 4.3), supernatants were harvested, centrifuged at $300\times g$ for 5 min and used for the quantification of IL-6, KIM-1 or NGAL, or stored at -20 °C for later measurement. Interleukin-6 was quantified using a commercially available EIA kit (Immunotools, Friesoythe, Germany; no. 31670069). KIM-1 was quantified using a commercially available EIA DuoSet (R&DSystems, Wiesbaden, Germany; no. DY1750). NGAL was quantified using a commercially available EIA DuoSet (R&DSystems, Wiesbaden, Germany; no. DY1757). All assays were processed as described by the manufacturer. In brief, the wells of 96-well microtiter plates were coated with the capture antibody overnight at room temperature. Nonspecific binding sites were blocked with blocking buffer for 1 h. The plates were then washed with PBS/0.05 % Tween and the standard (IL-6 assay: 8–500 pg/mL; KIM-1: 15.5–1000 pg/mL; NGAL: 78.1–5000 pg/mL), and the samples were added for 2 h at room temperature. All samples were diluted in assay buffer (IL-6: 1:25; KIM-1: 1:20; NGAL 1:20) and run in duplicate. The plates were washed and incubated with biotinylated detection antibody for 2 h at room temperature, washed again and incubated with horseradish-peroxidase-streptavidin for 30 min. After washing, TMB was added for 5–20 min and the substrate reaction was stopped and measured (450 vs. 620 nm). The data are calculated as ng/mL in the supernatant and presented as percent versus the related control.

4.9. Statistical Analysis

The data are expressed as mean $\pm$ SD. Analysis of variance with Dunnett's Multiple Comparison Test or Student's t-test were used for statistical analysis. Analyses were performed using Prism 5.0 (GraphPad Software, San Diego, CA, USA). p values < 0.05 were considered significant.

Author Contributions: Investigation, P.C.B. and J.F.; Conceptualization, P.C.B., B.K., R.S., and H.G.; Formal analysis, P.C.B., B.K., and J.F.; Writing, review, and editing, P.C.B., B.K., R.S., and H.G. All authors have read and agreed to the published version of the manuscript.

Funding: This work was supported by the Adolf-Messer-Stiftung, Bad Soden, Germany.

Acknowledgments: We thank Rita Schmitt-Prokopp and Michael Lein, SANA, Klinik für Urologie und Kinderurologie, Offenbach, Germany, for providing us with human renal tissue. We also thank Felix Chun, Klinik für Urologie, Goethe Universität, Frankfurt, Germany, for providing us with human renal tissue.

Conflicts of Interest: The authors declare no conflict of interest.

Abbreviations

AKI	Acute kidney injury
Dapa	Dapagliflozin
DAPI	4,6-diamino-2-phenylindole
DCF	2′,7′-dichlorofluorescein
EIA	Enzyme immune assay
Empa	Empagliflozin
FBS	Fetal bovine serum
HCT	Hydro-chloro-thiazide
HG	High glucose medium 199 (450 mg/dl)
IL-6	Interleukin-6
KIM-1	Kidney injury molecule-1
LDH	Lactate dehydrogenase
LG	Low glucose medium 199 (100 mg/dl)
NBDG-2	2-Deoxy-2-[(7-nitro-2,1,3-benzoxadiazol-7-yl)amino]-D-glucose
NGAL	Neutrophil gelatinase-associated lipocalin (Lipocalin-2)
PCR	Polymerase chain reaction
PTC	Primary human renal proximal tubular epithelial cells
SGLT	Sodium-glucose co-transporter
XTT	2,3-Bis-(2-Methoxy-4-Nitro-5-Sulfophenyl)-2*H*-Tetrazolium-5-Carboxanilide

References

1. Gerich, J.E. Role of the kidney in normal glucose homeostasis and in the hyperglycaemia of diabetes mellitus: Therapeutic implications. *Diabet. Med.* **2010**, *27*, 136–142. [CrossRef] [PubMed]
2. Vallon, V. The proximal tubule in the pathophysiology of the diabetic kidney. *Am. J. Physiol. Regul. Integr. Comp. Physiol.* **2011**, *300*, R1009–R1022. [CrossRef] [PubMed]
3. Faillie, J.-L. Pharmacological aspects of the safety of gliflozins. *Pharmacol. Res.* **2017**, *118*, 71–81. [CrossRef] [PubMed]
4. De Nicola, L.; Gabbai, F.B.; Liberti, M.E.; Sagliocca, A.; Conte, G.; Minutolo, R. Sodium/glucose cotransporter 2 inhibitors and prevention of diabetic nephropathy: Targeting the renal tubule in diabetes. *Am. J. Kidney Dis.* **2014**, *64*, 16–24. [CrossRef]
5. Bae, J.H.; Park, E.-G.; Kim, S.; Kim, S.G.; Hahn, S.; Kim, N.H. Effects of Sodium-Glucose Cotransporter 2 Inhibitors on Renal Outcomes in Patients with Type 2 Diabetes: A Systematic Review and Meta-Analysis of Randomized Controlled Trials. *Sci. Rep.* **2019**, *9*, 13009. [CrossRef]
6. Perkovic, V.; Jardine, M.J.; Neal, B.; Bompoint, S.; Heerspink, H.J.L.; Charytan, D.M.; Edwards, R.; Agarwal, R.; Bakris, G.; Bull, S.; et al. Canagliflozin and Renal Outcomes in Type 2 Diabetes and Nephropathy. *N. Engl. J. Med.* **2019**, *380*, 2295–2306. [CrossRef]
7. Mayer, G.J.; Wanner, C.; Weir, M.R.; Inzucchi, S.E.; Koitka-Weber, A.; Hantel, S.; von Eynatten, M.; Zinman, B.; Cherney, D.Z.I. Analysis from the EMPA-REG OUTCOME® trial indicates empagliflozin may assist in preventing the progression of chronic kidney disease in patients with type 2 diabetes irrespective of medications that alter intrarenal hemodynamics. *Kidney Int.* **2019**, *96*, 489–504. [CrossRef]
8. Heerspink, H.J.L.; Karasik, A.; Thuresson, M.; Melzer-Cohen, C.; Chodick, G.; Khunti, K.; Wilding, J.P.H.; Garcia Rodriguez, L.A.; Cea-Soriano, L.; Kohsaka, S.; et al. Kidney outcomes associated with use of SGLT2 inhibitors in real-world clinical practice (CVD-REAL 3): A multinational observational cohort study. *Lancet Diabetes Endocrinol.* **2020**, *8*, 27–35. [CrossRef]
9. Cianciolo, G.; de Pascalis, A.; Capelli, I.; Gasperoni, L.; Di Lullo, L.; Bellasi, A.; La Manna, G. Mineral and Electrolyte Disorders with SGLT2i Therapy. *JBMR Plus* **2019**, *3*, e10242. [CrossRef]
10. Di Lullo, L.; Mangano, M.; Ronco, C.; Barbera, V.; de Pascalis, A.; Bellasi, A.; Russo, D.; Di Iorio, B.; Cozzolino, M. The treatment of type 2 diabetes mellitus in patients with chronic kidney disease: What to expect from new oral hypoglycemic agents. *Diabetes Metab. Syndr.* **2017**, *11*, S295–S305. [CrossRef]

11. Perlman, A.; Heyman, S.N.; Matok, I.; Stokar, J.; Muszkat, M.; Szalat, A. Acute renal failure with sodium-glucose-cotransporter-2 inhibitors: Analysis of the FDA adverse event report system database. *Nutr. Metab. Cardiovasc. Dis.* **2017**, *27*, 1108–1113. [CrossRef] [PubMed]

12. Hassani-Ardakania, K.; Lipman, M.L.; Laporta, D.; Yu, O.H.Y. A Case of Severe Acute Kidney Injury Exacerbated by Canagliflozin in a Patient with Type 2 Diabetes. *Case Rep. Endocrinol.* **2019**. [CrossRef] [PubMed]

13. Pleros, C.; Stamataki, E.; Papadaki, A.; Damianakis, N.; Poulidaki, R.; Gakiopoulou, C.; Tzanakis, I. Dapagliflozin as a cause of acute tubular necrosis with heavy consequences: A case report. *CEN Case Rep.* **2018**, *7*, 17–20. [CrossRef] [PubMed]

14. FDA. *FDA Drug Safety Communication: FDA Strengthens Kidney Warnings for Diabetes Medicines Canagliflozin (Invokana, Invokamet) and Dapagliflozin (Farxiga, Xigduo XR) (06-14-2016)*; US Food and Drug Administration: Silver Spring, MD, USA, 2016.

15. Arzneimittelkommission der deutschen Ärzteschaft. *Drug Safety Mail No. 2019-064*; Bundesärztekammer: Berlin, Germany, 2019.

16. Hahn, K.; Ejaz, A.A.; Kanbay, M.; Lanaspa, M.A.; Johnson, R.J. Acute kidney injury from SGLT2 inhibitors: Potential mechanisms. *Nat. Rev. Nephrol.* **2016**, *12*, 711–712. [CrossRef] [PubMed]

17. Blaheta, R.A.; Franz, M.; Auth, M.K.; Wenisch, H.J.; Markus, B.H. A rapid non-radioactive fluorescence assay for the measurement of both cell number and proliferation. *J. Immunol. Methods* **1991**, *142*, 199–206. [CrossRef]

18. Hahn, K.; Kanbay, M.; Lanaspa, M.A.; Johnson, R.J.; Ejaz, A.A. Serum uric acid and acute kidney injury: A mini review. *J. Adv. Res.* **2017**, *8*, 529–536. [CrossRef]

19. Soltani, Z.; Rasheed, K.; Kapusta, D.R.; Reisin, E. Potential role of uric acid in metabolic syndrome, hypertension, kidney injury, and cardiovascular diseases: Is it time for reappraisal? *Curr. Hypertens. Rep.* **2013**, *15*, 175–181. [CrossRef]

20. Handler, J.S.; Kwon, H.M. Kidney cell survival in high tonicity. *Comp. Biochem. Physiol. A Physiol.* **1997**, *117*, 301–306. [CrossRef]

21. Cirillo, P.; Gersch, M.S.; Mu, W.; Scherer, P.M.; Kim, K.M.; Gesualdo, L.; Henderson, G.N.; Johnson, R.J.; Sautin, Y.Y. Ketohexokinase-dependent metabolism of fructose induces proinflammatory mediators in proximal tubular cells. *J. Am. Soc. Nephrol.* **2009**, *20*, 545–553. [CrossRef]

22. Mittal, M.; Siddiqui, M.R.; Tran, K.; Reddy, S.P.; Malik, A.B. Reactive oxygen species in inflammation and tissue injury. *Antioxid. Redox Signal.* **2014**, *20*, 1126–1167. [CrossRef]

23. Tousoulis, D.; Economou, E.K.; Oikonomou, E.; Papageorgiou, N.; Siasos, G.; Latsios, G.; Kokkou, E.; Mourouzis, K.; Papaioannou, S.; Deftereos, S.; et al. The Role and Predictive Value of Cytokines in Atherosclerosis and Coronary Artery Disease. *Curr. Med. Chem.* **2015**, *22*, 2636–2650. [CrossRef] [PubMed]

24. Mazzaferro, S.; Cianciolo, G.; De Pascalis, A.; Guglielmo, C.; Urena Torres, P.A.; Bover, J.; Tartaglione, L.; Pasquali, M.; La Manna, G. Bone, inflammation and the bone marrow niche in chronic kidney disease: What do we know? *Nephrol. Dial. Transpl.* **2018**, *33*, 2092–2100. [CrossRef] [PubMed]

25. Yao, D.; Wang, S.; Wang, M.; Lu, W. Renoprotection of dapagliflozin in human renal proximal tubular cells via the inhibition of the high mobility group box 1-receptor for advanced glycation end products-nuclear factor-κB signaling pathway. *Mol. Med. Rep.* **2018**, *18*, 3625–3630. [CrossRef] [PubMed]

26. Lee, W.-C.; Chau, Y.-Y.; Ng, H.-Y.; Chen, C.-H.; Wang, P.-W.; Liou, C.-W.; Lin, T.-K.; Chen, J.-B. Empagliflozin Protects HK-2 Cells from High Glucose-Mediated Injuries via a Mitochondrial Mechanism. *Cells* **2019**, *8*, 1085. [CrossRef]

27. Panchapakesan, U.; Pegg, K.; Gross, S.; Komala, M.G.; Mudaliar, H.; Forbes, J.; Pollock, C.; Mather, A. Effects of SGLT2 inhibition in human kidney proximal tubular cells—Renoprotection in diabetic nephropathy? *PLoS ONE* **2013**, *8*, e54442. [CrossRef]

28. Kim, J.H.; Ko, H.Y.; Wang, H.J.; Lee, H.; Yun, M.; Kang, E.S. Effect of Dapagliflozin, a Sodium-glucose Cotransporter-2 Inhibitor, on Gluconeogenesis in Proximal Renal Tubules. *Diabetes Obes. Metab.* **2019**. [CrossRef]

29. Smith, J.D.; Huang, Z.; Escobar, P.A.; Foppiano, P.; Maw, H.; Loging, W.; Yu, H.; Phillips, J.A.; Taub, M.; Ku, W.W. A Predominant Oxidative Renal Metabolite of Empagliflozin in Male Mice Is Cytotoxic in Mouse Renal Tubular Cells but not Genotoxic. *Int. J. Toxicol.* **2017**, *36*, 440–448. [CrossRef]

30. Uthman, L.; Homayr, A.; Juni, R.P.; Spin, E.L.; Kerindongo, R.; Boomsma, M.; Hollmann, M.W.; Preckel, B.; Koolwijk, P.; van Hinsbergh, V.W.M.; et al. Empagliflozin and Dapagliflozin Reduce ROS Generation and Restore NO Bioavailability in Tumor Necrosis Factor α-Stimulated Human Coronary Arterial Endothelial Cells. *Cell. Physiol. Biochem.* **2019**, *53*, 865–886. [CrossRef]

31. Chen, Y.-Y.; Wu, T.-T.; Ho, C.-Y.; Yeh, T.-C.; Sun, G.-C.; Kung, Y.-H.; Wong, T.-Y.; Tseng, C.-J.; Cheng, P.-W. Dapagliflozin Prevents NOX- and SGLT2-Dependent Oxidative Stress in Lens Cells Exposed to Fructose-Induced Diabetes Mellitus. *Int. J. Mol. Sci.* **2019**, *20*, 4357. [CrossRef]

32. Arora, M.K.; Singh, U.K. Oxidative stress: Meeting multiple targets in pathogenesis of diabetic nephropathy. *Curr. Drug Targets* **2014**, *15*, 531–538. [CrossRef]

33. Andreadou, I.; Efentakis, P.; Balafas, E.; Togliatto, G.; Davos, C.H.; Varela, A.; Dimitriou, C.A.; Nikolaou, P.-E.; Maratou, E.; Lambadiari, V.; et al. Empagliflozin Limits Myocardial Infarction in Vivo and Cell Death in Vitro: Role of STAT3, Mitochondria, and Redox Aspects. *Front. Physiol.* **2017**, *8*, 1077. [CrossRef] [PubMed]

34. Ninčević, V.; Omanović Kolarić, T.; Roguljić, H.; Kizivat, T.; Smolić, M.; Bilić Ćurčić, I. Renal Benefits of SGLT 2 Inhibitors and GLP-1 Receptor Agonists: Evidence Supporting a Paradigm Shift in the Medical Management of Type 2 Diabetes. *Int. J. Mol. Sci.* **2019**, *20*, 5831. [CrossRef] [PubMed]

35. Komala, M.G.; Panchapakesan, U.; Pollock, C.; Mather, A. Sodium glucose cotransporter 2 and the diabetic kidney. *Curr. Opin. Nephrol. Hypertens.* **2013**, *22*, 113–119. [CrossRef]

36. Secker, P.F.; Beneke, S.; Schlichenmaier, N.; Delp, J.; Gutbier, S.; Leist, M.; Dietrich, D.R. Canagliflozin mediated dual inhibition of mitochondrial glutamate dehydrogenase and complex I: An off-target adverse effect. *Cell Death Dis.* **2018**, *9*, 226. [CrossRef] [PubMed]

37. Dekkers, C.C.J.; Petrykiv, S.; Laverman, G.D.; Cherney, D.Z.; Gansevoort, R.T.; Heerspink, H.J.L. Effects of the SGLT-2 inhibitor dapagliflozin on glomerular and tubular injury markers. *Diabetes Obes. Metab.* **2018**, *20*, 1988–1993. [CrossRef] [PubMed]

38. Gonzalez-Vicente, A.; Cabral, P.D.; Hong, N.J.; Asirwatham, J.; Saez, F.; Garvin, J.L. Fructose reabsorption by rat proximal tubules: Role of Na+-linked cotransporters and the effect of dietary fructose. *Am. J. Physiol. Renal Physiol.* **2019**, *316*, F473–F480. [CrossRef]

39. Nakayama, T.; Kosugi, T.; Gersch, M.; Connor, T.; Sanchez-Lozada, L.G.; Lanaspa, M.A.; Roncal, C.; Perez-Pozo, S.E.; Johnson, R.J.; Nakagawa, T. Dietary fructose causes tubulointerstitial injury in the normal rat kidney. *Am. J. Physiol. Renal Physiol.* **2010**, *298*, F712–F720. [CrossRef]

40. Davies, M.J.; Trujillo, A.; Vijapurkar, U.; Damaraju, C.V.; Meininger, G. Effect of canagliflozin on serum uric acid in patients with type 2 diabetes mellitus. *Diabetes Obes. Metab.* **2015**, *17*, 426–429. [CrossRef]

41. Baer, P.C.; Nockher, W.A.; Haase, W.; Scherberich, J.E. Isolation of proximal and distal tubule cells from human kidney by immunomagnetic separation. Technical note. *Kidney Int.* **1997**, *52*, 1321–1331. [CrossRef]

42. Baer, P.C.; Bereiter-Hahn, J.; Schubert, R.; Geiger, H. Differentiation status of human renal proximal and distal tubular epithelial cells in vitro: Differential expression of characteristic markers. *Cells Tissues Organs* **2006**, *184*, 16–22. [CrossRef]

43. Baer, P.C.; Koch, B.; Hickmann, E.; Schubert, R.; Cinatl, J.; Hauser, I.A.; Geiger, H. Isolation, Characterization, Differentiation and Immunomodulatory Capacity of Mesenchymal Stromal/Stem Cells from Human Perirenal Adipose Tissue. *Cells* **2019**, *8*, 1346. [CrossRef] [PubMed]

44. EMA. Assessment Report-Empagliflozin-EMA/CHMP/137741/2014. Available online: https://www.ema.europa.eu/en/documents/assessment-report/jardiance-epar-public-assessment-report_en.pdf (accessed on 25 November 2019).

45. EMA. Assessment Report-Dapagliflozin-EMA/689976/2012. Available online: https://www.ema.europa.eu/en/documents/assessment-report/forxiga-epar-public-assessment-report_en.pdf (accessed on 25 November 2019).

46. Leira, F.; Louzao, M.C.; Vieites, J.M.; Botana, L.M.; Vieytes, M.R. Fluorescent microplate cell assay to measure uptake and metabolism of glucose in normal human lung fibroblasts. *Toxicol. In Vitro* **2002**, *16*, 267–273. [CrossRef]

47. Pfaffl, M.W. A new mathematical model for relative quantification in real-time RT-PCR. *Nucleic Acids Res.* **2001**, *29*, e45. [CrossRef] [PubMed]

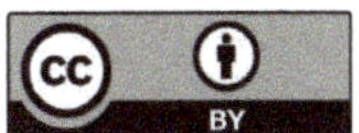

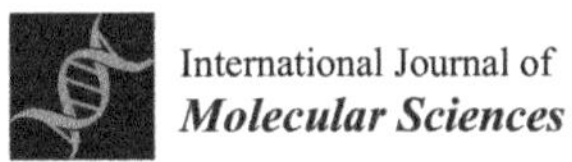

International Journal of
Molecular Sciences

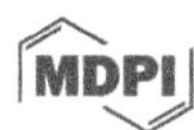

Article

LPS-Binding Protein Modulates Acute Renal Fibrosis by Inducing Pericyte-to-Myofibroblast Trans-Differentiation through TLR-4 Signaling

Giuseppe Castellano [1,*,†], Alessandra Stasi [1,†], Rossana Franzin [1], Fabio Sallustio [1,2], Chiara Divella [1], Alessandra Spinelli [1], Giuseppe Stefano Netti [3], Enrico Fiaccadori [4], Vincenzo Cantaluppi [5], Antonio Crovace [6], Francesco Staffieri [6], Luca Lacitignola [6], Giuseppe Grandaliano [3], Simona Simone [1], Giovanni Battista Pertosa [1] and Loreto Gesualdo [1]

[1] Nephrology, Dialysis and Transplantation Unit, Department of Emergency and Organ Transplantation, University of Bari, 70124 Bari, Italy
[2] Department of Basic Medical Sciences, Neuroscience and Sense Organs, University of Bari, 70124 Bari, Italy
[3] Nephrology, Dialysis and Transplantation Unit, Department of Medical and Surgical Sciences, University of Foggia, 71122 Foggia, Italy
[4] Nephrology Unit, Department of Medicine and Surgery, University of Parma, 43121 Parma, Italy
[5] Department of Translational Medicine, University of Piemonte Orientale, 28100 Novara, Italy
[6] Veterinary Surgery Unit, Department of Emergency and Organ Transplantation, University of Bari, 70010 Bari, Italy
* Correspondence: giuseppe.castellano@uniba.it; Tel.: +39-080-547-88-78
† These two authors equally contributed to the present study.

Received: 12 July 2019; Accepted: 24 July 2019; Published: 27 July 2019

Abstract: During sepsis, the increased synthesis of circulating lipopolysaccharide (LPS)-binding protein (LBP) activates LPS/TLR4 signaling in renal resident cells, leading to acute kidney injury (AKI). Pericytes are the major source of myofibroblasts during chronic kidney disease (CKD), but their involvement in AKI is poorly understood. Here, we investigate the occurrence of pericyte-to-myofibroblast trans-differentiation (PMT) in sepsis-induced AKI. In a swine model of sepsis-induced AKI, PMT was detected within 9 h from LPS injection, as evaluated by the reduction of physiologic PDGFRβ expression and the dysfunctional α-SMA increase in peritubular pericytes. The therapeutic intervention by citrate-based coupled plasma filtration adsorption (CPFA) significantly reduced LBP, TGF-β, and endothelin-1 (ET-1) serum levels, and furthermore preserved PDGFRβ and decreased α-SMA expression in renal biopsies. In vitro, both LPS and septic sera led to PMT with a significant increase in Collagen I synthesis and α-SMA reorganization in contractile fibers by both SMAD2/3-dependent and -independent TGF-β signaling. Interestingly, the removal of LBP from septic plasma inhibited PMT. Finally, LPS-stimulated pericytes secreted LBP and TGF-β and underwent PMT also upon TGF-β receptor-blocking, indicating the crucial pro-fibrotic role of TLR4 signaling. Our data demonstrate that the selective removal of LBP may represent a therapeutic option to prevent PMT and the development of acute renal fibrosis in sepsis-induced AKI.

Keywords: LPS-binding protein; fibrosis; pericyte; myofibroblast; endotoxemia-induced oliguric kidney injury

---

1. Introduction

Sepsis is a multi-organ disease and represents a systemic immune response to a bacterial infection. In critically ill patients, sepsis is the major cause of acute kidney injury (AKI) and is associated with high mortality or risk of chronic kidney disease (CKD) [1]. The pathophysiology of sepsis-induced AKI is complex and characterized by an overwhelming inflammatory response that leads to metabolic dysfunction, tubular damage, and microvascular dysfunction [2,3]. The most common bacteria involved in sepsis-induced

AKI are gram-negative, since their outer wall component, named lipopolysaccharide (LPS) or endotoxin, can activate a wide variety of cells through interaction with specific pattern recognition receptors (PRR), such as TLRs (toll-like receptors) [4]. In the kidney, LPS is mainly recognized by TLR4, which is expressed by tubular, endothelial cells [2,5] and pericytes [6]. The cellular response to endotoxin requires a shuttle protein—LPS-binding protein (LBP)—that brings LPS to TLR4 and maximizes intracellular signaling [7–12].

Renal pericytes are a large population of resident stromal cells lining the peritubular capillaries that stabilize the endothelium. Recently, Heng Zeng et al. evaluated the critical role of capillary pericytes in sepsis-associated vascular destabilization and leakage, which is crucial in the pathogenesis of end-organ dysfunction and septic shock [13,14]. Indeed, sepsis may cause microvascular hyper-permeability via disruption of pericyte/endothelial cell (EC) interactions. Furthermore, renal pericytes represent a major source of the pathological extracellular matrix [6]. Although pericytes do not have specific markers, the receptor tyrosin kinase PDGFRβ is considered a constitutive marker for renal pericyte isolation and characterization [15,16]. It has been extensively shown that after injury, PDGFRβ$^+$ pericytes are able to detach from the endothelium, and after migration and differentiation into α-SMA$^+$ myofibroblasts, may lead to interstitial fibrosis [17–21].

Renal fibrosis is the common, final process directed to repair tissue injury; however during sepsis-induced AKI overwhelming and persistent inflammation can lead to renal AKI. Despite recent developments in understanding the immunopathology of sepsis, therapeutic advances have been slow. Further protective therapies are based on the concept that increased levels of pro-inflammatory mediators or endotoxin are associated with the development of AKI, whereby their elimination can prevent sepsis-induced AKI. Indeed, elimination of cytokines and endotoxin is feasible by purification of blood in extracorporeal circuit, through a device (membrane, sorbent) where solute (toxins, cytokines) and fluid can be removed [22,23]. In a previous study, we observed a protective effect of coupled plasma filtration adsorption (CPFA) treatment on EC dysfunction and renal fibrosis; we demonstrated that this beneficial effect was due to the clearance of LBP, a soluble carrier of LPS [11,12].

Here, we investigate the involvement of LBP and TLR4 signalling in pericyte activation. We demonstrate the occurrence of pericyte-to-myofibroblast trans-differentiation (PMT) in a swine model of LPS-induced oliguric kidney. We elucidate that PMT is regulated by the cross-talk between TLR4 and TGF-β signaling and is mediated by common effectors (as SMADs proteins). We also show that CPFA treatment reduces PMT through a mechanism mediated by LBP removal, which might represent a potential strategy to prevent the occurrence of early fibrosis in patients with sepsis-induced AKI.

2. Results

2.1. Acute Induction of PMT in Endotoxemia-Induced Oliguric Kidney Injury

First, we analyzed the activation of renal pericytes in our model of LPS-induced AKI by immunohistochemistry analysis for PDGFRβ. In healthy and CPFA-treated healthy pigs (T9 CTR, T9 CPFA, Figure 1A), PDGFRβ$^+$ expression was detected in interstitial peritubular capillaries, in mesangial cells, and Bowman's capsule. 9 h after LPS infusion, we found a significant reduction of PDGFRβ expression in endotoxemic pigs at peritubular capillary level (T9 LPS) (Figure 1C); on the contrary, PDGFRβ expression of mesangial cells was not significantly down-regulated, as expected [21]. Interestingly, CPFA treatment significantly inhibited PDGFRβ downregulation (Figure 1A, T9 LPS CPFA and Figure 1C).

To investigate whether the PDGFRβ decrease could be associated with occurrence of PMT, we performed a double immunofluorescence for both PDGFRβ and α-SMA marker. In the CTR and CPFA groups (Figure 1B, T9 CTR, and T9 CPFA), PDGFRβ$^+$ pericytes were weakly positive for α-SMA, as expected. As shown in Figure 1B and calculated in Figure 1E, α-SMA positivity was predominately found on larger arterial wall (Figure 1B, T9 CTR, white arrow). In the septic pigs, 9 h after LPS infusion (T9 LPS), the phenotype of renal pericytes dramatically changed with a significant increase in α-SMA (Figure 1B, T9 LPS). The co-localization of these two markers (PDGFRβ/α-SMA) was more evident in arterioles, peritubular capillaries and mesangial cells (Figure 1B, T9 LPS), indicating that these cells acquired myofibroblast characteristics. After 9 h of adsorption treatment with CPFA, the number of PDGFRβ$^+$/α-SMA$^+$ cells in the peritubular capillaries was significantly reduced (Figure 1D), concurrent with the restoring of a physiological cellular phenotype (Figure 1B, T9 LPS CPFA).

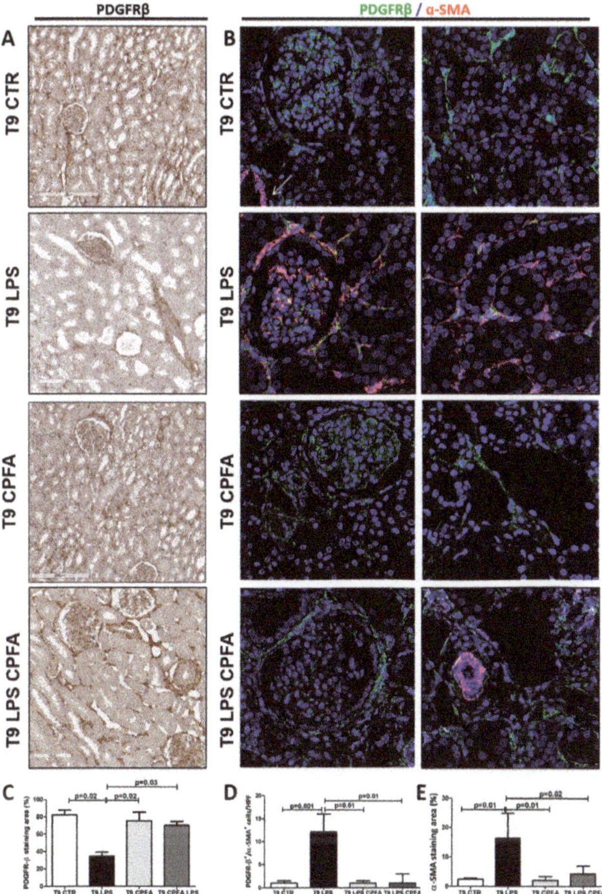

Figure 1. CPFA inhibited LPS-induced PDGFRβ down-regulation and pericyte-to-myofibroblast trans-differentiation (PMT) in endotoxemic pigs. (**A**) IHC (Immunohistochemistry) revealed a strong decrease in PDGFRβ expression at perivascular level after 9 h from LPS infusion (T9 LPS) compared to control (T9 CTR) and CPFA-treated healthy pigs (T9 CPFA). Renal biopsies of endotoxemic animals after CPFA treatment showed a preservation of PDGFRβ$^+$ cells (T9 LPS CPFA) Magnification 10x. (**B**) Pericytes were double-stained for PDGFRβ (green) and α-SMA marker (red) to further demonstrate the occurrence of PMT. In the interstitium of T9 CTR and T9 CPFA pigs, PDGFRβ$^+$/α-SMA$^+$ cells were rarely detectable. Nine h after LPS infusion, the number of these cells dramatically increased (T9 LPS). CPFA treatment reversed LPS-induced PMT, decreasing the number of these transitioning cells (T9 LPS CPFA) Magnification 630×. The fluorescent dye To-pro 3 was used to counterstain nuclei (blue)Quantitative analyses of PDGFRβ (**C**), PDGFRβ/ α-SMA double positive cells (**D**) and α-SMA staining (**E**) were obtained as described in the Methods section and expressed as median ± interquartile range (IQR) of five independent pigs for each group. (**D**) Results are expressed as median ± IQR of the numbers of PDGFRβ$^+$/α-SMA$^+$ cells/ high-power (×630) fields (HPF) of five independent pigs for each group. Results were statistically analyzed in GraphPad Prism. Statistically significant differences were assessed by the Mann–Whitney test. (**E**) Moreover, α-SMA expression (red-stained area) significantly increased in endotoxemic pigs (T9 LPS) and was reduced by CPFA treatment (T9 LPS CPFA). Magnification 630×.

2.2. LPS-Mediated Early Pericyte-to-Myofibroblast Trans-Differentiation (PMT)

To test whether LPS was directly involved in the trans-differentiation of pericytes in myofibroblast, we cultured human pericytes in presence of LPS. A significant increase of α-SMA protein expression was detected after 9 h from LPS stimulation compared to basal condition (LPS:3.9 $\pm$ 1.27 vs. basal:1.08 $\pm$ 0.5, $p = 0.03$) (Figure 2A).

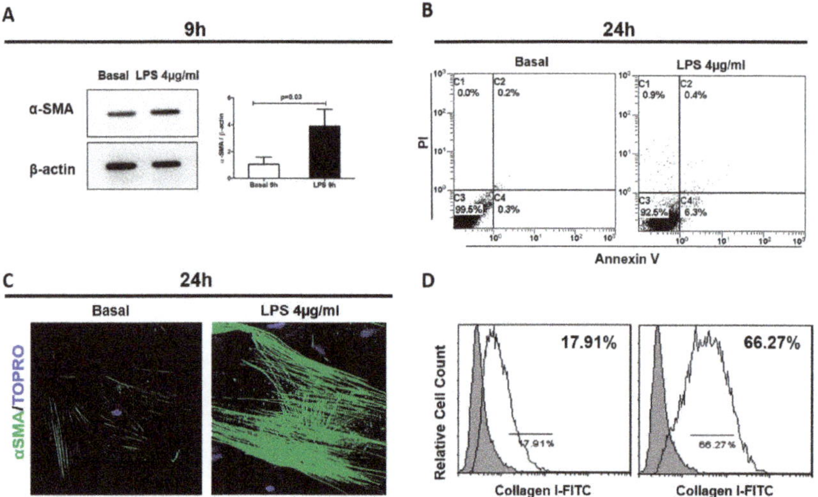

Figure 2. LPS mediated early PMT. Cultured pericytes were incubated with LPS 4 µg/mL, for 9 and 24 h. (**A**) WB analysis revealed a significant increase of α-SMA expression after 9 h of LPS stimulation, compared to basal level. β-actin protein expression was used for normalization. Data are expressed as mean $\pm$ standard deviation (SD) of three independent experiments and compared with the Student t test. 24 h of LPS exposure did not affect pericyte viability (**B**) and induced a remodeling of contractile α-SMA-stress fibers (**C**) and a protein increase of Collagen I (**D**). Results are representative of three independent experiments.

Moreover, we found that endotoxin exposure did not affect pericyte viability (Figure 2B) and LPS-stimulated pericytes changed their morphology to an elongated and spindle-like cell shape similar to that of fibroblasts. Under immunofluorescence analysis, pericytes showed high α-SMA expression localized in stress fibers, indicating the acquirement of a contractile phenotype (Figure 2C). Finally, flow cytometry analysis revealed that these changes were accompanied by increased Collagen I protein expression (Figure 2D). Collectively, these findings showed that LPS triggered PMT in vitro, indicating the differentiation towards a pro-fibrotic phenotype (Figure 2C,D).

2.3. LPS Binding Protein (LBP) Was Critical in LPS-Mediated PMT

Next, we investigated whether LPS/TLR4 signaling may be critical in mediating PMT during endotoxemia-induced AKI. Recently, we demonstrated in the same animal model that CPFA treatment prevented an LBP serum increase and that the removal of LBP drastically reduced the binding of LPS to TLR4 receptor [11]. We cultured pericytes in the presence of different swine sera for 9 h and 24 h (CTR, CPFA, LPS, and LPS CPFA). Firstly, we examined whether LBP and swine sera could affect pericyte viability. After 24 h of LBP-activation and incubation with swine sera, flow cytometry analysis showed that pericytes did not undergo apoptosis (Figure 3A).

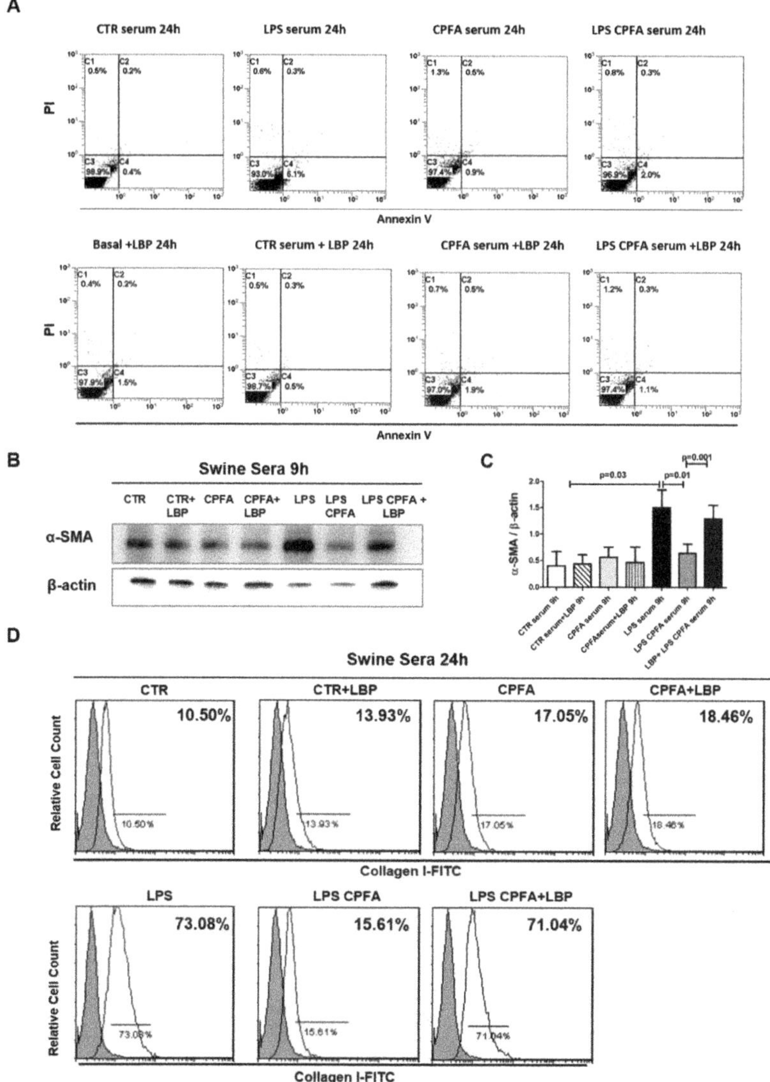

Figure 3. LBP was critical in LPS-mediated early PMT. Cultured pericytes were stimulated with LPS 4 µg/Ml or LBP 9 µg/Ml, or cultured in presence of different swine sera with/without LBP for the indicated time period. (**A**) Pericyte viability was evaluated by flow cytometry analysis (AnnV/PI). Cells did not undergo apoptosis. (**B,C**) WB analysis revealed a significant increase of α-SMA expression after 9 h of endotoxemic sera incubation. CPFA-treated septic sera (LPS CPFA) maintained the expression of α-SMA at low level as CPFA-treated healthy sera (CPFA group). Both in CTR and CPFA sera, the addition of exogenous LBP did not increase α-SMA expression. Remarkably, the addition of LBP in CPFA-treated endotoxemic sera (LPS CPFA) induced PMT like the untreated endotoxemic sera. β-actin protein expression was used for normalization. Data were shown as mean ± standard deviation (SD) and compared with the Student t test. (**D**) FACS (Fluorescence Activated Cell Sorting) showed a strong increase of Collagen I after 24 h of endotoxemic sera incubation compared to control. In accordance, CPFA-treated endotoxemic sera maintained Collagen I expression at basal level as CTR and CPFA group. Exogenous LBP supplementation in CTR and CPFA group did not stimulate Collagen I synthesis in pericytes. The LBP addition in LPS CPFA group completely reversed the effects of CPFA treatment, leading to PMT. Results are representative of three independent experiments.

Western blot analysis revealed a significant increase of α-SMA expression after incubation with LPS group sera compared to CTR group sera (data LPS vs. CTR) (Figure 3B,C). CPFA treatment restored the expression of α-SMA at CTR group level in pericytes (LPS CPFA: 0.6 ± 0.21 vs. LPS: 1.02 ± 0.22, p = 0.001). Moreover, CPFA-treated healthy sera maintained α-SMA expression at basal level as CTR group.

Flow cytometry analysis also showed a strong increase of Collagen I after 24 h of endotoxemic sera incubation compared to control, indicating that PMT resulted in active contribution to the synthesis of extracellular matrix components (Figure 3D). CPFA-healthy sera did not affect pericyte phenotype. In accordance, CPFA-treated endotoxemic sera maintained Collagen I expression at basal level.

In order to understand the molecular mechanism involved in the CPFA anti-fibrotic function on human pericyte, we reconstituted the swine group sera with LBP. Both in CTR and CPFA sera, the addition of exogenous LBP did not influence α-SMA and Collagen I expression. Remarkably, the addition of exogenous LBP in sera of LPS CPFA pigs completely reverted the CPFA protective effect. We detected that after LBP sera reconstitution, LPS CPFA group sera re-acquired the capacity to induce PMT in vitro, as shown by the increase of α-SMA and Collagen I protein expression (Figure 3B,D).

2.4. TLR4 Signaling Mediates PMT via Enhanced Canonical and Non-Canonical TGF-β Signaling

Next, to identify the signaling involved in PMT and directly activated by LBP/LPS/TLR4 we analyzed the early extracellular signal-regulated kinase 1 (ERK1) phosphorylation, a mediator that is common to TLR4 and pro-fibrotic TGF-β pathways. Regarding TGF-β pathway, we assessed the level of activation of the two different SMAD 2/3-dependent and SMAD2/3- independent signaling.

Pericytes were cultured with or without LPS or sera from LPS group for 5, 30, and 60 min. To analyze the intracellular signaling activated during the incubation, we studied pERK1 and pSMAD2/3 protein expression. Both LPS and endotoxemic sera significantly increased phosphorylation of SMAD2/3 and ERK1, demonstrating the involvement of both canonical SMAD2/3-dependent and non-canonical SMAD2/3-independent signaling, respectively. (Figure 4A–D).

Because we found the maximum increase of pERK1 and pSMAD2/3 level after 30 min of activation by LPS or incubation with septic serum, we decided to further analyze at this time point the potential effect of CPFA treatment on this signaling activation (Figure 4E,F). Compared to LPS group sera, the LPS CPFA group sera led to a significant downregulation of ERK1 and SMAD2/3. In line with the previous findings regarding α-SMA and collagen I protein expression (Figure 3B,D), the restoration of LBP serum significantly increased the phosphorylation of ERK1 and SMAD2/3. Otherwise, the addition of LBP in CTR and CPFA-treated healthy sera did not modify the phosphorylation of SMAD2/3 and ERK1 (Figure 4E,F, quantization in Figure 4G,H). All together, these data indicated that CPFA treatment was able to remove the serum components capable to induce the rapid ERK1 and SMAD2/3 phosphorylation during endotoxemia, and that LBP may be considered a key factor not only in LPS/TLR4 signaling but also in the pro-fibrotic activity of TGF-β pathway.

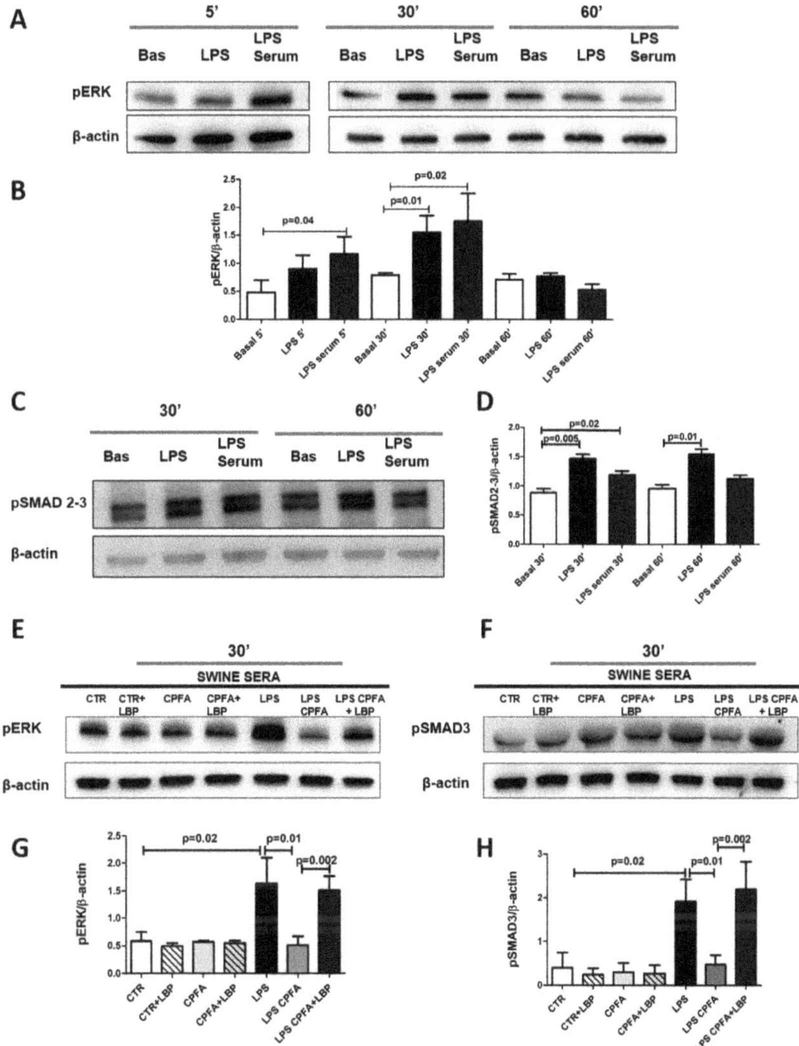

Figure 4. LPS and endotoxemic sera induced PMT by canonical TGF-β-SMAD2/3-dependent and non-canonical TGF-β-SMAD-independent signaling. (**A–D**) Pericytes were cultured with LPS or endotoxemic sera for 5, 30, and 60 min. Cell extracts were then used for WB analysis for pERK1 and pSMAD2/3. Both LPS and endotoxemic sera augmented SMAD2/3 and ERK1 phosphorylation, demonstrating the involvement of both canonical TGF-β-SMAD2/3-dependent and non-canonical TGF-β-SMAD-independent signaling. (**E–H**) Cultured pericytes were incubated in the presence of 1% of different swine sera for 30 min, with/without LBP (pre-treatment 1 h). CTR and CPFA-treated healthy sera maintained the phosphorylation of SMAD2/3 and ERK1 at basal level. Endotoxemic sera significantly increased phosphorylation of SMAD2/3 and ERK1. CPFA-treated endotoxemic sera reduced the phosphorylation of SMAD2/3 and ERK1 at basal level. The addition of LBP in CTR and CPFA-treated healthy sera did not augment phosphorylation of SMAD2/3 and ERK1. Otherwise, the addition of LBP in LPS CPFA sera reversed CPFA effects, increasing the activation of SMAD2/3 and ERK1. Results are representative of three independent experiments. Data are shown as mean ± standard deviation (SD) and compared with the Student t test.

2.5. CPFA Treatment Significantly Decreased Pro-Fibrotic Factors in Endotoxemic Pigs

Several reports have referred to an increase of circulating TGF-β in septic patients [24] and the involvement of Endothelin-1 (ET-1) in the pathogenesis of sepsis [25]. In addition, it is also known that TGF-β can amplify and further enhance LPS signaling [26] and ET-1 promotes the induction of the myofibroblast phenotype from vascular pericytes [27].

In line with these findings, in LPS group sera we found an increase of the TGF-β and ET-1 levels compared to CTR group after 9 h from LPS infusion. Interestingly, CPFA-treated endotoxemic pigs presented a significant reduction in TGF-β and ET-1 serum levels (Figure 5A,B).

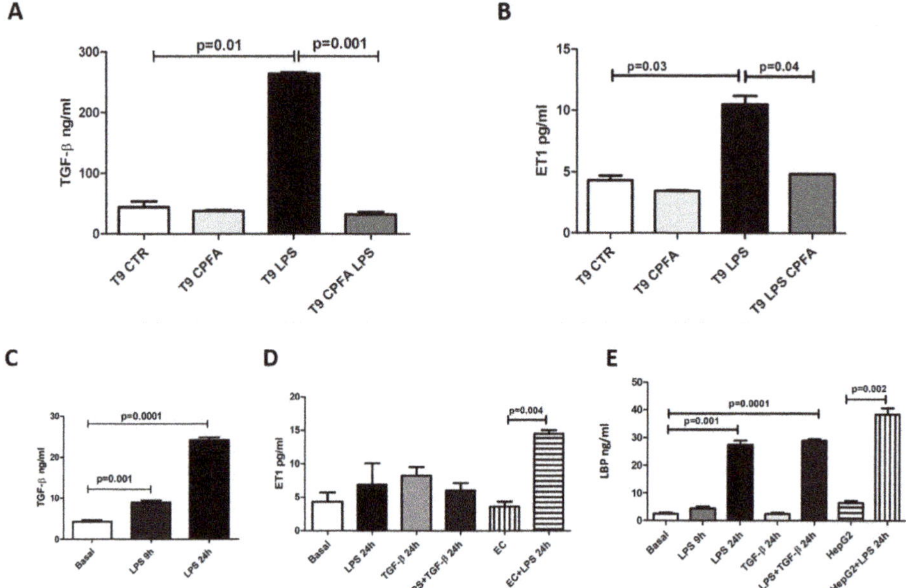

Figure 5. CPFA treatment modulated serum levels of TGF-β and ET-1, and LPS-stimulated pericytes secreted TGF-β and LBP. (**A,B**) Serum levels of TGF-β and ET-1 significantly increased after 9 h of LPS infusion compared to healthy pigs. Interestingly, CPFA-treated pigs presented a dramatic reduction in serum TGF-β and ET-1 levels. Data are expressed as median ± IQR of five independent pigs for each group. Statistically significant differences were assessed by the Mann–Whitney test. (**C–E**) cultured pericytes were stimulated with LPS and/or TGF-β, and their supernatants were analyzed by ELISA. Human endothelial cells (EC) and human liver hepatocellular cells (HepG2) were used as control positive for ET-1 and LBP synthesis, respectively.(**C**) LPS augmented TGF-β production in pericytes, particularly at 24 h. (**D**) LPS and/or TGF-β stimulation did not increase ET-1 production compared with EC treated with LPS for 24 h (positive control). (**E**) After 24 h from LPS stimulation, pericytes significantly increased LBP synthesis. Stimulation of pericytes with TGF-β alone did not influence LBP production. HepG2 stimulated with LPS for 24 h were used as positive control. Data were shown as mean ± standard deviation (SD) and compared with the Student t test.

In order to clarify the contribution of pericytes to circulating TGF-β, ET-1, and LBP serum release, we evaluated whether LPS exposition could influence their production in culture (Figure 5C–E).

Thereby, we stimulated pericytes with LPS and/or TGF-β for 9 h and 24 h and analyzed the pericyte culture supernatants by ELISA. Interestingly, LPS augmented TGF-β production, particularly at 24 h (LPS 24 h: 24.20 ± 1.51 vs. basal: 4.22 ± 0.88, $p = 0.001$) (Figure 5C). Otherwise, LPS and TGF- β, alone or in combination, did not induce ET-1 production by pericytes.

Because we have already demonstrated [11], in the same animal model, the increase of circulating LBP in endotoxemic pigs, we also evaluated the contribution of pericytes to LBP secretion. 24 h after LPS stimulation, we observed a significant increase of LBP with respect to basal level. Otherwise, TGF-β did not induce LBP synthesis in pericytes.

2.6. LBP-LPS Axis-Induced PMT was Characterized by Canonical and Non-Canonical TGF-β Signaling

First, we analyzed the effects of LBP alone or in presence of LPS. In vitro, we observed that LPS-stimulated pericytes contributed to LBP synthesis, which is known to maximize cellular response to endotoxin [11,12,28,29]. Stimulation of pericytes with LBP alone did not induce phenotypical changes in pericytes. Interestingly, pericytes treated with LBP and LPS in combination or with LBP, LPS, and TGF-β mixture additively increased Collagen I expression and decreased PDGFRβ marker more than LPS-stimulated pericytes. These data demonstrate that LBP is a cofactor of LPS that contributes to LPS signaling (Figure 6A).

Moreover, we observed that LPS-stimulated pericytes are associated with TGF-β secretion, which, in turn, can trigger or enhance PMT [19,21]. Thus, in order to selectively analyze the role of LPS/TLR4 signaling in inducing PMT, we blocked the TGF-β pathway by TGF-βR inhibition (Figure 6B). Pericytes were pre-treated with anti-TGF-βR -specific neutralizing antibody for 1 h followed by LPS and/or LBP stimulation for 24 h. As expected, LBP-stimulated pericytes did not modify their phenotype. Interestingly, we found that LPS or LBP/LPS-stimulated pericytes underwent PMT also following TGF-βR-blocking, as observed by a significant increase of collagen I expression and a decrease of PDGFRβ marker (Figure 6B). These data support the role of LBP-LPS axis in promoting PMT and fibrosis, independently from TGF-β.

Moreover, the anti-TGF-βR neutralizing antibody did not reduce phosphorylation of both ERK1/2 and SMAD3 (Figure 6C–F) mediated by LPS alone or in combination with LBP at 30 min. Stimulation of pericytes with LBP alone did not modify phosphorylation of both ERK1/2 and SMAD3. Collectively, these data indicated that in vitro LPS alone or in combination with LBP can promote both TGF-β canonical and non-canonical pathways, leading to fibrosis and collagen release independently from TGF-β receptor activation.

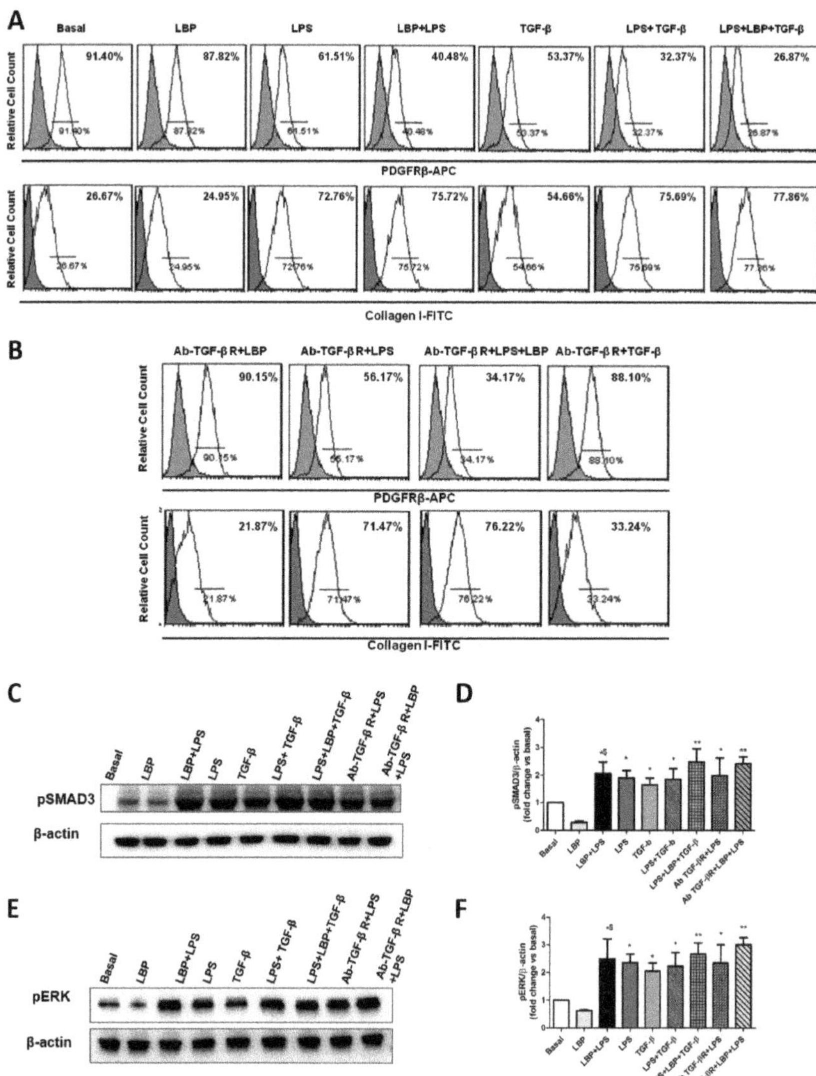

Figure 6. LBP-LPS axis induced PMT upon blocking TGF-βR. (**A**) Cultured pericytes were treated with LBP and/or LPS or TGF- β and with LBP, LPS, and TGF-β mixture for 24 h. LBP alone did not induce phenotypical changes in pericytes. Pericytes treated with LBP and LPS in combination or with LBP, LPS, and TGF-β mixture additively increased Collagen I expression and decreased PDGFRβ marker. (**B**) Pericytes were pretreated with anti-TGF-Br-specific neutralizing antibody for 1 h followed by LPS and/or LBP stimulation for 24 h. FACS analysis showed that pericytes acquired phenotypic change also upon TGF-βR-blocking. Results are representative of three independent experiments. (**C–F**) Pericytes were pretreated with anti-TGF-βR specific neutralizing antibody for 1 h followed by LPS and/or LBP for short stimulation time (30 min). Pretreatment of pericytes with anti-TGF-βR antibody did not reduce LPS and LPS/LBP-induced phosphorylation of both SMAD3 (**C,D**) and ERK1/2 (**E,F**) at 30 min. Results are representative of three independent experiments. Data are shown as mean ± standard deviation (SD) and compared with the Student t test (**D,F**: * $p < 0.05$, ** $p \leq 0.005$, versus basal level; $^{\$}$ $p < 0.05$ versus LBP).

3. Discussion

In this paper, we demonstrated for the first time the occurrence of PMT in a swine model of LPS-induced oliguric kidney. We elucidated that the PMT is regulated by the cross-talk between the TLR-4 and TGF-β signaling and mediated by common intracellular pathways. We also showed that CPFA treatment reduced the PMT through a mechanism mediated by LBP removal [11], which might represent a potential strategy to prevent early fibrosis in patients with sepsis-induced AKI.

Pericytes are mesenchymal-derived cells that stabilize endothelial cells, regulate capillary blood flow, and perform various functions throughout the cellular body [30]. Recent evidence has suggested the prominent role of renal pericytes in scar-forming myofibroblasts generation during CKD [17,18,31] as well as early phases of AKI [21]. Our data demonstrate that renal pericytes are activated also in acute settings such as LPS induced AKI; in vivo and in vitro PMT occurred already after 9 h from LPS activation, with reduced expression of the specific marker PDGFRβ and expression myofibroblast markers α-SMA. Interestingly, in the same swine model of LPS-induced kidney injury, we previously showed that endothelial to mesenchymal transition also contributes to kidney fibrosis [11,12]. Endothelial cells lose their functions and switch from a quiescent to an activated state, acquiring fibroblast phenotype. Taken together, these data indicated pericytes and endothelial cells as the main contributors in the acute induction of renal fibrosis in endotoxemia-induced oliguric kidney injury.

Hyperdinamic renal circulation and an exacerbated inflammatory response without significant evidence of acute tubular necrosis have been extensively characterized in sepsis-induced AKI [32]. In this scenario, the mechanisms involved are attributed to invading microorganisms and their products, known as pathogen-associated molecular patterns (PAMPs), which activate immune cells and renal resident cells by a broad spectrum of PPRs, including TLRs. In particular, LPS, a critical structural component of the outer wall of gram-negative bacteria, is considered the main PAMP and is specifically recognized by TLR-4 [4,33,34]. TLR4 mediates pro-inflammatory and pro-fibrotic pathways, leading to fibroblast accumulation during renal injury [15,35–38]. Moreover, TLR4-deficient mice were protected from kidney fibrosis with reduced α-SMA protein expression and less tubulointerstitial fibrosis [39]. Recent evidence has demonstrated that TLR4-MyD88-dependent pathway activates not only immune signaling but simultaneously fibrogenesis in pericytes, contributing to matrix deposition and pathology in AKI [6]. Activation of TLR-4 leads to the stimulation of both MyD88-dependent and a MyD88-indipendent pathway that lead to downstream activation of the IKK complex, mitogen-activated protein kinase (MAPK), and phosphatidylinositol 3-kinase (PI3K)/Akt pathways [40].

Our results demonstrated that LPS induced PMT with the acquirement of α-SMA contractile stress fibers and the secretion of ECM products as Collagen I, by triggering TGF-β canonical and non-canonical pathway [41–47]. Indeed, LPS increased phosphorylation of SMAD2/3 and ERK1, suggesting that acute PMT was induced, respectively, by canonical TGF-β-SMAD-dependent and non-canonical TGF-β-SMAD-independent signaling. (Figure A1)

Moreover, our study showed that LPS can directly induce SMAD2/3 phosphorylation in a TGF-β independent manner. LPS-stimulated pericytes secreted TGF-β and underwent PMT also following TGF-β receptor-blocking, pointing out the pro-fibrotic role of TLR4 signaling. Since LPS may modulate TGF-β synthesis in pericytes, we speculated that LPS/TLR4 signaling contributes to further accumulation of TGF-β, amplifying LPS signaling and developing a self-sustaining positive feedback loop that initiates collagen accumulation and leads to renal fibrosis progression. As LPS and TGF-β additively triggered PMT process in vitro, we suggest that this endotoxin can amplify the responsiveness of pericytes to TGF-β stimulation. Our data are in line with other papers showing that the activation of TLR4 signaling enhanced the sensitivity of fibroblasts to the stimulatory effect of TGF-β, activating SMAD signaling and down-regulating anti-fibrotic antagonist BAMBI [48].

Among the different factors involved in TLR-4 signaling, LBP seems to be crucial in enhancing and amplifying cellular response to endotoxin [11,12,28,29]. In vivo, the binding of LPS to TLR-4 requires a carrier protein—LBP—an acute phase protein, synthesized by hepatocytes and released into the bloodstream after gram-negative infection. During the acute inflammatory response, LBP blood levels increase and amplify the host response to infection, even at low concentrations of endotoxin [7,9,10,49]. LBP alone has no effect on the development of tissue injury but serves as a key modulator of cellular and systemic responses to LPS. Moreover, many different types of cells in several organs such as lungs, kidneys, and liver contribute to LBP synthesis, maximizing the local parenchymal inflammation [50]. Here, we showed that pericytes release LBP, as well as TGF-β, in response to LPS. These secretory capacities of pericytes in response to LPS may be particularly important for their contribution to kidney fibrosis.

Moreover, pericytes treated with LBP in combination with LPS and TGF-β significantly amplified PMT process respect to LPS-stimulated pericytes. Our findings are consistent with published data showing that LBP functions as a "biological taxi service" [51] for transporting endotoxin in blood and facilitating LPS binding to TLR-4 maximizing inflammatory response on host cells.

Accordingly with our previous study, in the same swine model of LPS-induced oliguric kidney injury, endotoxemic pigs with high levels of LBP were prone to inflammation, endothelial dysfunction, early development of fibrosis, and increased risk of mortality [11].

Thus, targeting TLR signaling may confer a novel therapeutic strategy for renal fibrosis in early and end-stage renal disease. Until now, soluble receptors and monoclonal antibodies used to block the interaction of LPS and other ligands with TLR-4 did not have any efficacy [52]. Extracorporeal elimination techniques have been proposed as a possible approach for cytokine elimination to improve the clinical conditions of septic patients. Recently, we have demonstrated the beneficial effects of CPFA treatment in LPS-induced oliguric kidney injury. CPFA is a technique of blood purification in which systemic blood circulates through a plasmafilter that separates plasma from whole blood, allowing the non-selective removal of inflammatory mediators through the adsorption resin cartridge [53]. In our previous study, in the same swine model, we demonstrated that the removal of LBP by CPFA, rather than endotoxin, impaired the development of endothelial to mesenchymal transition and prevented the acute development of tubulo-interstitial fibrosis [11]. Accordingly, here we have found that the in vivo removal of LBP strongly reduces LPS binding to TLR4 and the subsequent pericyte activation; moreover, in vitro supplementation of exogenous LBP in treated endotoxemic sera induced the early development of PMT through the activation of TLR-4 signaling and both SMAD dependent and independent TGF-β- signal transduction. On the basis of our results, the in vivo blocking of LBP, rather than endotoxin, may significantly reduce the intracellular signaling regulating pericyte dysfunction and kidney fibrosis (Figure A2). Other studies with knockout mice for LBP are needed to underline the potential benefit of LBP blockade in endotoxemic kidney injury.

Furthermore, we observed that CPFA treatment was critical in modulating TGF-β serum level in endotoxemic pigs, suggesting the efficacy of adsorption treatments in preventing kidney fibrosis and the subsequent progression to CKD.

ET-1 is also of interest, since it is able to promote the induction of myofibroblast differentiation from vascular pericytes contributing to fibrotic disorders in several organs and tissues. It has been described as an important factor both in renal pathophysiology and kidney diseases. Accordingly, we showed a significant increase of ET-1 in endotoxemic pigs that could contribute to phenotypical changes in pericytes. We also demonstrated for the first time that CPFA treatment reduced ET-1 sera levels, thus regulating the pro-fibrotic process. However, pericytes did not contribute to ET-1 synthesis, and we supposed that other cells like glomerular endothelial cells [27] could be the main source for this factor.

In conclusion, our data suggest that in the early phase of LPS-induced AKI, renal pericytes contribute to renal fibrosis and kidney failure. Extracorporeal treatment by CPFA decrease PMT and might affect fibrosis progression, thereby counteracting the long-term effect of sepsis-induced AKI.

4. Materials and Methods

4.1. Animal Model

Animal studies were carried out under protocol approved by Ethical Committee of the Italian Ministry of Health, Prot. N823/2016-PR (2016, approved on 2 September 2016). Briefly, endotoxemia was induced in pig by intravenous infusion of a saline solution containing 300 µg/kg of LPS (lipopolisaccharide membrane of escherichia coli), as described previously [11]. Pigs were divided into four groups: control (CTR, healthy pigs, $n = 7$), CPFA (CPFA-treated healthy pigs, $n = 7$), LPS (endotoxemic pigs, $n = 7$), and LPS CPFA (CPFA-treated endotoxemic pigs, $n = 7$). CTR and CPFA pigs received 10 mL of sterile saline solution.

CPFA treatment was performed for 6 h, as previously described [11]. Animals were sacrificed after 9 h from LPS/saline infusion or after 6 h CPFA treatment (T9).

4.2. Collection of Samples

Renal biopsies were performed at the start of experimental procedure (T0) and at different intervals from saline or LPS infusion until death (T9). A portion of each biopsy was fixed in buffered formalin (4%) for 12 h and embedded in paraffin by using standard procedures as previously described [11]. Swine sera were collected at T0, at intermediate time points, and at T9 from an arterial blood catheter.

4.3. Cell Culture

Human placental-derived pericytes (PromoCell, Heidelberg, Germany) were grown in Serum-Free Pericyte Growth Medium (PromoCell) at 5% CO2 and 37 °C [21]. Human umbilical vein endothelial cells (HUVEC, EC) and Human Hepato Cancer cells (HepG2) were purchased from American Type Culture Collection (ATCC-LGC Standards S.r.l., Sesto San Giovanni, Milan, Italy). EC and HepG2 were maintained in their recommended medium, EndGro (Merck Millipore, Darmstadt, Germany) and DMEM high-glucose medium supplemented with 10% Fetal Bovine serum (FBS), 100 U/mL penicillin, 0.1 mg/mL streptomycin, 2 mM L-glutamine (Sigma Aldrich, Milan, Italy), respectively. When cells became confluent, they were stimulated with LPS 4 µg/mL (E. Coli O111:B4, Sigma-Aldrich, Milan, Italy), LPS Binding Protein (LBP, HycultBiotech, Uden, The Netherlands) 9 µg/mL [11], and TGF-β1 10 ng/mL (Biovision, San Francisco, CA, USA). Moreover cells were incubated in the presence of 1% of different swine sera with/without LPS Binding Protein (LBP), 9 µg/mL [11], for the indicated time period. All experiments were performed at early P3–P5 passages. For TGF-βR inhibition assay, pericytes were pre-treated with mouse monoclonal anti-TGF-βR (Abcam, Cambridge, UK) at 5–10–20–25–30 µg/mL for 1 h before the TGF-β (10 ng/mL) exposition (Figure A2). The concentration used for TGF-βR blocking before LPS (4 µg/mL) and/or LBP (9 µg/mL) stimulation was 20 µg/mL.

4.4. Immunohistochemistry (IHC)

Renal sections underwent deparaffination and heat-mediated antigen retrieval as previously described [11]. Sections were incubated with the primary antibody PDGFRβ (Abcam, Cambridge, MA, USA) and detected by the Peroxidase/DAB Dako Real EnVision Detection System ((Dako, Glostrup, Denmark). Negative controls were obtained by incubation with a control irrelevant antibody. Images were acquired by Aperio ScanScope CS2 device, and signals were analyzed with the ImageScope V12.1.0.5029 (Aperio Technologies, Vista, CA, USA).

4.5. Confocal Laser Scanning Microscopy

Swine paraffin-embedded renal sections and cultured pericytes were stained or double stained for α-SMA (Santa Cruz Biotechnologies, Santa Cruz, CA, USA) and PDGFRβ (Abcam, Cambridge, MA, USA) as previously described [21]. All the antibodies cross-reacted with pig tissue. For immunofluorescence microscopy on cultured pericytes, 5×10^4 cells were seeded on a cover slip, grown to 70% confluence, and then stimulated with LPS 4 µg/mL. After stimulation, cells were fixed in 3.7% paraformaldehyde for 5 min. To counterstain nuclei of renal tissue and cells, we used the fluorescent dye TO-PRO-3 (Molecular Probes, Eugene, OR, USA). Image acquisition was performed with confocal microscope Leica TCS SP2 (Leica, Wetzlar, Germany). The number of PDGFRβ+/α-SMA+ cells was quantified in at least 10 high-power (×630) fields (HPF)/sections by two independent observers. The final counts were the mean of the two measures. In no case was interobserver variability higher than 20%.

4.6. Detection of Viable and Apoptotic Pericytes by Flow Cytometry Analysis (FACS)

Apoptotic and viable pericytes were evaluated with Annexin V(Ann V)–fluorescein isothiocyanate (FITC) and propidium iodide (PI) according to manufacturers' instructions (Beckman Coulter, Brea, CA, USA). Three independent experiments were performed. Data were obtained using a FC500 flow cytometer (Beckman Coulter, Brea, CA, USA) and analyzed by Kaluza software.

4.7. Immunophenotypic Analysis

After stimulations, pericytes were permeabilized with IntraPrep kit (Instrumentation Laboratory) and incubated with APC-conjugated anti-PDGFRβ (LSBio, Seattle, WA, USA) and FITC-conjugated anti-collagen I (Millipore, Millimarck, Germany) as previously described [21]. Data were analyzed with FC500 (Beckman Coulter, Brea, CA, USA) and Kaluza software. This assay was done in triplicate. The area of positivity was determined by using an isotype-matched mAb, and, in total, 10^4 events for each sample were acquired. Data were obtained by using a FC500 (Beckman Coulter) flow cytometer and analyzed with Kaluza software. Three independent experiments were performed.

4.8. ELISA for TGF-β, ET-1, and LBP

TGF-β (ELISA; Enzo Life Sciences, Farmingdale, NY, USA) and ET-1 (ELISA; R&D Systems, Minneapolis, MN, USA) levels in swine sera and in cell culture supernatants were measured by a commercially available enzyme-linked immunosorbent assay (ELISA).

LBP levels were revealed in cell culture supernatants were measured by ELISA kit from HycultBiotech (Uden, The Netherlands).

4.9. Protein Extraction and Western Blotting

The cell monolayer was rapidly rinsed twice with ice-cold PBS and lysed in RIPA buffer (1 mM PMSF, 5 mM EDTA, 1 mM sodium orthovanadate, 150 mM sodium chloride, 8 µg/mL leupeptin, 1.5% Nonidet P-40, and 20 mM tris-HCl (pH 7.4)) with phosphatase and protease inhibitors. The samples (30 µg of proteins) were separated in 4–15% polyacrylamide gel and then transferred to PVDF membrane (0.2 mM) by Trans-Blot Turbo (BioRad, Hercules, CA, USA). After blocking in BSA at 5%, the membranes were probed with the following primary antibodies: pSMAD2/3 (Abcam), pSMAD3 (Cell Signaling, Danvers, MA, USA), and pERK (Cell Signaling) extracellular signal regulated kinases (ERK) α-SMA (Santa Cruz Biotechnology, Inc.), and then with secondary antibody (hrp-conjugated, Abcam). The same membranes were incubated with mouse monoclonal anti-βactin antibody (1:20,000; Sigma). Immune complexes were detected by the ECL chemiluminescence system (Amersham Pharmacia, Little Chalfont, UK), according to the manufacturer's instructions. The chemiluminescent blots were acquired by Chemidoc and analyzed using Image J software. Each experiments was repeated three times.

4.10. Statistical Analysis

Animal data were expressed as median±interquartile range (IQR) and compared with a Mann–Whitney test. For FACS analysis and western blot, data were shown as mean ± standard deviation (SD) and compared with the Student t test. A *p* value < 0.05 was considered statistically significant. All analyses were performed by using GraphPad Prism 5.0 (GraphPad software, Inc., San Diego, CA, USA).

Author Contributions: G.C. and A.S. (Alessandra Stasi). are equal first authors. G.C. provided new analytic tools, designed and supervised the research and drafted the manuscript. A.S. (Alessandra Stasi) planned the research, coordinated the study, performed most experiments, and drafted the manuscript. R.F. contributed to design most experiments, analyzed the respective data, and drafted the manuscript. F.S. (Fabio Sallustio) participated in the design of the study and assisted in vitro experiments and in manuscript preparation. C.D. participated in the immunolabeling and confocal microscopy of renal sections and contributed to data analysis. A.S. (Alessandra Spinelli). participated in the coordination of the study and assisted in in vitro experiments. G.S.N. contributed to the in vivo swine model and performed statistical analysis of clinical parameters. E.F. participated in the design of the study and helped to draft the manuscript. V.C. participated in the coordination of the study and assisted in manuscript preparation. A.C., F.S. (Francesco Staffieri), and L.L. carried out all surgical procedures of the animal model and helped to revise the manuscript. G.G., S.S., and G.B.P. participated in the design of the study and critically revised the manuscript. L.G. participated in the coordination of the study and assisted in manuscript preparation.

Funding: This study was supported by University of Bari "Aldo Moro", the Italian Ministry of Health (Giovani Ricercatori 2011-2012, GR-2011-02351027, granted to GC). LG was supported by a Regional Strategic Grant, Apulia Region (PSR 094).

Acknowledgments: We thank Eustacchio Montemurno for technical assistance in image editing.

Conflicts of Interest: The authors declare no conflict of interest.

Abbreviations

PMT	Pericyte-to-Myofibroblast Trans-differentiation
LBP	LPS Binding Protein
AKI	Acute Kidney Injury
HepG2	Human Hepato Cancer Cells
CKD	Chronic Kidney Disease
CPFA	Citrate-Based Coupled Plasma Filtration Adsorption
EC	Endothelial Cell
WB	Western Blot
TLR-4	Toll Like Receptor-4
ET-1	Endothelin-1
LPS	Lipopolysaccharide
PRR	Pattern Recognition Receptors
Ab	Antibody
TGF-βR	TGF-βReceptor
Ab-TGF-βR	Antibody Anti-TGF-βReceptor

Appendix A

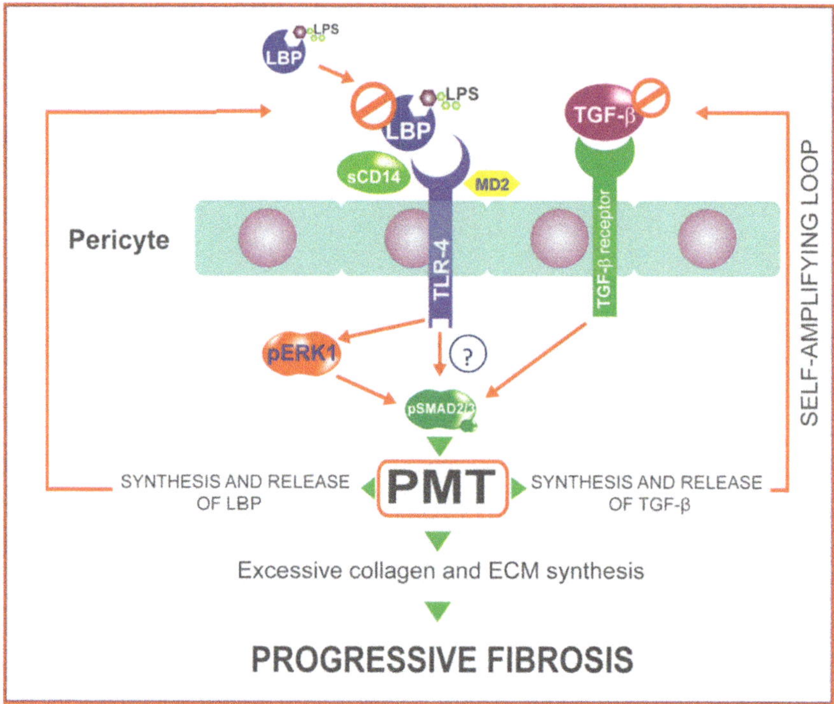

Figure A1. CPFA reduced activation of pericytes and PMT by LBP and TGF-β removal from septic sera. Pericyte TLR4 signaling might contribute to further accumulation of TGF-β and LBP, developing a self-sustaining feed-forward loop that amplifies and maintains renal fibrosis. Disrupting persistent TLR4 signaling activation by the removal of LBP and other molecules as TGF-β represents a potential novel strategy for breaking the cycle of progressive fibrosis.

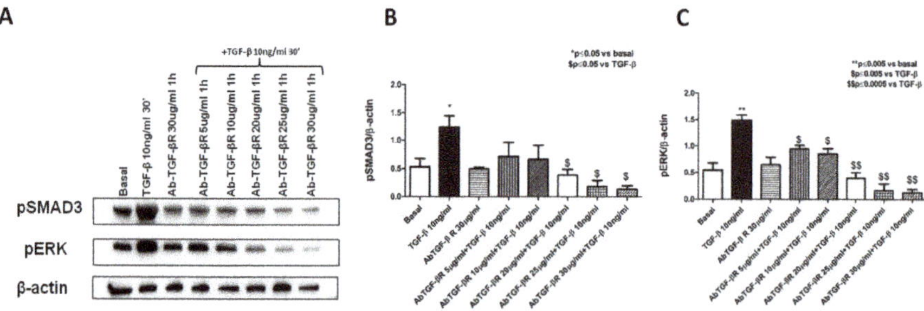

Figure A2. TGF-βR inhibition assay. (**A–C**) Pericytes were pre-treated with mouse monoclonal anti-TGF-βR at 5-10-20-25-30 μg/mL for 1 h before the TGF-β (10 ng/mL) exposition for 30 min. Pretreatment of pericytes with anti-TGF-βR antibody at 20 μg/mL is sufficient to significantly reduce TGF-β-induced phosphorylation of SMAD3 and ERK.

References

1. Gómez, H.; Kellum, J.A. Sepsis-induced acute kidney injury. *Curr. Opin. Crit. Care* **2016**, *22*, 546–553. [CrossRef] [PubMed]

2. Zarbock, A.; Gomez, H.; Kellum, J.A. Sepsis-induced acute kidney injury revisited: Pathophysiology, prevention and future therapies. *Curr. Opin. Crit. Care* **2014**, *20*, 588–595. [CrossRef] [PubMed]

3. Fenhammar, J.; Rundgren, M.; Hultenby, K.; Forestier, J.; Taavo, M.; Kenne, E.; Weitzberg, E.; Eriksson, S.; Ozenci, V.; Wernerson, A.; et al. Renal effects of treatment with a TLR4 inhibitor in conscious septic sheep. *Crit. Care* **2014**, *18*, 488. [PubMed]

4. Lu, Y.-C.; Yeh, W.-C.; Ohashi, P.S. LPS/TLR4 signal transduction pathway. *Cytokine* **2008**, *42*, 145–151. [CrossRef] [PubMed]

5. Schouten, M.; Wiersinga, W.J.; Levi, M.; van der Poll, T. Inflammation, endothelium, and coagulation in sepsis. *J. Leukoc. Biol.* **2008**, *83*, 536–545. [CrossRef] [PubMed]

6. Leaf, I.A.; Nakagawa, S.; Johnson, B.G.; Cha, J.J.; Mittelsteadt, K.; Guckian, K.M.; Gomez, I.G.; Altemeier, W.A.; Duffield, J.S. Pericyte MyD88 and IRAK4 control inflammatory and fibrotic responses to tissue injury. *J. Clin. Investig.* **2017**, *127*, 321–334. [CrossRef] [PubMed]

7. Peri, F.; Piazza, M.; Calabrese, V.; Damore, G.; Cighetti, R. Exploring the LPS/TLR4 signal pathway with small molecules. *Biochem. Soc. Trans.* **2010**, *38*, 1390–1395. [CrossRef] [PubMed]

8. Park, B.S.; Lee, J.-O. Recognition of lipopolysaccharide pattern by TLR4 complexes. *Exp. Mol. Med.* **2013**, *45*, e66. [CrossRef] [PubMed]

9. Opal, S.M.; Scannon, P.J.; Vincent, J.L.; White, M.; Carroll, S.F.; Palardy, J.E.; Parejo, N.A.; Pribble, J.P.; Lemke, J.H. Relationship between plasma levels of lipopolysaccharide (LPS) and LPS-binding protein in patients with severe sepsis and septic shock. *J. Infect. Dis.* **1999**, *180*, 1584–1589. [CrossRef]

10. Villar, J.; Pérez-Méndez, L.; Espinosa, E.; Flores, C.; Blanco, J.; Muriel, A.; Basaldúa, S.; Muros, M.; Blanch, L.; Artigas, A.; et al. Serum lipopolysaccharide binding protein levels predict severity of lung injury and mortality in patients with severe sepsis. *PLoS ONE* **2009**, *4*, e6818. [CrossRef]

11. Castellano, G.; Stasi, A.; Intini, A.; Gigante, M.; Di Palma, A.M.; Divella, C.; Netti, G.S.; Prattichizzo, C.; Pontrelli, P.; Crovace, A.; et al. Endothelial dysfunction and renal fibrosis in endotoxemia-induced oliguric kidney injury: Possible role of LPS-binding protein. *Crit. Care* **2014**, *18*, 520. [CrossRef] [PubMed]

12. Stasi, A.; Intini, A.; Divella, C.; Franzin, R.; Montemurno, E.; Grandaliano, G.; Ronco, C.; Fiaccadori, E.; Pertosa, G.B.; Gesualdo, L.; et al. Emerging role of Lipopolysaccharide binding protein in sepsis-induced acute kidney injury. *Nephrol. Dial. Transplant.* **2016**, *32*, 24–31. [CrossRef] [PubMed]

13. Goldenberg, N.M.; Steinberg, B.E.; Slutsky, A.S.; Lee, W.L. Broken barriers: A new take on sepsis pathogenesis. *Sci. Transl. Med.* **2011**, *3*, 88ps25. [CrossRef]

14. Page, A.V.; Liles, W.C. Biomarkers of endothelial activation/dysfunction in infectious diseases. *Virulence* **2013**, *4*, 507–516. [CrossRef] [PubMed]

15. Chen, Y.-T.; Chang, F.-C.; Wu, C.-F.; Chou, Y.-H.; Hsu, H.-L.; Chiang, W.-C.; Shen, J.; Chen, Y.-M.; Wu, K.-D.; Tsai, T.-J.; et al. Platelet-derived growth factor receptor signaling activates pericyte–myofibroblast transition in obstructive and post-ischemic kidney fibrosis. *Kidney Int.* **2011**, *80*, 1170–1181. [CrossRef] [PubMed]

16. Wang, N.; Deng, Y.; Liu, A.; Shen, N.; Wang, W.; Du, X.; Tang, Q.; Li, S.; Odeh, Z.; Wu, T.; et al. Novel Mechanism of the Pericyte-Myofibroblast Transition in Renal Interstitial Fibrosis: Core Fucosylation Regulation. *Sci. Rep.* **2017**, *7*, 16914. [CrossRef] [PubMed]

17. Lin, S.-L.; Kisseleva, T.; Brenner, D.A.; Duffield, J.S. Pericytes and Perivascular Fibroblasts Are the Primary Source of Collagen-Producing Cells in Obstructive Fibrosis of the Kidney. *Am. J. Pathol.* **2008**, *173*, 1617–1627. [CrossRef]

18. Grgic, I.; Duffield, J.S.; Humphreys, B.D. The origin of interstitial myofibroblasts in chronic kidney disease. *Pediatr. Nephrol.* **2012**, *27*, 183–193. [CrossRef]

19. Wu, C.-F.; Chiang, W.-C.; Lai, C.-F.; Chang, F.-C.; Chen, Y.-T.; Chou, Y.-H.; Wu, T.-H.; Linn, G.R.; Ling, H.; Wu, K.-D.; et al. Transforming growth factor β-1 stimulates profibrotic epithelial signaling to activate pericyte-myofibroblast transition in obstructive kidney fibrosis. *Am. J. Pathol.* **2013**, *182*, 118–131. [CrossRef]

20. Kuppe, C.; Kramann, R. Role of mesenchymal stem cells in kidney injury and fibrosis. *Curr. Opin. Nephrol. Hypertens.* **2016**, *25*, 372–377. [CrossRef]

21. Castellano, G.; Franzin, R.; Stasi, A.; Divella, C.; Sallustio, F.; Pontrelli, P.; Lucarelli, G.; Battaglia, M.; Staffieri, F.; Crovace, A.; et al. Complement activation during ischemia/reperfusion injury induces pericyte-to-myofibroblast transdifferentiation regulating peritubular capillary Lumen Reduction Through pERK Signaling. *Front. Immunol.* **2018**, *9*, 1002. [CrossRef] [PubMed]

22. Ronco, C.; D'Intini, V.; Bellomo, R.; Ricci, Z.; Bonello, M.; Ratanarat, R.; Salvatori, G.; Bordoni, V.; Andricos, E.; Brendolan, A. Rationale for the use of extracorporeal treatments for sepsis. *Anesteziol. Reanimatol.* **2005**, *2*, 87–91.

23. Ronco, C.; Brendolan, A.; Dan, M.; Piccinni, P.; Bellomo, R.; De Nitti, C.; Inguaggiato, P.; Tetta, C. Adsorption in sepsis. *Kidney Int. Suppl.* **2000**, *76*, S148–S155. [CrossRef] [PubMed]

24. de Pablo, R.; Monserrat, J.; Reyes, E.; Díaz, D.; Rodríguez-Zapata, M.; de la Hera, A.; Prieto, A.; Alvarez-Mon, M. Sepsis-induced acute respiratory distress syndrome with fatal outcome is associated to increased serum transforming growth factor beta-1 levels. *Eur. J. Intern. Med.* **2012**, *23*, 358–362. [CrossRef] [PubMed]

25. Freeman, B.D.; Machado, F.S.; Tanowitz, H.B.; Desruisseaux, M.S. Endothelin-1 and its role in the pathogenesis of infectious diseases. *Life Sci.* **2014**, *118*, 110–119. [CrossRef] [PubMed]

26. Bhattacharyya, S.; Kelley, K.; Melichian, D.S.; Tamaki, Z.; Fang, F.; Su, Y.; Feng, G.; Pope, R.M.; Budinger, G.R.S.; Mutlu, G.M.; et al. Toll-Like Receptor 4 Signaling Augments Transforming Growth Factor-β Responses. *Am. J. Pathol.* **2013**, *182*, 192–205. [CrossRef] [PubMed]

27. Rodríguez-Pascual, F.; Busnadiego, O.; González-Santamaría, J. The profibrotic role of endothelin-1: Is the door still open for the treatment of fibrotic diseases? *Life Sci.* **2014**, *118*, 156–164. [CrossRef]

28. Dunzendorfer, S.; Lee, H.-K.; Soldau, K.; Tobias, P.S. Toll-like receptor 4 functions intracellularly in human coronary artery endothelial cells: Roles of LBP and sCD14 in mediating LPS responses. *FASEB J.* **2004**, *18*, 1117–1119. [CrossRef]

29. Tran, M.; Tam, D.; Bardia, A.; Bhasin, M.; Rowe, G.C.; Kher, A.; Zsengeller, Z.K.; Akhavan-Sharif, M.R.; Khankin, E.V.; Saintgeniez, M.; et al. PGC-1α promotes recovery after acute kidney injury during systemic inflammation in mice. *J. Clin. Investig.* **2011**, *121*, 4003–4014. [CrossRef]

30. Kennedy-Lydon, T.M.; Crawford, C.; Wildman, S.S.P.; Peppiatt-Wildman, C.M. Renal pericytes: Regulators of medullary blood flow. *Acta Physiol.* **2013**, *207*, 212–225. [CrossRef]

31. Kramann, R.; Schneider, R.K.; DiRocco, D.P.; Machado, F.; Fleig, S.; Bondzie, P.A.; Henderson, J.M.; Ebert, B.L.; Humphreys, B.D. Perivascular Gli1+ progenitors are key contributors to injury-induced organ fibrosis. *Cell Stem Cell* **2015**, *16*, 51–66. [CrossRef] [PubMed]

32. Langenberg, C.; Wan, L.; Egi, M.; May, C.N.; Bellomo, R. Renal blood flow in experimental septic acute renal failure. *Kidney Int.* **2006**, *69*, 1996–2002. [CrossRef] [PubMed]

33. Anders, H.-J.; Banas, B.; Schlöndorff, D. Signaling danger: Toll-like receptors and their potential roles in kidney disease. *J. Am. Soc. Nephrol.* **2004**, *15*, 854–867. [CrossRef] [PubMed]

34. Dauphinee, S.M.; Karsan, A. Lipopolysaccharide signaling in endothelial cells. *Lab. Investig.* **2006**, *86*, 9–22. [CrossRef] [PubMed]

35. Bonventre, J.V.; Yang, L. Cellular pathophysiology of ischemic acute kidney injury. *J. Clin. Investig.* **2011**, *121*, 4210–4221. [CrossRef] [PubMed]

36. Souza, A.C.P.; Tsuji, T.; Baranova, I.N.; Bocharov, A.V.; Wilkins, K.J.; Street, J.M.; Alvarez-Prats, A.; Hu, X.; Eggerman, T.; Yuen, P.S.T.; et al. TLR4 mutant mice are protected from renal fibrosis and chronic kidney disease progression. *Physiol. Rep.* **2015**, *3*, e12558. [CrossRef]

37. Zhang, Y.; Su, X.; Zou, F.; Xu, T.; Pan, P.; Hu, C. Toll-like receptor-4 deficiency alleviates chronic intermittent hypoxia-induced renal injury, inflammation, and fibrosis. *Sleep Breath.* **2019**, *23*, 503–513. [CrossRef]

38. Jiang, H.; Qu, P.; Wang, J.-W.; Li, G.-H.; Wang, H.-Y. Effect of NF-κB inhibitor on Toll-like receptor 4 expression in left ventricular myocardium in two-kidney-one-clip hypertensive rats. *Eur. Rev. Med. Pharmacol. Sci.* **2018**, *22*, 3224–3233.

39. Campbell, M.T.; Hile, K.L.; Zhang, H.; Asanuma, H.; Vanderbrink, B.A.; Rink, R.R.; Meldrum, K.K. Toll-Like Receptor 4: A Novel Signaling Pathway During Renal Fibrogenesis. *J. Surg. Res.* **2011**, *168*, e61–e69. [CrossRef]

40. Tanimura, N.; Saitoh, S.; Matsumoto, F.; Akashi-Takamura, S.; Miyake, K. Roles for LPS-dependent interaction and relocation of TLR4 and TRAM in TRIF-signaling. *Biochem. Biophys. Res. Commun.* **2008**, *368*, 94–99. [CrossRef]

41. Sato, M.; Muragaki, Y.; Saika, S.; Roberts, A.B.; Ooshima, A. Targeted disruption of TGF-beta1/Smad3 signaling protects against renal tubulointerstitial fibrosis induced by unilateral ureteral obstruction. *J. Clin. Investig.* **2003**, *112*, 1486–1494. [CrossRef] [PubMed]

42. Carthy, J.M. TGFβ signaling and the control of myofibroblast differentiation: Implications for chronic inflammatory disorders. *J. Cell. Physiol.* **2018**, *233*, 98–106. [CrossRef] [PubMed]

43. Derynck, R.; Zhang, Y.E. Smad-dependent and Smad-independent pathways in TGF-β family signalling. *Nature* **2003**, *425*, 577–584. [CrossRef]

44. Li, J.H.; Huang, X.R.; Zhu, H.-J.; Oldfield, M.; Cooper, M.; Truong, L.D.; Johnson, R.J.; Lan, H.Y. Advanced glycation end products activate Smad signaling via TGF-beta-dependent and independent mechanisms: Implications for diabetic renal and vascular disease. *FASEB J.* **2004**, *18*, 176–178. [CrossRef] [PubMed]

45. Mori, Y.; Ishida, W.; Bhattacharyya, S.; Li, Y.; Platanias, L.C.; Varga, J. Selective inhibition of activin receptor-like kinase 5 signaling blocks profibrotic transforming growth factor beta responses in skin fibroblasts. *Arthritis Rheum.* **2004**, *50*, 4008–4021. [CrossRef]

46. Meng, X.-M.; Huang, X.R.; Xiao, J.; Chung, A.C.K.; Qin, W.; Chen, H.; Lan, H.Y. Disruption of Smad4 impairs TGF-β/Smad3 and Smad7 transcriptional regulation during renal inflammation and fibrosis in vivo and in vitro. *Kidney Int.* **2012**, *81*, 266–279. [CrossRef]

47. Gu, H.; Mickler, E.A.; Cummings, O.W.; Sandusky, G.E.; Weber, D.J.; Gracon, A.; Woodruff, T.; Wilkes, D.S.; Vittal, R. Crosstalk between TGF-β1 and complement activation augments epithelial injury in pulmonary fibrosis. *FASEB J.* **2014**, *28*, 4223–4234. [CrossRef]

48. Bhattacharyya, S.; Midwood, K.S.; Yin, H.; Varga, J. Toll-Like Receptor-4 Signaling Drives Persistent Fibroblast Activation and Prevents Fibrosis Resolution in Scleroderma. *Adv. Wound Care* **2017**, *6*, 356–369. [CrossRef]

49. Jerala, R. Structural biology of the LPS recognition. *Int. J. Med. Microbiol.* **2007**, *297*, 353–363. [CrossRef]

50. Wang, S.C.; Klein, R.D.; Wahl, W.L.; Alarcon, W.H.; Garg, R.J.; Remick, D.G.; Su, G.L. Tissue Coexpression of LBP and CD14 mRNA in a Mouse Model of Sepsis. *J. Surg. Res.* **1998**, *76*, 67–73. [CrossRef]

51. Stromberg, L.R.; Mendez, H.M.; Kubicek-Sutherland, J.Z.; Graves, S.W.; Hengartner, N.W.; Mukundan, H. Presentation matters: Impact of association of amphiphilic LPS with serum carrier proteins on innate immune signaling. *PLoS ONE* **2018**, *13*, e0198531. [CrossRef] [PubMed]

52. Webster, N.R.; Galley, H.F. Immunomodulation in the critically ill. *Br. J. Anaesth.* **2009**, *103*, 70–81. [CrossRef] [PubMed]

53. Bellomo, R.; Wan, L.; Langenberg, C.; May, C. Septic Acute Kidney Injury: New Concepts. *Nephron Exp. Nephrol.* **2008**, *109*, e95–e100. [CrossRef] [PubMed]

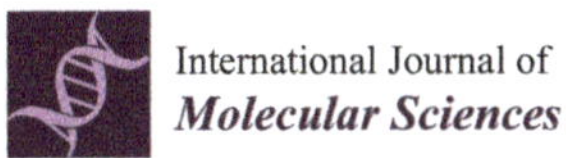

International Journal of
Molecular Sciences

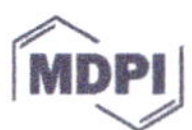

Article

Targeting ROS and cPLA2/COX2 Expressions Ameliorated Renal Damage in Obese Mice with Endotoxemia

Jia-Feng Chang [1,2,3,4,5,†], Jih-Chen Yeh [2,6,†], Chun-Ta Ho [2], Shih-Hao Liu [7], Chih-Yu Hsieh [1,2], Ting-Ming Wang [8,9], Shu-Wei Chang [10], I-Ta Lee [11], Kuo-Yang Huang [12], Jen-Yu Wang [4] and Wei-Ning Lin [4,*]

1 Division of Nephrology, Department of Internal Medicine, En Chu Kong Hospital, New Taipei City 237, Taiwan
2 Renal Care Joint Foundation, New Taipei City 220, Taiwan
3 Department of Nursing, Yuanpei University of Medical Technology, Hsinchu 300, Taiwan
4 Graduate Institution of Biomedical and Pharmaceutical Science, College of Medicine, Fu Jen Catholic University, New Taipei City 242, Taiwan
5 Division of Nephrology, Department of Internal Medicine, Shuang Ho Hospital, Taipei Medical University, New Taipei City 235, Taiwan
6 Department of Dentistry, Far Eastern Memorial Hospital, New Taipei City 220, Taiwan
7 Division of Pathology, En-Chu-Kong Hospital, New Taipei City 237, Taiwan
8 Department of Orthopaedic Surgery, School of Medicine, National Taiwan University, Taipei 106, Taiwan
9 Department of Orthopaedic Surgery, National Taiwan University Hospital, Taipei 106, Taiwan
10 Department of Civil Engineering, National Taiwan University, Taipei 106, Taiwan
11 School of Dentistry, College of Oral Medicine, Taipei Medical University, Taipei 110, Taiwan
12 Graduate Institute of Pathology and Parasitology, National Defense Medical Center, Taipei 114, Taiwan
* Correspondence: 081551@mail.fju.edu.tw; Tel.: +886-2-2905-3398; Fax: +886-2-2905-3412
† These authors contributed equally to this work.

Received: 27 August 2019; Accepted: 4 September 2019; Published: 6 September 2019

Abstract: Obesity is associated with metabolic endotoxemia, reactive oxygen species (ROS), chronic inflammation, and obese kidney fibrosis. Although the fat–intestine–kidney axis has been documented, the pathomechanism and therapeutic targets of obese kidney fibrosis remain unelucidated. To mimic obese humans with metabolic endotoxemia, high-fat-diet-fed mice (HF group) were injected with lipopolysaccharide (LPS) to yield the obese kidney fibrosis–metabolic endotoxemia mouse model (HL group). Therapeutic effects of ROS, cytosolic phospholipases A2 (cPLA2) and cyclooxygenase-2 (COX-2) inhibitors were analyzed with a quantitative comparison of immunohistochemistry stains and morphometric approach in the tubulointerstitium of different groups. Compared with basal and HF groups, the HL group exhibited the most prominent obese kidney fibrosis, tubular epithelial lipid vacuoles, and lymphocyte infiltration in the tubulointerstitium. Furthermore, inhibitors of nonspecific ROS, cPLA2 and COX-2 ameliorated the above renal damages. Notably, the ROS-inhibitor-treated group ameliorated not only oxidative injury but also the expression of cPLA2 and COX-2, indicating that ROS functions as the upstream signaling molecule in the inflammatory cascade of obese kidney fibrosis. ROS acts as a key messenger in the signaling transduction of obese kidney fibrosis, activating downstream cPLA2 and COX-2. The given antioxidant treatment ameliorates obese kidney fibrosis resulting from a combined high-fat diet and LPS—ROS could serve as a potential therapeutic target of obese kidney fibrosis with metabolic endotoxemia.

Keywords: obese kidney fibrosis; endotoxemia; ROS; cPLA2 and COX-2

---

1. Introduction

The worldwide increase in the prevalence of obesity has occurred in parallel with an increasing prevalence of chronic diseases, including diabetes mellitus, hypertension, cardiovascular diseases and chronic kidney disease (CKD) [1]. In light of this, the focus of World Kidney Day 2017 is kidney disease and obesity. It is found that the increase of BMI positively related to the presence and development of low estimated glomerular filtration rate and the incidence of end-stage renal disease [2]. Even metabolically healthy obesity is not a harmless condition—the phenotype of obese humans, no matter the abnormalities of metabolism, is reversely correlated with renal function [3]. In addition, the fat–intestine–kidney axis has a pivotal position in the mechanism of obese kidney disease, involving metabolic endotoxemia (ME) from intestinal dysbiosis, reactive oxygen species (ROS), systemic inflammation, and progressive renal fibrosis [4]. The rupture of the epithelial barrier results in the translocation of endotoxin and changes in the microbiome, which correlate to the occurrence of inflammation [5]. The evaluation of blood bacterial DNA shows that *Proteobacteria phylum*, *Gammaproteobacteria* class, and *Enterobacteriaceae* and *Pseudomonadaceae* families are more abundant in the CKD group compared with healthy controls [6]. Furthermore, there is elevated plasma lipopolysaccharide (LPS)-binding protein in hemodialysis patients with metabolic syndrome and obesity [7]. These studies suggested that LPS, also called endotoxin, functioned as a linker between the gut microbiome and CKD.

Emerging evidence indicates that prostaglandin (PG) pathways intricately interact with diabetes, metabolic syndrome, CKD progression, and cardiovascular events [8]. In a fatty rat model, renal cyclooxygenase-2 (COX-2) protein expression was accentuated and correlated with metabolic abnormalities [9]. Furthermore, a myriad of studies showed inhibition of cytoplasmic phospholipase A2 (cPLA2) and downstream signals attenuate renal injury [10–13]. Initiation of the PG signaling pathway usually occurs with the release of arachidonic acids from phospholipids within membranes by cPLA2. The subsequent conversion of arachidonic acid into PG is facilitated by COX-2, leading to inflammation and fibrosis in the kidney. Indeed, compared with healthy controls, renal tissues in CKD groups exhibit higher expressions of fibroblasts and the *COX-2* gene [14]. Although cPLA2 and eicosanoids contributed to renal oxidative stress, inflammation, and end-organ damage [15], eradication of bone-marrow-derived cPLA2 attenuated the eicosanoid storm and renal fibrosis [16].

Intracellular redox imbalance plays important roles in the pathogenesis of CKD. Plasma cells of CKD patients show activation of NF-κB and up-regulated expression of pro-inflammatory and pro-oxidant genes, as well as down-regulation of Nrf2-associated antioxidant gene expression [14]. Similarly, the nephrotoxic agent, aristolochic acid I, increases protein abundance of the NADPH oxidase subunits NOX4, $p47^{phox}$, $p22^{phox}$ and 3-nitrotyrosine in rats within 8 to 24 weeks [17]. Moreover, upregulation of intracellular ROS promotes the expression of inflammatory genes, including *cPLA2* and *COX-2* [18,19]. In fact, ameliorating oxidative stress via modulating forkhead box class O1 (FOXO1) expression attenuated high glucose-induced renal proximal tubular cell injury [20].

Despite previously documented implications, the pathomechanism and therapeutic targets of obese kidney fibrosis (OKF) remain unelucidated. To mimic obese humans with ME, we developed a combined high-fat-diet-fed (HF) and lipopolysaccharide (LPS)-treated mouse model to explore inflammatory signaling pathways of OKF. We hypothesized that OKF is involved in ROS generations, activating downstream cPLA2 and COX-2, resulting in progressive tubulointerstitial fibrosis. Thus, ROS could serve as a potential therapeutic target of OKF. Quantitative comparison of immunohistochemical (IHC) staining and morphometric approach were used to test this hypothesis.

2. Results

2.1. HF Mice with ME Exhibit the Most Prominent Renal Fibrosis, Depositions of Lipid Vacuoles in Tubular Epithelium, and Lymphocyte Infiltration in Tubulointerstitium

Recent evidence indicates that adipose tissue inflammation in obesity and metabolic syndrome is not strictly a macrophage-dependent phenomenon. Lymphocytes, especially T cells, infiltrate the adipose tissue and mediate the inflammatory response. The infiltration of T effector cells precedes the accumulation of macrophages in adipose tissue and reducing regulatory T cells during obesity are thought to contribute to the development of adipose tissue inflammation [21]. Deposition of lipid vacuoles (LV) in proximal tubular epithelial cells are the typical features of fatty kidneys [22,23], and renal fibrosis is a hallmark and common outcome across all kinds of progressive CKD [24]. To investigate human obese kidney fibrosis with metabolic endotoxemia, we used an experimental rodent model, fed a high-fat diet with LPS injection (called the OKF-ME model) (Figure 1). In accordance with previous studies [22,23], our high-fat diet course induced shedding of renal tubule epithelial cells, tubular LV deposition and increased lymphocyte infiltration in renal tubulointerstitium with or without LPS treatment at week 15 (Figure 2A). Compared with the basal group and HF mice, the HL group exhibited the most prominent fibrosis (Figure 2B), tubular LV accumulation (Figure 2C), and lymphocyte infiltration in tubulointerstitium (Figure 2D). Current data demonstrate that HF and ME result in not only renal tubule injury but also tubulointerstitial inflammation and fibrosis.

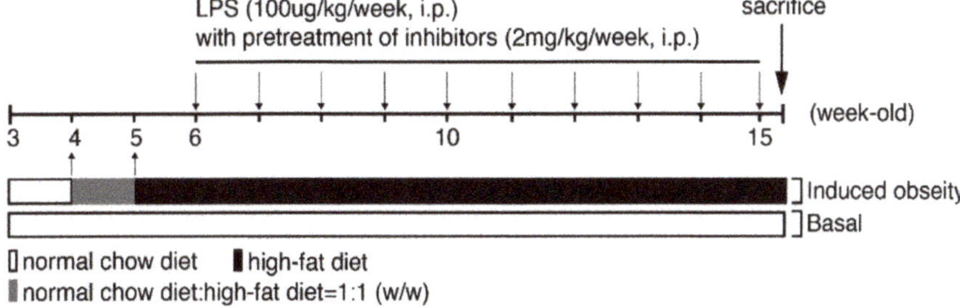

Figure 1. Model of obese kidney fibrosis with metabolic endotoxemia (OKF-ME). Mice were randomized into three groups: normal chow-fed control group (basal group), high-fat diet-fed group (HF group), and high-fat diet-fed group with lipopolysaccharides (LPS) treatment (HL group). The HL group was induced with LPS (100 µg/kg/week intraperitoneal (i.p.) injection) as the working model of OKF-ME.

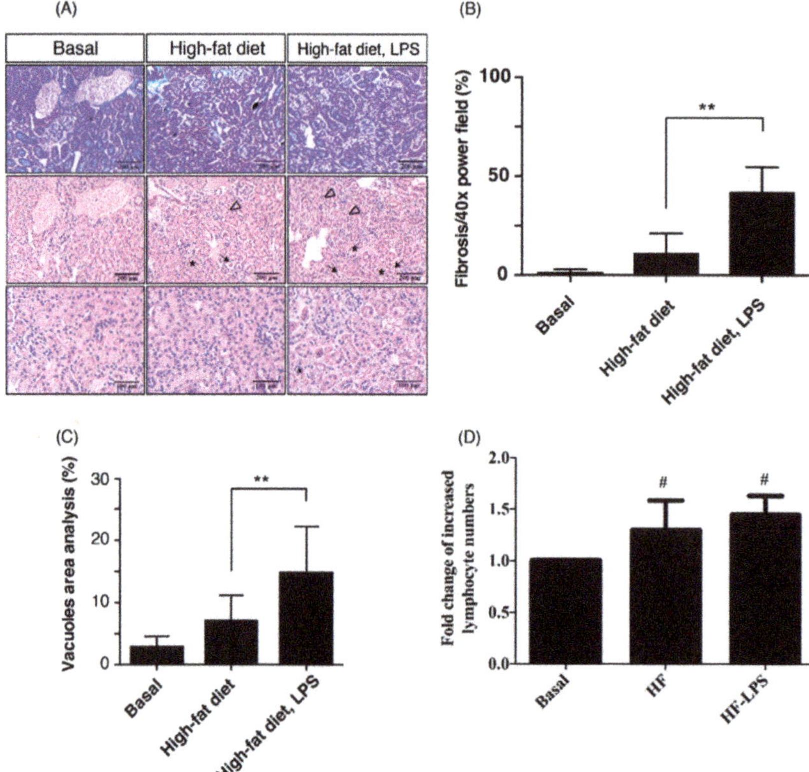

Figure 2. HF mice with ME exhibit the most prominent renal fibrosis, depositions of lipid vacuoles in tubular epithelium, and lymphocyte infiltration in tubulointerstitium. (**A**) Mice were scarified at the end of treatment, and kidney tissues were extracted for histological staining (Haematoxylin and Eosin and Masson's trichrome staining). Compared with the basal group and HF mice, the HL group exhibited the most prominent renal fibrosis, depositions of lipid vacuoles in tubular epithelium, and lymphocyte infiltration in the tubulointerstitium. Black hollow triangles indicate shedding of tubules. Black arrows indicate infiltration of lymphocytes. Stars indicate lipid vacuoles. Scale bars in the panels are 200 μm or 100 μm as indicated. Quantification analyses were performed by ImageJ software for (**B**) fibrosis area (**C**) lipid vacuoles and (**D**) lymphocyte number. Data are expressed as mean ± SD ($n = 8$); ** $p < 0.01$, to compare the differences between the two indicated groups. # $p < 0.05$, compared with the basal group.

2.2. *Inhibitors of ROS, cPLA2, and COX-2 Attenuate the Tubulointerstitial Fibrosis in HF Mice with ME*

As we had already proven that HF and ME result in tubulointerstitial fibrosis, we aimed to investigate the underlying mechanism and inflammatory signaling pathways of OKF. Our previous research has contributed a mechanistic insight of uremic lung injury in a CKD mouse model, showing that ROS activates downstream PG pathways and recruits leukocytes to injured sites [25]. Furthermore, recent studies reported inhibitions of ROS and cPLA2/COX-2 ameliorates renal damages [10–13]. Nonetheless, therapeutic effects of the above inhibitors on OKF remain unclear. To investigate which factor mediated the progression of OKF, N-acetylcysteine (NAC; ROS scavenger), AACOCF3 (AAC; cPLA2 inhibitor), and NS-398 (COX-2 inhibitor) were used. Our results demonstrate significant fibrosis was found in juxtamedullary to medullar regions of HF and HL groups (Figure 3A). In corresponding fibrotic regions, the HL/NAC group exhibited residual renal tubular structures, suggesting that the above fibrotic process was attenuated (Figure 3A, zoom-in region). Under high-power magnification, evident epithelioid tubular-like cells were also seen in corresponding fibrotic regions in the HL/NS-398 group (Figure 3A, zoom-in region), indicating tissue repair after inflammation. In contrast with the severe tubularinterstitial fibrosis in the HL group, inhibitor-treated groups of NAC, AAC and NS-398 attenuated such injury (Figure 3A, yellow dotted line regions). To compare therapeutic effects of inhibitors, the HL/NAC and HL/NS-398 group presented the lowest degree of OKF after quantification analysis for fibrotic area verses total tissue area (%) (Figure 3B). Indeed, the results of Sirius Red stain confirmed that the HL groups contained the strongest red staining of fibrosis and treatment of NAC, AAC or NS398 alleviated the fibrotic staining (Supplementary Data 1). After quantification analysis to determine the area of vacuoles, the HL/NAC group exerted the lowest degree of LV deposition in the tubular epithelium (Figure 3C).

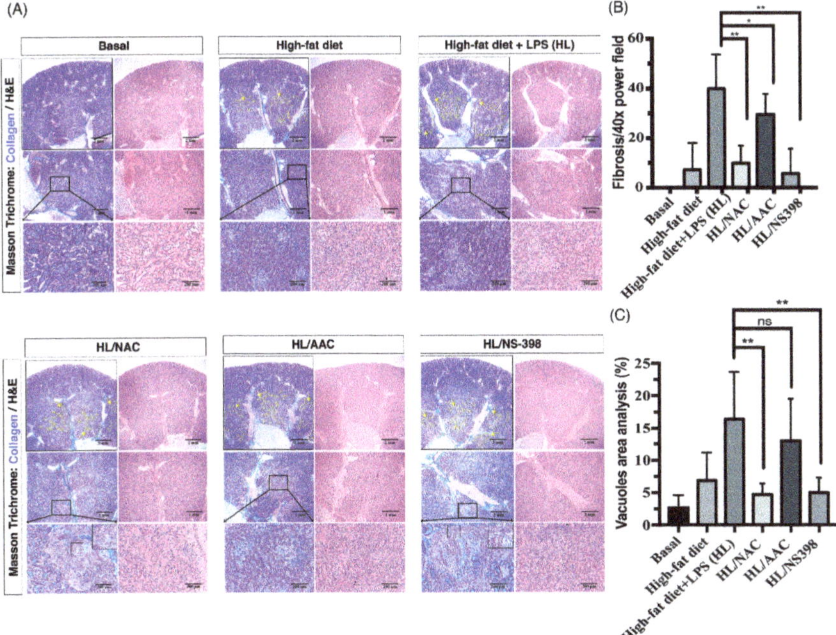

Figure 3. Inhibitors of reactive oxygen species (ROS), cPLA2, and COX-2 attenuate the tubulointerstitial fibrosis in HF mice with ME. (**A**) The HL group exerts the most significant collagen deposition and tubulointerstitial fibrosis in the juxtamedullary to medullar regions. In corresponding fibrotic regions, the HL/N-acetylcysteine (NAC) group exhibited residual renal tubular structures, suggesting that the above fibrotic process was attenuated (zoom-in region). Under high-power magnification, evident epithelioid tubular-like cells were also visible in corresponding fibrotic regions in the HL/NS-398 group (zoom-in region), indicating tissue repair after inflammation. In contrast with the profound tubularinterstitial fibrosis in HL group, inhibitor-treated groups of NAC, AACOCF3 (AAC) and NS-398 attenuated such injury (yellow dotted line regions). The fibrosis area was marked by yellow dotted lines. Yellow arrows indicated the borderline of the fibrosis area. Scale bars are 2 mm, 1mm and 200 μm in the panels. (**B**) To compare the therapeutic effects of inhibitors, the HL/NAC and HL/NS-398 group presented the lowest degree of OKF after quantification analysis for the fibrotic area verses total tissue area (%). (**C**) After quantification analysis for the area of vacuoles, the HL/NAC group exerted the lowest degree of lipid vacuole deposition in the tubular epithelium. Quantification analysis was performed by image J. Data are expressed as mean ± SD ($n = 8$); * $p < 0.05$; and ** $p < 0.01$ to compare the differences between the two indicated groups. ns, not significant.

2.3. Scavengers of Non-Specific ROS Attenuate Not Only Oxidative Injury But Also Downstream Pathways of cPLA2 and COX-2 in Obese Kidney Fibrosis with Metabolic Endotoxemia

As we have proven, ROS, cPLA2 and COX-2 were involved in OKF with ME, the key messenger of signal transduction pathways in the OKF mechanism remain unclear. Given that ROS could function as a short-lived intracellular second messenger in signaling transduction [25–27], we hypothesized that ROS could function as an upstream signal transducer in cPLA2 and COX-2-mediated inflammatory pathways. To investigate it further, expressions of 8-hydroxy-2'-deoxyguanosine (8-OHdG), a derivative of oxidized deoxyguanosine, was evaluated as an indicator of oxidative damages. Results of IHC assay showed that there is an increased expression of 8-OHdG in the HL group (HF mice with ME) and treatment of NAC (scavenger of ROS) reduced the stain density of 8-OHdG in the HL/NAC group (Figure 4A,B). On the aspects of cPLA2 and COX-2 expression, as expected, the HL group (HF mice with ME) exerted the highest expression of cPLA2 and COX-2, which were ameliorated by AACOCF3 (AAC, inhibitor of cPLA2) and NS-398 (inhibitor of COX-2), respectively (Figure 5). Notably, the NAC-treated group ameliorated not only oxidative injury but also expressions of cPLA2 and COX-2 after the quantification analysis (Figure 5C,D), indicating that ROS acts as the upstream signal in the inflammatory cascades of OKF. Western blot was further used to confirm the results of IHC. As shown in the Supplementary Data 2, HL-induced expression of cPLA2 and COX-2 were attenuated by treatment of AAC, NAC or NS-398, separately. Collectively, ROS serves as a key pro-inflammatory signal to activate PG pathways, and ultimately, leads to OKF.

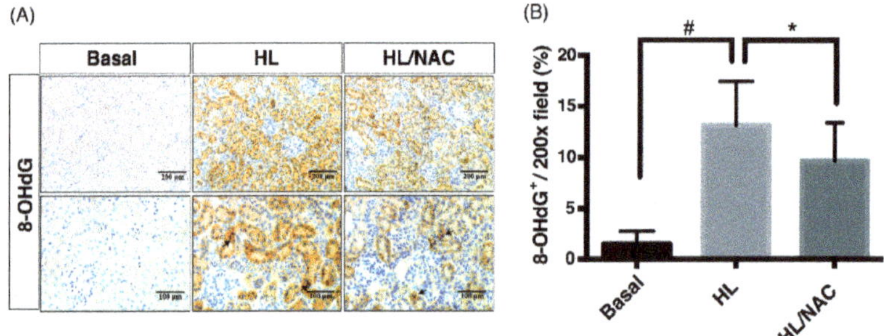

Figure 4. Scavengers of non-specific ROS attenuate oxidative injury in obese kidney fibrosis with metabolic endotoxemia. (**A**) Immunohistochemical staining methods were used to detect expressions of 8-OHdG. The HL group (HF mice with ME) exerts the highest expression of 8-OHdG, which was ameliorated by NAC. Scale bars are 200 μm or 100 μm in the panels. (**B**) Quantification analysis was performed by imageJ software. Data are expressed as mean ± SD ($n = 8$); * $p < 0.05$, # $p < 0.01$, to compare the differences between the two indicated groups.

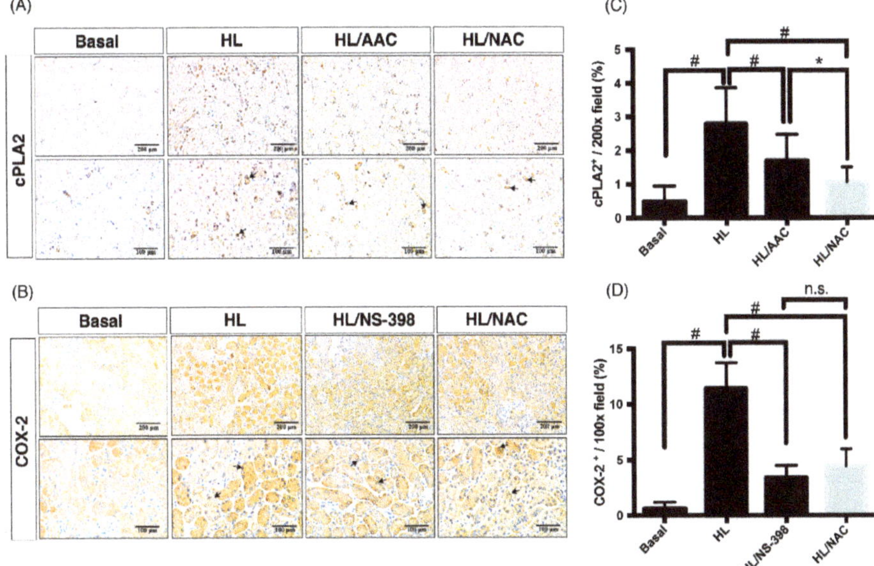

Figure 5. Scavengers of non-specific ROS reduced expression of cPLA2 and COX-2 in obese kidney fibrosis with metabolic endotoxemia. Immunohistochemical staining methods were used to detect expressions of (**A**) cPLA2, and (**B**) COX-2. The HL group (HF mice with ME) exerts the highest expression of cPLA2 and COX-2, which were ameliorated by NAC, AACCOCFS (AAC), and NS-398, respectively. Scale bars in the panels are 200 μm or 100 μm. (**C,D**) Quantification analysis indicated that ROS acts as the upstream key signal in the inflammatory cascades of OKF. Quantification analysis as performed by ImageJ software. Data are expressed as mean ± SD ($n = 8$); * $p < 0.05$, # $p < 0.01$, to compare the differences between the two indicated groups. n.s., not significant.

3. Discussion

In the present study, an OKF-ME mouse model was developed to demonstrate how a high-fat diet and LPS impair kidneys, providing a mechanical insight into OKF. Through testing the effects of ROS and cPLA2/COX-2 inhibitors, major breakthroughs were achieved, and the new findings markedly advance our understanding of OKF process.

3.1. The Fat–Intestine–Kidney Axis

The fat–intestine–kidney axis is the foundation stone of OKF, and underlying mechanisms are increasingly recognized through both human and animal models [4]. The role of an HF diet in promoting an obesogenic gut microbiota is undergoing confirmation, and gut dysbiosis can direct host storage of lipids in adipose tissue [28]. It has become more evident that the gut microbiota is altered in obesity, leading to activation of the LPS-toll-like receptor 4 (TLR4) axis and modulation of the intestinal barrier integrity [29]. Thus, intestinal dysbiosis in obesity has recently been recognized as a key environmental factor driving metabolic diseases, and ME via the increased paracellular transport of LPS is believed to contribute to chronic high-grade inflammation [30,31]. Studies in mice demonstrated that a HF diet or LPS infusion induced a two- to threefold increase in circulating LPS levels, contributing to the development of obesity and increased insulin resistance [32,33], and vice versa, LPS and TLR4 initiate a well-characterized signaling cascade that elicits intricate pro-oxidant and pro-inflammatory pathways in obesity [34]. A high LPS concentration is found in patients with type 2 diabetes [35], which is termed ME and reduced by the administration of hypoglycemic agents with potential anti-inflammatory effects [36]. Continuous administration of LPS resulted in recruiting inflammatory cells, activating mTOR signaling, tubular injury and collagen deposition in mice kidneys [37]. By contrast, the administration of antioxidants protects renal blood flow in LPS-treated animal models [38]. Recently, adipose-specific PLA2 have received attention for potential anti-obesity and anti-diabetic roles. Both genetic and pharmacological inhibition of particular PLA2s has resulted in obesity-resistant mouse models, suggesting a potential to develop new drugs [39]. In addition, COX-2 has long been believed to play a role in the inflammatory process as a result of obesity with an HF diet [9,40]. Given the role of PG pathways and oxidative stress in the etiology of obesity-induced renal injuries, the fat–intestine–kidney axis may intricately interact with ROS, cPLA2 and COX-2 in OKF progression. Current data suggest a healthy lifestyle—including antioxidant foods and the avoidance of excessive dietary fat intake—may ensure a friendly gut microbiota and positively affect prevention and treatment of various metabolic disorders.

3.2. Therapeutic Targets of ROS, cPLA2 and COX-2 in Kidney Diseases

Renal tubules are the main structure of the kidney and can be subjected to a variety of damage, including hypoxia, proteinuria, toxins, metabolic disorders, inflammation and oxidative stress [41]. Thus, tubular epithelial damage plays a pivotal role in renal fibrinogenesis [42,43], and PG pathways are crucial homeostatic modulators of kidney function [3]. Through the effects of cPLA2 in the initial stage, membrane phospholipids release arachidonic acid. In the following stepwise conversion of arachidonic acid by COX enzymes and PGE synthase, the major product of PGE2 is elevated and responsible for not only cardiovascular risks but also renal diseases [8]. Recent studies have shown that cPLA2 enhances proliferation and de-differentiation in human renal tubular epithelial cells [44], and silencing cPLA2 expression in knock-out (KO) mice is able to ameliorate pro-inflammatory eicosanoids production, inflammatory cell recruitment, and severity of fibrosis [16]. In another mouse model of high-carbohydrate high-fat-diet-induced obesity, the cPLA2 inhibitor treatment attenuated visceral adiposity and improved most features of metabolic syndrome, including insulin sensitivity, glucose intolerance, and cardiovascular abnormalities [10]. A considerable amount of literature reported that cPLA2 is a useful therapeutic target for diverse diseases. There are a number of concerns in using cPLA2 as a therapeutic target, especially because most of the studies are based on disease models comparing cPLA2 wild type (WT) and KO mice, which may not accurately reflect processes contributing to human diseases. This is apparent from the differences between mice and humans as a consequence of cPLA2 deficiency, e.g., cPLA2 is the first regulatory enzyme in the pathway for the production of numerous lipid mediators. Although, targeting cPLA2 may be beneficial in some diseases where COX metabolites contribute to diseases, such as asthma and arthritis [45]. However, PGs regulate labor and birth in humans, and an important source of PGs is amnion fibroblasts in fetal membranes [46,47]. Considering the essential roles of cPLA2 in human health, particularly for maintenance of the small intestine and female reproduction, is also a concern for targeting cPLA2 in OKF. Moreover, selective COX-2 inhibitors used in the rat model of an HF diet improved insulin sensitivity and TNFα mRNA expression [40]. Nonetheless, the nephrotoxic effect of COX-2 inhibitor for CKD patients is another concern in clinical practice.

Our research indicates ROS serve as a predisposition factor of OKF and thus a therapeutic target, activating downstream PG pathways and tubulointerstitial fibrosis. In contrast with PG inhibitors, NAC can easily be applied to a clinical therapeutic strategy, because a large oral dose of antioxidant is well tolerated without systemic side effects. Notably, the origin, the kinetics, and the localization of ROS generation all influence responses of T lymphocytes and inflammatory cells [48]. Shen Y et al. reported that the administration of NAC significantly mitigated oxidative and fibrotic responses resulting from angiotensin-II upregulation in the obstructed kidneys of mice, including expressions of fibronectin, collagen I, α-SMA and TGF-β [13].

We recognize several limitations of our study. In the first place, endogenous plasma creatinine levels and creatinine clearance as a tool to evaluate renal function were not evaluated in our mouse model. Difficulties have included the lack of an accurate, reproducible method to estimate renal function in conscious mice, problems obtaining sufficient blood volume and precisely timed urine collections repeatedly. Next, further parameters of tubulointerstitial injury in our OKF mouse models were not provided, e.g., neutrophil gelatinase-associated lipocalin, transforming growth factor beta, and alpha-smooth muscle actin. From the perspectives of nephrologists and pathologists, whereas the single method of Masson's trichrome staining can easily and convincingly diagnose tubulointerstitial fibrosis in routine clinical practice of human renal biopsies.

In conclusion, our research has contributed a mechanistic insight into OKF-ME, showing that a high-fat diet and ME impair kidneys through lipid deposition in the tubular epithelium, recruiting lymphocytes, triggering ROS to activate downstream PG pathways, and ultimately, tubulointerstitial fibrosis (Figure 6). ROS may serve as a predisposition factor of PG inflammatory pathways and OKF. We also elucidate that non-specific antioxidant NAC attenuates a high-fat diet and ME-induced renal inflammation and fibrosis. The protective effects are superior to cPLA2 and COX-2 inhibitors. This potential therapeutic target can easily be applied to clinical practice, because a large oral dose of NAC is well tolerated without systemic side effects. In light of the growing prevalence of obesity worldwide with an increasing trend in total medicare expenditures, the organ-protective effects of NAC should be tested in OKF patients who are in urgent need of new therapeutics. Several important issues in this research merit further discussion.

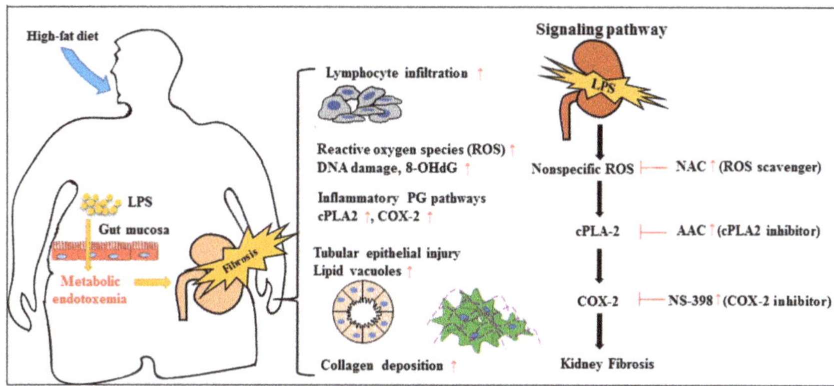

Figure 6. Potential mechanisms of obese kidney fibrosis induced by the fat–intestine–kidney axis. The schematic diagram has contributed a mechanistic insight into obese kidney fibrosis (OKF) with metabolic endotoxemia (ME). A high-fat diet leads to intestinal dysbiosis and hyperpermeability, favoring translocation of microbiome-derived lipopolysaccharide (LPS) to the bloodstream. A high-fat diet and ME impair kidneys through lipid deposition in the tubular epithelium, recruiting lymphocytes, triggering ROS to activate downstream prostaglandin pathways, and ultimately tubulointerstitial fibrosis. ROS may serve as predisposition factors and thus therapeutic targets in the prevention of OKF-ME. Different levels of the inhibitors' activity are indicated as red arrows.

4. Materials and Methods

4.1. Materials

Most materials and methods were previously described [25]. Other materials utilized in this study can be purchased from Santa Cruz Biotechnology (Santa Cruz, CA, USA) or Sigma (St. Louis, MO, USA), including the inhibitor of cPLA2 (AACOCF3 (AAC)/Arachidonyltrifluoromethane), COX-2 (NS-398/N-[2-(cyclohexyloxy)-4-nitrophenyl] methanesulfonamide), and nonspecific ROS (NAC/N-Acetyl L-Cysteine).

4.2. Creating Animal Models to Mimic Obese Kidney Fibrosis (OKF) in Humans

A WT C57BL/6NCrlBltw mouse was provided by BioLASCO Taiwan Co., Ltd. (Taipei, Taiwan). The study was approved by the Animal Care and Use Committee of the Fu Jen Laboratory Animal Center (IACUC number: A10603; 1, March, 2017). All animals were handled according to the guidelines of the Animal Care Committee of Fu Jen Catholic University and NIH Guides for the Care and Use of Laboratory Animals. Animals were maintained in a temperature-controlled room (22 °C) under 12 h light–dark cycles. One week after arrival, four-week-old mice were divided into different groups. The control group received continuous feeding of a normal chow (Lactamin, Stockholm, Sweden). The HF group was first fed with a mix of a high-fat diet (#D12492, Research Diets, New Brunswick, NJ) and normal chow ($w:w$ = 1:1) for diet adaptation for one week, then a complete high-fat diet course was given for the next 10 weeks. To create the animal model of OKF with ME, six-week-old mice that were fed with a high-fat diet were injected with LPS (10 μg/kg/week, intraperitoneal (i.p.) injection) as the HL group. If inhibitors were used, various inhibitors (2 mg/kg/week, i.p.) were injected one hour before LPS injection as inhibitor-treated groups. Mice were then sacrificed at the age of fifteen weeks, and kidneys were quickly removed and preserved in formalin for paraffin embedment for further analyses.

4.3. Tissue Preparation for Histopathological Evaluation of H&E Stain

Mice were anaesthetized via the inhalation of isoflurane and euthanized by cervical dislocation. Kidneys were removed and fixed in 10% formalin. Specimens were embedded in paraffin and sliced into 2–3 μm in thickness. Subsequently, the kidney tissues were stained with Hematoxylin-eosin (H&E stain). The images were captured using a Nikon Digital Camera Microscope (Nikon, Tokyo, Japan).

4.4. Masson's Trichrome Staining Method

Masson's trichrome staining method was used to determine the extent of collagen deposition and fibrosis in mouse kidney tissues. In the corresponding area, H&E staining of the adjacent paraffin section was performed for comparisons of tissue morphology. The experiments were conducted as follows: sections were first deparaffinized and rehydrated in ethanol/water solutions then post-fixed with Bouin's solution for 1 h at room temperature. The fixation buffer was removed, and slides were stained with iron hematoxylin, Biebrich scarlet-acid fuchsin, and phosphomolybdic-phosphotungstic acid sequentially for 10 min per stain. Slides were then stained with Aniline blue. Finally, slides were washed in 10% acetate solution for 3–5 min and mounted in the mounting medium for observations to be made.

4.5. Immunohistochemistry Staining Method

Immunohistochemistry (IHC) was performed manually or automatically with an autostainer (BenchMark XT, Ventana Medical Systems Inc., Tucson, AZ, USA). For the manual protocol, paraffin sections were first deparaffinized and rehydrated in ethanol/water solutions. Epitopes on tissue were then retrieved with Heat-Induced Epitope Retrieval (HIER) in citrate buffer (0.01 M, pH 6.0). For blocking endogenous peroxidase activity, sections were treated with 3% hydrogen peroxide for 30 min in the dark. To reduce non-specific primary antibody binding, Blocking Buffer (DAKO) was used for one hour at room temperature. Sections were then incubated with primary antibodies at 4 °C overnight. Rabbit anti-mouse COX-2, anti-human cPLA2, and anti-8-OHdG polyclonal antibodies were purchased from Santa Cruz Biotechnology (SC-1747-R, SC-7891, and SC-139586, Santa Cruz, CA, USA). Afterward, staining was detected with a DAKO polymer system. For image acquisitions, three random high-power magnification fields were obtained in each sample by a Nikon Digital Camera Microscope (Nikon, Tokyo, Japan). All slides were reviewed by a blinded pathologist (Dr. Shih-Hao Liu), and the area percentage of staining in a 200× power magnification field were analyzed by NIH ImageJ software (Version 1.47, Bethesda, MD, USA).

4.6. Statistical Analysis of Data

All data are expressed as the mean ± SD using the GraphPad Prism Program (GraphPad, San Diego, CA, USA). Quantitative data were analyzed with a non-paired Student's t-test. The significance threshold was set at 5% ($p < 0.05$). All of the experiments were performed at least three times.

Supplementary Materials: The following are available online at http://www.mdpi.com/1422-0067/20/18/4393/s1.

Author Contributions: J.-F.C. and W.-N.L. were responsible for study design, data interpretation, study supervision, and manuscript draft. C.-T.H., S.-H.L. and C.-Y.H. assisted with digital analysis for immunohistochemistry staining and morphometric analysis in histopathology. J.-Y.W. assisted the protein extraction. J.-C.Y., S.-W.C., T.-M.W., I.-T.L., and K.-Y.H. were responsible for writing and revision of the manuscript.

Funding: This work was supported by the En Chu Kong Hospital (ECKH10602); Renal Care Joint Foundation; Fu Jen Catholic University Research Foundation (A0103017 and A0106010); the grant of NTU-CC-107L891102 and MOST 107-2218-E-002-064.

Conflicts of Interest: The authors declare that they have no conflict of interest.

Abbreviations

CKD	chronic kidney disease
COX-2	cyclooxygenase-2
cPLA2	cytosolic phospholipases A2
HF group	high-fat diet-fed group injected with lipopolysaccharide
IHC	immunohistochemistry
LPS	lipopolysaccharide
ME	metabolic endotoxemia
OKF	obese kidney fibrosis
PG	prostaglandin
ROS	reactive oxygen species

References

1. Stenvinkel, P.; Zoccali, C.; Ikizler, T.A. Obesity in CKD—What should nephrologists know? *J. Am. Soc. Nephrol.* **2013**, *24*, 1727–1736. [CrossRef]

2. Kovesdy, C.P.; Furth, S.L.; Zoccali, C.; on Behalf of the World Kidney Day Steering Committee. Obesity and Kidney Disease: Hidden Consequences of the Epidemic. *Am. J. Hypertens.* **2017**, *30*, 328–336. [CrossRef]

3. Jung, C.H.; Lee, M.J.; Kang, Y.M.; Hwang, J.Y.; Kim, E.H.; Park, J.Y.; Kim, H.K.; Lee, W.J. The risk of chronic kidney disease in a metabolically healthy obese population. *Kidney Int.* **2015**, *88*, 843–850. [CrossRef]

4. Câmara, N.O.S.; Iseki, K.; Kramer, H.; Liu, Z.-H.; Sharma, K. Kidney disease and obesity: Epidemiology, mechanisms and treatment. *Nat. Rev. Nephrol.* **2017**, *13*, 181. [CrossRef]

5. Hobby, G.P.; Karaduta, O.; Dusio, G.F.; Singh, M.; Zybailov, B.L.; Arthur, J.M. Chronic Kidney Disease and the Gut Microbiome. *Am. J. Physiol. Renal Physiol.* **2019**. [CrossRef]

6. Shah, N.B.; Allegretti, A.S.; Nigwekar, S.U.; Kalim, S.; Zhao, S.; Lelouvier, B.; Servant, F.; Serena, G.; Thadhani, R.I.; Raj, D.S.; et al. Blood Microbiome Profile in CKD: A Pilot Study. *Clin. J. Am. Soc. Nephrol. CJASN* **2019**. [CrossRef]

7. Lim, P.S.; Chang, Y.K.; Wu, T.K. Serum Lipopolysaccharide-Binding Protein is Associated with Chronic Inflammation and Metabolic Syndrome in Hemodialysis Patients. *Blood Purif.* **2019**, *47*, 28–36. [CrossRef]

8. Nasrallah, R.; Hassouneh, R.; Hébert, R.L. PGE2, kidney disease, and cardiovascular risk: Beyond hypertension and diabetes. *J. Am. Soc. Nephrol.* **2016**, *27*, 666–676. [CrossRef]

9. Komers, R.; Zdychova, J.; Cahova, M.; Kazdova, L.; Lindsley, J.N.; Anderson, S. Renal cyclooxygenase-2 in obese Zucker (fatty) rats. *Kidney Int.* **2005**, *67*, 2151–2158. [CrossRef]

10. Iyer, A.; Lim, J.; Poudyal, H.; Reid, R.C.; Suen, J.Y.; Webster, J.; Prins, J.B.; Whitehead, J.P.; Fairlie, D.P.; Brown, L. An inhibitor of phospholipase A2 group IIA modulates adipocyte signaling and protects against diet-induced metabolic syndrome in rats. *Diabetes* **2012**, *61*, 2320–2329. [CrossRef]

11. Jia, Z.; Zhang, Y.; Ding, G.; Heiney, K.M.; Huang, S.; Zhang, A. Role of COX-2/mPGES-1/prostaglandin E2 cascade in kidney injury. *Mediat. Inflamm.* **2015**, *2015*, 147894. [CrossRef]

12. Câmara, N.O.; Martins, J.O.; Landgraf, R.G. Emerging roles for eicosanoids in renal diseases. *Curr. Opin. Nephrol. Hypertens.* **2009**, *18*, 21–27. [CrossRef]

13. Shen, Y.; Miao, N.-J.; Xu, J.-L.; Gan, X.-X.; Xu, D.; Zhou, L.; Xue, H.; Zhang, W.; Lu, L.-M. N-acetylcysteine alleviates angiotensin II-mediated renal fibrosis in mouse obstructed kidneys. *Acta Pharmacol. Sin.* **2016**, *37*, 637. [CrossRef]

14. Chen, D.Q.; Cao, G.; Chen, H.; Liu, D.; Su, W.; Yu, X.Y.; Vaziri, N.D.; Liu, X.H.; Bai, X.; Zhang, L.; et al. Gene and protein expressions and metabolomics exhibit activated redox signaling and wnt/beta-catenin pathway are associated with metabolite dysfunction in patients with chronic kidney disease. *Redox Biol.* **2017**, *12*, 505–521. [CrossRef]

15. Khan, N.S.; Song, C.Y.; Thirunavukkarasu, S.; Fang, X.R.; Bonventre, J.V.; Malik, K.U. Cytosolic Phospholipase A2alpha Is Essential for Renal Dysfunction and End-Organ Damage Associated with Angiotensin II-Induced Hypertension. *Am. J. Hypertens.* **2016**, *29*, 258–265. [CrossRef]

16. Montford, J.R.; Lehman, A.M.B.; Bauer, C.D.; Klawitter, J.; Klawitter, J.; Poczobutt, J.M.; Scobey, M.; Weiser-Evans, M.; Nemenoff, R.A.; Furgeson, S.B. Bone marrow-derived cPLA2α contributes to renal fibrosis progression. *J. Lipid Res.* **2018**, *59*, 380–390. [CrossRef]

17. Zhao, Y.Y.; Wang, H.L.; Cheng, X.L.; Wei, F.; Bai, X.; Lin, R.C.; Vaziri, N.D. Metabolomics analysis reveals the association between lipid abnormalities and oxidative stress, inflammation, fibrosis, and Nrf2 dysfunction in aristolochic acid-induced nephropathy. *Sci. Rep.* **2015**, *5*, 12936. [CrossRef]

18. Chen, H.M.; Yang, C.M.; Chang, J.F.; Wu, C.S.; Sia, K.C.; Lin, W.N. AdipoR-increased intracellular ROS promotes cPLA2 and COX-2 expressions via activation of PKC and p300 in adiponectin-stimulated human alveolar type II cells. *Am. J. Physiol. Lung Cell Mol. Physiol.* **2016**, *311*, L255–L269. [CrossRef]

19. Hsu, P.S.; Lin, C.M.; Chang, J.F.; Wu, C.S.; Sia, K.C.; Lee, I.T.; Huang, K.Y.; Lin, W.N. Participation of NADPH Oxidase-Related Reactive Oxygen Species in Leptin-Promoted Pulmonary Inflammation: Regulation of cPLA2alpha and COX-2 Expression. *Int. J. Mol. Sci.* **2019**, *20*, 1078. [CrossRef]

20. Ji, L.; Wang, Q.; Huang, F.; An, T.; Guo, F.; Zhao, Y.; Liu, Y.; He, Y.; Song, Y.; Qin, G. FOXO1 Overexpression Attenuates Tubulointerstitial Fibrosis and Apoptosis in Diabetic Kidneys by Ameliorating Oxidative Injury via TXNIP-TRX. *Oxidative Med. Cell. Longev.* **2019**, *2019*, 3286928. [CrossRef]

21. Reilly, S.M.; Saltiel, A.R. Adapting to obesity with adipose tissue inflammation. *Nat. Rev. Endocrinol.* **2017**, *13*, 633. [CrossRef]

22. De Vries, A.P.; Ruggenenti, P.; Ruan, X.Z.; Praga, M.; Cruzado, J.M.; Bajema, I.M.; D'Agati, V.; Lamb, H.J.; Barlovic, D.P.; Hojs, R. Fatty kidney: Emerging role of ectopic lipid in obesity-related renal disease. *Lancet Diabetes Endocrinol.* **2014**, *2*, 417–426. [CrossRef]

23. Jiang, T.; Wang, Z.; Proctor, G.; Moskowitz, S.; Liebman, S.E.; Rogers, T.; Lucia, M.S.; Li, J.; Levi, M. Diet-induced obesity in C57BL/6J mice causes increased renal lipid accumulation and glomerulosclerosis via a sterol regulatory element-binding protein-1c-dependent pathway. *J. Biol. Chem.* **2005**, *280*, 32317–32325. [CrossRef]

24. Zhou, D.; Liu, Y. Renal fibrosis in 2015: Understanding the mechanisms of kidney fibrosis. *Nat. Rev. Nephrol.* **2016**, *12*, 68. [CrossRef]

25. Chang, J.-F.; Liang, S.-S.; Thanasekaran, P.; Chang, H.-W.; Wen, L.-L.; Chen, C.-H.; Liou, J.-C.; Yeh, J.-C.; Liu, S.-H.; Dai, H.-M. Translational Medicine in Pulmonary-Renal Crosstalk: Therapeutic Targeting of p-Cresyl Sulfate Triggered Nonspecific ROS and Chemoattractants in Dyspneic Patients with Uremic Lung Injury. *J. Clin. Med.* **2018**, *7*, 266. [CrossRef]

26. Droge, W. Free radicals in the physiological control of cell function. *Physiol. Rev.* **2002**, *82*, 47–95. [CrossRef]

27. Finkel, T. Signal transduction by reactive oxygen species in non-phagocytic cells. *J. Leukoc. Biol.* **1999**, *65*, 337–340. [CrossRef]

28. Wong, A.C.; Vanhove, A.S.; Watnick, P.I. The interplay between intestinal bacteria and host metabolism in health and disease: Lessons from Drosophila melanogaster. *Dis. Models Mech.* **2016**, *9*, 271–281. [CrossRef]

29. Musso, G.; Gambino, R.; Cassader, M. Obesity, diabetes, and gut microbiota: The hygiene hypothesis expanded? *Diabetes Care* **2010**, *33*, 2277–2284. [CrossRef]

30. Marchesi, J.R.; Adams, D.H.; Fava, F.; Hermes, G.D.; Hirschfield, G.M.; Hold, G.; Quraishi, M.N.; Kinross, J.; Smidt, H.; Tuohy, K.M. The gut microbiota and host health: A new clinical frontier. *Gut* **2016**, *65*, 330–339. [CrossRef]

31. Rosas-Villegas, A.; Sánchez-Tapia, M.; Avila-Nava, A.; Ramírez, V.; Tovar, A.; Torres, N. Differential effect of sucrose and fructose in combination with a high fat diet on intestinal microbiota and kidney oxidative stress. *Nutrients* **2017**, *9*, 393. [CrossRef]

32. Cani, P.D.; Amar, J.; Iglesias, M.A.; Poggi, M.; Knauf, C.; Bastelica, D.; Neyrinck, A.M.; Fava, F.; Tuohy, K.M.; Chabo, C. Metabolic endotoxemia initiates obesity and insulin resistance. *Diabetes* **2007**, *56*, 1761–1772. [CrossRef]

33. Cani, P.D.; Bibiloni, R.; Knauf, C.; Waget, A.; Neyrinck, A.M.; Delzenne, N.M.; Burcelin, R. Changes in gut microbiota control metabolic endotoxemia-induced inflammation in high-fat diet–induced obesity and diabetes in mice. *Diabetes* **2008**, *57*, 1470–1481. [CrossRef]

34. Boutagy, N.E.; McMillan, R.P.; Frisard, M.I.; Hulver, M.W. Metabolic endotoxemia with obesity: Is it real and is it relevant? *Biochimie* **2016**, *124*, 11–20. [CrossRef]

35. Creely, S.J.; McTernan, P.G.; Kusminski, C.M.; Khanolkar, M.; Evans, M.; Louise Harte, A.; Kumar, S. Lipopolysaccharide activates an innate immune system response in human adipose tissue in obesity and type 2 diabetes. *Am. J. Physiol.-Endocrinol. Metabol.* **2007**, *292*, E740–E747. [CrossRef]

36. Mohanty, P.; Aljada, A.; Ghanim, H.; Hofmeyer, D.; Tripathy, D.; Syed, T.; Al-Haddad, W.; Dhindsa, S.; Dandona, P. Evidence for a potent antiinflammatory effect of rosiglitazone. *J. Clin. Endocrinol. Metab.* **2004**, *89*, 2728–2735. [CrossRef]

37. Chen, H.; Zhu, J.; Liu, Y.; Dong, Z.; Liu, H.; Liu, Y.; Zhou, X.; Liu, F.; Chen, G. Lipopolysaccharide induces chronic kidney injury and fibrosis through activation of mTOR signaling in macrophages. *Am. J. Nephrol.* **2015**, *42*, 305–317. [CrossRef]

38. Magder, S.; Parthenis, D.; Ghouleh, I. Preservation of Renal Blood Flow by the Antioxidant EUK-134 in LPS-Treated Pigs. *Int. J. Mol. Sci.* **2015**, *16*, 6801–6817. [CrossRef]

39. Abbott, M.J.; Tang, T.; Sul, H.S. The role of phospholipase A2-derived mediators in obesity. *Drug Discov. Today Disease Mech.* **2010**, *7*, e213–e218. [CrossRef]

40. Hsieh, P.S.; Jin, J.S.; Chiang, C.F.; Chan, P.C.; Chen, C.H.; Shih, K.C. COX-2-mediated inflammation in fat is crucial for obesity-linked insulin resistance and fatty liver. *Obesity* **2009**, *17*, 1150–1157. [CrossRef]

41. Liu, B.-C.; Tang, T.-T.; Lv, L.-L.; Lan, H.-Y. Renal tubule injury: A driving force toward chronic kidney disease. *Kidney Int.* **2018**, *93*, 568–579. [CrossRef]

42. Grande, M.T.; Sánchez-Laorden, B.; López-Blau, C.; De Frutos, C.A.; Boutet, A.; Arévalo, M.; Rowe, R.G.; Weiss, S.J.; López-Novoa, J.M.; Nieto, M.A. Snail1-induced partial epithelial-to-mesenchymal transition drives renal fibrosis in mice and can be targeted to reverse established disease. *Nat. Med.* **2015**, *21*, 989. [CrossRef]

43. Lovisa, S.; LeBleu, V.S.; Tampe, B.; Sugimoto, H.; Vadnagara, K.; Carstens, J.L.; Wu, C.-C.; Hagos, Y.; Burckhardt, B.C.; Pentcheva-Hoang, T. Epithelial-to-mesenchymal transition induces cell cycle arrest and parenchymal damage in renal fibrosis. *Nat. Med.* **2015**, *21*, 998. [CrossRef]

44. Montford, J.R.; Lehman, A.M.; Scobey, M.S.; Weiser-Evans, M.C.; Nemenoff, R.A.; Furgeson, S.B. Cytosolic phospholipase A2α increases proliferation and de-differentiation of human renal tubular epithelial cells. *Prostaglandins Lipid Mediat.* **2016**, *126*, 1–8. [CrossRef]

45. Hegen, M.; Sun, L.; Uozumi, N.; Kume, K.; Goad, M.E.; Nickerson-Nutter, C.L.; Shimizu, T.; Clark, J.D. Cytosolic phospholipase A2α–deficient mice are resistant to collagen-induced arthritis. *J. Exp. Med.* **2003**, *197*, 1297–1302. [CrossRef]

46. Challis, J.R.; Matthews, S.G.; Gibb, W.; Lye, S.J. Endocrine and paracrine regulation of birth at term and preterm. *Endocr. Rev.* **2000**, *21*, 514–550. [CrossRef]

47. Challis, J.R.; Sloboda, D.M.; Alfaidy, N.; Lye, S.J.; Gibb, W.; Patel, F.A.; Whittle, W.L.; Newnham, J.P. Prostaglandins and mechanisms of preterm birth. *Reprod. Camb.* **2002**, *124*, 1–17. [CrossRef]

48. Belikov, A.V.; Schraven, B.; Simeoni, L. T cells and reactive oxygen species. *J. Biomed. Sci.* **2015**, *22*, 85. [CrossRef]

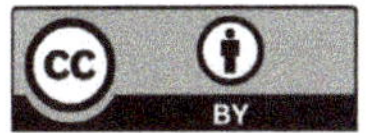

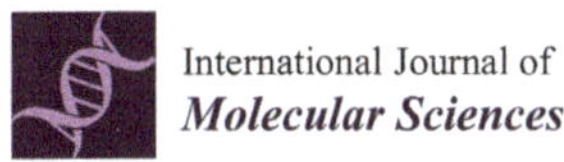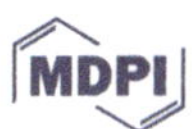

International Journal of
Molecular Sciences

Review

Kidney Cells Regeneration: Dedifferentiation of Tubular Epithelium, Resident Stem Cells and Possible Niches for Renal Progenitors

Nadezda V. Andrianova [1,2], Marina I. Buyan [1], Ljubava D. Zorova [2,3], Irina B. Pevzner [2,3], Vasily A. Popkov [2,3], Valentina A. Babenko [2,3], Denis N. Silachev [2,3], Egor Y. Plotnikov [2,3,4,*] and Dmitry B. Zorov [2,3,*]

[1] Faculty of Bioengineering and Bioinformatics, Lomonosov Moscow State University, 119992 Moscow, Russia; andnadya12@gmail.com (N.V.A.); marinanenart@gmail.com (M.I.B.)

[2] A.N. Belozersky Institute of Physico-Chemical Biology, Lomonosov Moscow State University, 119992 Moscow, Russia; lju_2003@list.ru (L.D.Z.); irinapevzner@mail.ru (I.B.P.); popkov.vas@gmail.com (V.A.P.); nucleus-90@yandex.ru (V.A.B.); silachevdn@belozersky.msu.ru (D.N.S.)

[3] V.I. Kulakov National Medical Research Center of Obstetrics, Gynecology and Perinatology, 117997 Moscow, Russia

[4] Sechenov First Moscow State Medical University, Institute of Molecular Medicine, 119991 Moscow, Russia

* Correspondence: plotnikov@belozersky.msu.ru (E.Y.P.); zorov@belozersky.msu.ru (D.B.Z.); Tel.: +7-495-939-5944 (E.Y.P.)

Received: 29 November 2019; Accepted: 12 December 2019; Published: 15 December 2019

Abstract: A kidney is an organ with relatively low basal cellular regenerative potential. However, renal cells have a pronounced ability to proliferate after injury, which undermines that the kidney cells are able to regenerate under induced conditions. The majority of studies explain yielded regeneration either by the dedifferentiation of the mature tubular epithelium or by the presence of a resident pool of progenitor cells in the kidney tissue. Whether cells responsible for the regeneration of the kidney initially have progenitor properties or if they obtain a "progenitor phenotype" during dedifferentiation after an injury, still stays the open question. The major stumbling block in resolving the issue is the lack of specific methods for distinguishing between dedifferentiated cells and resident progenitor cells. Transgenic animals, single-cell transcriptomics, and other recent approaches could be powerful tools to solve this problem. This review examines the main mechanisms of kidney regeneration: dedifferentiation of epithelial cells and activation of progenitor cells with special attention to potential niches of kidney progenitor cells. We attempted to give a detailed description of the most controversial topics in this field and ways to resolve these issues.

Keywords: renal stem cells; differentiation; scattered tubular cells; papilla; niches

---

1. Introduction

Despite the fact that the kidney has relatively low basal cellular regenerative potential, tubular epithelial cells have a pronounced ability to proliferate after injury [1]. However, the complexity of the renal tissue in mammals and the low rate of cell renewal makes it difficult to study kidney regeneration mechanisms. In this regard, there is still no consensus on what cells are responsible for the recovery of tubular epithelium after injury [2]. A number of hypotheses have been proposed about the nature of regenerative potential in the kidney tissue. The majority of studies assign the basis of such regenerative potential either to the dedifferentiation of the mature tubular epithelium or to the presence of a resident pool of progenitor cells in the kidney tissue [3,4].

The hypothesis of dedifferentiation as a mechanism of renal tissue restoration was based on the analysis of proliferation after ischemia/reperfusion (I/R) or exposure to damaging agents showing that more than half of all tubular epithelium becomes positively stained for proliferation markers (PCNA, Ki-67, BrdU) [5–8]. In addition, some morphological changes were observed in the tubular epithelial cells, which together with the aforementioned data was interpreted as dedifferentiation of these cells [9]. Furthermore, cells indicated the appearance of markers of an embryonic kidney, which could be assumed as a return to a less differentiated state [10–12]. Since then, a lot of evidence has been accumulated about the dominant role of dedifferentiation in the restoration of renal tissue after injury, including data obtained in transgenic animals.

Subsequently, there was additional evidence indicating the possible existence of a population of progenitor cells (so-called scattered tubular cells, STCs) in the adult kidney which had a more pronounced regenerative potential than differentiated tubular epithelium [13–15]. These cells were initially found in the kidneys of rodents [13] and then they were also described in humans [16,17]. Human kidneys have become a very convenient object for progenitor cells studying due to the presence of specific marker CD133 with glycosylated epitope being a "gold standard" to consider these cells as progenitor cells in humans [16,18], as well as in some other mammals [19,20]. Lack of this marker in rodents forces to use other markers for identification of the progenitor population there and determines the need for experiments with transgenic animals expressing fluorescent markers in progenitor cells [21]. A large number of such markers have been proposed (Tables 1 and 2), which apparently characterize the population of progenitor cells in both human and rodent kidneys [22–24].

Table 1. Conventional markers used for the detection of progenitor cells or the dedifferentiation of tubular epithelial cells. Markers, which are used for progenitor cells detection, are partially different for human and rodent kidneys. Foxm1 is the only marker specific for dedifferentiation. Other markers are used both for dedifferentiated cells and progenitor cells and not selective. Empty fields indicate that the marker was not reported for specified conditions.

	Marker	Progenitor Cells		Dedifferentiation
		Human	*Rodents*	
	ALDH1	[18,25]	-	-
	BrdU retention	Not applicable	[13,26–28]	-
	CD24	[16–18,25,29–31]	[15]	-
	CD44	[30,32]	[33]	-
	CD73	[30,32]	-	-
	CD133	[16–18,29–32,34]	Not applicable	-
Markers of progenitor cells	C-kit	-	[14,35]	-
	Musculin	-	[36]	-
	NCAM1	[37]	-	-
	NFATc1	-	[38]	-
	S100A6	[16,18,25]	-	-
	Sall1	[25,37]	[39]	-
	Sca-1	-	[14,15,35,36,40]	-
	SIX2	[37,41]	-	-
Marker of dedifferentiation	Foxm1	-	-	[42,43]
	Nestin	[44]	[35]	[45]
Non-selective markers	Pax-2	[25,30,32,34,37,44]	[14,33,35,46]	[8,11,47–49]
	Sox9	-	[50]	[42,51]
	Vimentin	[16–18,25,30,31,44]	[13,14,26,33,35]	[9,42,47,48,52,53]

Table 2. Markers of progenitor cells located in the papilla of human or rodent kidney.

Marker	The Papilla of Human Kidney	The Papilla of Rodent Kidney
BrdU retention	Not applicable	[27,54–59]
CD133	[60,61]	Not applicable
mTert	-	[59]
Nestin	[60,61]	[55,62]
Oct4	[60,61]	-
Pax-2	[61]	-
Sca-1	-	[63]
Troy/TNFRSF19	-	[64]
Vimentin	[61]	-
Zfyve27	-	[65]

The identification of cells responsible for the restoration of tubular epithelium is in the scope of regenerative medicine [66,67]. This review examines the main mechanisms of kidney regeneration: dedifferentiation of the epithelium and activation of progenitor cells with special attention to potential niches of kidney progenitor cells. We attempted to give a detailed description of the most controversial issues in this area. In particular, we considered issues based on defects of techniques involved in the detection of progenitor cells and on the inability of discrimination of tubular epithelium proliferation from progenitor cells preexistence.

2. Dedifferentiation or Recruitment of Progenitor Cells?

2.1. Dedifferentiation

In the kidneys of adult organisms, a renewal rate the cell population is very slow, however, it dramatically enhances after injury [5]. Staining for various proliferative markers, for example, proliferating cell nuclear antigen (PCNA), Ki-67, and evaluating the accumulation of probes such as bromodeoxyuridine (BrdU) showed that injury-induced cell proliferation in the kidney tissue is not associated with some specific regeneration centers, but goes stochastically [7,8]. In this regard, the first hypothesis explaining the restoration of lost renal cells was the dedifferentiation of the tubular epithelium [5,68]. For a long time, it was believed that any renal epithelial cell has a regenerative potency in response to injury [9,69,70].

After exposure to a damaging factor, a peak of proliferation in the kidney tissue was observed usually occurring on the 2nd day, whereas normal epithelial morphology is normally restored within 5–7 days after challenge [1]. Histological analysis of the kidney tissue distinguishes 4 stages of the regeneration process. At the first stage, the death of tubular epithelium is observed, occurring by apoptosis, necrosis, or another death mode, and it is usually accompanied by an inflammatory reaction. In the second stage, survived tubular cells exhibit changes in normal differentiated epithelial phenotypes, such as a loss of brush border, tubular flattening, and rapid loss of cell polarity [71,72]. During this stage, cells undergo epithelial-mesenchymal transition, detected by overexpression of vimentin, which is a marker of mesenchymal cells [9,52]. The third phase is associated with increased levels of growth factors, such as IGF1, HGF, FGFs, and enhanced proliferation of a majority of kidney cells [73]. Growth factors stimulate cells in the G_0 phase and promote their entry into the cell cycle [74]. The regeneration process is terminated after the recovery of the normal morphology of epithelial cells and restoration of nephron function [75]. Thus, regeneration through dedifferentiation refers to the sequence of histological changes including loss of mature epithelium morphology, epithelial-mesenchymal transition, proliferation to replace lost cells, and re-differentiation [5].

S3 segment of the proximal tubule located near the cortico-medullary junction is known as the most vulnerable part of the nephron [76,77]. Remarkably, the S3 segment also exhibits the most pronounced proliferation after injury compared to other segments of the nephron [78]. Therefore, the majority of studies investigating mechanisms of kidney regeneration are focused on this particular area. Double staining with chlorodeoxyuridine (CldU) and antibodies against Ki-67 revealed that within 48 h after I/R more than 55% of the cells, mainly in the S3 segment, reentered the cell cycle or even passed the S phase [8].

There is a direct histological confirmation of the dedifferentiation of tubular epithelium. In the injured tubules, dividing cells were detected revealing both epithelial and proliferative markers [52,69]. Particularly, dividing cells in the S3 segment of proximal tubules and in the distal tubules had a basolateral expression of Na-K-ATPase (a marker of terminal epithelial differentiation) at the same level as neighboring non-proliferating cells [69], and cells survived after injury carrying intact nuclei actively proliferated and expressed vimentin. Paradoxically, actively proliferating cells continued the expression of Kim-1 [79], a well-known marker of the injured proximal tubular epithelium [80]. Usually, around 35–50% of survived kidney cells begin to express this protein in response to injury [81]. In a strange way, the co-expression of an alarming damaging factor Kim-1 with proliferative factor vimentin in tubular cells after an injury has been currently interpreted as evidence for the proliferation of injured epithelium [8]. It is unclear, whether it reflects the compensatory mechanism for replenishment renal loss of functionality, although it seems dangerous for the organism to reproduce damaged cells.

In addition to vimentin, during kidney regeneration markers specific to kidney development appeared, i.g., Pax-2, and neural cell adhesion molecule 1 (NCAM1). Transcription factor Pax-2 is almost not expressed in adult kidneys, except the collecting ducts and papilla [11]. However, after ischemic or nephrotoxic kidney injury, Pax-2 expression is significantly increased in the survived tubular epithelium, indicating the appearance of cells with immature phenotype [11,49]. NCAM1 is widely represented during nephrogenesis, but it is not detected in the differentiated tubular epithelium [49]. However, upon injury or isolation of kidney cells for culturing, epithelium starts to express NCAM1 again [37]. NCAM1-positive cells exhibit features of epithelial-mesenchymal transformation and possess robust clonal capacity, adopting a progenitor phenotype [82].

Similarly to Pax-2 and NCAM1, another marker of dedifferentiation, Sox9, is actively involved in embryogenesis [51], but is not presented in the kidney tissue of adult organisms [83]. Sox9 expression increases by more than 20-fold 24 h after I/R and its elevated level persists up to 30 days after injury [51]. Over 40% of Sox9-positive cells also express Ki-67 and locate in a scattered-like manner, mainly in the proximal tubules. Sox9+ cells co-express injury markers, neutrophil gelatinase-associated lipocalin (NGAL) and Kim-1, which may indicate that these cells represent injured epithelium. In addition, experiments were performed using lineage tracing showed that Sox9+ cells really contributed to kidney regeneration [51].

In addition, nestin, the protein belonging to intermediate filaments, was recently proposed as a marker of dedifferentiation. After subtotal nephrectomy, the expression of nestin was increased in epithelial cells bordering the injured area [45]. These cells actively proliferated, so the expression of nestin was suggested as a dedifferentiation-associated feature.

2.2. Progenitor Cells

2.2.1. Progenitor Cells in Rodent Kidneys

The first assumption of the presence of progenitor cells in the kidneys arose in the study of Maeshima et al. [13]. In this study, adult intact rats were treated with BrdU, which accumulated in cells in the S-phase [84]. Analysis of kidney cells was conducted 2 weeks after the end of the 7-days BrdU administration and allowed to identify cells with the slow cell cycle. These cells were scattered among other cells of the proximal and distal tubules, so they later became known as scattered tubular cells (STCs), or label-retaining cells (LRCs). To detect possible progenitor properties of LRCs, rats were exposed to I/R, and it was revealed that the number of BrdU+ cells significantly increased 24 h after I/R, most of them were located in 2-cell clusters and expressed PCNA. These cells expressed vimentin as well, and at day 10 began to express E-cadherin (a marker of differentiated epithelium) [85]. Similar data on the presence of LRCs were obtained in newborn mice in which BrdU+ cells were located mainly in the S3 segment and in the papilla [28].

In addition to label retention, these presumably progenitor cells have a more pronounced regenerative potential than non-LRCs. For example, on a three-dimensional gel substrate, they formed tubule-like or tubulocystic structures in response to growth factors treatment [26]. When transplanted into the metanephric kidney, these cells were embedded into epithelial components of a nephron, including proximal tubules, where they demonstrated 3.5–13 times higher proliferative potential [15]. Cells isolated from the S3 segment of adult rat kidneys were able to reconstruct a three-dimensional kidney-like structure in vitro, having all parts of the nephron, including the glomerulus, tubules, and collecting ducts [35]. Moreover, S3-segment cells injected into adult kidney right after ischemia were found in the cortex and medulla confirming their participation in regeneration [14]. However, despite implantation into the kidney tissue, these cells did not cause any significant physiological effects on kidney function estimated by serum creatinine and urea.

A comparative analysis of human and rat renal progenitor cells revealed a population of human scattered tubular cells with a small amount of cytoplasm and mitochondria, without a brush border, which was positive for CD24, CD133 and other progenitors markers [16]. No similar cells with atypical morphology were found in intact rats. The study of renal progenitor cells in rats is complicated by the lack of specific expression of CD24 and glycosylated form of CD133, therefore the search was carried out by the staining for vimentin and CD44 which is another marker for stemness. While absent in intact tissue, vimentin-positive cells with atypical morphology appeared de novo after unilateral ureteral obstruction. The cells (appeared in areas with severe tubules damage) were located singly or in chains of cells and did not have a brush border [16]. However, the emergence of progenitor cells de novo may be only the result of the dedifferentiation.

A similar situation was observed for transcription factor Sox9, which sometimes is used as a marker of progenitor STCs in mice [50]. For a number of tissues, Sox9 is considered to characterize the population of progenitor cells, for example, in hair follicles, retina, and nerve tissue [12,86,87]. However, in renal tissue, cells begin to actively express Sox9 only after injury. Therefore, although they possess many features of progenitor cells (expression of CD133 and Lgr4, the ability to differentiate into adipogenic, osteogenic and chondrogenic cultures), their appearance can be attributed only to dedifferentiation of some renal cells [50].

Sall1, CD24, Sca-1, and nestin have also been proposed as markers of renal progenitor cells. Sall1 is a transcription factor involved in nephrogenesis [88]. Analysis of its expression in the adult kidney revealed that about 0.5% of all cells contained Sall1 located mainly in the cortico-medullary junction [39]. After I/R, 90% of Sall1-positive cells started to proliferate and 5% of these cells showed asymmetric cell division with one of the two adjacent Sall1-positive cells. CD24 is a glycoprotein that is selectively expressed in immature cells of different tissues and it is almost absent in differentiated cells [89]. The presence of this marker was shown in the population of progenitor cells in rodent kidneys [15], however, it is not always possible to obtain its specific staining [16]. Another important marker is Sca-1, which was initially detected as a marker of hematopoietic stem cells until its association with renal progenitor cells was shown [14,15,36,40]. Finally, the aforementioned nestin, intermediate filaments protein, unambiguously associated with progenitor cells in nervous tissue [90], was also found in the cells of some kidney compartments, which are considered as niches for progenitor cells, particularly, the papilla and cortico-medullary junction [62].

In a recent study, the analysis of kidney progenitor cells was performed using transgenic mice with doxycycline-induced random labeling of all tubular epithelial cells by permanent recombination of a single-color-encoding gene [46]. Analysis carried out 30 days after an acute kidney injury (AKI) showed that tubules consisted of clones of cells with the same color and mainly located in the S3 segment of the kidney. Calculations based on the percentage of differently colored clones demonstrated that only a small number of epithelial cells underwent mitosis after I/R, most of them were Pax-2-positive. During regeneration, these cells formed single-colored clones of more than 10 cells. Only Pax-2+ cells fully passed the mitotic cycle, whereas the rest of the tubular epithelium has undergone an endoreplication cycle [46].

Further evidence for the presence of progenitor cells pool in rodent kidneys came from the study of Rinchevich et al. using the so-called rainbow mice [91]. These mice express multicolored reporter constructs allowing to detect cells with segment-specific clonogenic and proliferative potential. One month after the induction of reporter protein expression in intact mice, the clones were observed as small groups of 2–3 cells with the same color. After a longer period, the clones increased to groups consisting of more than 8 cells and they were located both in the cortical substance and in the medulla, in particular, the papilla. The findings showed that tubulogenesis exists in the adult kidney and only a subset of adult epithelial cells was responsible for it. The number of clones of the same color increased after I/R, and most of them (60%) were found in the cortical substance. Thus, this study proved the presence of a functional population of renal progenitor cells [91]. However, it still remains unclear whether these cells belong to a separate pool or they originate from the epithelium transiently acquiring a progenitor phenotype [92].

2.2.2. Progenitor Cells in Human Kidneys

After the discovery of progenitor cells in rodent kidneys, there were studies demonstrating the existence of such cells in human kidneys [27,32]. A population of cells with morphology and progenitor properties different from normal epithelial cells was isolated in the proximal tubules. The main markers of this population were CD24, CD133, and vimentin, and cells were scattered throughout the proximal tubule in the normal human kidney [16]. If compared to conventional epithelial cells, these cells contained less cytoplasm, fewer mitochondria, and had no brush border [16]. The average number of progenitor cells in the cortical substance of the human kidney was estimated at 0.5–4% [17,32] or slightly more (3%–12%) [31]. Most CD133+ cells in the human kidney are located in the S3 segment of the proximal tubules [27,93]. It is noteworthy that this region is most susceptible to damaging factors, but at the same time, it has a remarkable capacity to rerestore its structure and function [77,94].

A convenient feature of human kidney progenitor cells, absent in similar rodent cells, is the presence of CD133, a specific marker of undifferentiated cells. Although CD133 is abundant in both immature and differentiated cells, specific glycosylated epitopes (CD133/1 and CD133/2) have been found only on immature cells in humans [95,96], such as hematopoietic stem/progenitor cells and tissue-specific progenitor cells [97]. The glycosylated form of CD133 has been shown to be expressed in S-shaped bodies in the fetal kidney and co-expressed with Ki-67 [93]. Thus, CD133 is a widely used marker of progenitor cells, however, when staining for this antigen, it is very important to monitor the specificity of antibodies, to exclusively recognize the epitope related to undifferentiated cells only [98]. For confirmation of the results of CD133 detection, cells often are examined for CD24, which usually co-expresses with CD133 [99].

It has been shown that cells positive for CD24/CD133 in various parts of the nephron can be considered as a population of resident progenitor cells. They have the ability to expansion, self-renewal, and epithelial differentiation both in vitro and in vivo [16,17,31,32]. In culture, they are able to differentiate into tubular, osteogenic, neuronal, adipose cells and to repair tubular structures [100]. In vitro, they have the ability to form spheres, which is a specific feature of stem cells [18] and to proliferate for a long time without signs of cell senescence [25]. These cells contain fewer mitochondria than conventional epithelial cells [16], which was confirmed by electron microscopy using gold-conjugated vimentin antibodies, as well as by double immunofluorescence staining for CD133 and mitochondrial markers [31]. However, despite the reduced mitochondrial content, CD133+ cells demonstrate increased Bcl-2 expression [16,18]. CD133 itself is known to participate in glucose uptake [101], and stem cells, in general, are prone to anaerobic metabolism [102]. Probably, the combination of these factors explains the increased resistance of these cells to apoptosis [17].

In addition, cells expressing CD24 and CD133 have a pronounced regenerative potential when administered to mice with severe combined immunodeficiency (SCID) exposed to I/R [100]. A population of human CD133+ papillary cells also possesses a profound nephroprotective potential when administered to rats subjected to glycerol-induced acute tubular damage. It provides restoration of kidney function, preventing tubular necrosis and stimulating proliferation of their own resident cells [30]. CD133+ cells also show signs of proliferation in the renal biopsy material from patients suffering renal insults [17,31]. Despite the fact that the high proliferative activity of putative progenitor cells has been widely shown, it should be kept in mind that cells can behave in vitro in a completely different way than in the organism [48]. For example, human CD133+ cells injected after kidney injury have been shown to be implanted into the tubules of embryonic kidneys, but not in adult rat kidneys [103].

It was found that, apart from CD24 and CD133, another 49 proteins were expressed in the kidney in the same scattered pattern [16]. Among them, there are already mentioned Pax-2 and Sox9, however, colocalization with CD24 or CD133 was shown only for vimentin, S100A6 and several other proteins, e.g., aldehyde dehydrogenase 1 [18]. Recently, a transcriptional profile of CD133+ cells was obtained by RNA sequencing [25]. Overexpression of CD24, PAX-2, vimentin, aldehyde dehydrogenase 1, S100A6, as well as of some other markers were detected.

The existence of progenitor cells distributed in the kidney in a scattered-like manner raises the question of their origin in the process of nephrogenesis [17]. CD133 and CD24 are expressed under kidney development, with the main cluster located in the urinal pole of Bowman's capsule, and a small portion located in the distal tubules in the junction with the glomerulus. It is assumed that during the growth of the kidney, the cells spread and formed the STCs observed in the adult kidney [104]. This once again proves the indissoluble connection of STCs of tubules with the population of glomerular parietal cells, which are recognized as a pool of progenitor cells for podocytes and contain the same markers as STCs [105].

2.3. State of the Art

Thus, there is still a discussion about the genuine nature of the regenerating mechanisms in the adult kidneys of humans and other mammals [1]. The main problem is the lack of specific methods and unique markers for distinguishing between dedifferentiation and progenitor cells' preexistence [2]. For instance, vimentin, which in some studies used as a marker of dedifferentiation and epithelial-mesenchymal transition [9], is also overexpressed in the population of cells defined as progenitors [5].

A similar discussion is going around Kim-1 [106], which is a common marker of the injured proximal tubular epithelium [79,80]. For a long time, the coexpression of vimentin and Kim-1 in the same cells was considered as strict evidence of the dedifferentiation of the injured epithelium as a regenerative mechanism [79]. However, several studies showed that progenitor cells also express Kim-1 after injury [16,18]. To resolve the issue, transgenic mice were created expressing a fluorescent construct under the Kim-1 promoter [42]. The study revealed that Kim-1 was not expressed in renal cells of intact animals. Therefore Kim-1 could not be a marker of the resident progenitor cells. After I/R, in the kidney tissue, clones of cells were found expressing Kim-1, vimentin, Sox9, and Ki67, that was interpreted as a return to the dedifferentiated state rather than a proliferation of resident tubular progenitors. In addition, in this study transcription factor, Foxm1 was described as a new potential marker of dedifferentiated kidney cells [42]. Foxm1 was overexpressed in the injured proximal tubular epithelium, especially in the S3 segment.

The identification of embryonic kidney markers does not resolve the existing contradictions. On the one hand, markers that take part in the process of nephrogenesis should presumably appear during dedifferentiation [1]. On the other hand, a population of progenitor cells, if exists, may also express neonatal kidney markers [23]. For instance, Pax-2 overexpression has been suggested as an argument in favor of the dedifferentiation of mature tubular epithelium after injury [11]. However, in the intact kidney, a population of Pax-2+ cells was also found, which constituted about 10% of cells in the S3 segment [46].

A similar situation occurs around Sox9 [1], initially proposed as a marker of dedifferentiated epithelium due to its expression during nephrogenesis [51]. After an injury, Sox9 colocalized with markers of injured tubular epithelium, such as NGAL and Kim-1 [51]. However, in the intact adult kidney, Sox9-positive cells were found representing a small population of scattered cells that started to proliferate after injury [50], suggesting Sox9 more likely associated with progenitors.

It still remains unclear whether the population of progenitor cells differs from mature tubular epithelium by the number of mitochondria. On the one hand, in adult rat kidney, STCs were characterized by a large number of mitochondria [107]. On the other, in human kidneys, it was found that STCs had a small amount of these organelles [16,31]. Since the content of mitochondria has a very strong effect on cell metabolism, accurate information about the number of these organelles in progenitor cells could help in the development of methods for affecting these cells.

There is a serious limitation in studying renal progenitor cells due to using CD133 as a key marker of undifferentiated cells in human kidneys [108]. Firstly, the glycosylated epitope of CD133 is present in the kidneys of humans, primates, and pigs, but it is absent in rodents [109], which are the main experimental animals. Secondly, the level of glycosylation depends on the stage of cell differentiation [98]. Therefore, the usage of antibodies recognizing CD133 outside the glycosylated epitope can lead to incorrect results [96]. So it is crucial to monitor the specificity of antibodies to the glycosylated epitope in order to selectively determine the pool of progenitor cells. Finally, CD133 antigenic specificity may not only be a limitation of the technique but also indicates differences in the mechanism for kidney regeneration in humans and rodents [2]. For instance, it has been suggested that in humans, progenitor cells could preexist in the tubules, while, in rodents, dedifferentiation might predominate as the main regeneration mechanism [16]. However, this hypothesis was questioned by the detection of progenitor cells in rodent kidneys using other markers [38,50,64].

Thus, the majority of studies support the idea that after injury, the adult kidneys acquire a population of cells with pronounced regenerative potential. However, it remains unclear whether these cells arose from dedifferentiated epithelial cells or from the preexisting population of progenitor cells. The current views on these mechanisms are summarized in Figure 1.

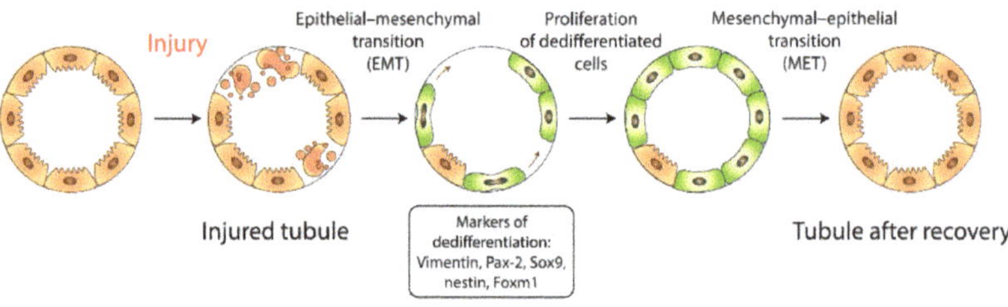

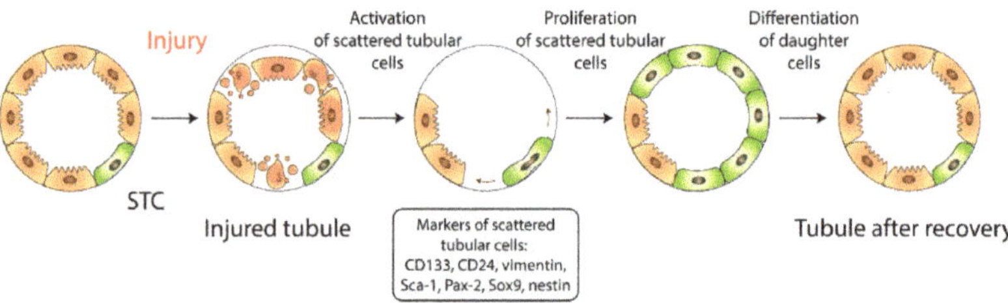

Figure 1. Two major putative mechanisms of kidney tissue regeneration: dedifferentiation of tubular epithelial cells and proliferation of resident renal progenitors with subsequent differentiation.

3. Renal Papilla as a Niche for Progenitor Cells

Morphologically, papilla belongs to the inner layer of renal medulla and plays a crucial role in urine concentration due to residing Henle's loop of juxtamedullary nephrons [110]. Some studies suggest papilla as a putative niche for progenitor cells [55,62,111]. This hypothesis is based on the presence of a large number of cells with the slow cell cycle in the papilla and those cells carrying markers of progenitor cells [2]. Moreover, the papilla is a place with unique conditions that are simultaneously hyperosmotic and hypoxic [112]. The hypoxic microenvironment is a distinguishing feature for stem cell niches in the other organs, such as bone marrow and brain [113]. Papilla cells along with STCs in proximal tubules express progenitor cell markers, for instance, glycated CD133 in human kidneys or nestin in rodent kidneys, and these cells change their properties during tissue regeneration [30,61,62]. Furthermore, papilla cells are positive for embryonic kidney markers, for instance, Pax-2 [11] and TNFRSF19 [64], even in intact adult kidneys.

Papilla as a niche for progenitor cells was suggested in 2004 by Oliver et al., who tried to discover renal resident progenitor cells and outline their properties [55]. The research was based on the observation that organ-specific adult stem cells in a number of tissues have a slow cell cycle that can be detected by retention of BrdU, which integrates into DNA molecule during replication [84]. The study was performed on neonatal rats and mice, which are characterized by the ongoing process of nephrogenesis for a few days after birth. Newborn rodents were injected with BrdU solution, and label retention was estimated 2 months later in the kidney tissue. As a result, in papilla, a population of LRCs was found, with a slow cell cycle, which resided mostly in interstitium although some of them were colocalized with markers of tubular epithelial cells. These LRCs were not bone marrow-derived or belong to endothelial cells. However, after I/R, BrdU-positive cells were absent in the cortex and medulla, which refuted the hypothesis about LRCs migration towards injured areas of the kidney [55].

However, the BrdU labeling assay has several restrictions. The assay mechanism bases on the ability of bromodeoxyuridine to replace thymidine during replication with such replacements being detected by specific antibodies [84]. Label levels slowly decrease in the daughter cells when cells divide after label withdraw. Due to the slow cycle, stem and progenitor cells contain the label for a longer time [114]. However, all cells in S-phase accumulate BrdU during its administration that is the main limitation of the assay [7].

As a result of limitations with BrdU labeling assay, there were attempts to detect progenitor cells in the papilla using lineage tracing in transgenic mice expressing green fluorescent protein (GFP)-fused histone protein (H2B-GFP) under tetracycline-sensitive promotor [115]. The assay was based on the high stability of H2B-GFP protein in the cells with a slow cycle. Consequently, stimulation of its expression before the mice's birth resulted in the detection of cells with a slow cycle even within months after birth [58]. This assay confirmed that cells with slow cycles were located mainly in the papilla, but not in the outer medulla or cortex. Moreover, GFP-positive cells migrated toward the upper part of the papilla where these cells formed chain-like structures of proliferating cells positive for Ki-67 [58].

The population of papilla stem cells was also found in transgenic mice expressing GFP under the nestin promoter [90]. Nestin is considered to be a marker of progenitor cells, including the kidney [60,116]. Those mice had GFP-positive cells mainly in the papilla, and only a small amount was located in the cortico-medullary junction [62]. In the study, evidence was found that GFP-positive cells migrate from the papilla to cortex [90]. The main limitation of the model was a constitutive nestin expression in the adult podocytes and in some endotheliocytes [117,118]. Furthermore, nestin expression in podocytes has been shown to rise during some pathological conditions [119,120].

One more approach for detecting cells with a slow cell cycle is in using mTert-GFP as a reporter system, thus labeling telomerase-expressing embryonic stem cells [59]. On the one hand, such a reporter was chosen because telomerase is a biomarker of stem cells. On the other hand, knockout of mTert leads to the increased severity of AKI, which is believed to be associated with inhibiting of mTert-expressing renal progenitor cell population [121]. The majority of GFP+ cells were observed in the papilla (about 10% of all papillary cells); a small amount was detected in the outer medulla, but not in the cortex. Colocalization with the other cell type-specific proteins showed that mTert was expressed primarily in epithelial cells [59].

Based on the suggestion that papillary progenitor cells have the same cell markers as other tissues progenitor cells GFP-positive cells from H2B-GFP transgenic mice were obtained by fluorescence-activated cell sorting (FACS), and their specific markers were defined. Only protrudin (Zfyve27) demonstrated selective expression in the papilla and it was absent in the other kidney areas [65]. Protrudin-positive cells appeared not to contribute to normal kidney maintenance, however, after severe kidney injury, cells started to proliferate and generate long tubular segments located preferentially in the kidney medulla [65]. Additionally, these cells had many morphological characteristics specific to migratory cells [122].

Considering this data, it was suggested that different kidney areas might have different progenitor cell pools [65] (Figure 2). For instance, papillary LRCs could be activated only in response to severe injury and they restore mainly epithelium in the medulla. This suggestion correlates with the experiments performed on the other epithelial tissues which showed the existence of progenitor cell pools responding to damaging factors being responsible for restoring anatomically various parts of an organ [123,124].

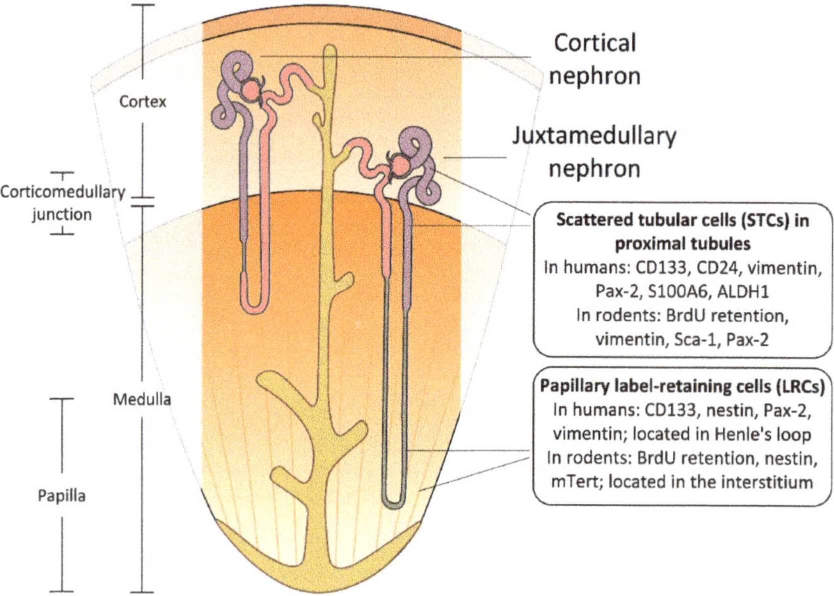

Figure 2. Major suggested niches of renal progenitor cells based on the immunophenotyping with specific surface markers and label retention approach. There are two putative niches for progenitor cells: proximal tubules (especially their S3-segments) and papilla. Progenitor cells in human and rodents kidneys are characterized by slightly different markers listed in Table 2. It is worth noting some differences in the location of progenitor cells: in the papilla of rodent kidney, label-retaining cells (LRCs) reside in the interstitium, while in human kidneys these progenitors constitute the Henle's loop among differentiated cells of the nephron.

Interestingly, papillary progenitor cells were found both in rodents [55,62] and human kidneys [60,61], but with some differences in the localization of the cells. In rodents, a preferential interstitial localization of progenitor cells was observed [55,58,62], while human progenitors were found primarily inside Henle's loops [60]. Both in rodents and humans, these cells were colocalized with the conventional progenitor cell markers. It was shown that CD133+ and nestin+ cells in Henle's loop were located both in the papilla and cortex of the human kidneys. CD133+ cells obtained from the human papilla actively proliferated; after injection into mice embryonic kidney, they integrated into tubules and were involved in tubulogenesis [60]. Similarly, rodent papilla contained cells expressing nestin and telomerase [59,62,125], and papillary cells from pig kidneys were positive for progenitor cells markers CD24 and CD133, and they had myogenic, osteogenic, and adipogenic differentiation potential [111].

To date, the involvement of the papillary cells in kidney regeneration is not fully understood. Whether it is achieved through progenitors migration and integration into tubules, or through paracrine mechanisms is not clear. Hypothesis about proliferation and migration of progenitors daughter cells are based on almost 9 fold decrease of LRCs in papilla 3 weeks after I/R injury [55]. However, in GFP-nestin mice such a decrease in LRCs was not shown after I/R [62]. The question is: why so many papillary LRCs lose BrdU label after injury, whereas only a fraction of them proliferate after injury, and apoptosis is not observed in this area [114].

The migration of papillary LRCs was confirmed in the single study using GFP-nestin mice when papillary nestin-GFP+ cells migrated to cortex and medulla after I/R [62]. Other studies with more evidence-based data demonstrated that migration is limited by the medulla [58,65]. Moreover, the mTert-GFP mouse model showed no evidence of the migration of mTert LRCs from the papilla in response to injury [59]. Humphreys et al. reiterated the study with BrdU administration during nephrogenesis; LRCs in their experiments neither migrated during repair from I/R nor selectively proliferated in those conditions [8]. Furthermore, Ki-67 staining in kidneys of mice injected with CldU during infancy showed that LRCs did not demonstrate proliferation after injury in the cortex and medulla [8]. "Chains" of proliferating Ki-67+ cells found in upper papilla did not colocalize with CldU-positive cells. However, despite the negative results with LRCs, Humphreys et al. did not refute that papilla cells might affect other cells via the paracrine mechanisms [54].

Thus, various methods indicated that kidney papilla contains a cell population with a slow cell cycle involved in regeneration processes in the other parts of the kidney [8,28,55]. However, the biological significance of the long-term BrdU-retaining population is not fully understood yet. These cells could be a population that differentiated in the kidney as early as during embryogenesis and then have never proliferated for any reason. On the other hand, LRCs rapidly exit the cell cycle and undergo much fewer divisions than tubular epithelium thus having more significant regenerative capacity after injury [56]. Due to a large number of contradictions in this area, it is difficult to accept unambiguously that a kidney papilla is a niche of progenitor cells. Further experiments are required to clarify the biological significance of this renal papillary cell population and to identify possible mechanisms of its role in regeneration.

4. Potential Approaches Affecting Kidney Regeneration

A discussion around the presence of progenitor cells in the kidneys of adult organisms appears from the requests of regenerative medicine, because if such cells exist, it would be possible to develop approaches selectively enhancing kidney regeneration [66]. The development of such approaches is possible in the case of dedifferentiation as the main mechanism of regeneration, as well. However, the presence of a pool of progenitors with specific markers and their own physiological characteristics increases the chances to find a successful strategy. Therefore, numerous studies are focused on searching and phenotyping these cells [67].

One of the cell therapy approaches is the use of resident progenitor cells obtained from the kidney by isolation, cultivation and subsequent transplantation (autologous or allogeneic) in the injured organ. Such design is frequently described in the experimental works performed on rodents. Recent studies showed that cells could integrate into the tubules of neonatal and adult kidneys, and then either directly or indirectly could influence the regeneration of renal tissue through the paracrine mechanisms [15–17,35]. However, not in all studies the real improvement of the organ functions was achieved [33]. It is known that cell therapy with resident kidney progenitor cells reduces the activation of apoptosis and inflammation [126], improves angiogenesis [127], reduces fibrosis [128,129], and even increases animal survival after kidney injury [130].

On the other hand, attempts are continuing to develop approaches for affecting resident progenitor cells, for example, to increase the activity of glomerular parietal cells, which are known to be progenitors of podocytes. Some compounds, such as glycogen synthase kinases 3-α and -β (GSK3s) inhibitor 6-bromoindirubin-3-oxime (BIO) [131], notch signaling inhibitors [132], interferon [133], steroids [134], and some others enhanced the proliferation of parietal cells and mediated their differentiation into podocytes in vitro [135]. Perhaps, compounds exist that would selectively affect STC or other possible pools of progenitor cells.

However, it should be taken into account that excessive activation of kidney progenitor cells could have unwanted side effects on organ function. For instance, the above-mentioned activation of parietal cells is observed in glomerulonephritis and diabetic nephropathy and does not lead to a positive outcome. Excessive proliferation can generate lesions of cells, extracapillary crescentic glomerulonephritis, collapsing glomerulopathy, tip lesions, and ultimately these processes compromise the normal functioning of the glomerulus [136].

5. Summary

Obviously, a kidney has a pronounced regenerative potential, however, its cellular basis is still not fully understood. No doubt that some renal cells are responsible for the regeneration of the kidney, but whether these cells initially have progenitor properties or they obtain a "progenitor phenotype" during dedifferentiation after an injury, still stays the main question. The major stumbling block in resolving the issue is the lack of specific methods for distinguishing between dedifferentiated cells and resident progenitor cells [2]. The complexity of the morphological structure of the kidney and the evidence of the existence of populations of different progenitor cells led to the suggestion that different parts of the kidney may have various progenitor cell pools. Another hypothesis is that diverse cell populations are activated in response to different damaging stimuli [137]. Finally, it is possible that two mechanisms of regeneration may coexist in the kidney, complement and compensate each other [2,92].

Transgenic animals are a powerful tool to solve this problem, as well as new methods, for example, single-cell transcriptomics, which has already been successfully used to study the kidney recovery after injury [43,138]. It is hoped that the application of these approaches will soon lead to the discovery of the true source of regenerative potential in the kidney and allow regenerative medicine to choose targeted methods for renal tissue regeneration after injury.

Funding: This study was supported by the Russian science foundation (grant 18-15-00058, the study of dedifferentiation in AKI) and the Russian Foundation for basic research (grant 19-29-04090, kidney progenitor cell research).

Acknowledgments: The authors are very thankful to Anastasia V. Balakireva for her valuable help with the illustrations.

Conflicts of Interest: The authors declare no conflict of interest.

Abbreviations

I/R	Ischemia/reperfusion
AKI	Acute kidney injury
STCs	Scattered tubular cells
LRCs	Label-retaining cells

References

1. Little, M.H.; Kairath, P. Does Renal Repair Recapitulate Kidney Development? *J. Am. Soc. Nephrol.* **2017**, *28*, 34–46. [CrossRef] [PubMed]
2. Huling, J.; Yoo, J.J. Comparing adult renal stem cell identification, characterization and applications. *J. Biomed. Sci.* **2017**, *24*, 32. [CrossRef] [PubMed]
3. Eymael, J.; Smeets, B. Origin and fate of the regenerating cells of the kidney. *Eur. J. Pharmacol.* **2016**, *790*, 62–73. [CrossRef] [PubMed]
4. Kramann, R.; Kusaba, T.; Humphreys, B.D. Who regenerates the kidney tubule? *Nephrol. Dial. Transplant.* **2015**, *30*, 903–910. [CrossRef] [PubMed]
5. Bonventre, J. V Dedifferentiation and proliferation of surviving epithelial cells in acute renal failure. *J. Am. Soc. Nephrol.* **2003**, *14* (Suppl. 1), S55–S61. [CrossRef]
6. Ledda-Columbano, G.M.; Columbano, A.; Coni, P.; Curto, M.; Faa, G.; Pani, P. Cell proliferation in rat kidney induced by 1,2-dibromoethane. *Toxicol. Lett.* **1987**, *37*, 85–90. [CrossRef]
7. Iatropoulos, M.J.; Williams, G.M. Proliferation markers. *Exp. Toxicol. Pathol.* **1996**, *48*, 175–181. [CrossRef]
8. Humphreys, B.D.; Czerniak, S.; DiRocco, D.P.; Hasnain, W.; Cheema, R.; Bonventre, J. V Repair of injured proximal tubule does not involve specialized progenitors. *Proc. Natl. Acad. Sci. USA* **2011**, *108*, 9226–9231. [CrossRef]
9. Witzgall, R.; Brown, D.; Schwarz, C.; Bonventre, J.V. Localization of proliferating cell nuclear antigen, vimentin, c-Fos, and clusterin in the postischemic kidney. Evidence for a heterogenous genetic response among nephron segments, and a large pool of mitotically active and dedifferentiated cells. *J. Clin. Invest.* **1994**, *93*, 2175–2188. [CrossRef]
10. Barker, N.; Rookmaaker, M.B.; Kujala, P.; Ng, A.; Leushacke, M.; Snippert, H.; van de Wetering, M.; Tan, S.; Van Es, J.H.; Huch, M.; et al. Lgr5+ve Stem/Progenitor Cells Contribute to Nephron Formation during Kidney Development. *Cell Rep.* **2012**, *2*, 540–552. [CrossRef]
11. Imgrund, M.; Gröne, E.; Gröne, H.J.; Kretzler, M.; Holzman, L.; Schlöndorff, D.; Rothenpieler, U.W. Re-expression of the developmental gene Pax-2 during experimental acute tubular necrosis in mice. *Kidney Int.* **1999**, *56*, 1423–1431.
12. Poché, R.A.; Furuta, Y.; Chaboissier, M.C.; Schedl, A.; Behringer, R.R. Sox9 is expressed in mouse multipotent retinal progenitor cells and functions in Müller Glial cell development. *J. Comp. Neurol.* **2008**, *510*, 237–250. [CrossRef] [PubMed]
13. Maeshima, A.; Yamashita, S.; Nojima, Y. Identification of renal progenitor-like tubular cells that participate in the regeneration processes of the kidney. *J. Am. Soc. Nephrol.* **2003**, *14*, 3138–3146. [CrossRef] [PubMed]
14. Kitamura, S.; Yamasaki, Y.; Kinomura, M.; Sugaya, T.; Sugiyama, H.; Maeshima, Y.; Makino, H. Establishment and characterization of renal progenitor like cells from S3 segment of nephron in rat adult kidney. *FASEB J.* **2005**, *19*, 1789–1797. [CrossRef] [PubMed]
15. Challen, G.A.; Bertoncello, I.; Deane, J.A.; Ricardo, S.D.; Little, M.H. Kidney Side Population Reveals Multilineage Potential and Renal Functional Capacity but also Cellular Heterogeneity. *J. Am. Soc. Nephrol.* **2006**, *17*, 1896–1912. [CrossRef]
16. Smeets, B.; Boor, P.; Dijkman, H.; Sharma, S.V.; Jirak, P.; Mooren, F.; Berger, K.; Bornemann, J.; Gelman, I.H.; Floege, J.; et al. Proximal tubular cells contain a phenotypically distinct, scattered cell population involved in tubular regeneration. *J. Pathol.* **2013**, *229*, 645–659. [CrossRef]
17. Angelotti, M.L.; Ronconi, E.; Ballerini, L.; Peired, A.; Mazzinghi, B.; Sagrinati, C.; Parente, E.; Gacci, M.; Carini, M.; Rotondi, M.; et al. Characterization of renal progenitors committed toward tubular lineage and their regenerative potential in renal tubular injury. *Stem Cells* **2012**, *30*, 1714–1725. [CrossRef]
18. Lindgren, D.; Boström, A.K.; Nilsson, K.; Hansson, J.; Sjölund, J.; Möller, C.; Jirström, K.; Nilsson, E.; Landberg, G.; Axelson, H.; et al. Isolation and characterization of progenitor-like cells from human renal proximal tubules. *Am. J. Pathol.* **2011**, *178*, 828–837. [CrossRef]
19. Berger, K.; Moeller, M.J. Mechanisms of epithelial repair and regeneration after acute kidney injury. *Semin. Nephrol.* **2014**, *34*, 394–403. [CrossRef]
20. Romagnani, P. Family portrait: Renal progenitor of Bowman's capsule and its tubular brothers. *Am. J. Pathol.* **2011**, *178*, 490–493. [CrossRef]

21. Meyer-Schwesinger, C. The Role of Renal Progenitors in Renal Regeneration. *Nephron* **2016**, *132*, 101–109. [CrossRef]

22. Gupta, S.; Rosenberg, M.E. Do stem cells exist in the adult kidney? *Am. J. Nephrol.* **2008**, *28*, 607–613. [CrossRef] [PubMed]

23. McCampbell, K.K.; Wingert, R.A. Renal stem cells: fact or science fiction? *Biochem. J.* **2012**, *444*, 153–168. [CrossRef] [PubMed]

24. Marcheque, J.; Bussolati, B.; Csete, M.; Perin, L. Concise Reviews: Stem Cells and Kidney Regeneration: An Update. *Stem Cells Transl. Med.* **2019**, *8*, 82–92. [CrossRef] [PubMed]

25. Brossa, A.; Papadimitriou, E.; Collino, F.; Incarnato, D.; Oliviero, S.; Camussi, G.; Bussolati, B. Role of CD133 Molecule in Wnt Response and Renal Repair. *Stem Cells Transl. Med.* **2018**, *7*, 283–294. [CrossRef] [PubMed]

26. Maeshima, A.; Sakurai, H.; Nigam, S.K. Adult kidney tubular cell population showing phenotypic plasticity, tubulogenic capacity, and integration capability into developing kidney. *J. Am. Soc. Nephrol.* **2006**, *17*, 188–198. [CrossRef] [PubMed]

27. Kim, K.; Lee, K.M.; Han, D.J.; Yu, E.; Cho, Y.M. Adult stem cell-like tubular cells reside in the corticomedullary junction of the kidney. *Int. J. Clin. Exp. Pathol.* **2008**, *1*, 232–241.

28. Kim, J.; Kim, J.I.; Na, Y.K.; Park, K.M. Intra-renal slow cell-cycle cells contribute to the restoration of kidney tubules injured by ischemia/reperfusion. *Anat. Cell Biol.* **2011**, *44*, 186. [CrossRef]

29. Sallustio, F.; De Benedictis, L.; Castellano, G.; Zaza, G.; Loverre, A.; Costantino, V.; Grandaliano, G.; Schena, F.P. TLR2 plays a role in the activation of human resident renal stem/progenitor cells. *FASEB J.* **2009**, *24*, 514–525. [CrossRef]

30. Grange, C.; Moggio, A.; Tapparo, M.; Porta, S.; Camussi, G.; Bussolati, B. Protective effect and localization by optical imaging of human renal CD133+ progenitor cells in an acute kidney injury model. *Physiol. Rep.* **2014**, *2*, e12009. [CrossRef]

31. Hansson, J.; Hultenby, K.; Cramnert, C.; Pontén, F.; Jansson, H.; Lindgren, D.; Axelson, H.; Johansson, M.E. Evidence for a morphologically distinct and functionally robust cell type in the proximal tubules of human kidney. *Hum. Pathol.* **2014**, *45*, 382–393. [CrossRef]

32. Bussolati, B.; Bruno, S.; Grange, C.; Buttiglieri, S.; Deregibus, M.C.; Cantino, D.; Camussi, G. Isolation of renal progenitor cells from adult human kidney. *Am. J. Pathol.* **2005**, *166*, 545–555. [CrossRef]

33. Gupta, S.; Verfaillie, C.; Chmielewski, D.; Kren, S.; Eidman, K.; Connaire, J.; Heremans, Y.; Lund, T.; Blackstad, M.; Jiang, Y.; et al. Isolation and characterization of kidney-derived stem cells. *J. Am. Soc. Nephrol.* **2006**, *17*, 3028–3040. [CrossRef] [PubMed]

34. Loverre, A.; Capobianco, C.; Ditonno, P.; Battaglia, M.; Grandaliano, G.; Schena, F.P. Increase of proliferating renal progenitor cells in acute tubular necrosis underlying delayed graft function. *Transplantation* **2008**, *85*, 1112–1119. [CrossRef] [PubMed]

35. Kitamura, S.; Sakurai, H.; Makino, H. Single adult kidney stem/progenitor cells reconstitute three-dimensional nephron structures in vitro. *Stem Cells* **2015**, *33*, 774–784. [CrossRef] [PubMed]

36. Hishikawa, K.; Marumo, T.; Miura, S.; Nakanishi, A.; Matsuzaki, Y.; Shibata, K.; Ichiyanagi, T.; Kohike, H.; Komori, T.; Takahashi, I.; et al. Musculin/MyoR is expressed in kidney side population cells and can regulate their function. *J. Cell Biol.* **2005**, *169*, 921–928. [CrossRef]

37. Buzhor, E.; Omer, D.; Harari-Steinberg, O.; Dotan, Z.; Vax, E.; Pri-Chen, S.; Metsuyanim, S.; Pleniceanu, O.; Goldstein, R.S.; Dekel, B. Reactivation of NCAM1 defines a subpopulation of human adult kidney epithelial cells with clonogenic and stem/progenitor properties. *Am. J. Pathol.* **2013**, *183*, 1621–1633. [CrossRef]

38. Langworthy, M.; Zhou, B.; de Caestecker, M.; Moeckel, G.; Baldwin, H. NFATc1 identifies a population of proximal tubule cell progenitors. *J. Am. Soc. Nephrol.* **2009**, *20*, 311–321. [CrossRef]

39. Abedin, M.J.; Imai, N.; Rosenberg, M.E.; Gupta, S. Identification and characterization of Sall1-expressing cells present in the adult mouse kidney. *Nephron. Exp. Nephrol.* **2011**, *119*, e75–e82. [CrossRef]

40. Iwatani, H.; Ito, T.; Imai, E.; Matsuzaki, Y.; Suzuki, A.; Yamato, M.; Okabe, M.; Hori, M. Hematopoietic and nonhematopoietic potentials of Hoechst low /side population cells isolated from adult rat kidney. *Kidney Int.* **2004**, *65*, 1604–1614.

41. Da Sacco, S.; Thornton, M.E.; Petrosyan, A.; Lavarreda-Pearce, M.; Sedrakyan, S.; Grubbs, B.H.; De Filippo, R.E.; Perin, L. Direct Isolation and Characterization of Human Nephron Progenitors. *Stem Cells Transl. Med.* **2017**, *6*, 419–433. [CrossRef]

42. Chang-Panesso, M.; Kadyrov, F.F.; Lalli, M.; Wu, H.; Ikeda, S.; Kefaloyianni, E.; Abdelmageed, M.M.; Herrlich, A.; Kobayashi, A.; Humphreys, B.D. FOXM1 drives proximal tubule proliferation during repair from acute ischemic kidney injury. *J. Clin. Invest.* **2019**, *129*. [CrossRef]

43. Kirita, Y.; Chang-Panesso, M.; Humphreys, B.D. Recent Insights into Kidney Injury and Repair from Transcriptomic Analyses. *Nephron* **2019**. [CrossRef] [PubMed]

44. Ye, Y.; Wang, B.; Jiang, X.; Hu, W.; Feng, J.; Li, H.; Jin, M.; Ying, Y.; Wang, W.; Mao, X.; et al. Proliferative capacity of stem/progenitor-like cells in the kidney may associate with the outcome of patients with acute tubular necrosis. *Hum. Pathol.* **2011**, *42*, 1132–1141. [CrossRef] [PubMed]

45. Wen, D.; Ni, L.; You, L.; Zhang, L.; Gu, Y.; Hao, C.M.; Chen, J. Upregulation of nestin in proximal tubules may participate in cell migration during renal repair. *Am. J. Physiol. Ren. Physiol.* **2012**, *303*. [CrossRef] [PubMed]

46. Lazzeri, E.; Angelotti, M.L.; Peired, A.; Conte, C.; Marschner, J.A.; Maggi, L.; Mazzinghi, B.; Lombardi, D.; Melica, M.E.; Nardi, S.; et al. Endocycle-related tubular cell hypertrophy and progenitor proliferation recover renal function after acute kidney injury. *Nat. Commun.* **2018**, *9*. [CrossRef] [PubMed]

47. Lin, F.; Moran, A.; Igarashi, P. Intrarenal cells, not bone marrow-derived cells, are the major source for regeneration in postischemic kidney. *J. Clin. Invest.* **2005**, *115*, 1756–1764. [CrossRef] [PubMed]

48. Kusaba, T.; Lalli, M.; Kramann, R.; Kobayashi, A.; Humphreys, B.D. Differentiated kidney epithelial cells repair injured proximal tubule. *Proc. Natl. Acad. Sci. USA* **2014**, *111*, 1527–1532. [CrossRef]

49. Villanueva, S.; Céspedes, C.; Vio, C.P. Ischemic acute renal failure induces the expression of a wide range of nephrogenic proteins. *Am. J. Physiol. Regul. Integr. Comp. Physiol.* **2006**, *290*, R861–R870. [CrossRef]

50. Kang, H.M.; Huang, S.; Reidy, K.; Han, S.H.; Chinga, F.; Susztak, K. Sox9-Positive Progenitor Cells Play a Key Role in Renal Tubule Epithelial Regeneration in Mice. *Cell Rep.* **2016**. [CrossRef]

51. Kumar, S.; Liu, J.; Pang, P.; Krautzberger, A.M.; Reginensi, A.; Akiyama, H.; Schedl, A.; Humphreys, B.D.; McMahon, A.P. Sox9 Activation Highlights a Cellular Pathway of Renal Repair in the Acutely Injured Mammalian Kidney. *Cell Rep.* **2015**, *12*, 1325–1338. [CrossRef]

52. Fujigaki, Y.; Goto, T.; Sakakima, M.; Fukasawa, H.; Miyaji, T.; Yamamoto, T.; Hishida, A. Kinetics and characterization of initially regenerating proximal tubules in S3 segment in response to various degrees of acute tubular injury. *Nephrol. Dial. Transplant.* **2006**, *21*, 41–50. [CrossRef]

53. Gröne, H.J.; Weber, K.; Gröne, E.; Helmchen, U.; Osborn, M. Coexpression of keratin and vimentin in damaged and regenerating tubular epithelia of the kidney. *Am. J. Pathol.* **1987**, *129*, 1–8. [PubMed]

54. Humphreys, B.D.; Valerius, M.T.; Kobayashi, A.; Mugford, J.W.; Soeung, S.; Duffield, J.S.; McMahon, A.P.; Bonventre, J.V. Intrinsic Epithelial Cells Repair the Kidney after Injury. *Cell Stem Cell* **2008**, *2*, 284–291. [CrossRef] [PubMed]

55. Oliver, J.A.; Maarouf, O.; Cheema, F.H.; Martens, T.P.; Al-Awqati, Q. The renal papilla is a niche for adult kidney stem cells. *J. Clin. Invest.* **2004**. [CrossRef] [PubMed]

56. Adams, D.C.; Oxburgh, L. The long-term label retaining population of the renal papilla arises through divergent regional growth of the kidney. *Am. J. Physiol. Physiol.* **2009**, *297*, F809–F815. [CrossRef]

57. Liu, X.; Liu, H.; Sun, L.; Chen, Z.; Nie, H.; Sun, A.; Liu, G.; Guan, G. The role of long-term label-retaining cells in the regeneration of adult mouse kidney after ischemia/reperfusion injury. *Stem Cell Res. Ther.* **2016**, *7*. [CrossRef]

58. Oliver, J.A.; Klinakis, A.; Cheema, F.H.; Friedlander, J.; Sampogna, R.V.; Martens, T.P.; Liu, C.; Efstratiadis, A.; Al-Awqati, Q. Proliferation and migration of label-retaining cells of the kidney papilla. *J. Am. Soc. Nephrol.* **2009**, *20*, 2315–2327. [CrossRef]

59. Song, J.; Czerniak, S.; Wang, T.; Ying, W.; Carlone, D.L.; Breault, D.T.; Humphreys, B.D. Characterization and fate of telomerase-expressing epithelia during kidney repair. *J. Am. Soc. Nephrol.* **2011**, *22*, 2256–2265. [CrossRef]

60. Ward, H.H.; Romero, E.; Welford, A.; Pickett, G.; Bacallao, R.; Gattone, V.H.; Ness, S.A.; Wandinger-Ness, A.; Roitbak, T. Adult human CD133/1(+) kidney cells isolated from papilla integrate into developing kidney tubules. *Biochim. Biophys. Acta* **2011**, *1812*, 1344–1357. [CrossRef]

61. Bussolati, B.; Moggio, A.; Collino, F.; Aghemo, G.; D'Armento, G.; Grange, C.; Camussi, G. Hypoxia modulates the undifferentiated phenotype of human renal inner medullary CD133+ progenitors through Oct4/miR-145 balance. *Am. J. Physiol. Renal Physiol.* **2012**, *302*, F116–F128. [CrossRef]

62. Patschan, D.; Michurina, T.; Shi, H.K.; Dolff, S.; Brodsky, S.V.; Vasilieva, T.; Cohen-Gould, L.; Winaver, J.; Chander, P.N.; Enikolopov, G.; et al. Normal distribution and medullary-to-cortical shift of Nestin-expressing cells in acute renal ischemia. *Kidney Int.* **2007**, *71*, 744–754. [CrossRef]

63. Dekel, B.; Zangi, L.; Shezen, E.; Reich-Zeliger, S.; Eventov-Friedman, S.; Katchman, H.; Jacob-Hirsch, J.; Amariglio, N.; Rechavi, G.; Margalit, R.; et al. Isolation and characterization of nontubular Sca-1+Lin-multipotent stem/progenitor cells from adult mouse kidney. *J. Am. Soc. Nephrol.* **2006**, *17*, 3300–3314. [CrossRef] [PubMed]

64. Schutgens, F.; Rookmaaker, M.B.; Blokzijl, F.; Van Boxtel, R.; Vries, R.; Cuppen, E.; Verhaar, M.C.; Clevers, H. Troy/TNFRSF19 marks epithelial progenitor cells during mouse kidney development that continue to contribute to turnover in adult kidney. *Proc. Natl. Acad. Sci. USA* **2017**, *114*, E11190–E11198. [CrossRef] [PubMed]

65. Oliver, J.A.; Sampogna, R.V.; Jalal, S.; Zhang, Q.-Y.; Dahan, A.; Wang, W.; Shen, T.H.; Al-Awqati, Q. A Subpopulation of Label-Retaining Cells of the Kidney Papilla Regenerates Injured Kidney Medullary Tubules. *Stem Cell Rep.* **2016**, *6*, 757–771. [CrossRef] [PubMed]

66. Aggarwal, S.; Moggio, A.; Bussolati, B. Concise Review: Stem/Progenitor Cells for Renal Tissue Repair: Current Knowledge and Perspectives. *Stem Cells Transl. Med.* **2013**, *2*, 1011–1019. [CrossRef] [PubMed]

67. Pleniceanu, O.; Omer, D.; Harari-Steinberg, O.; Dekel, B. Renal lineage cells as a source for renal regeneration. *Pediatr. Res.* **2018**, *83*, 267–274. [CrossRef] [PubMed]

68. Houghton, D.C.; Hartnett, M.; Campbell-Boswell, M.; Porter, G.; Bennett, W. A light and electron microscopic analysis of gentamicin nephrotoxicity in rats. *Am. J. Pathol.* **1976**, *82*, 589.

69. Vogetseder, A.; Karadeniz, A.; Kaissling, B.; Hir, M. Le Tubular cell proliferation in the healthy rat kidney. *Histochem. Cell Biol.* **2005**, *124*, 97–104. [CrossRef]

70. Vogetseder, A.; Palan, T.; Bacic, D.; Kaissling, B.; Le Hir, M. Proximal tubular epithelial cells are generated by division of differentiated cells in the healthy kidney. *Am. J. Physiol. Cell Physiol.* **2007**, *292*, C807–C813. [CrossRef]

71. Molitoris, B.A.; Hoilien, C.A.; Dahl, R.; Ahnen, D.J.; Wilson, P.D.; Kim, J. Characterization of ischemia-induced loss of epithelial polarity. *J. Membr. Biol.* **1988**, *106*, 233–242. [CrossRef]

72. Solez, K.; Morel-Maroger, L.; Sraer, J.D. The morphology of "acute tubular necrosis" in man: analysis of 57 renal biopsies and a comparison with the glycerol model. *Medicine (Baltimore)* **1979**, *58*, 362–376. [CrossRef]

73. Schena, F.P. Role of growth factors in acute renal failure. *Kidney Int. Suppl.* **1998**, *66*, S11-5. [PubMed]

74. El Sabbahy, M.; Vaidya, V.S. Ischemic kidney injury and mechanisms of tissue repair. *Wiley Interdiscip. Rev. Syst. Biol. Med.* **2011**, *3*, 606–618. [CrossRef] [PubMed]

75. Devarajan, P.; Mishra, J.; Supavekin, S.; Patterson, L.T.; Steven Potter, S. Gene expression in early ischemic renal injury: clues towards pathogenesis, biomarker discovery, and novel therapeutics. *Mol. Genet. Metab.* **2003**, *80*, 365–376. [CrossRef] [PubMed]

76. Spiegel, D.M.; Shanley, P.F.; Molitoris, B.A. Mild ischemia predisposes the S3 segment to gentamicin toxicity. *Kidney Int.* **1990**, *38*, 459–464. [CrossRef] [PubMed]

77. Sekine, M.; Monkawa, T.; Morizane, R.; Matsuoka, K.; Taya, C.; Akita, Y.; Joh, K.; Itoh, H.; Hayashi, M.; Kikkawa, Y.; et al. Selective depletion of mouse kidney proximal straight tubule cells causes acute kidney injury. *Transgenic Res.* **2012**, *21*, 51–62. [CrossRef] [PubMed]

78. Vogetseder, A.; Picard, N.; Gaspert, A.; Walch, M.; Kaissling, B.; Le Hir, M. Proliferation capacity of the renal proximal tubule involves the bulk of differentiated epithelial cells. *Am. J. Physiol. Physiol.* **2008**, *294*, C22–C28. [CrossRef]

79. Ichimura, T.; Hung, C.C.; Yang, S.A.; Stevens, J.L.; Bonventre, J.V. Kidney injury molecule-1: a tissue and urinary biomarker for nephrotoxicant-induced renal injury. *Am. J. Physiol. Physiol.* **2004**, *286*, F552–F563. [CrossRef]

80. Ichimura, T.; Bonventre, J.V.; Bailly, V.; Wei, H.; Hession, C.A.; Cate, R.L.; Sanicola, M. Kidney injury molecule-1 (KIM-1), a putative epithelial cell adhesion molecule containing a novel immunoglobulin domain, is up-regulated in renal cells after injury. *J. Biol. Chem.* **1998**, *273*, 4135–4142. [CrossRef]

81. Berger, K.; Bangen, J.-M.; Hammerich, L.; Liedtke, C.; Floege, J.; Smeets, B.; Moeller, M.J. Origin of regenerating tubular cells after acute kidney injury. *Proc. Natl. Acad. Sci. USA* **2014**, *111*, 1533–1538. [CrossRef]

82. Romagnani, P.; Rinkevich, Y.; Dekel, B. The use of lineage tracing to study kidney injury and regeneration. *Nat. Rev. Nephrol.* **2015**, *11*, 420–431. [CrossRef]

83. Chaboissier, M.C.; Kobayashi, A.; Vidal, V.I.P.; Lützkendorf, S.; van de Kant, H.J.G.; Wegner, M.; de Rooij, D.G.; Behringer, R.R.; Schedl, A. Functional analysis os Sox8 and Sox9 during sex determination in the mouse. *Development* **2004**, *131*, 1891–1901. [CrossRef] [PubMed]

84. Cavanagh, B.L.; Walker, T.; Norazit, A.; Meedeniya, A.C.B. Thymidine analogues for tracking DNA synthesis. *Molecules* **2011**, *16*, 7980–7993. [CrossRef] [PubMed]

85. Piepenhagen, P.A.; Peters, L.L.; Lux, S.E.; Nelson, W.J. Differential expression of Na+-K+-ATPase, ankyrin, fodrin, and E- cadherin along the kidney nephron. *Am. J. Physiol. Cell Physiol.* **1995**, *269*, C1417–C1432. [CrossRef] [PubMed]

86. Nowak, J.A.; Polak, L.; Pasolli, H.A.; Fuchs, E. Hair follicle stem cells are specified and function in early skin morphogenesis. *Cell Stem Cell* **2008**, *3*, 33–43. [CrossRef] [PubMed]

87. Cheung, M.; Briscoe, J. Neural crest development is regulated by the transcription factor Sox9. *Development* **2003**, *130*, 5681–5693. [CrossRef] [PubMed]

88. Yamashita, K.; Sato, A.; Asashima, M.; Wang, P.C.; Nishinakamura, R. Mouse homolog of SALL1, a causative gene for Townes-Brocks syndrome, binds to A/T-rich sequences in pericentric heterochromatin via its C-terminal zinc finger domains. *Genes Cells* **2007**, *12*, 171–182. [CrossRef] [PubMed]

89. Shirasawa, T.; Akashi, T.; Sakamoto, K.; Takahashi, H.; Maruyama, N.; Hirokawa, K. Gene expression of CD24 core peptide molecule in developing brain and developing non-neural tissues. *Dev. Dyn.* **1993**, *198*, 1–13. [CrossRef]

90. Mignone, J.L.; Kukekov, V.; Chiang, A.S.; Steindler, D.; Enikolopov, G. Neural Stem and Progenitor Cells in Nestin-GFP Transgenic Mice. *J. Comp. Neurol.* **2004**, *469*, 311–324. [CrossRef]

91. Rinkevich, Y.; Montoro, D.T.; Contreras-Trujillo, H.; Harari-Steinberg, O.; Newman, A.M.; Tsai, J.M.; Lim, X.; Van-Amerongen, R.; Bowman, A.; Januszyk, M.; et al. In vivo clonal analysis reveals lineage-restricted progenitor characteristics in mammalian kidney development, maintenance, and regeneration. *Cell Rep.* **2014**. [CrossRef]

92. Chang-Panesso, M.; Humphreys, B.D. Cellular plasticity in kidney injury and repair. *Nat. Rev. Nephrol.* **2017**, *13*, 39–46. [CrossRef]

93. Kim, K.; Park, B.-H.; Ihm, H.; Kim, K.M.; Jeong, J.; Chang, J.W.; Cho, Y.M. Expression of stem cell marker CD133 in fetal and adult human kidneys and pauci-immune crescentic glomerulonephritis. *Histol. Histopathol.* **2011**, *26*, 223–232. [PubMed]

94. Lieberthal, W.; Nigam, S.K. Acute renal failure. I. Relative importance of proximal vs. distal tubular injury. *Am. J. Physiol.* **1998**, *275*, F623–F632. [CrossRef] [PubMed]

95. Kemper, K.; Sprick, M.R.; De Bree, M.; Scopelliti, A.; Vermeulen, L.; Hoek, M.; Zeilstra, J.; Pals, S.T.; Mehmet, H.; Stassi, G.; et al. The AC133 epitope, but not the CD133 protein, is lost upon cancer stem cell differentiation. *Cancer Res.* **2010**, *70*, 719–729. [CrossRef] [PubMed]

96. Angelotti, M.L.; Lazzeri, E.; Lasagni, L.; Romagnani, P. Only anti-CD133 antibodies recognizing the CD133/1 or the CD133/2 epitopes can identify human renal progenitors. *Kidney Int.* **2010**, *78*, 620–621. [CrossRef] [PubMed]

97. Corbeil, D.; Röper, K.; Hellwig, A.; Tavian, M.; Miraglia, S.; Watt, S.M.; Simmons, P.J.; Peault, B.; Buck, D.W.; Huttner, W.B. The human AC133 hematopoietic stem cell antigen is also expressed in epithelial cells and targeted to plasma membrane protrusions. *J. Biol. Chem.* **2000**, *275*, 5512–5520. [CrossRef]

98. Mizrak, D.; Brittan, M.; Alison, M.R. CD 133: Molecule of the moment. *J. Pathol.* **2008**, *214*, 3–9. [CrossRef]

99. Romagnani, P.; Remuzzi, G. CD133+ renal stem cells always co-express CD24 in adult human kidney tissue. *Stem Cell Res.* **2014**, *12*, 828–829. [CrossRef]

100. Sagrinati, C.; Netti, G.S.; Mazzinghi, B.; Lazzeri, E.; Liotta, F.; Frosali, F.; Ronconi, E.; Meini, C.; Gacci, M.; Squecco, R.; et al. Isolation and characterization of multipotent progenitor cells from the Bowman's capsule of adult human kidneys. *J. Am. Soc. Nephrol.* **2006**, *17*, 2443–2456. [CrossRef]

101. Chen, H.; Luo, Z.; Dong, L.; Tan, Y.; Yang, J.; Feng, G.; Wu, M.; Li, Z.; Wang, H. CD133/prominin-1-mediated autophagy and glucose uptake beneficial for hepatoma cell survival. *PLoS ONE* **2013**, *8*, e56878. [CrossRef]

102. Rehman, J. Empowering self-renewal and differentiation: The role of mitochondria in stem cells. *J. Mol. Med.* **2010**, *88*, 981–986. [CrossRef]

103. Santeramo, I.; Perez, Z.H.; Illera, A.; Taylor, A.; Kenny, S.; Murray, P.; Wilm, B.; Gretz, N. Human kidney-derived cells ameliorate acute kidney injury without engrafting into renal tissue. *Stem Cells Transl. Med.* **2017**. [CrossRef] [PubMed]

104. Romagnani, P.; Lasagni, L.; Remuzzi, G. Renal progenitors: An evolutionary conserved strategy for kidney regeneration. *Nat. Rev. Nephrol.* **2013**, *9*, 137–146. [CrossRef] [PubMed]

105. Shankland, S.J.; Freedman, B.S.; Pippin, J.W. Can podocytes be regenerated in adults? *Curr. Opin. Nephrol. Hypertens.* **2017**, *26*, 154–164. [CrossRef] [PubMed]

106. Humphreys, B.D. Kidney injury, stem cells and regeneration. *Curr. Opin. Nephrol. Hypertens.* **2014**, *23*, 25–31. [CrossRef]

107. Forbes, M.S.; Thornhill, B.A.; Galarreta, C.I.; Chevalier, R.L. A population of mitochondrion-rich cells in the pars recta of mouse kidney. *Cell Tissue Res.* **2016**, *363*, 791–803. [CrossRef]

108. Bussolati, B.; Camussi, G. Therapeutic use of human renal progenitor cells for kidney regeneration. *Nat. Rev. Nephrol.* **2015**. [CrossRef]

109. Romagnani, P. Of mice and men: The riddle of tubular regeneration. *J. Pathol.* **2013**, *229*, 641–644. [CrossRef]

110. Vanslambrouck, J.; Li, J.; Little, M.H. The renal papilla: An enigma in damage and repair. *J. Am. Soc. Nephrol.* **2011**, *22*, 2145–2147. [CrossRef]

111. Burmeister, D.M.; McIntyre, M.K.; Montgomery, R.K.; Gómez, B.I.; Dubick, M.A. Isolation and Characterization of Multipotent CD24+ Cells From the Renal Papilla of Swine. *Front. Med.* **2018**, *5*. [CrossRef]

112. Pannabecker, T.L.; Layton, A.T. Targeted delivery of solutes and oxygen in the renal medulla: role of microvessel architecture. *Am. J. Physiol. Renal Physiol.* **2014**, *307*, F649–F655. [CrossRef]

113. Mohyeldin, A.; Garzón-Muvdi, T.; Quiñones-Hinojosa, A. Oxygen in stem cell biology: A critical component of the stem cell niche. *Cell Stem Cell* **2010**, *7*, 150–161. [CrossRef] [PubMed]

114. Humphreys, B.D. Slow-Cycling Cells in Renal Papilla: Stem Cells Awaken? *J. Am. Soc. Nephrol.* **2009**. [CrossRef] [PubMed]

115. Tumbar, T.; Guasch, G.; Greco, V.; Blanpain, C.; Lowry, W.E.; Rendl, M.; Fuchs, E. Defining the epithelial stem cell niche in skin. *Science* **2004**, *303*, 359–363. [CrossRef] [PubMed]

116. Wiese, C.; Rolletschek, A.; Kania, G.; Blyszczuk, P.; Tarasov, K.V.; Tarasova, Y.; Wersto, R.P.; Boheler, K.R.; Wobus, A.M. Nestin expression-A property of multi-lineage progenitor cells? *Cell. Mol. Life Sci.* **2004**. [CrossRef] [PubMed]

117. Chen, J.; Boyle, S.; Zhao, M.; Su, W.; Takahashi, K.; Davis, L.; DeCaestecker, M.; Takahashi, T.; Brever, M.D.; Hao, C.M. Differential expression of the intermediate filament protein nestin during renal development and its localization in adult podocytes. *J. Am. Soc. Nephrol.* **2006**, *17*, 1283–1291. [CrossRef]

118. Kirik, O.V.; Korzhevskii, D.E. Expression of neural stem cell marker nestin in the kidney of rats and humans. *Bull. Exp. Biol. Med.* **2009**, *147*, 539–541. [CrossRef]

119. Zou, J.; Yaoita, E.; Watanabe, Y.; Yoshida, Y.; Nameta, M.; Li, H.; Qu, Z.; Yamamoto, T. Upregulation of nestin, vimentin, and desmin in rat podocytes in response to injury. *Virchows Arch.* **2006**, *448*, 485–492. [CrossRef]

120. Perry, J.; Ho, M.; Viero, S.; Zheng, K.; Jacobs, R.; Thorner, P.S. The intermediate filament nestin is highly expressed in normal human podocytes and podocytes in glomerular disease. *Pediatr. Dev. Pathol.* **2007**, *10*, 369–382. [CrossRef]

121. Westhoff, J.H.; Schildhorn, C.; Jacobi, C.; Hömme, M.; Hartner, A.; Braun, H.; Kryzer, C.; Wang, C.; Von Zglinicki, T.; Kränzlin, B.; et al. Telomere shortening reduces regenerative capacity after acute kidney injury. *J. Am. Soc. Nephrol.* **2010**, *21*, 327–336. [CrossRef]

122. Ridley, A.J.; Schwartz, M.A.; Burridge, K.; Firtel, R.A.; Ginsberg, M.H.; Borisy, G.; Parsons, J.T.; Horwitz, A.R. Cell Migration: Integrating Signals from Front to Back. *Science* **2003**, *302*, 1704–1709. [CrossRef]

123. Solanas, G.; Benitah, S.A. Architecture of the Interfolliculer epidermis. *Nat. Rev. Mol. Cell Biol.* **2013**, *14*, 737–748. [CrossRef] [PubMed]

124. Yousefi, M.; Li, L.; Lengner, C.J. Hierarchy and Plasticity in the Intestinal Stem Cell Compartment. *Trends Cell Biol.* **2017**, *27*, 753–764. [CrossRef] [PubMed]

125. Wang, J.; Lin, G.; Alwaal, A.; Zhang, X.; Wang, G.; Jia, X.; Banie, L.; Villalta, J.; Lin, C.S.; Lue, T.F. Kinetics of Label Retaining Cells in the Developing Rat Kidneys. *PLoS ONE* **2015**. [CrossRef] [PubMed]

126. Gupta, A.K.; Jadhav, S.H.; Tripathy, N.K.; Nityanand, S. Fetal kidney cells can ameliorate ischemic acute renal failure in rats through their anti-inflammatory, anti-apoptotic and anti-oxidative effects. *PLoS ONE* **2015**, *10*. [CrossRef] [PubMed]

127. Gupta, A.K. Fetal kidney stem cells ameliorate cisplatin induced acute renal failure and promote renal angiogenesis. *World J. Stem Cells* **2015**, *7*, 776. [CrossRef] [PubMed]

128. Aggarwal, S.; Grange, C.; Iampietro, C.; Camussi, G.; Bussolati, B. Human CD133 + Renal Progenitor Cells Induce Erythropoietin Production and Limit Fibrosis after Acute Tubular Injury. *Sci. Rep.* **2016**, *6*. [CrossRef]

129. Chen, C.; Chou, K.; Fang, H.; Hsu, C.; Huang, W.; Huang, C.; Huang, C.; Chen, H.; Lee, P. Progenitor-like cells derived from mouse kidney protect against renal fibrosis in a remnant kidney model via decreased endothelial mesenchymal transition. *Stem Cell Res. Ther.* **2015**, *6*. [CrossRef]

130. Lee, P.T.; Lin, H.H.; Jiang, S.T.; Lu, P.J.; Chou, K.J.; Fang, H.C.; Chiou, Y.Y.; Tang, M.J. Mouse kidney progenitor cells accelerate renal regeneration and prolong survival after ischemic injury. *Stem Cells* **2010**, *28*, 573–584. [CrossRef]

131. Lasagni, L.; Angelotti, M.L.; Ronconi, E.; Lombardi, D.; Nardi, S.; Peired, A.; Becherucci, F.; Mazzinghi, B.; Sisti, A.; Romoli, S.; et al. Podocyte Regeneration Driven by Renal Progenitors Determines Glomerular Disease Remission and Can Be Pharmacologically Enhanced. *Stem Cell Rep.* **2015**, *5*, 248–263. [CrossRef]

132. Lasagni, L.; Ballerini, L.; Angelotti, M.L.; Parente, E.; Sagrinati, C.; Mazzinghi, B.; Peired, A.; Ronconi, E.; Becherucci, F.; Bani, D.; et al. Notch activation differentially regulates renal progenitors proliferation and differentiation toward the podocyte lineage in glomerular disorders. *Stem Cells* **2010**, *28*, 1673–1685. [CrossRef]

133. Migliorini, A.; Angelotti, M.L.; Mulay, S.R.; Kulkarni, O.O.; Demleitner, J.; Dietrich, A.; Sagrinati, C.; Ballerini, L.; Peired, A.; Shankland, S.J.; et al. The antiviral cytokines IFN-α and IFN-β modulate parietal epithelial cells and promote podocyte loss: Implications for IFN toxicity, viral glomerulonephritis, and glomerular regeneration. *Am. J. Pathol.* **2013**, *183*, 431–440. [CrossRef] [PubMed]

134. Zhang, J.; Pippin, J.W.; Krofft, R.D.; Naito, S.; Liu, Z.H.; Shankland, S.J. Podocyte repopulation by renal progenitor cells following glucocorticoids treatment in experimental FSGS. *Am. J. Physiol. Ren. Physiol.* **2013**, *304*, 1375–1389. [CrossRef] [PubMed]

135. Becherucci, F.; Mazzinghi, B.; Allinovi, M.; Angelotti, M.L.; Romagnani, P. Regenerating the kidney using human pluripotent stem cells and renal progenitors. *Expert Opin. Biol. Ther.* **2018**. [CrossRef] [PubMed]

136. Lasagni, L.; Romagnani, P. Glomerular Epithelial Stem Cells: The Good, The Bad, and The Ugly. *J. Am. Soc. Nephrol.* **2010**, *21*, 1612–1619. [CrossRef] [PubMed]

137. Gheisari, Y.; Nassiri, S.M.; Arefian, E.; Ahmadbeigi, N.; Azadmanesh, K.; Jamali, M.; Jahanzad, I.; Zeinali, S.; Vasei, M.; Soleimani, M. Severely damaged kidneys possess multipotent renoprotective stem cells. *Cytotherapy* **2010**, *12*. [CrossRef]

138. Wilson, P.C.; Humphreys, B.D. Kidney and organoid single-cell transcriptomics: the end of the beginning. *Pediatr. Nephrol.* **2019**. [CrossRef]

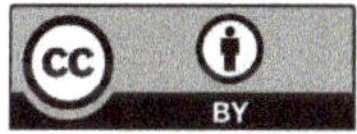

International Journal of
Molecular Sciences

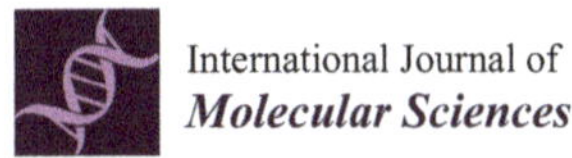
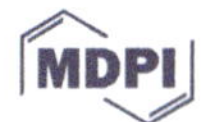

Review

Cell Death in the Kidney

Giovanna Priante *, Lisa Gianesello, Monica Ceol, Dorella Del Prete and Franca Anglani

Kidney Histomorphology and Molecular Biology Laboratory, Clinical Nephrology, Department of
Medicine - DIMED, University of Padua, via Giustiniani 2, 35128 Padova, Italy
* Correspondence: giovanna.priante@unipd.it; Tel.: +39-0498212993

Received: 31 May 2019; Accepted: 18 July 2019; Published: 23 July 2019

Abstract: Apoptotic cell death is usually a response to the cell's microenvironment. In the kidney, apoptosis contributes to parenchymal cell loss in the course of acute and chronic renal injury, but does not trigger an inflammatory response. What distinguishes necrosis from apoptosis is the rupture of the plasma membrane, so necrotic cell death is accompanied by the release of unprocessed intracellular content, including cellular organelles, which are highly immunogenic proteins. The relative contribution of apoptosis and necrosis to injury varies, depending on the severity of the insult. Regulated cell death may result from immunologically silent apoptosis or from immunogenic necrosis. Recent advances have enhanced the most revolutionary concept of regulated necrosis. Several modalities of regulated necrosis have been described, such as necroptosis, ferroptosis, pyroptosis, and mitochondrial permeability transition-dependent regulated necrosis. We review the different modalities of apoptosis, necrosis, and regulated necrosis in kidney injury, focusing particularly on evidence implicating cell death in ectopic renal calcification. We also review the evidence for the role of cell death in kidney injury, which may pave the way for new therapeutic opportunities.

Keywords: apoptosis; necrosis; regulated necrosis; kidney injury; tubular injury; glomerular injury

---

1. Introduction

While naturally occurring cell death had already been observed many years ago, it was long considered a passive phenomenon and seen as an unavoidable endpoint of biological systems. Cells can remain stationary, supporting the relationships between an organ's structure and function, or they can proliferate, sometimes becoming hypertrophic, or they can die. Regulation of the homeostatic balance between cell proliferation and cell death is important to the development and maintenance of multicellular organisms.

The historical concept of programmed cell death has been associated with apoptosis because it is considered a form of suicide, based on a genetic mechanism. Any cell death other than apoptosis has generally been called "accidental cell death" [1]. Necrosis has consequently been described as accidental cell death [2] rather than as the result of definite pathways. The classic definition of necrosis is not really appropriate, because it does not always indicate a particular form of cell death. The term is often used to refer to changes secondary to cell death by any mechanism, including apoptosis. Many insults induce apoptosis at lower doses and necrosis at higher doses. Depending on the stimulus, apoptosis and necrosis could lie on a continuum of cell death, so the two forms are not mutually exclusive, and can coexist in many pathological conditions.

Cell death by apoptosis usually occurs in response to the cell's microenvironment, and it is as fundamental to cellular and tissue physiology as cell division and differentiation. Attention to this form of cell death was prompted primarily by its crucial role in the normal embryonic development of higher vertebrates and in maintaining normal tissue homeostasis [3–6] by controlling cell numbers and eliminating nonfunctioning, damaged, or misplaced cells. As a result, and given that there are both pro- and anti-cell-death genes, the apoptotic pathway has been equated to programmed cell death (PCD). PCD is described as cell death occurring at a definite point in time during physiological development, based on an embedded genetic program that works like a clock. Because most examples of PCD happen by apoptosis, and apoptosis appears to be programmed by molecular events in the cell, the two terms are often used interchangeably. A now well-accepted concept of PCD includes clear examples that are not apoptosis, however [7–9]. Indeed, PCD can result in either a lytic or a nonlytic morphology, depending on the signaling pathway, whereas apoptosis is a nonlytic and typically immunologically silent form of cell death. Programmed lytic cell death is highly inflammatory, and necrosis is distinguished from apoptosis because of the related inflammatory response due to the rupture of the plasma membrane and release of intracellular content, including cellular organelles and highly immunogenic proteins (Figure 1).

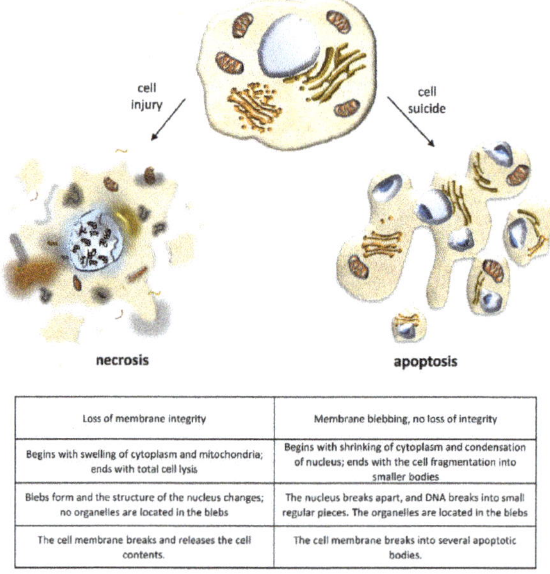

Loss of membrane integrity	Membrane blebbing, no loss of integrity
Begins with swelling of cytoplasm and mitochondria; ends with total cell lysis	Begins with shrinking of cytoplasm and condensation of nucleus; ends with the cell fragmentation into smaller bodies
Blebs form and the structure of the nucleus changes; no organelles are located in the blebs	The nucleus breaks apart, and DNA breaks into small regular pieces. The organelles are located in the blebs
The cell membrane breaks and releases the cell contents.	The cell membrane breaks into several apoptotic bodies.

Figure 1. Changes in cell morphology that distinguish apoptosis from necrosis.

It has now been established that necrosis is not an accidental, passive, unregulated form of cell death, but like apoptosis, it can be governed by a "regulated" mechanism, meaning a death with the classic morphological features of necrosis but genetically determined [5,10,11].

At a molecular level, the best-characterized pathway of regulated necrosis (RN) is necroptosis, a receptor-interacting protein kinase (RIPK)-based necrotic cell death [9,12–15]. Several other specialized forms of regulated necrosis have been described, however, such as ferroptosis [16], pyroptosis [17], parthanatos [18,19], mitochondrial permeability transition-dependent regulated necrosis (MPT-RN) [20], pyronecrosis [21,22], and NETosis, a process based on the rapid release of so-called neutrophil extracellular traps (NETs) [23]. All of these cell death pathways occur independently of an RIPK, or they can occur in the presence of RIPK inhibitors, often highlighting overlapping functions and pathways. Thus, cell death, be it by apoptosis or necrosis, is now considered to be regulated cell death (RCD) rather than a PCD. RCD implies an active participation of the cell in its own death through the activation of a genetically encoded death program, which specifies the means for starting a process that leads to the point of no return. Autophagy is a newly described, highly regulated cell death typified by the markers of a specific pathway [24], and it is as necessary as apoptosis for keeping the kidney healthy.

It is very important to be aware that every cell is "programmed" to die in response to an appropriate stimulus. Disruption of the signaling pathways or aberrant triggering of the processes that regulate physiological cell death due to extracellular causes, infections, toxins and toxicants, gene mutations, etc., may lead to abnormal cell functioning, which can become manifest in a wide array of human diseases. Gaining further insight into cell death mechanisms and a better understanding of the molecular processes involved will lead to a better characterization of a disease's etiology and pathogenesis. Cell death pathways can also be manipulated, targeting their clinical management as a way to develop new treatment approaches.

2. Kidney Injury and Cell Death

Although the term apoptosis was first introduced in the early 1970s by Kerr et al. [25], Glucksmann et al. had already described the morphological alterations associated with the process in kidney cells in the early 1950s [26].

It is now well accepted that apoptosis is an integral part of normal kidney functioning. As in other tissues, there is no inflammatory response in apoptotic cells, and their smaller fragments (apoptotic bodies) in the kidney providing these bodies are promptly ingested by neighboring cells and are degraded in lysosomes or eliminated via the tubular lumen. In fact, various types of cells may be involved in this tissue maintenance process, including epithelial cells. Phagocytes recognize and engulf apoptotic cells before their membrane is damaged, protecting surrounding tissues and cells from the damaging effects of the release of intracellular contents. If apoptotic cells are not ingested by phagocytes or epithelia, however, the cells proceed to a necrotic phase (called secondary necrosis), and their contents can spill into the extracellular space, causing inflammation and leading to inflammation-mediated kidney injury. Attempts to interfere with apoptosis (by certain caspase inhibitors, for instance) may trigger necrosis and consequent inflammation-mediated kidney injury [27].

The rate of apoptosis in the kidney is particularly intense in the developmental age [28–31]. Given the complexity of the renal microenvironment, cell death in the kidney is decoded in terms of the organ as a whole, not separately by its tubular, glomerular, interstitial, or endothelial compartments. Like all complex organisms, moreover, the kidney needs a physiological cell death modality: cell proliferation and cell death are strictly linked to keep the overall number of cells constant, eliminating cells that are damaged or no longer necessary at each stage of development, based on endogenous or exogenous factors. Developing kidneys are known not only to contain apoptotic cells [28,32], but also to express high levels of several apoptosis-related genes [33–39].

The mature mammalian kidney is a quiescent organ with little or no mitotic activity, and little or no apoptosis has been found in adult human kidneys. Thus, the nephrogenesis process (the formation of new nephrons) is limited to the period of embryonic development in humans. However, the mature kidney is capable of cellular proliferation, and in certain circumstances renal cells (like differentiated neurons) can divide. Several observations now point to the existence of adult kidney stem cells being implicated in both homeostatic tissue maintenance and functional recovery after injury [40–48].

In the case of injury in the adult kidney, cell death may occur in different compartments (the tubular and glomerular) and different types of cells, including the proximal and distal tubular cells and endothelial and glomerular cells [27]. Renal cell death is central to the pathophysiology of renal diseases. Renal cell loss is rarely a consequence of apoptosis, but rather of regulated necrosis, or simply the flushing of detached living cells.

Several common renal insults have been shown to disrupt kidney autophagy, including ischemia, toxic injury, and inflammation. Dysregulated, excessive, or defective autophagy is implicated in numerous disease states. Dysregulated autophagy leads to chronic inflammation and autoimmune diseases. Excessive autophagy can contribute to the expansion of malignant cells in renal cell cancer. Insufficient autophagy is a result of renal ischemia and facilitates cell death [49]. The death rate of renal cells might be abnormally high in nephropathies, promoting cell loss, as in acute tubular necrosis (ATN), acute rejection, necrotizing glomerulonephritis, or renal atrophy. Conversely, the cell death rate may drop (with an abnormal accumulation of cells) in cases of proliferative glomerulonephritis, polycystic renal disease, and neoplasia, for instance [50–53].

2.1. Tubular Cell Injury

Cell death in renal disease has been investigated primarily through the mechanism of tubular damages. In acute renal failure, cell death may be a direct consequence of exposure to harmful stimuli. Many renal insults, such as toxic injury or ischemia, mainly affect tubular epithelial cells and the metabolically very active proximal tubular segment in particular. Tubules are responsible for the reabsorption and secretion of several solutes, and injury to this nephron segment is the main mediator of acute kidney injury (AKI), which determines a rapid decline in renal function.

Apoptosis increases in the event of an acute unilateral ureteral obstruction (UUO) due to a physical obstruction or congenital anomalies. This causes renal growth impairment and tubular atrophy, primarily in the distal tubular epithelium, but also in the proximal renal tubules, resulting in hydronephrosis and renal failure [54–59]. Stretching, ischemia, and oxidative stress following ureteral obstruction are primary causes of tubular cell apoptosis. Increased apoptosis also activates cell infiltration, interstitial cell proliferation, and interstitial fibrosis [59–61]. Intriguingly, mild injury triggers apoptosis, and tubulointerstitial atrophy after UUO results from cell deletion by apoptosis. This leads to phagocytosis of the apoptotic bodies by neighboring tubular cells and direct apoptotic cell shedding into the tubular lumen, reestablishing homeostasis. When injury is severe, however, necrosis is more likely to be the dominant model of cell loss [61–64].

Renal ischemia followed by reperfusion (I/R) initiates apoptosis in the proximal tubular cells [27, 65–67]. I/R injury is known to be caused by ischemia, and then recovery of the blood flow unexpectedly worsens the damage. Renal tubular epithelial cell apoptosis is the key pathophysiological alteration occurring in I/R, and it defines the extent of the damage to kidney function. I/R injury is related to several inflammatory reactions, among which endothelial cell activation, the expression of adhesion molecules, the adhesion, aggregation and activation of leukocytes and platelets, the production of oxygen free radicals, and cellular calcium increase, as well as with the apoptosis mediated by these processes. AKI caused by I/R is a clinical syndrome that prompts kidney dysfunction and leads to a high mortality rate [68,69].

The consecutively hypoxic and oxidative stress evoked by renal I/R has been shown to enhance autophagy in several rodent models. The role of autophagy after renal I/R injury is still debated, however, and both protective and detrimental properties have been proposed [70].

Apoptosis seems to be common in post-transplant acute and chronic renal failure due to I/R injury [71–77]. In acute rejection, apoptosis occurs in the renal tubular epithelium, leading to tubular atrophy [78]. Chronic renal allograft rejection develops gradually, suggesting persistent low-grade injury, with a sustained and irreversible loss of renal function accompanied by clinical signs of proteinuria and hypertension [79,80].

During chronic kidney disease (CKD), the depletion of tubular cells by apoptosis gradually increases, contributing to the tubular atrophy and renal fibrosis associated with the progression of CKD [56,81–85]. Necrosis occurs in CKD as well, and the relative involvement of the two death mechanisms in cell loss depends on the balance of regulatory events. The dynamics of cell death during the early and intermediate stages of CKD have remained unclear, however. In an animal model that mimicked the progression of CKD in humans (rats undergoing subtotal nephrectomy), the authors demonstrated that both necrosis and apoptosis caused tubular injury. Since the RIPK3-regulated pathway was predominant with respect to the caspase-3 regulated pathway, the authors concluded that necrosis was the primary mechanism mediating renal tubular epithelial cell loss in the early and intermediate stages of chronic renal damage [86].

Tubular atrophy and tubular epithelial cell apoptosis have a role in diabetic kidney disease, although vascular and glomerular injuries are considered the main features of this condition [87–89]. Hyperglycemia triggers the generation of free radicals and oxidative stress in the tubular cells, and reactive oxygen species (ROS) are well-known important mediators of several biological responses, including proliferation, extracellular matrix deposition, and apoptosis [90].

Evidence of apoptosis has also been found in toxic renal exposure. The large luminal membrane surface area of proximal tubular cells makes them particularly susceptible to toxicants. Both toxicants and natural toxins are associated with altered renal apoptosis and affect several cellular factors. Studies with arsenic trioxide showed that low quantities of this agent prompted Bax/Bak-dependent apoptosis, while higher doses triggered MPT and apoptotic/necrotic cell death [91]. Thes studies showed that different cell death modalities may coexist within the same injury and that interference with specific signaling pathways or critical cell functions might result in cell killing by a distinct process. Various heavy metals induce apoptosis in renal cells via diverse mechanisms and molecular pathways [92–98]. For example, free cadmium accumulates in mitochondria, blocking the respiratory chain and culminating in mitochondrial dysfunction and the release of free radicals, which triggers caspase cascade and apoptosis. Antineoplastic agents are among the drugs that can trigger renal epithelial cell apoptosis. Cisplatin induces apoptosis in already low concentrations, resulting in cell loss, and this effect appears to be mediated by the generation of ROS. Oxidative damage to mitochondrial lipids and proteins increases with caspase-3 activity [27,99–101]. Moreover, the disruption of intracellular Ca^{2+} homeostasis or the induction of mild oxidative stress might mediate the apoptosis-inducing effects of these chemicals. In rat renal proximal tubules, cytochalasin D and dithiothreitol also caused apoptosis with associated cytoskeletal disorganization [102,103]. Antibiotics may have the potential to induce apoptosis, too. Gentamicin was found to induce apoptosis in renal distal tubules in the acute phase of injury and in the proximal tubules during the recovery phase [104,105]. Natural toxins from contaminated food and water supplies also pose a potential risk of renal apoptosis [106].

2.2. Glomerular Cell Injury

Cell death has also been documented in the diseased glomerulus [107–111]. Harrison et al. [107] were the first to report finding apoptotic bodies in human glomerulonephritis based on light and electron microscopy of kidney biopsies.

Apoptosis in glomerulonephritis appears to reduce hypercellularity during the repair process, controlling the size of the glomerular population and clearing excess cells. Apoptosis is required for the recovery of normal glomerular function [109,110,112,113]. In an experimental model of glomerulonephritis, however, the number of apoptotic glomerular cells was found to increase with the progression of glomerulosclerosis [114]. Apoptotic cell accumulation in the glomeruli has also been found to correlate with the glomerular sclerosis index and apoptotic index (the number of apoptotic cells divided by the number of normal cells) and with a decline in kidney function [114,115]. These results suggest that apoptosis is one of the mechanisms of glomerular cell depletion during progressive glomerulosclerosis.

In proliferative glomerulonephritis, on the other hand, the lack of a compensatory increase in cell death gives rise to an accumulation of cells, with glomerular hypercellularity due to mesangial and endocapillary cell proliferation [108,116–119]. During the chronic proliferative stage of systemic lupus erythematosus (SLE), apoptotic cells' number declines, while the number of proliferating cells increases, resulting in an imbalance in tissue homeostasis. An impaired removal of apoptotic bodies also indirectly contributes to the pathogenesis of SLE. Histone-bound DNA complexes, which have high affinity for the glomerular basement membrane, are carried out from apoptotic cells and accumulated in the glomerulus, triggering an immune response and causing glomerular damage [120–129].

In crescentic glomerulonephritis (CGN), disease progression is related to fibrosis of the glomerular crescents and renal interstitium. A number of different cell types, such as epithelial cells, fibroblasts, monocytes and macrophages, have been involved in the development of glomerular crescents and their progression to fibrosis. Proliferating macrophages as well as proliferating parietal epithelial cells seem to be the master contributors to this type of lesion [130–132], however, indicating that the glomerular proliferative index is more important than apoptosis alone in CGN.

Idiopathic nephrotic syndrome is the result of podocyte impairment. Basement membrane denuding and podocyte detachment and loss have been implicated in several human nephrotic syndromes, including focal and segmental glomerulosclerosis, minimal change disease, glomerulonephritis, and diabetic nephropathy [133–136]. Remarkably, not only resident glomerular cells but also infiltrating leukocytes might be eliminated by apoptosis in the glomeruli. Indeed, apoptotic bodies have been found to be particularly prominent in glomeruli containing numerous neutrophils, proving that apoptosis is a homeostatic mechanism that enables hypercellular glomeruli to return to normal [108–110,137,138].

2.3. Necrosis/Regulated Necrosis and the Kidney

Renal cortical necrosis is the death of tissue in the outer portion of the kidney (cortex) resulting from the blockage of the small arteries supplying blood to the cortex, and it causes AKI. The cause is usually a significantly diminished renal arterial perfusion secondary to vascular spasm, microvascular injury, or intravascular coagulation. Renal cortical necrosis is generally extensive, though focal and localized forms do occur. In most cases, the medulla, the juxtamedullary cortex, and a thin rim of subcapsular cortex are spared [139].

Renal papillary necrosis is a disorder in which all or part of the renal papillae die. It is characterized by coagulative necrosis of the renal medullary pyramids and papillae brought on by several associated conditions and toxins synergistically promoting the onset of ischemia. Renal papillary necrosis can lead to secondary infection of desquamated necrotic foci, stone formation, and/or the separation and eventual sloughing of papillae, resulting in acute urinary tract obstruction. The clinical course of renal papillary necrosis depends on the degree of vascular impairment, the presence of associated causal factors, the patient's general health, any bilateral involvement, and specifically, the number of papillae affected [140].

The biochemical signaling pathways that trigger necrosis have been investigated in detail in recent years. It is now clear that RN is a genetically driven process that strongly contributes to the pathophysiology of kidney injury.

Cell death by RN involves RIPK pathway-mediated rupture of the plasma membrane caused by a complement-related membrane attack complex, exotoxins, or cytotoxic T cells. Necrotic cell death is thus accompanied by the release of immunogenic cellular components collectively known as damage-associated molecular patterns (DAMPs) [141,142], which cause severe tissue damage, leading to systemic inflammation and organ injury or failure. Immune cell necrosis (i.e., NETosis or pyroptosis) is another component of necrotic renal lesions. This means that any causal factors triggering the RN signal pathways and the release of inflammatory mediators could be mutually enhancing and self-amplifying, leading to further renal cell loss, kidney atrophy, and scarring. The extremely proinflammatory effect of necrosis is very important in the kidney transplantation setting and in AKI, when inflammation occurs mostly together with renal cell necrosis (necroinflammation), as in necrotizing glomerulonephritis, thrombotic microangiopathy, and ATN [143,144]. RN modalities such as necroptosis, ferroptosis, parthanatos, and MPT-RN may be mechanistically distinct, but their damage to tubular segments and multicellular functional units may be synchronized, because otherwise they would only kill single cells in the tubular compartment [67,145–148]. Interestingly, the localization of tubular injury may differ in the several forms of renal damage. For example, tubular injury is variable in ischemic lesions, acting on short pieces of the proximal straight tubule and focal areas of the ascending limb of Henle's loop. In toxic forms, tubular damage is more continuous along all segments of the proximal tubule.

In the early phases of I/R injury, reduced oxygen supply to metabolically active tubular epithelial cells lowers oxidative metabolism and depletes cell supplies of high-energy phosphate compounds. Reperfusion restores the oxygen supply and improves oxygen radical formation, resulting in mitochondrial impairment. Neutrophil infiltration participates in this process via NET formation and further histone release into the extracellular space due to tubular cell necrosis [143,149]. The innate immune response arises soon after I/R injury and involves neutrophils, natural killer cells, and macrophages. Together with the tubular epithelial cells, macrophages produce proinflammatory cytokines, thus contributing to injury. The histones released kill more tubular cells through direct cytotoxic effects, possibly interfering with normal mitochondrial function or altering lysosome function, thus resulting in cell membrane alteration and disorganized protein synthesis. The mechanism of histone cytotoxicity is probably due to the polycationic nature of histones and their capacity to bind to the anionic moiety cell walls [149]. Moreover, histones that are immunologically inert when they are within the nucleus exert DAMP effects once released into the extracellular space [143]. Concomitant with the injury, there is shedding of viable and necrotic cells into the tubular lumen, and as the lesion progresses, cell proliferation could also intensify in an effort to replace neighboring cells and repair tubular cell injury [150].

In immune complex diseases such as crescent glomerulonephritis, renal vasculitis, or antiglomerular basement membrane disease, cell necrosis triggers massive glomerular inflammation with cytokine and chemokine expression, together with the release of dangerous intracellular molecules. The influx of neutrophils accelerates this process, with a subsequent inflammatory response (NETosis) in the capillaries of the glomerular tuft. This loop triggers a massive parietal epithelial cell hyperplasia, followed by basement membrane rupture and plasma leakage from disrupted glomerular capillaries and then crescent formation [151–154].

In either tubular or glomerular injury, a mild form of the same insult can lead to apoptosis, while a severe form can lead to necrosis. The pathway followed by the cell therefore depends on both the nature and the severity of the insult, sometimes evolving from an apoptotic to a necrotic form of cell death.

2.4. Cell Death and Crystal Nephropathies

The kidney is susceptible to crystal formation, as mineral secretion and urine concentration favor supersaturation, which can give rise to several acute and chronic kidney disorders related to crystal deposition or formation inside the kidney, referred to as crystal or crystalline nephropathies and renal stone disease [155–160].

Tubular crystallopathies result from precipitates inside the tubular lumen. The dynamics of crystal deposition determine the outcomes of kidney injury, i.e., AKI or CKD. A sudden onset of crystal formation causes cell necrosis and inflammation leading to AKI, whereas a chronic dynamic of crystal formation causes plugs in distal tubules or collecting ducts, leading to persistent tubule obstruction and hence CKD.

Apart from the urine concentration of both minerals and regulators of crystallization, the different types of crystal-induced renal disease are determined not only by the physicochemical properties of the crystals but also by the type of signaling pathway triggered by the crystals. Once crystals have formed in the tubular lumen, they contribute to kidney injury mainly through a direct or indirect cytotoxic effect, the underlying molecular mechanisms of which are largely unknown. Furthermore, crystals elicit inflammation and inflammation-driven cell necrosis in an auto-amplifying loop that is referred to as necroinflammation [143].

Calcium oxalate, calcium phosphate, and other crystals of various composition are known to be capable of inducing cell death, especially in renal proximal tubule cells [155]. Their effect might depend on their size. Nanosized crystals primarily cause apoptotic cell death, whereas micron-sized crystals cause necrotic cell death. Nanosized crystals may be internalized and transferred into lysosomes, thus causing damage that can trigger apoptosis. Alternatively, crystals can pass through pores into the nucleus, prompting DNA cleavage into regular fragments, an important characteristic of apoptotic cell death.

Micron-sized crystals on cells may cause irregular injury of the cell membrane and local strong physical stress, resulting in necrotic cell death. Released inflammatory factors by necrotic cells lead to cell membrane rupture that in turn causes an imbalance in cell osmotic pressure and consequently the sudden massive destruction of lysosomes accompanied by hydrolytic enzyme release [157].

Various crystals can also enter cells via a process of phagocytosis [159,161]. Phagosomes fuse with lysosomes in an attempt to digest the crystals. However, either amorphous calcium released by lysosomes into the cytosol or indigestible lysosome particles trigger necroptosis.

Crystals deposited in the kidneys act as intrarenal DAMPs, promoting intrarenal inflammation and contributing to further tubular injury and subsequent renal dysfunction [100,162]. These molecules can activate Toll-like receptors, which results in inflammasome activation in immune renal cells. Tubular cell necroptosis or ferroptosis due to calcium oxalate internalization can contribute to promoting inflammation [147,148]. Crystal-induced DAMPs also include histones that in large amounts are released into extracellular space by necrotic cells. Due to their strong basic charge, histones can potentially disrupt plasma membranes of neighboring intact cells, a process that increases the number of dying tubular cells and thus aggravates kidney injury [149,160].

The importance of cell death in pathological soft tissue calcification is well documented [163]. Such calcifications usually consist of calcium phosphate salts (including hydroxyapatite), but they sometimes contain calcium oxalates, too, as in calcium nephrolithiasis. In the kidney, the presence of necrotic tubular cells has been associated with renal cortical calcification, a rare condition usually due to severe cortex destruction and any condition causing acute and prolonged shock [164]. The role of cell death in the more common medullary nephrocalcinosis - microscopic renal crystal deposition in the tubular lumen (intratubular nephrocalcinosis) or interstitium (interstitial nephrocalcinosis) -, frequently associated with nephrolithiasis remains unclear. In two in vitro models of nephrocalcinosis obtained by exposing wild-type or Glial cell-derived neurotrophic factor (GDNF)-silenced human renal tubular cells to an osteogenic medium, it was recently shown that apoptosis and necroptosis respectively triggered renal cell calcification even before calcium phosphate crystal deposition [165,166] and mimicked vascular cell calcification [167–170]. The authors speculated that if cell death is an important event in the pathogenesis of renal ectopic calcification, any damage that shifts the balance between cell survival and cell death toward the latter could (in conjunction with a particular renal milieu) give rise to interstitial nephrocalcinosis and ultimately to kidney stones [171].

3. Targeting Renal Cell Death

In the undeniably complex picture of the mechanisms involved in cell death, under certain conditions, markers of apoptosis and necrosis may be found simultaneously, meaning that more than one cell death mechanism can be activated at the same time [146,172–174]. While there may be signs of different cell death pathways being involved, one pathway is usually the fastest and most effective. It is important to understand the interplay between different cell death pathways, especially with a view toward targeting these pathways for therapeutic purposes.

Elucidating the precise mechanisms behind cell death is essential to the development of new drugs. Numerous cellular factors have been proposed to regulate cell death response following a variety of induction mechanisms in numerous cell types, but the role of many of these factors depends both on the signal triggering a given cell death process and on the type of cell in which the response is induced.

Apoptosis and RN are characterized by distinct morphological, cell biological, and biochemical features. These two forms of cell death can occur at the same time in the same kidney compartment. They are not mutually exclusive and coexist in many renal pathological conditions [27,67,175]. The occurrence of either may depend on the intensity of the triggering events. For instance, renal ischemia may kill cells by either apoptosis or necrosis. The proportion of cells killed by each mechanism may also vary from one individual to another, because a part of the cell population predetermined to die by apoptosis might be rescued by interference with the genetic program, or apoptotic cells and their debris might be rapidly removed by phagocytes. Alternatively, apoptosis may cause secondary necrosis, as in prolonged kidney injury, in which case the plasma membrane of apoptotic cells may break down, thus acquiring a necrotic morphology.

Apoptosis occurs in three different phases: Initiation, effector, and final. The initiation phase is dependent upon stimuli, and two pathways can be identified, either extrinsic or intrinsic. In the extrinsic (death receptor-mediated) pathway, the ligation of death receptors determines the enrolment and activation of caspase-8. Caspase-8 further activates downstream caspases leading to apoptosis. Caspase-8 also triggers the intrinsic pathway to intensify the apoptotic cascade and inhibits necroptosis (Figure 2). In the intrinsic (mitochondrial) pathway, pro-apoptotic Bcl-2 family proteins Bax and

Bak create pores on the mitochondrial outer membrane, determining the release of apoptogenic factors, such as Cytochrome *c* (Cyt C). In the cytosol, Cyt C binds to and stimulates conformational modifications in the adaptor protein Apaf-1, thus leading to the enrolment and activation of caspase-9. Caspase-9 further activates executioner caspases to elicit apoptosis. Notably, other components of the Bcl-2 protein family, such as Bcl-xL and Bcl-2, prevents pore formation in healthy cells by binding to Bax and Bak. Initiating factors include Tumor necrosis factor (TNF) receptors and ligands, growth factors, and changes in the extracellular matrix. Oxidative stress plays an important role in renal apoptosis. Either by acting as signal transduction molecules or by directly causing cellular damage, ROS activate apoptosis at multiple steps in the cell death pathway and lead to the damage of cellular macromolecules, including DNA, proteins, and lipids [27,91] (Figure 2).

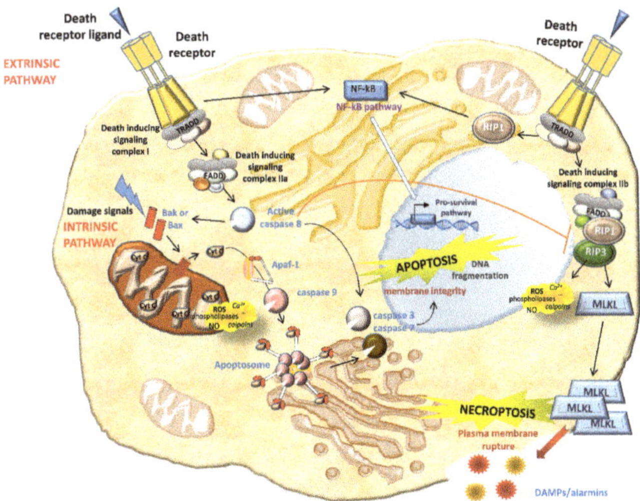

Figure 2. Overview of key molecular pathways of apoptosis and necroptosis. Apoptosis can start via intrinsic pathways (perturbation of intracellular homeostasis) or extrinsic pathways (death receptor binding). In the former case, cell stress leads directly (or via mediators, such as Bax and Bak) to mitochondrial outer membrane permeabilization, resulting in the release of apoptogenic factors, including Cytochrome *c*, which binds Apaf-1 to stimulate caspase-9 via apoptosomes. Bcl-2-related proteins induce apoptosis (e.g., Bax) or protect against it (e.g., Bcl-2). As for the extrinsic pathway, death receptor binding guides the recruitment of adapter proteins such as TRADD (TNFR-associated death domain), forming complex I. While complex I promotes cell survival via NF-κB activation, its transition to a secondary cytosolic complex, complex II, mediates cell death. Complex II is formed through the association of complex I with FADD (Fas-associated death domain). The formation of complex IIa promotes the activation of apoptosis in a caspase-8-dependent manner. Upon inhibition of caspase 8, complex IIb promotes necroptosis. Caspase-8 or caspase-9 activation subsequently triggers executioner caspases, such as caspase-3, -6, and -7. The cleavage of receptor-interacting protein kinase (RIPK) 1 and 3 by caspase-8 leads to apoptosis, whereas their phosphorylation triggers necroptosis in conditions of caspase-8 inhibition. RIPK1 and RIPK3 activation in turn causes the recruitment of the executioner mixed-lineage kinase domain-like protein (MLKL), which is phosphorylated by RIPK3 and initiates structural changes, leading to its insertion into the plasma membrane and channel formation. MLK channels increase Na⁺ influx, osmotic pressure, and membrane rupture, ending in cell death. Membrane rupture promotes the release of intracellular contents and endogenous damage-associated molecular patterns (DAMPs) and/or preformed proinflammatory molecules (alarmins). Through RIPK1 kinase activity, a wide range of necrotic mediators are activated in the execution phase of necrotic cell death, including reactive oxygen species (ROS), calcium (Ca²⁺), calpains, cathepsins, phospholipases, and ceramide.

In the final phase, which is common in extrinsic and intrinsic pathways, apoptotic cells show cytoplasmic shrinkage, chromatin condensation (pyknosis), nuclear fragmentation (karyorrhexis), and plasma membrane blebbing, culminating with the formation of apoptotic bodies. Since initiators and effectors of apoptosis are often unique to a particular cell or induction mode and take action upstream from the final common phase, cells committed to an apoptotic pathway may be rescued by specific therapeutic interventions. Several therapies targeting the apoptotic pathway have shown beneficial effects in many in vitro and in vivo models. Caspase inhibitors, such as z-VAD (z-Val-Ala-Asp fluoromethyl ketone), reduced apoptosis and improved organ function in several AKI models [176, 177]. TDZD-8 (4-benzyl-2-methyl-1,2,4-thiadiazolidine-3,5-dione), a pharmacological inhibitor of the powerful proapoptotic kinase GSK3β (glycogen synthase kinase 3 beta), reduces proximal tubular epithelial cell apoptosis and has positive influences on the kidney by inhibiting inflammation and increasing renal cell proliferation [178,179]: This makes it a rational option in human trials designed to prevent or treat AKI (Figure 3).

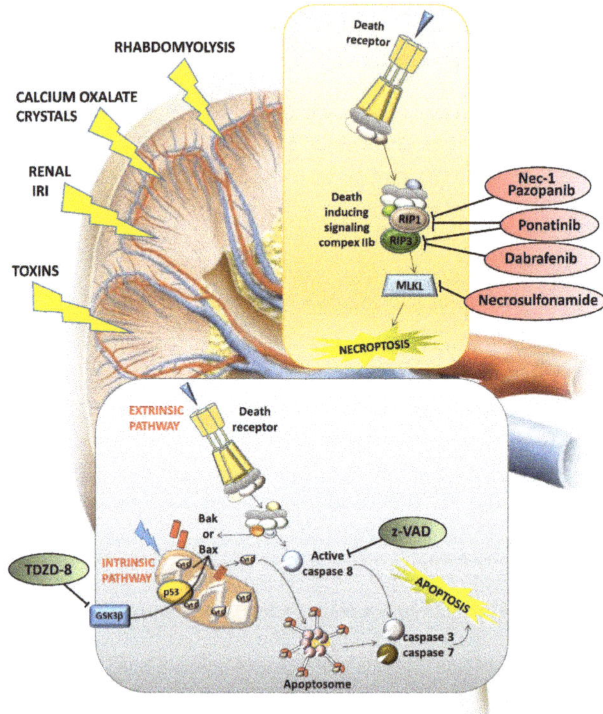

Figure 3. Targeting apoptosis and necroptosis in kidney lesions. Different kidney lesions activate different cell death modalities: z-VAD (z-Val-Ala-Asp fluoromethyl ketone) has been found to protect renal function, and the effect of the pan-caspase inhibitor z-VAD on experimental renal ischemia-reperfusion (I/R) injury was to reduce serum urea levels, thereby preventing inflammation. TDZD-8 (4-benzyl-2-methyl-1,2,4-thiadiazolidine-3,5-dione) has been found to inhibit ischemia-induced activation of GSK3β (glycogen synthase kinase 3 beta), Bax, and caspase 3, thus ameliorating tubular and epithelial cell damage and significantly protecting renal function.

RN may interact with apoptosis at various molecular and cellular levels, but both forms of cell death involve pathological changes in the mitochondria. In renal and other cells, the mitochondria are crucial sites for integrating intrinsic and extrinsic apoptotic signals. Bax, a known classic pro-apoptotic protein taking effect via mitochondrial membrane permeabilization, has been shown to regulate

MPT-RN as well, again by affecting mitochondrial dynamics [180]. It is important to bear in mind, however, that mitochondria are not involved in some RN pathways [20]. Necroptosis is generally considered a mitochondrion-independent form of RN. Very recent studies, however, have shown that in TNF-induced necroptosis, ROS induction was RIPK3-dependent and well correlated with necroptosis. Using mitochondrial respiration inhibitors and mitochondrial depletion, the authors showed that a TNF-induced increment of aerobic respiration accounted for ROS induction in necroptosis [181]. As they are the point where cell injury and death converge, the mitochondria may be promising targets for therapy.

Similarly to extrinsic apoptosis, necroptosis begins with the activation of death receptors such as Fas and TNF-α receptor 1 (Figure 2). Provided that caspase-8 (a key inhibitor of necrosis) is inactive, RIPK1 activates RIPK3, which in turn activates the mixed-lineage kinase domain-like protein (MLKL). MLKL oligomerizes and translocates to the plasma membrane, determining membrane rupture. RIPK1 is thought to be essential to necrosis induced by the Fas ligand and TNF- α. Necrostatin-1 (Nec-1) is an RIPK1 inhibitor that prevents the death of TNF-α-treated Fas-associated death domain (FADD)-deficient cells [182,183] (Figure 3). In addition to Nec-1, a number of necroptosis inhibitors have been reported [184–192], and some of them have been approved by the Food and drug administration (FDA), such as dabrafenib (a selective RIPK3 inhibitor), pazopanib (for RIPK1), and ponatinib (for both RIPK1 and RIPK3) [189,190] (Figure 3). In light of the multiple initiating pathways upstream, manipulating downstream necroptosis mediators such as MLKL may be more effective [182] (Figure 3). Although necroptosis inhibitors have been used in clinical trials, there are several issues to consider. These drugs may be useful, given their current clinical use as anticancer agents, but whether their toxicity-related side effects are admissible for patients with necroptosis-associated renal diseases remains to be seen. Many necroptosis inhibitors have yet to be extensively explored, so the efficacy and safety of these potential drugs should be further validated. Necroptosis also prompts the release of unprocessed intracellular contents, such as DAMPs or various preformed proinflammatory molecules (alarmins) stored inside the cell [142,193–195]. These proinflammatory molecules activate innate immunity, prompting the production of more proinflammatory cytokines and consequently more necrosis in renal tissue. If not opposed at an early stage, this self-amplifying process can lead to systemic inflammation and remote organ injury or even organ failure. In theory, the RN pathways can therefore be targeted therapeutically to block these inflammatory agents, and this should suffice to slow and even cancel RN [16,182,196–198]. It is essential to consider a combination of therapies capable of blocking multiple regulated cell death pathways, either simultaneously or at different time points, to ensure cell survival and renal function.

Necroptosis and apoptosis undoubtedly coexist in the pathophysiological process of AKI. Despite the limitations of separating the two cell death pathways, therapeutic interventions that primarily inhibit apoptosis have the potential to minimize renal dysfunction and accelerate recovery after AKI. The effectiveness of anti-apoptosis therapies has confirmed the contribution of apoptosis to AKI, which should not be neglected. Preclinical studies have identified several pathways resulting in RN that could be modulated successfully in AKI in vivo by drugs or interventions targeting the molecular pathways. In practice, specific therapies need to intercept events occurring upstream from cell death, so early intervention is essential. Unfortunately, this strategy might not be feasible in a large proportion of cases, because AKI is usually asymptomatic in the early stage.

4. Conclusions

Despite the difficulties of classifying cell death modalities in categorized patterns, great efforts have been made in recent years to do so in kidney injury. The description of new regulated cell death modalities, the realization that they may coexist in the same organ, and the discovery of inhibitors of the various types of cell death have raised hopes for therapeutic interventions in diseases characterized by massive cell death, such as AKI. Unfortunately, there have been no changes in clinical practice to date because it is difficult to translate these results into clinical trials in the absence of convincing preclinical evidence.

Author Contributions: G.P., L.G., M.C., D.D.P., and F.A. contributed to the literature review and critically reviewed manuscript drafting, each author in his/her specific field of expertise. G.P. conceived of the manuscript structure, wrote the manuscript, and prepared the table and figures. F.A. conceived of the manuscript structure, supervised its writing, and thoroughly reviewed all content.

Conflicts of Interest: The authors have no conflicts of interest to disclose.

References

1. Bessis, M. Studies on cell agony and death: An attempt at classification. In *Ciba Foundation Symposium - Cellular Injury*; de Reuck, A.V.S., Knight, J., Eds.; J&A Churchill: London, UK, 1964; ISBN 978-04-7072-277-0.

2. Green, D.R. *Means to an End: Apoptosis and Other Cell Death Mechanisms*, 1st ed.; Cold Spring Harbor Laboratory Press: Cold Spring Harbor, NY, USA, 2010; ISBN 978-08-7969-888-1.

3. Lynch, M.P.; Nawaz, S.; Gerschenson, L.E. Evidence for soluble factors regulating cell death and cell proliferation in primary cultures of rabbit endometrial cells grown on collagen. *Proc. Natl. Acad. Sci. USA* **1986**, *83*, 4784–4788. [CrossRef] [PubMed]

4. Fuchs, Y.; Steller, H. Programmed cell death in animal development and disease. *Cell* **2011**, *147*, 742–758. [CrossRef] [PubMed]

5. Galluzzi, L.; Bravo-San Pedro, J.M.; Vitale, I.; Aaronson, S.A.; Abrams, J.M.; Adam, D.; Alnemri, E.S.; Altucci, L.; Andrews, D.; Annicchiarico-Petruzzelli, M.; et al. Essential versus accessory aspects of cell death: Recommendations of the NCCD 2015. *Cell Death Differ.* **2015**, *22*, 58–73. [CrossRef] [PubMed]

6. Green, D.R. *Cell Death: Apoptosis and Other Means to an End*, 2nd ed.; Cold Spring Harbor Laboratory Press: Cold Spring Harbor, NY, USA, 2018; ISBN 978-16-2182-214-1.

7. Schwartz, L.M.; Smith, S.W.; Jones, M.E.; Osborne, B.A. Do all programmed cell deaths occur via apoptosis? *Proc. Natl Acad. Sci. USA* **1993**, *90*, 980–984. [CrossRef] [PubMed]

8. Taylor, R.C.; Cullen, S.P.; Martin, S.J. Apoptosis: Controlled demolition at the cellular level. *Nat. Rev. Mol. Cell Biol.* **2008**, *9*, 231–241. [CrossRef] [PubMed]

9. Jorgensen, I.; Rayamajhi, M.; Miao, E.A. Programmed cell death as a defence against infection. *Nat. Rev. Immunol.* **2017**, *17*, 151–164. [CrossRef] [PubMed]

10. Vanden Berghe, T.; Linkermann, A.; Jouan-Lanhouet, S.; Walczak, H.; Vandenabeele, P. Regulated necrosis: The expanding network of non-apoptotic cell death pathways. *Nat. Rev. Mol. Cell Biol* **2014**, *15*, 135–147. [CrossRef]

11. Galluzzi, L.; Kepp, O.; Krautwald, S.; Kroemer, G.; Linkermann, A. Molecular mechanisms of regulated necrosis. *Semin Cell Dev. Biol.* **2014**, *35*, 24–32. [CrossRef]

12. Tait, S.W.; Oberst, A.; Quarato, G.; Milasta, S.; Haller, M.; Wang, R.; Karvela, M.; Ichim, G.; Yatim, N.; Albert, M.L.; et al. Widespread mitochondrial depletion via mitophagy does not compromise necroptosis. *Cell Reports* **2013**, *5*, 878–885. [CrossRef]

13. Vanden Berghe, T.; Hassannia, B.; Vandenabeele, P. An outline of necrosome triggers. *Cell Mol. Life Sci.* **2016**, *73*, 2137–2152. [CrossRef]

14. Dillon, C.P.; Tummers, B.; Baran, K.; Green, D.R. Developmental checkpoints guarded by regulated necrosis. *Cell Mol. Life Sci.* **2016**, *73*, 2125–2136. [CrossRef] [PubMed]

15. Dondelinger, Y.; Darding, M.; Bertrand, M.J.M.; Walczak, H. Poly-ubiquitination in TNFR1-mediated necroptosis. *Cell Mol. Life Sci.* **2016**, *73*, 2165–2176. [CrossRef] [PubMed]

16. Dixon, S.J.; Lemberg, K.M.; Lamprecht, M.R.; Skouta, R.; Zaitsev, E.M.; Gleason, C.E.; Patel, D.N.; Bauer, A.J.; Cantley, A.M.; Yang, W.S.; et al. Ferroptosis: An iron-dependent form of nonapoptotic cell death. *Cell* **2012**, *149*, 1060–1072. [CrossRef] [PubMed]

17. Jorgensen, I.; Miao, E.A. Pyroptotic cell death defends against intracellular pathogens. *Immunol. Rev.* **2015**, *265*, 130–142. [CrossRef] [PubMed]

18. Andrabi, S.A.; Dawson, T.L.; Dawson, V.L. Mitochondrial and nuclear cross talk in cell death: Parthanatos. *Ann. NY Acad. Sci.* **2008**, *1147*, 233–241. [CrossRef] [PubMed]

19. Gibson, B.; Kraus, W. New insights into the molecular and cellular functions of poly(ADP-ribose) and PARPs. *Nature Rev. Mol. Cell Biol.* **2012**, *13*, 411–424. [CrossRef]

20. Galluzzi, L.; Kepp, O.; Kroemer, G. Mitochondrial regulation of cell death: A phylogenetically conserved control. *Microb. Cell* **2016**, *3*, 101–108. [CrossRef]

21. Cookson, B.T.; Brennan, M.A. Pro-inflammatory programmed cell death. *Trends Microbiol* **2001**, *9*, 113–114. [CrossRef]

22. Fink, S.L.; Cookson, B.T. Caspase-1-dependent pore formation during pyroptosis leads to osmotic lysis of infected host macrophages. *Cell Microbiol.* **2006**, *8*, 1812–1825. [CrossRef]

23. Remijsen, Q.; Kuijpers, T.W.; Wirawan, E.; Lippens, S.; Vandenabeele, P.; Vanden Berghe, T. Dying for a cause: NETosis, mechanisms behind an antimicrobial cell death modality. *Cell Death Differ.* **2011**, *18*, 581–588. [CrossRef]

24. Galluzzi, L.; Maiuri, M.C.; Vitale, I.; Zischka, H.; Castedo, M.; Zitvogel, L.; Kroemer, G. Cell death modalities: Classification and pathophysiological implications. *Cell Death Differ.* **2007**, *147*, 1237–1243. [CrossRef] [PubMed]

25. Kerr, J.F.; Wyllie, A.H.; Currie, A.R. Apoptosis: A basic biological phenomenon with wide-ranging implications in tissue kinetics. *Br. J. Cancer* **1972**, *26*, 239–257. [CrossRef] [PubMed]

26. Glucksmann, A. Cell deaths in normal verebrate ontogeny. *Biol. Rev.* **1951**, *26*, 59–86. [CrossRef] [PubMed]

27. Havasi, A.; Borkan, S.C. Apoptosis and acute kidney injury. *Kidney Int.* **2011**, *80*, 29–40. [CrossRef]

28. Koseki, C.; Herzlinger, D.; al-Awqati, Q. Apoptosis in metanephric development. *J. Cell Biol.* **1992**, *119*, 1327–1333. [CrossRef]

29. Meier, P.; Finch, A.; Evan, G. Apoptosis in development. *Nature* **2000**, *407*, 796–801. [CrossRef]

30. Bard, J.B. Growth and death in the developing mammalian kidney: Signals, receptors and conversations. *Bioessays* **2002**, *24*, 72–82. [CrossRef]

31. Bouchard, M. Transcriptional control of kidney development. *Differentiation* **2004**, *72*, 295–306. [CrossRef]

32. Coles, H.S.R.; Burne, J.F.; Raff, M.C. Large scale normal cell death in the developing rat kidney and its reduction by epidermal growth factor. *Development* **1993**, *118*, 777–784.

33. Lebrun, D.P.; Warncke, R.A.; Cleary, M.L. Expression of bcl-2 in fetal tissues suggests a role in morphogenesis. *Am. J. Pathol.* **1993**, *142*, 743–753.

34. Lu, Q.L.; Poulsom, R.; Wong, L.; Hanby, A.M. Bcl-2 expression in adult and embryonic non hematopietic tissues. *J. Pathol.* **1993**, *169*, 431–437. [CrossRef] [PubMed]

35. Saifudeen, Z.; Dipp, S.; El-Dahr, S.S. A role for p53 in terminal epithelial cell differentiation. *J. Clin. Invest.* **2002**, *109*, 1021–1030. [CrossRef] [PubMed]

36. Ewings, K.E.; Wiggins, C.M.; Cook, S.J. Bim and the pro-survival Bcl-2 proteins: Opposites attract, ERK repels. *Cell Cycle* **2007**, *6*, 2236–2240. [CrossRef] [PubMed]

37. Saifudeen, Z.; Dipp, S.; Stefkova, J.; Yao, X.; Lookabaugh, S.; El-Dahr, S.S. p53 regulates metanephric development. *J. Am. Soc. Nephrol.* **2009**, *20*, 2328–2337. [CrossRef] [PubMed]

38. El-Dahr, S.; Hilliard, S.; Aboudehen, K.; Saifudeen, Z. The MDM2-p53 pathway: Multiple roles in kidney evelopment. *Pediatr. Nephrol.* **2014**, *29*, 621–627. [CrossRef] [PubMed]

39. Ho, J. The regulation of apoptosis in kidney development: Implications for nephron number and pattern? *Front. Pediatr.* **2014**, *2*, 128. [CrossRef] [PubMed]

40. Bussolati, B.; Bruno, S.; Grange, C.; Buttiglieri, S.; Deregibus, M.C.; Cantino, D.; Camussi, G. Isolation of renal progenitor cells from adult human kidney. *Am. J. Pathol.* **2005**, *166*, 545–555. [CrossRef]

41. Kitamura, S.; Yamasaki, Y.; Kinomura, M.; Sugaya, T.; Sugiyama, H.; Maeshima, Y.; Makino, H. Establishment and characterization of renal progenitor like cells from S3 segment of nephron in rat adult kidney. *FASEB J.* **2005**, *19*, 1789–1797. [CrossRef]

42. Dekel, B.; Zangi, L.; Shezen, E.; Reich-Zeliger, S.; Eventov-Friedman, S.; Katchman, H.; Jacob-Hirsch, J.; Amariglio, N.; Rechavi, G.; Margalit, R.; et al. Isolation and characterization of non tubular sca-1+lin_multipotent stem/progenitor cells from adult mouse kidney. *J. Am. Soc. Nephrol.* **2006**, *17*, 3300–3314. [CrossRef]

43. Gupta, S.; Verfaillie, C.; Chmielewski, D.; Kren, S.; Eidman, K.; Connaire, J.; Heremans, Y.; Lund, T.; Blackstad, M.; Jiang, Y.; et al. Isolation and characterization of kidney-derived stem cells. *J. Am. Soc. Nephrol.* **2006**, *17*, 3028–3040. [CrossRef]

44. Maeshima, A.; Sakurai, H.; Nigam, S.K. Adult kidney tubular cell population showing phenotypic plasticity, tubulogenic capacity, and integration capability into developing kidney. *J. Am. Soc. Nephrol.* **2006**, *17*, 188–198. [CrossRef] [PubMed]

45. Humphreys, B.D.; Bonventre, J.V. Mesenchymal Stem Cells in Acute Kidney Injury. *Annu Rev. Med.* **2008**, *59*, 311–325. [CrossRef] [PubMed]

46. Chou, Y.H.; Pan, S.Y.; Yang, C.H.; Lin, S.L. Stem cells and kidney regeneration. *J. Formos Med. Assoc.* **2014**, *113*, 201–209. [CrossRef] [PubMed]

47. Lam, A.Q.; Bonventre, J.V. Regenerating the nephron with human pluripotent stem cells. *Curr Opin Organ. Transplant.* **2015**, *20*, 187–192. [CrossRef] [PubMed]

48. Thomasova, D.; Anders, H.J. Cell cycle control in the kidney. *Nephrol Dial. Transplant.* **2015**, *30*, 1622–1630. [CrossRef] [PubMed]

49. Havasi, A.; Dong, Z. Autophagy and Tubular Cell Death in the Kidney. *Semin. Nephrol.* **2016**, *36*, 174–188. [CrossRef]

50. Gobe, G.C.; Axeisen, R.A. Genesís of renal tubular atrophy in experimental hydronephrosis in the rat. *Lab. Invest.* **1987**, *56*, 273–281.

51. Gobe, G.C.; Axelson, R.A.; Searle, J.W. Cellular events in experimental unilateral ischemic renal atrophy and in regeneration after contralateral nephrectomy. *Lab. Invest.* **1990**, *63*, 770–779.

52. Todd, D.; Yang, G.; Brown, R.W.; Cao, J.; D'Agati, V.; Thompson, T.S.; Truong, L.D. Apoptosis in renal cell carcinoma: Detection by in situ end-labeling of fragmented DNA and correlation with other prognostic factors. *Hum. Pathol.* **1996**, *27*, 1012–1017. [CrossRef]

53. Tannapfel, A.; Hahn, H.A.; Katalinic, A.; Fietkau, R.J.; Kuhn, R.; Wittekind, C.W. Incidence of apoptosis, cell proliferation and p53 expression in renal cell carcinomas. *Anticancer Res.* **1997**, *17*, 1155–1162.

54. Kennedy, W.A., II; Stenberg, A.; Lackgren, G.; Hensle, T.W.; Sawczuk, I.S. Renal tubular apoptosis after partial ureteral obstruction. *J. Urol.* **1994**, *152*, 658–664. [CrossRef]

55. Truong, L.D.; Petrusevska, G.; Yang, G.; Gurpinar, T.; Shappell, S.; Lechago, J.; Rouse, D.; Suki, W.N. Cell apoptosis and proliferation in experimental chronic obstructive uropathy. *Kidney Int.* **1996**, *50*, 200–207. [CrossRef] [PubMed]

56. Kennedy, W.A., 2nd; Buttyan, R.; Garcia-Montes, E.; D'Agati, V.; Olsson, C.A.; Sawczuk, I.S. Epidermal growth factor suppresses renal tubular apoptosis following ureteral obstruction. *Urology* **1997**, *49*, 973–980. [CrossRef]

57. Klahr, S.; Morrissey, J. Obstructive nephropathy and renal fibrosis. *Am. J. Physiol. Renal Physiol.* **2002**, *283*, F861–F875. [CrossRef] [PubMed]

58. Jang, H.S.; Padanilam, B.J. Simultaneous deletion of Bax and Bak is required to prevent apoptosis and interstitial fibrosis in obstructive nephropathy. *Am. J. Physiol Renal Physiol.* **2015**, *309*, F540–F550. [CrossRef] [PubMed]

59. Nilsson, L.; Madsen, K.; Krag, S.; Frokiaer, J.; Jensen, B.L.; Norregaard, R. Disruption of cyclooxygenase type 2 exacerbates apoptosis and renal damage during obstructive nephropathy. *Am. J. Physiol. Renal Physiol.* **2015**, *309*, F1035–F1048. [CrossRef]

60. Docherty, N.G.; O'Sullivan, O.E.; Healy, D.A.; Fitzpatrick, J.M.; Watson, R.W. Evidence that inhibition of tubular cell apoptosis protects against renal damage and development of fibrosis following ureteric obstruction. *Am. J. Physiol. Renal Physiol. 2006* **2006**, *290*, F4–F13. [CrossRef]

61. Mei, W.; Peng, Z.; Lu, M.; Liu, C.; Deng, Z.; Xiao, Y.; Liu, J.; He, Y.; Yuan, Q.; Yuan, X.; et al. Peroxiredoxin 1 inhibits the oxidative stress induced apoptosis in renal tubulointerstitial fibrosis. *Nephrology* **2015**, *20*, 832–842. [CrossRef]

62. Saikumar, P.; Venkatachalam, M.A. Role of apoptosis in hypoxic/ischemic damage in the kidney. *Semin Nephrol.* **2003**, *23*, 511–521. [CrossRef]

63. Luo, S.; Rubinsztein, D.C. Apoptosis blocks Beclin 1-dependent autophagosome synthesis: An effect rescued by Bcl-xL. *Cell Death Differ.* **2010**, *17*, 268–277. [CrossRef]

64. Xu, Y.; Ruan, S.; Wu, X.; Chen, H.; Zheng, K.; Fu, B. Autophagy and apoptosis in tubular cells following unilateral ureteral obstruction are associated with mitochondrial oxidative stress. *Int. J. Mol. Med.* **2013**, *31*, 628–636. [CrossRef] [PubMed]

65. Schumer, M.; Colombel, M.C.; Sawczuk, I.S.; Gobé, G.; Connor, J.; O'Toole, K.M.; Olsson, C.A.; Wise, G.J.; Buttyan, R. Morphologic, biochemical, and molecular evidence of apoptosis during the reperfusion phase after brief periods of renal ischemia. *Am. J. Pathol.* **1992**, *140*, 831–838. [PubMed]

66. Price, P.M.; Hodeify, R. A possible mechanism of renal cell death after ischemia/reperfusion. *Kidney Int.* **2012**, *81*, 720–721. [CrossRef] [PubMed]

67. Linkermann, A.; Chen, G.; Dong, G.; Kunzendorf, U.; Krautwald, S.; Dong, Z. Regulated cell death in AKI. *J. Am. Soc. Nephrol.* **2014**, *25*, 2689–2701. [CrossRef] [PubMed]

68. Hoste, E.A.; Clermont, G.; Kersten, A.; Venkataraman, R.; Angus, D.C.; De Bacquer, D.; Kellum, J.A. RIFLE criteria for acute kidney injury are associated with hospital mortality in critically ill patients: A cohort analysis. *Crit Care* **2006**, *10*, R73:1-73-10. [CrossRef] [PubMed]

69. Kellum, J.A.; Unruh, M.L.; Murugan, R. Acute kidney injury. *BMJ Clin. Evid.* **2011**, *2011*, 2001:1–2001:36. [CrossRef] [PubMed]

70. Decuypere, J.P.; Ceulemans, L.J.; Agostinis, P.; Monbaliu, D.; Naesens, M.; Pirenne, J.; Jochmans, I. Autophagy and the Kidney: Implications for Ischemia-Reperfusion Injury and Therapy. *Am. J. Kidney Dis.* **2015**, *66*, 699–709. [CrossRef] [PubMed]

71. Olsen, S.; Burdick, J.F.; Keown, P.A.; Wallace, A.C.; Racussen, L.C.; Solez, K. Primary acute renal failure ("acute tubular necrosis") in the transplanted kidney: Morphology and pathogenesis. *Medicine (Baltimore)* **1989**, *68*, 173–187. [CrossRef]

72. Ito, H.; Kasagi, N.; Shomori, K.; Osaki, M.; Adachi, H. Apoptosis in the human allografted kidney. Analysis by terminal deoxynucleotidyl transferase-mediated DUTP-botin nick end labeling. *Transplantation* **1995**, *60*, 794–798. [CrossRef] [PubMed]

73. Kato, S.; Akasaka, Y.; Kawamura, S. Fas antigen expression and its relationship with apoptosis in transplanted kidney. *Pathol. Int.* **1997**, *47*, 230–237. [CrossRef]

74. Seron, D.; Moreso, F.; Bover, J.; Condom, E.; Gil-Vernet, S.; Canas, C.; Fulladosa, X.; Torras, J.; Carrera, M.; Grinyo, J.M.; et al. Early protocol renal allograft biopsies and graft outcome. *Kidney Int.* **1997**, *51*, 310–316. [CrossRef] [PubMed]

75. Castaneda, M.P.; Swiatecka-Urban, A.; Mitsnefes, M.M.; Feuerstein, D.; Kaskel, F.J.; Tellis, V.; Devarajan, P. Activation of mitochondrial apoptotic pathways in human renal allografts after ischemiareperfusion injury. *Transplantation* **2003**, *76*, 50–54. [CrossRef] [PubMed]

76. Sanz, A.B.; Santamaría, B.; Ruiz-Ortega, M.; Egido, J.; Ortiz, A. Mechanisms of Renal Apoptosis in Health and Disease. *J. Am. Soc. Nephrol.* **2008**, *19*, 1634–1642. [CrossRef] [PubMed]

77. Pallet, N.; Dieudé, M.; Cailhier, J.; Hébert, M. The Molecular Legacy of Apoptosis in Transplantation. *Am. J. Transplant.* **2012**, *12*, 1378–1384. [CrossRef] [PubMed]

78. Bonegio, R.; Lieberthal, W. Role of apoptosis in the pathogenesis of acute renal failure. *Curr. Opin. Nephrol. Hypertens* **2002**, *11*, 301–308. [CrossRef] [PubMed]

79. Foster, M.C.; Wenham, P.W.; Rowe, P.A.; Burden, R.P.; Morgan, A.G.; Cotton, R.E.; Blamey, R.W. The late results of renal transplantation and the importance of chronic rejection as a cause of graft loss. *Ann. R Coll Surg. Engl.* **1989**, *71*, 44–47. [PubMed]

80. Laine, J.; Etelamaki, P.; Holmberg, C.; Dunkel, L. Apoptotic cell death in human chronic renal allograft rejection. *Transplantation* **1997**, *63*, 101–105. [CrossRef]

81. Thomas, G.L.; Yang, B.; Wagner, B.E.; Savill., J.; El Nahas, A.M. Cellular apoptosis and proliferation in experimental renal fibrosis. *Nephrol Dial. Transplant.* **1998**, *13*, 2216–2226. [CrossRef]

82. Schelling, J.R.; Nkemere, N.; Kopp, J.B.; Cleveland, R.P. Fas-dependent fratricidal apoptosis is a mechanism of tubular epithelial cell deletion in chronic renal failure. *Lab. Invest.* **1998**, *78*, 813–824.

83. Khan, S.; Cleveland, R.P.; Koch, C.J.; Schelling, J.R. Hypoxia induces renal tubular epithelial cell apoptosis in chronic renal disease. *Lab. Invest.* **1999**, *79*, 1089–1099.

84. Choi, Y.J.; Baranowska-Daca, E.; Nguyen, V.; Kpji, T.; Ballantyne, C.M.; Sheikh-Hamand, D.; Suki, W.N.; Truong, L.D. Mechanism of chronic obstructive uropathy: Increased expression of apoptosis-promoting molecules. *Kidney Int.* **2000** 58, 1481–1491. [CrossRef]

85. Yang, B.; Johnson, T.S.; Thomas, G.L.; Watson, P.F.; Wagner, B.; Skill, N.J.; Haylor, J.L.; El Nahas, A.M. Expression of apoptosis related genes and proteins in experimental chronic renal scarring. *J. Am. Soc. Nephrol.* **2001**, *12*, 275–288. [PubMed]

86. Zhu, Y.; Cui, H.; Xia, Y.; Gan, H. RIPK3-Mediated Necroptosis and Apoptosis Contributes toRenal Tubular Cell Progressive Loss and ChronicKidney Disease Progression in Rats. *PLoS ONE* **2016**, *11*, e0156729. [CrossRef]

87. Barnes, D.J.; Pinto, J.R.; Davison, A.M.; Cameron, J.S.; Grunfeld, J.P.; Kerr, D.N.S.; Ritz, E.; Viberti, G.C. The patient with diabetes mellitus. In *Oxford Textbook of Clinical Nephrology*, 2nd ed.; Turner, N., Turner, N.N., Lameire, N., Goldsmith, D.J., Winearls, C.G., Himmelfarb, J., Remuzzi, G., Eds.; Oxford university Press: Oxford, UK, 1998; pp. 723–775. ISBN 978-01-9959-254-8.

88. Bamri-Ezzine, S.; Ao, Z.J.; Londoño, I.; Gingras, D.; Bendayan, M. Apoptosis of Tubular Epithelial Cells in Glycogen Nephrosis During Diabetes. *Lab. Invest.* **2003**, *83*, 1069–1080. [CrossRef] [PubMed]

89. Habib, S.L. Diabetes and renal tubular cell apoptosis. *World J. Diabetes* **2013**, *4*, 27–30. [CrossRef] [PubMed]

90. Martindale, J.L.; Holbrook, N.J. Cellular response to oxidative stress: Signaling for suicide and survival. *J. Cell Physiol.* **2002**, *192*, 1–15. [CrossRef] [PubMed]

91. Orrenius, S.; Nicotera, P.; . Zhivotovsky, B. Cell Death Mechanisms and Their Implications in Toxicology. *Toxicological Sci.* **2011**, *119*, 3–19. [CrossRef]

92. Hamada, T.; Nakano, S.; Iwai, S.; Tanimoto, A.; Ariyoshi, K.; Koide, O. Pathological study on beagles after long-term oral administration of cadmium. *Toxicol. Pathol.* **1991**, *19*, 138–147. [CrossRef]

93. Hamada, T.; Tanimoto, A.; Iwai, S.; Fujiwara, H.; Sasaguri, Y. Cytopathological changes induced by cadmium-exposure in canine proximal tubular cells: A cytochemical and ultrastructural study. *Nephron* **1994**, *68*, 104–111. [CrossRef]

94. Duncan-Achanzar, K.B.; Jones, J.T.; Burke, M.F.; Carter, D.E.; Laird, H.E., II. Inorganic mercury chloride-induced apoptosis in the cultured porcine renal cell line LLC-PK1. *J. Pharmacol. Exp. Ther.* **1996**, *277*, 1726–1732.

95. Nath, K.A.; Croatt, A.J.; Likely, S.; Behrens, T.W.; Warden, D. Renal oxidant injury and oxidant response induced by mercury. *Kidney Int.* **1996**, *50*, 1032–1043. [CrossRef] [PubMed]

96. Sabath, E.; Robles-Osorio, M.L. Renal health and the environment: Heavy metal nephrotoxicity. *Nefrologia* **2012**, *32*, 279–286. [CrossRef] [PubMed]

97. Yuan, G.; Dai, S.; Yin, Z.; Lu, H.; Jia, R.; Xu, J.; Song, X.; Li, L.; Shu, Y.; Zhao, X.; et al. Sub-chronic lead and cadmium co-induce apoptosis protein expression in liver and kidney of rats. *Int J. Clin. Exp. Pathol.* **2014**, *7*, 2905–2914. [PubMed]

98. Eid, R.A. Apoptosis of Rat Renal Cells by Organophosphate Pesticide, Quinalphos: Ultrastructural Study. *Saudi J. Kidney Dis. Transpl.* **2017**, *28*, 725–736. [PubMed]

99. Lieberthal, W.; Triaca, V.; Levine, J. Mechanisms of death induced by cisplatin in proximal tubular epithelial cells: Apoptosis vs. necrosis. *Am. J. Physiol.* **1996**, *270*, F700–F708. [CrossRef] [PubMed]

100. Miller, R.P.; Tadagavadi, R.K.; Ramesh, G.; Reeves, W.B. Mechanisms of Cisplatin Nephrotoxicity. *Toxins (Basel)* **2010**, *2*, 2490–2518. [CrossRef] [PubMed]

101. Ortiz, A.; Lorz, C.; Catalán, M.P.; Danoff, T.M.; Yamasaki, Y.; Egido, J.; Neilson, E.G. Expression of apoptosis regulatory proteins in tubular epithelium stressed in culture or following acute renal failure. *Kidney Int.* **2000**, *57*, 969–981. [CrossRef]

102. Van de Water, B.; Kruidering, M.; Nagelkerke, J.F. F-actin disorganization in apoptotic cell death of cultured rat renal proximal tubular cells. *Am. J. Physiol.* **1996**, *270*, F593–F603. [CrossRef]

103. Desouza, M.; Gunning, P.W.; Stehn, J.R. The actin cytoskeleton as a sensor and mediator of apoptosis. *Bioarchitecture* **2012**, *2*, 75–87. [CrossRef]

104. Nouwen, E.J.; Verstrepen, W.A.; Buyssens, N.; Zhu, M.Q.; De Broe, M.E. Hyperplasia, hypertrophy, and phenotypic alterations in the distal nephron after acute proximal tubular injury in the rat. *Lab. Invest.* **1994**, *70*, 479–493.

105. Abuelezz, S.A.; Hendawy, N.; Abdel Gawad, S. Alleviation of renal mitochondrial dysfunction and apoptosis underlies the protective effect of sitagliptin in gentamicin-induced nephrotoxicity. *J. Pharm. Pharmacol.* **2016**, *68*, 523–532. [CrossRef] [PubMed]

106. Vervaet, B.A.; D'Haese, P.C.; Verhulst, A. Environmental toxin-induced acute kidney injury. *Clin. Kidney J.* **2017**, *10*, 747–758. [CrossRef] [PubMed]

107. Harrison, D.J. Cell death in the diseased glomerulus. *Histopathology* **1998**, *12*, 679–683. [CrossRef]

108. Savill, J.; Smith, J.; Sarraf, C.; Ren, Y.; Abbott, F.; Rees, A. Glomerular mesangial cells and inflammatory macrophages ingest neutrophils undergoing apoptosis. *Kidney Int.* **1992**, *42*, 924–936. [CrossRef] [PubMed]

109. Baker, A.J.; Mooney, A.; Hughes, J.; Lombardi, D.; Johnson, R.J.; Savill, J. Mesangial cell apoptosis: The major mechanism for resolution of glomerular hypercellularity in experimental mesangial proliferative nephritis. *J. Clin. Invest.* **1994**, *94*, 2105–2116. [CrossRef] [PubMed]

110. Shimizu, A.; Kitamura, H.; Masuda, Y.; Ishizaki, M.; Sugisaki, Y.; Yamanaka, N. Apoptosis in the repair process of experimental proliferative glomerulonephritis. *Kidney Int.* **1995**, *47*, 114–121. [CrossRef] [PubMed]

111. Jung, D.S.; Lee, S.H.; Kwak, S.J.; Li, J.J.; Kim, D.H.; Nam, B.Y.; Kang, H.Y.; Chang, T.I.; Park, J.T.; Han, S.H.; et al. Apoptosis occurs differentially according to glomerular size in diabetic kidney disease. *Nephrol Dial. Transplant.* **2012**, *27*, 259–266. [CrossRef] [PubMed]

112. Savill, J. Apoptosis and the kidney. *J. Am. Soc. Nephrol* **1994**, *5*, 12–21.

113. Takemura, T.; Murakami, K.; Miyazato, H.; Yagi, K.; Yoshioka, K. Expression of Fas antigen and Bcl-2 in human glomerulonephritis. *Kidney Int* **1995**, *48*, 1886–1892. [CrossRef]

114. Sugiyama, H.; Kashihara, N.; Makino, H.; Yamasaki, Y.; Ota, A. Apoptosis in glomerular sclerosis. *Kidney Int* **1996**, *49*, 103–111. [CrossRef]

115. Shimizu, A.; Kitamura, H.; Masuda, Y.; Ishizaki, M.; Sugisaki, Y.; Yamanaka, N. Glomerular capillary regeneration and endothelial cell apoptosis in both reversible and progressive models of glomerulonephritis. *Contrib Nephrol* **1996**, *118*, 29–40. [PubMed]

116. Shimizu, A.; Masuda, Y.; Kitamura, H.; Ishizaki, M.; Sugisaki, Y.; Yamanaka, N. Apoptosis in progressive crescentic glomerulonephritis. *Lab. Invest.* **1996**, *74*, 941–951. [PubMed]

117. Soto, H.; Mosquera, J.; Rodriguez, I.B.; Henriquez, L.A.; Roche, C.; Pinto, A. Apoptosis in proliferative glomerulonephritis: Decreased apoptosis expression in lupus nephritis. *Nephrol Dial. Transplant.* **1997**, *12*, 273–280. [CrossRef] [PubMed]

118. Savill, J. Regulation of glomerular cell number by apoptosis. *Kidney Int* **1999**, *56*, 1216–1222. [CrossRef] [PubMed]

119. Ruiz, P.; Soares, M.F. Acute postinfectious glomerulonephritis: An immune response gone bad? *Hum. Pathol* **2003**, *34*, 1–2. [CrossRef] [PubMed]

120. Schmiedeke, T.M.; Stockl, F.W.; Weber, R.; Sugisaki, Y.; Batsford, S.R.; Vogt, A. Histones have high affinity for the glomerular basement membrane. Relevance for immune complex formation in lupus nephritis. *J. Exp. Med.* **1989**, *169*, 1879–1894. [CrossRef] [PubMed]

121. Vogt, A.; Schmiedeke, T.; Stockl, F.; Sugisaki, Y.; Mertz, A.; Batsford, S. The role of cationic proteins in the pathogenesis of immune complex glomerulonephritis. *Nephrol Dial. Transplant.* **1990**, *5*, 6–9. [CrossRef]

122. Schmiedeke, T.; Stoeckl, F.; Muller, S.; Sugisaki, Y.; Batsford, S.; Woitas, R.; Vogt, A. Glomerular immune deposits in murine lupus models may contain histones. *Clin. Exp. Immunol* **1992**, *90*, 453–458. [CrossRef]

123. Stockl, F.; Muller, S.; Batsford, S.; Schmiedeke, T.; Waldherr, R.; Andrassy, K.; Sugisaki, Y.; Nakabayashi, K.; Nagasawa, T.; Rodriguez- Iturbe, B.; et al. A role for histones and ubiquitin in lupus nephritis? *Clin. Nephrol* **1994**, *41*, 10–17.

124. Kuenkele, S.; Beyer, T.D.; Voll, R.E.; Kalden, J.R.; Herrmann, M. Impaired clearance of apoptotic cells in systemic lupus erythematosus: Challenge of T and B cell tolerance. *Curr Rheumatol Rep.* **2003**, *5*, 175–177. [CrossRef]

125. Dieker, J.W.; van der Vlag, J.; Berden, J.H. Deranged removal of apoptotic cells: Its role in the genesis of lupus. *Nephrol Dial. Transplant.* **2004**, *19*, 282–285. [CrossRef] [PubMed]

126. Gaipl, U.S.; Voll, R.E.; Sheriff, A.; Franz, S.; Kalden, J.R.; Herrmann, M. Impaired clearance of dying cells in systemic lupus erythematosus. *Autoimmun Rev.* **2005**, *4*, 189–194. [CrossRef] [PubMed]

127. Kalaaji, M.; Mortensen, E.; Jorgensen, L.; Olsen, R.; Rekvig, O.P. Nephritogenic lupus antibodies recognize glomerular basement membrane-associated chromatin fragments released from apoptotic intraglomerular cells. *Am. J. Pathol* **2006**, *168*, 1779–1792. [CrossRef] [PubMed]

128. Gaipl, U.S.; Sheriff, A.; Franz, S.; Munoz, L.E.; Voll, R.E.; Kalden, J.R.; Herrmann, M. Inefficient clearance of dying cells and autoreactivity. *Curr Top. Microbiol Immunol* **2006**, *305*, 161–176. [PubMed]

129. Chen, R.; Kang, R.; Fan, X.G.; Tang, D. Release and activity of histone in diseases. *Cell Death Dis* **2014**, *5*, e1370:1-1370:9. [CrossRef] [PubMed]

130. Holzman, B.L.; Wiggins, R.C. Glomerular crescent formation. *Semin Nephrol* **1991**, *11*, 346–353. [PubMed]

131. Ophascharoensuk, V.; Pippin, J.W.; Gordon, K.L.; Shankland, S.J.; Couser, W.G.; Johnson, R.J. Role of intrinsic renal cells versus infiltrating cells in glomerular crescent formation. *Kidney Int* **1998**, *54*, 416–425. [CrossRef] [PubMed]

132. Su, H.; Chen, S.; He, F.F.; Wang, Y.M.; Bondzie, P.; Zhang, C. New Insights into Glomerular Parietal Epithelial Cell Activation and Its Signaling Pathways in Glomerular Diseases. *Biomed. Res. Int* **2015**, *2015*, 318935:1–318935:8. [CrossRef] [PubMed]

133. Cohen, A.H.; Mampaso, F.; Zamboni, L. Glomerular podocyte degeneration in human renal disease. *Lab. Invest.* **1977**, *37*, 30–42. [PubMed]

134. Susztak, K.; Raff, A.C.; Schiffer, M.; Böttinger, E.P. Glucose-induced reactive oxygen species cause apoptosis of podocytes and podocyte depletion at the onset of diabetic nephropathy. *Diabetes* **2006**, *55*, 225–233. [CrossRef] [PubMed]

135. Tharaux, P.L.; Huber, T.B. How Many Ways Can a Podocyte Die? *Semin Nephrol* **2012**, *32*, 394–404. [CrossRef] [PubMed]

136. Burlaka, I.; Nilsson, L.M.; Scott, L.; Holtbäck, U.; Eklöf, A.C.; Fogo, A.B.; Brismar, H.; Aperia, A. Prevention of apoptosis averts glomerular tubular disconnection and podocyte loss in proteinuric. kidney disease. *Kidney Int* **2016**, *90*, 135–148. [CrossRef] [PubMed]

137. Bagchus, W.M.; Hoedemaeker, P.J.; Rozing, J.; Bakker, W.W. Glomerulonephritis induced by monoclonal anti-Thy 1.1 antibodies. A sequential histological and ultrastructural study in the rat. *Lab. Invest.* **1986**, *55*, 680–687. [PubMed]

138. Wörnle, M.; Schmid, H.; Merkle, M.; Banas, B. Effects of chemokines on proliferation and apoptosis of human mesangial cells. *BMC Nephrology* **2004**, *5*, 8:1–8:14. [CrossRef] [PubMed]

139. Prakash, J.; Singh, V.P. Changing picture of renal cortical necrosis in acute kidney injury in developing country. *World J. Nephrol* **2015**, *4*, 480–486. [CrossRef] [PubMed]

140. Brix, A.E. Renal papillary necrosis. *Toxicol Pathol* **2002**, *30*, 672–674. [CrossRef] [PubMed]

141. Kono, H.; Rock, K.L. How dying cells alert the immune system to danger. *Nat. Rev. Immunol* **2008**, *8*, 279–289. [CrossRef]

142. Kaczmarek, A.; Vandenabeele, P.; Krysko, D.V. Necroptosis: The release of damage-associated molecular patterns and its physiological relevance. *Immunity* **2013**, *38*, 209–223. [CrossRef]

143. Mulay, S.R.; Linkermann, A.; Anders, H.J. Necroinflammation in kidney disease. *J. Am. Soc. Nephrol* **2016**, *27*, 27–39. [CrossRef]

144. Sarhan, M.; von Mässenhausen, A.; Hugo, C.; Oberbauer, R.; Linkermann, A. Immunological consequences of kidney cell death. *Cell Death Dis* **2018**, *9*, 114:1–114:15. [CrossRef]

145. Linkermann, A.; Bräsen, J.H.; Himmerkus, N.; Liu, S.; Huber, T.B.; Kunzendorf, U.; Krautwald, S. Rip1 (receptor-interacting protein kinase 1) mediates necroptosis and contributes to renal ischemia/reperfusion injury. *Kidney Int* **2012**, *81*, 751–761. [CrossRef] [PubMed]

146. Linkermann, A.; Bräsen, J.H.; Darding, M.; Jin, M.K.; Sanz, A.B.; Heller, J.O.; De Zen, F.; Weinlich, R.; Ortiz, A.; Walczak, H.; et al. Two independent pathways of regulated necrosis mediate ischemia-reperfusion injury. *Proc. Natl. Acad. Sci. USA* **2013**, *110*, 12024–12029. [CrossRef] [PubMed]

147. Linkermann, A.; Skouta, R.; Himmerkus, N.; Mulay, S.R.; Dewitz, C.; De Zen, F.; Prokai, A.; Zuchtriegel, G.; Krombach, F.; Welz, P.S.; et al. Synchronized renal tubular cell death involves ferroptosis. *Proc. Natl. Acad. Sci. USA* **2014**, *111*, 16836–16841. [CrossRef] [PubMed]

148. Mulay, S.R.; Desay, J.; Kumar, S.V.R.; Eberhard, J.N.; Thomasova, D.; Romoli, S.; Grigorescu, M.; Kulkarni, O.P.; Popper, B.; Vielhauer, V.; et al. Cytotoxicity of crystals involves RIPK3- MLKL-mediated necroptosis. *Nat. Commun* **2016**, *7*, 10274:1–10274:15. [CrossRef] [PubMed]

149. Allam, R.; Kumar, S.V.; Darisipudi, M.N.; Anders, H.J. Extracellular histones in tissue injury and inflammation. *J. Mol. Med. (Berl)* **2014**, *92*, 465–472. [CrossRef] [PubMed]

150. Humphreys, B.D.; Valerius, M.T.; Kobayashi, A.; Mugford, J.W.; Soeung, S.; Duffield, J.S.; McMahon, A.P.; Bonventre, J.V. Intrinsic epithelial cells repair the kidney after injury. *Cell Stem Cell* **2008**, *2*, 284–291. [CrossRef] [PubMed]

151. Bonsib, S.M. Glomerular basement membrane necrosis and crescent organization. *Kidney Int* **1988**, *33*, 966–974. [CrossRef]

152. Smeets, B.; Angelotti, M.L.; Rizzo, P.; Dijkman, H.; Lazzeri, E.; Mooren, F.; Ballerini, L.; Parente, E.; Sagrinati, C.; Mazzinghi, B.; et al. Renal progenitor cells contribute to hyperplastic lesions of podocytopathies and crescentic glomerulonephritis. *J. Am. Soc. Nephrol* **2009**, *20*, 2593–2603. [CrossRef]

153. Schreiber, A.; Xiao, H.; Jennette, J.C.; Schneider, W.; Luft, F.C.; Kettritz, R. C5a receptor mediates neutrophil activation and ANCA-induced glomerulonephritis. *J. Am. Soc. Nephrol* **2009**, *20*, 289–298. [CrossRef]

154. Ryu, M.; Migliorini, A.; Miosge, N.; Gross, O.; Shankland, S.; Brinkkoetter, P.T.; Hagmann, H.; Romagnani, P.; Liapis, H.; Anders, H.J. Plasma leakage through glomerular basement membrane ruptures triggers the proliferation of parietal epithelial cells and crescent formation in non-inflammatory glomerular injury. *J. Pathol* **2012**, *228*, 482–494. [CrossRef]

155. Schepers, M.S.; van Ballegooijen, E.S.; Bangma, C.H.; Verkoelen, C.F. Crystals cause acute necrotic cell death in renal proximal tubule cells, but not in collecting tubule cells. *Kidney Int* **2005**, *68*, 1543–1553. [CrossRef] [PubMed]

156. Mulay, S.R.; Evan, A.; Anders, H.J. Molecular mechanisms of crystal-related kidney inflammation and injury. Implications for cholesterol embolism, crystalline nephropathies and kidney stone disease. *Nephrol Dial. Transplant.* **2014**, *29*, 507–514. [CrossRef] [PubMed]

157. Sun, X.Y.; Ouyang, J.M. New view in cell death mode: Effect of crystal size in renal epithelial cells. *Cell Death Dis* **2015**, *6*, e2013:1-2013:3. [CrossRef] [PubMed]

158. Sun, X.Y.; Ouyang, J.M.; Yu, K. Shape-dependent cellular toxicity on renal epithelial cells and stone risk of calcium oxalate dihydrate crystals. *Sci Rep.* **2017**, *7*, 7250:1–7250:13. [CrossRef] [PubMed]

159. Honarpisheh, M.; Foresto-Neto, O.; Desai, J.; Steiger, S.; Gómez, L.A.; Popper, B.; Boor, P.; Anders, H.J.; Mulay, S.R. Phagocytosis of environmental or metabolic crystalline particles induces cytotoxicity by triggering necroptosis across a broad range of particle size and shape. *Sci Rep.* **2017**, *7*, 15523:1–15523:11. [CrossRef] [PubMed]

160. Mulay, S.R.; Anders, H.J. Crystal nephropathies: Mechanisms of crystal-induced kidney injury. *Nat. Rev. Nephrol* **2017**, *13*, 226–240. [CrossRef] [PubMed]

161. Sun, X.Y.; Gan, Q.Z.; Ouyang, J.M. Calcium oxalate toxicity in renal epithelial cells: The mediation of crystal size on cell death mode. *Cell Death Discov* **2015**, *1*, 15055:1–15055:8. [CrossRef] [PubMed]

162. Mulay, S.R.; Kulkarni, O.P.; Rupanagudi, K.V.; Migliorini, A.; Darisipudi, M.N.; Vilaysane, A.; Muruve, D.; Shi, Y.; Munro, F.; Liapis, H.; et al. Calcium oxalate crystals induce renal inflammation by NLRP3-mediated IL-1beta secretion. *J. Clin. Invest.* **2013**, *123*, 236–246. [CrossRef]

163. Kirsch, T. Determinants of pathological mineralization. *Curr Opin Rheumatol* **2006**, *18*, 174–180. [CrossRef]

164. Schepens, D.; Verswijvel, G.; Kuypers, D.; Vanrenterghem, Y. Renal cortical nephrocalcinosis. *Nephrol Dial. Transplant.* **2000**, *15*, 1080–1082. [CrossRef]

165. Priante, G.; Quaggio, F.; Gianesello, L.; Ceol, M.; Cristofaro, R.; Terrin, L.; Furlan, C.; Del Prete, D.; Anglani, F. Caspase-independent programmed cell death triggers Ca2PO4 deposition in an in vitro model of nephrocalcinosis. *Biosci Rep.* **2018**, *38*, BSR20171228:1-BSR20171228:19. [CrossRef] [PubMed]

166. Priante, G.; Ceol, M.; Gianesello, L.; Furlan, C.; Del Prete, D.; Anglani, F. Human proximal tubular cells can form calcium phosphate deposits in osteogenic culture: Role of cell death and osteoblast-like transdifferentiation. *Cell Death Discov* **2019**, *5*, 57:1–57:14. [CrossRef]

167. Proudfoot, D.; Skepper, J.N.; Hegyi, L.; Bennett, M.R.; Shanahan, C.M.; Weissberg, P.L. Apoptosis regulates human vascular calcification in vitro: Evidence for initiation of vascular calcification by apoptotic bodies. *Circ Res* **2000**, *87*, 1055–1062. [CrossRef] [PubMed]

168. Giachelli, C.M. Vascular calcification mechanisms. *J. Am. Soc. Nephrol* **2004**, *15*, 2959–2964. [CrossRef] [PubMed]

169. Evrard, S.; Delanaye, P.; Kamel, S.; Cristol, J.P.; Cavalier, E. Vascular calcification: From pathophysiology to biomarkers. *Clin. Chim Acta* **2015**, *438*, 401–414. [CrossRef] [PubMed]

170. Leopold, J.A. Vascular calcification: Mechanisms of vascular smooth muscle cell calcification. *Trends Cardiovasc Med.* **2015**, *25*, 267–274. [CrossRef]

171. Priante, G.; Mezzabotta, F.; Cristofaro, R.; Quaggio, F.; Ceol, M.; Gianesello, L.; Del Prete, D.; Anglani, F. Cell death in ectopic calcification of the kidney. *Cell Death Dis* **2019**, *10*, 466. [CrossRef]

172. Unal-Cevik, I.; Kilinç, M.; Can, A.; Gürsoy-Ozdemir, Y.; Dalkara, T. Apoptotic and necrotic death mechanisms are concomitantly activated in the same cell after cerebral ischemia. *Stroke* **2004**, *35*, 2189–2194. [CrossRef]

173. Zychlinsky, A.; Zheng, L.M.; Liu, C.; Young, J.D. Cytolytic lymphocytes induce both apoptosis and necrosis in target celis. *J. Immunol* **1991**, *146*, 393–400.

174. Vanden Berghe, T.; Vanlangenakker, N.; Parthoens, E.; Deckers, W.; Devos, M.; Festjens, N.; Guerin, C.J.; Brunk, U.T.; Declercq, W.; Vandenabeele, P. Necroptosis, necrosis and secondary necrosis converge on similar cellular disintegration features. *Cell Death Differ.* **2010**, *17*, 922–930. [CrossRef]

175. Wang, S.; Zhang, C.; Hu, L.; Yang, C. Necroptosis in acute kidney injury: A shedding light. *Cell Death Dis* **2016**, *7*, e2125:1-2125:9. [CrossRef] [PubMed]

176. Homsi, E.; Janino, P.; de Faria, J.B. Role of caspases on cell death, inflammation, and cell cycle in glycerol-induced acute renal failure. *Kidney Int* **2006**, *69*, 1385–1392. [CrossRef] [PubMed]

177. Servais, H.; Ortiz, A.; Devuyst, O.; Denamur, S.; Tulkens, P.M.; Mingeot-Leclercq, M.P. Renal cell apoptosis induced by nephrotoxic drugs: Cellular and molecular mechanisms and potential approaches to modulation. *Apoptosis* **2008**, *13*, 11–32. [CrossRef] [PubMed]

178. Nelson, P.J.; Cantley, L. GSK3beta plays dirty in acute kidney injury. *J. Am. Soc. Nephrol* **2010**, *21*, 199–200. [CrossRef] [PubMed]

179. Wang, Z.; Havasi, A.; Gall, J.; Bonegio, R.; Li, Z.; Mao, H.; Schwartz, J.H.; Borkan, S.C. GSK3beta promotes apoptosis after renal ischemic injury. *J. Am. Soc. Nephrol* **2010**, *21*, 284–294. [CrossRef] [PubMed]

180. Whelan, R.S.; Konstantinidis, K.; Wei, A.C.; Chen, Y.; Reyna, D.E.; Jha, S.; Yang, Y.; Calvert, J.W.; Lindsten, T.; Thompson, C.B.; et al. Bax regulates primary necrosis through mitochondrial dynamics. *Proc. Natl. Acad. Sci. USA* **2012**, *109*, 6566–6571. [CrossRef]

181. Qiu, X.; Zhang, Y.; Han, J. RIP3 is an upregulator of aerobic metabolism and the enhanced respiration by necrosomal RIP3 feeds back on necrosome to promote necroptosis. *Cell Death & Differentiation* **2018**, *25*, 821–824.

182. Teng, X.; Degterev, A.; Jagtap, P.; Xing, X.; Choi, S.; Denu, R.; Yuan, J.; Cuny, G.D. Structure-activity relationship study of novel necroptosis inhibitors. *Bioorg Med. Chem Lett* **2005**, *15*, 5039–5044. [CrossRef]

183. Degterev, A.; Hitomi, J.; Germscheid, M.; Ch'en, I.L.; Korkina, O.; Teng, X.; Abbott, D.; Cuny, G.D.; Yuan, C.; Wagner, G.; et al. Identification of RIP1 kinase as a specific cellular target of necrostatins. *Nat. Chem Biol* **2008**, *4*, 313–321. [CrossRef]

184. Sun, L.; Wang, H.; Wang, Z.; He, S.; Chen, S.; Liao, D.; Wang, L.; Yan, J.; Liu, W.; Lei, X.; et al. Mixed lineage kinase domain-like protein mediates necrosis signaling downstream of RIP3 kinase. *Cell* **2012**, *148*, 213–227. [CrossRef]

185. Kaiser, W.J.; Sridharan, H.; Huang, C.; Mandal, P.; Upton, J.W.; Gough, P.J.; Sehon, C.A.; Marquis, R.W.; Bertin, J.; Mocarski, E.S. Toll-like receptor 3-mediated necrosis via TRIF, RIP3, and MLKL. *J. Biol Chem* **2013**, *288*, 31268–31279. [CrossRef] [PubMed]

186. Harris, P.A.; Bandyopadhyay, D.; Berger, S.B.; Campobasso, N.; Capriotti, C.A.; Cox, J.A.; Dare, L.; Finger, J.N.; Hoffman, S.J.; Kahler, K.M.; et al. Discovery of small molecule RIP1 kinase inhibitors for the treatment of pathologies associated with necroptosis. *ACS Med. Chem Lett* **2013**, *4*, 1238–1243. [CrossRef] [PubMed]

187. Hildebrand, J.M.; Tanzer, M.C.; Lucet, I.S.; Young, S.N.; Spall, S.K.; Sharma, P.; Pierotti, C.; Garnier, J.M.; Dobson, R.C.; Webb, A.I.; et al. Activation of the pseudokinase MLKL unleashes the four-helix bundle domain to induce membrane localization and necroptotic cell death. *Proc. Natl. Acad. Sci. USA* **2014**, *111*, 15072–15077. [CrossRef] [PubMed]

188. Weng, D.; Marty-Roix, R.; Ganesan, S.; Proulx, M.K.; Vladimer, G.I.; Kaiser, W.J.; Mocarski, E.S.; Pouliot, K.; Chan, F.K.; Kelliher, M.A.; et al. Caspase-8 and RIP kinases regulate bacteria-induced innate immune responses and cell death. *Proc. Natl. Acad. Sci. USA* **2014**, *111*, 7391–7396. [CrossRef] [PubMed]

189. Mandal, P.; Berger, S.B.; Pillay, S.; Moriwaki, K.; Huang, C.; Guo, H.; Lich, J.D.; Finger, J.; Kasparcova, V.; Votta, B.; et al. RIP3 induces apoptosis independent of pronecrotic kinase activity. *Mol. Cell* **2014**, *56*, 481–495. [CrossRef]

190. Li, J.X.; Feng, J.M.; Wang, Y.; Li, X.H.; Chen, X.X.; Su, Y.; Shen, Y.Y.; Chen, Y.; Xiong, B.; Yang, C.H.; et al. The B-Raf(V600E) inhibitor dabrafenib selectively inhibits RIP3 and alleviates acetaminophen-induced liver injury. *Cell Death Dis* **2014**, *5*, e1278:1-1278:11. [CrossRef]

191. Fauster, A.; Rebsamen, M.; Huber, K.V.; Bigenzahn, J.W.; Stukalov, A.; Lardeau, C.H.; Scorzoni, S.; Bruckner, M.; Gridling, M.; Parapatics, K.; et al. A cellular screen identifies ponatinib and pazopanib as inhibitors of necroptosis. *Cell Death Dis* **2015**, *6*, e1767:1-1767:10. [CrossRef]

192. Rodriguez, D.A.; Weinlich, R.; Brown, S.; Guy, C.; Fitzgerald, P.; Dillon, C.P.; Oberst, A.; Quarato, G.; Low, J.; Cripps, J.G.; et al. Characterization of RIPK3-mediated phosphorylation of the activation loop of MLKL during necroptosis. *Cell Death Differ.* **2016**, *23*, 76–88. [CrossRef]

193. Oppenheim, J.J.; Yang, D. Alarmins: Chemotactic activators of immune responses. *Curr Opin Immunol* **2005**, *17*, 359–365. [CrossRef]

Int. J. Mol. Sci. **2019**, *20*, 3598

194. Chan, J.K.; Roth, J.; Oppenheim, J.J.; Tracey, K.J.; Vogl, T.; Feldmann, M.; Horwood, N.; Nanchahal, J. Alarmins: Awaiting a clinical response. *J. Clin. Invest.* **2012**, *122*, 2711–2719. [CrossRef]

195. Silke, J.; Rickard, J.A.; Gerlic, M. The diverse role of RIP kinases in necroptosis and inflammation. *Nat. Immunol* **2015**, *16*, 689–697. [CrossRef] [PubMed]

196. Linkermann, A.; Hackl, M.J.; Kunzendorf, U.; Walczak, H.; Krautwald, S.; Jevnikar, A.M. Necroptosis in immunity and ischemia-reperfusion injury. *Am. J. Transplant.* **2013**, *13*, 2797–2804. [CrossRef] [PubMed]

197. Linkermann, A.; Green, D.R. Necroptosis. *N Engl J. Med.* **2014**, *370*, 455–465. [CrossRef] [PubMed]

198. Degterev, A.; Linkermann, A. Generation of small molecules to interfere with regulated necrosis. *Cell Mol. Life Sci.* **2016**, *73*, 2251–2267. [CrossRef] [PubMed]

International Journal of
Molecular Sciences

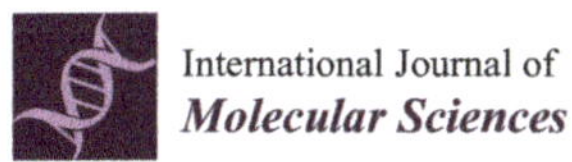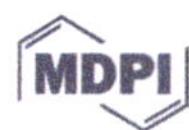

Review

Pigment Nephropathy: Novel Insights into Inflammasome-Mediated Pathogenesis

Kurt T. K. Giuliani [1,2,3], Andrew J. Kassianos [1,2,3,4], Helen Healy [1,2,3] and Pedro H. F. Gois [1,2,3,*]

1   Kidney Health Service, Royal Brisbane and Women's Hospital, Brisbane, QLD 4029, Australia;
    Kurt.Giuliani@uqconnect.edu.au (K.T.K.G.); Andrew.Kassianos@qimrberghofer.edu.au (A.J.K.);
    Helen.Healy@health.qld.gov.au (H.H.)
2   Conjoint Kidney Research Laboratory, Chemical Pathology—Pathology Queensland,
    Brisbane, QLD 4029, Australia
3   Faculty of Medicine, University of Queensland, Brisbane, QLD 4006, Australia
4   Institute of Health and Biomedical Innovation/School of Biomedical Sciences, Queensland University
    of Technology, Brisbane, QLD 4059, Australia
*   Correspondence: Pedro.FrancaGois@health.qld.gov.au; Tel.: +61-7-3362-0488

Received: 29 March 2019; Accepted: 17 April 2019; Published: 23 April 2019

Abstract: Pigment nephropathy is an acute decline in renal function following the deposition of endogenous haem-containing proteins in the kidneys. Haem pigments such as myoglobin and haemoglobin are filtered by glomeruli and absorbed by the proximal tubules. They cause renal vasoconstriction, tubular obstruction, increased oxidative stress and inflammation. Haem is associated with inflammation in sterile and infectious conditions, contributing to the pathogenesis of many disorders such as rhabdomyolysis and haemolytic diseases. In fact, haem appears to be a signalling molecule that is able to activate the inflammasome pathway. Recent studies highlight a pathogenic function for haem in triggering inflammatory responses through the activation of the nucleotide-binding domain-like receptor protein 3 (NLRP3) inflammasome. Among the inflammasome multiprotein complexes, the NLRP3 inflammasome has been the most widely characterized as a trigger of inflammatory caspases and the maturation of interleukin-18 and -1β. In the present review, we discuss the latest evidence on the importance of inflammasome-mediated inflammation in pigment nephropathy. Finally, we highlight the potential role of inflammasome inhibitors in the prophylaxis and treatment of pigment nephropathy.

Keywords: rhabdomyolysis; pigment nephropathy; haem; NLRP3 inflammasome; acute kidney injury

1. Introduction

Haem complexes consist of an Fe atom which is coordinated within the centre of a heterocyclic ring known as a protoporphyrin [1]. Haem-containing proteins are a large class of metalloproteins that play a pivotal role in maintaining basic biological functions [2]. Their broad activities range from mitochondrial electron transfer, oxygen transport and storage to signal transduction and control of gene expression [2].

Among the different haem group variants, haem a, b and c are the main biological types [3,4]. Of the haem variants, haem b is the most abundant form and is present biologically within myoglobin and haemoglobin, whilst haem a and c are present in cytochromes. Haem function as a prosthetic group in haemoproteins and are essential for reversible oxygen binding and transport [5,6]. However, under pathological conditions, an excess of circulating free haem may be highly cytotoxic and result in tissue damage, including within the kidney [3,6].

Pigment nephropathy (PN) is an acute decline in kidney function following the breakdown and deposition of endogenous haem pigment-containing proteins (myoglobin, haemoglobin) within renal tissue [7]. Both myoglobin and haemoglobin are freely filtered by glomeruli and when oxidised, release their haem moiety into the urinary space [8,9]. However, within the nephron, excess haem pigments may cause renal vasoconstriction, tubular obstruction, increased oxidative stress and inflammation [10–13].

Inflammation is an essential response of the innate immune system to harmful stimuli [14]. Haem is associated with inflammation in sterile and infectious conditions, contributing to the pathogenesis of many disorders such as rhabdomyolysis and haemolytic diseases [15]. There is an increasing body of evidence that haem trigger the inflammasome signalling cascade and ultimately, the innate immune response [16,17].

In the present review, we discuss the potential role of inflammasome activation as a driver of inflammation in PN. We explore the rationale of translating small molecule inhibitors of inflammasome activation already in clinical use, for diseases outside the kidney, in the prevention and treatment of PN.

2. The Nucleotide-Binding domain-Like Receptor Protein 3 (NLRP3) Inflammasome

The inflammasomes are a family of cytosolic signalling complexes with a central role in the activation of innate immune responses via the maturation and secretion of pro-inflammatory cytokines (interleukin (IL)-1β and IL-18) [18]. In particular, the nucleotide-binding domain-like receptor protein 3 (NLRP3) inflammasome, an extensively characterized inflammasome family member, is widely implicated in a variety of renal injuries, including acute and chronic kidney disease (CKD) [19–21]; oxalate and uric acid crystal nephropathy [22,23]; and diabetic nephropathies [24]. Inflammasomes respond to a diverse range of pathogen-associated molecular patterns (PAMPs) and endogenously derived damage-associated molecular patterns (DAMPs) via a suite of pattern recognition receptors (PRR). Of particular note, endogenous particulate matter, such as haem [16,17], monosodium urate (MSU) [25], oxalate [23,26] and cholesterol crystals [27,28] have all been identified as potent triggers of NLRP3 inflammasome activation and the subsequent release of pro-inflammatory cytokines [24].

Recently, Liston and Masters [29] proposed a mechanism of inflammasome activation in addition to the PAMP-DAMP axis. This mechanism responds to a loss of homeostasis via 'homeostasis-altering molecular processes' (HAMPs). They hypothesized that the PAMP-DAMP-HAMP axis was, collectively, likely to be sufficient for effective immunity and that deficiencies in this axis may cause the pathological inflammatory activation observed in sterile injury [29]. Examples of HAMPs which activate the inflammasome are perturbed membrane potential through K^+ efflux and Ca^{2+} influx [30], extracellular adenosine triphosphate (ATP) [31–33], and mitochondrial damage through reactive oxygen species (ROS) [34], altered mitochondrial membrane potential ($\Delta\Psi_m$) [35] and oxidised mitochondrial DNA (mtDNA) [36]. While their activation triggers may be diverse, the signalling pathways of inflammasome activation can be categorized into either canonical or non-canonical activation.

2.1. Canonical Inflammasome Activation

Following the detection of PAMPs or DAMPs (Signal 1) by PRRs, the NLRP3 inflammasome is canonically activated in an orchestrated cascade of signals [37], see Figure 1. The transmembrane protein family of Toll-like receptors (TLRs) play an important role as PRRs, activating the downstream signalling cascade. This signalling cascade is known as the "priming" phase of inflammasome activation. Once primed, the nuclear factor kappa-light-chain-enhancer of activated B cells (NF-κB) signalling complex translocates to the cell nucleus where it promotes the upregulation of NLRP3 and immature forms of IL-1β and IL-18 [38].

Following the priming phase, a second signal (Signal 2) is required to elicit the activation of the inflammasome, see Figure 1b. These signals can include interrupted phagocytosis [39], extracellular ATP [31–33], K^+ and Ca^{2+} flux [39–41], endoplasmic reticulum stress [42], mitochondrial ROS [34], $\Delta\Psi_m$ [35] and the release of oxidised mtDNA [36]. Particulate matter are also potent secondary signals which can activate the NLRP3 inflammasome via cell-surface contact [39]. The mechanism for detection of these PAMP/DAMP/HAMPs by NLRP3 remains poorly understood.

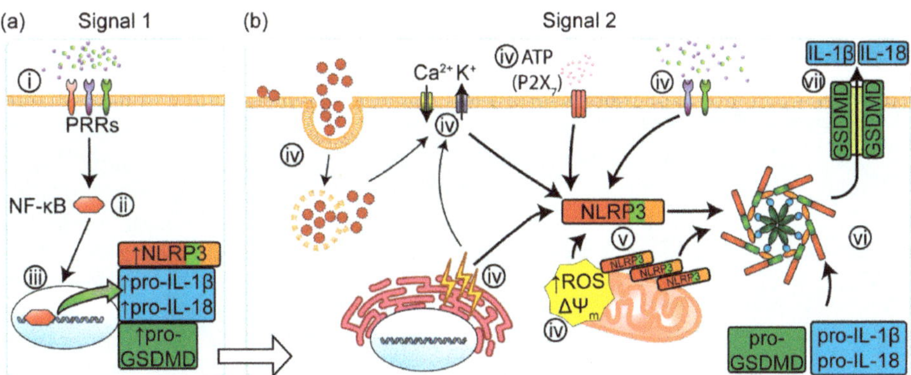

Figure 1. The canonical inflammasome activation signalling cascade is initiated by signal 1 PAMPs and DAMPs. (**a**) Signal 1 elicits the activation of PRRs on the cell surface (i). The activation of PRRs results in a downstream signalling cascade, triggering the translocation of NF-κB into the nucleus (ii), where NF-κB upregulates the expression of NLRP3, pro-GSDMD, pro-IL-1β and pro-IL-18 (iii). (**b**) Signal 2 is provided by an array of PAMPs, DAMPs and HAMPs (iv), including arrested phagocytosis, perturbed membrane potential ($\Delta\Psi_m$), endoplasmic reticulum stress, extracellular ATP, and mitochondrial dysfunction. NLPR3 proteins which have co-localized to the mitochondria (v) are ideally located to rapidly respond to these markers of cellular stress. NLRP3 then oligomerizes with ASC and pro-Caspase-1, forming the NLRP3 inflammasome complex (vi). Caspase-1 undergoes self-cleavage whilst bound to the inflammasome complex (vi), driving the post-translational processing of IL-1β, IL-18 and GSDMD. Once cleaved, GSDMD proteins self-oligomerize to form pores in the cell membrane (vii), allowing for the rapid release of IL-1β and IL-18. In addition, these GSDMD pores may also drive cell-death via pyroptosis. ASC: Apoptosis-associated Speck-like protein containing a Caspase-activation-and-recruitment domain; PRR: pattern recognition receptor; PAMP: pathogen-associated molecular pattern; DAMP: damage-associated molecular pattern; nuclear factor kappa-light-chain-enhancer of activated B cells: NF-κB; NLRP3: nucleotide-binding domain-like receptor protein 3; IL: interleukin; GSDMD: Gasdermin D; ROS: reactive oxygen species; $\Delta\Psi_m$: mitochondrial membrane potential.

Once activated by these molecular signalling patterns, NLRP3 proteins self-oligomerize and nucleate the formation of the NLRP3 inflammasome complex. This inflammasome complex consists of the NLRP3 protein, the ASC (Apoptosis-associated Speck-like protein containing a Caspase-activation-and-recruitment domain) adaptor protein and pro-caspase-1. Boucher, et al. [43] recently showed that pro-caspase-1 proteins dimerize following their recruitment to the inflammasome complex, before self-cleaving into an active state. The transiently active caspase-1 dimer undergoes additional cleavage, forming a proteolytically active holoenzyme with the inflammasome, capable of processing the pro-inflammatory cytokines IL-1β and IL-18 into their active forms [18,43]. Caspase-1 also cleaves Gasdermin-D (GSDMD) into its active form. Active GSDMD translocates to the cell membrane and forms GSDMD pores in the plasma membrane, driving pyroptosis and the consequent rapid release of IL-1β and IL-18 into the surrounding extracellular micro-environment [44–48].

2.2. Non-Canonical Inflammasome Activation

Non-canonical activation of the inflammasome differs in that it is dependent on caspase-11 (murine) or caspase-4 (human) activity [49–51]. Gram-negative bacteria-derived PAMPs are established triggers of non-canonical activation, directly sensed by and activating caspase-11/-4 [51]. Active caspase-11/-4 proteolytically cleave pro-GSDMD into its active state, effecting cell death by pyroptosis [49,50]. Kayagaki, et al. [50] showed that murine caspase-11 also triggers an NLRP3-inflammasome response through an as-yet-to-be identified mechanism, resulting in the release of IL-1β and IL-18 [50]. In humans, caspase-4 is required for the maturation and release of IL-18 via a non-canonical inflammasome pathway [51]. However, the role of non-canonical inflammasome activation in kidney disease remains to be elucidated.

2.3. Inflammasomes in the Kidney

Inflammasome activation is a key driver of the pathobiology in a variety of murine models and human etiologies of acute kidney injury (AKI) and CKD. Several murine studies investigating NLRP3 function, using small-molecule inflammasome-specific inhibitors or gene knockout models, have provided strong evidence for inflammasome activity in renal tissue injury. Specifically, *Nlrp3*[-/-], *Asc*[-/-] and *Casp1*[-/-] knock-out models have less kidney tissue damage and disease phenotype in unilateral ureteral obstruction (UUO) [52,53], diabetic kidney disease (DKD) [54] and crystal nephropathy [23,26]. However, the PAMPs/DAMPs/HAMPs that trigger inflammasome activation in these models are under active investigation.

Elevated soluble uric acid levels have been reported in the obstructed kidney of UUO mice [53]. Uric acid is an established activator of the inflammasome [55]. Furthermore, ROS derived from the activity of xanthine oxidase (XO), an enzyme which produces uric acid via purine catabolism, has also been reported to elicit an inflammasome response [56]. Allopurinol is a widely prescribed pharmaceutical used in the treatment of gout and directly inhibits XO activity. Notably, UUO mice treated with allopurinol exhibit less NLRP3 and IL-1β expression within the UUO kidney compared to untreated UUO controls [53]. These studies suggest a dual protective role for allopurinol by inhibiting both uric acid production and XO activity, thus preventing inflammasome activation.

Shahzad, et al. [54] reported NLRP3 activation in podocytes, an important cell type in the glomerular filtration barrier, in a murine DKD model [54]. Interestingly, this study demonstrated increased IL-1β and IL-18 expression within plasma and renal cortical extracts of diabetic animals, correlating with the functional kidney biomarker urine albumin/creatinine ratio [54].

IL-1β and IL-18 are produced by infiltrating hematopoietic cells, such as dendritic cells (DC) and macrophages, in mouse kidneys [57]. Supporting this concept, DC depletion in a crystal-induced model of murine renal fibrosis, resulted in reduced fibrosis and improved kidney function [20]. Furthermore, a similar outcome was achieved by treatment with a specific small molecule NLRP3 inflammasome inhibitor (MCC950; detailed below in Section 6.1) that blocked NLRP3 activation in kidney DC, reduced IL-1β and IL-18 production and inhibited the progression of renal fibrosis [20].

In contrast to these murine studies, the examination of inflammasome-mediated renal pathology in humans is less extensive. Whilst human proximal tubular epithelial cells (PTEC) appear to have the necessary inflammasome-related machinery, there is a paucity of evidence for its activation, particularly, whether these cells secrete IL-1β and IL-18 [58]. Intriguingly Kim, et al. [58] recently described an inflammasome-independent role for NLRP3 in human PTEC. In this study, hypoxic injury to PTEC increased NLRP3 expression independent of ASC, caspase-1, and IL-1β. Instead, the NLRP3 protein bound to the mitochondrial antiviral signal (MAVS), resulting in mitochondrial dysfunction (increased mitochondrial ROS) and cell death [58]. There is also emerging evidence that human tubular cells in acute oxalate nephropathy undergo a form of regulated cell death termed necroptosis. Products of necroptosis include DAMPs with the capacity to activate the canonical inflammasome pathway in innate immune cells (DC, macrophages) within the tubulointerstitium [20]. Our group has indeed shown increased numbers of activated human DC within the tubulointerstitium of fibrotic kidney biopsies, accumulating adjacent to injured PTEC [59].

The kidneys play a major role in maintaining homeostasis and regulating blood pressure. Renal inflammation and fibrosis are well-known contributing factors in the pathogenesis of hypertension [60]. In a murine model of salt-induced hypertension, NLRP3 inhibition by treatment with MCC950 reduced hypertension and heart rate, in addition to reduced inflammasome priming, inflammatory cytokines, kidney immune cell infiltration and kidney fibrosis [60]. Nevertheless, the specific mechanisms by which the inflammasome contributes to systemic hypertension are still unclear. Furthermore, the inflammasome-dependent interactions between specialized renal parenchymal and innate immune cells, in particular, the role of NLRP3 signalling in driving the pathobiology of human PN, remains to be elucidated.

3. Haem Catabolism and Role in Immune-Mediated Pathology

Excess haem pigments are highly cytotoxic in the kidney, leading to oxidative stress and inflammation under injurious conditions [61,62]. Our understanding of immune-mediated pathological conditions is that oxidative stress and inflammation are interdependent processes rather than discrete pathways of injury [63].

Free haem catalyses the formation of highly toxic free radicals—hydroxyl radicals (OH·)—from hydrogen peroxide (H_2O_2) via the Fenton reaction. Under homeostatic conditions, excess free cellular haem is catabolized by haem oxygenases (HO)—stress-responsive HO-1 and constitutive HO-2, as summarized in Figure 2. Catabolism of free haem by HO leads to the production of: (1) carbon monoxide (CO); (2) biliverdin (BV), that is converted by biliverdin reductase (BVR) to the antioxidant bilirubin; and (3) the release of labile Fe, which is promptly bound to ferritin (FtH), collectively preventing cellular oxidative stress [64–66]. However, under pathological conditions, the accumulation of intracellular free haem can exceed the rate of haem degradation by the HO-1 isoenzyme. Furthermore, levels of cellular Fe can be greater than the scavenging capacity of FtH. When this occurs, free haem and/or labile Fe accumulate in cells and drive oxidative stress in the micro-environment. The uncontrolled generation of free radicals and the subsequent imbalance between reactive metabolites and endogenous anti-oxidants constitutes the stress response and ultimately lead to cellular damage and inflammation.

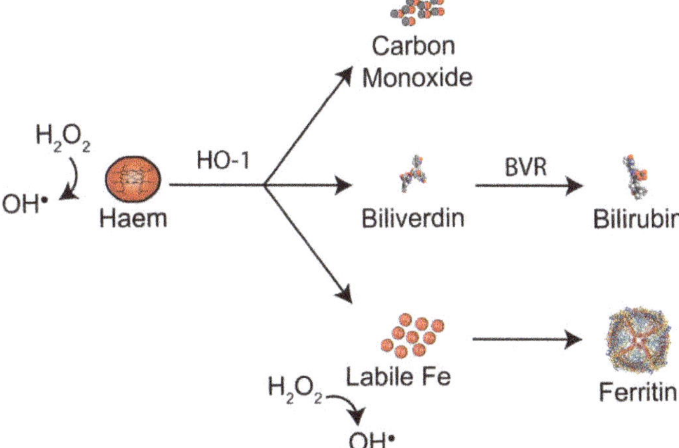

Figure 2. Haem catabolism by HO-1 produces equimolar amounts of carbon monoxide, Biliverdin and labile iron. Biliverdin is converted to bilirubin by biliverdin reductase. Labile Fe can produce ROS, but is rapidly bound to ferritin. Ferritin (PBD ID: 5Z8U) image generated using the RCSB PDB NGL viewer [67]. BVR: Bilirubin reductase; HO-1: Haem oxygenase-1.

Haem directly regulates inflammatory leukocyte migration and retention in vitro and in vivo [68]. In rodent models, intraperitoneal and intrapleural injection of haem results in dose-dependent neutrophil migration into the respective body compartments [68,69]. Haem inhibits neutrophil apoptosis, resulting in the accumulation of neutrophils at sites of haem deposition, and drives expression of proinflammatory cytokines [69–71]. Haem has also been reported to induce surface expression of adhesion molecules—i.e., intercellular adhesion molecule-1 (ICAM-1), vascular adhesion molecule-1 (VCAM-l) and endothelial leukocyte adhesion molecule (E-selectin)—in human endothelial cells, thereby driving the adhesion/retention of leukocytes [72].

Recent evidence suggests haem can trigger activation of innate immune cells via the NLRP3 inflammasome. Dutra et al. showed that haem activation of the NLRP3 inflammasome in bone marrow macrophages was dependent on NADPH oxidases, K^+ efflux and generation of mitochondrial ROS [8]. Notably, NLRP3 activation was independent of haem internalization, lysosomal damage and cell death [8]. Inflammasome activity within immortalized human endothelial cells in response to haem has also been reported in vitro, where haem was sufficient to induce significantly increased IL-1β mRNA transcripts and cytokine release [16]. Intriguingly, HO-1 activity appears to attenuate NLRP3 activity. However, this may be an indirect consequence of haem catabolism by HO-1, rather than direct interactions between HO-1 and NLRP3 [73]. Although recent studies suggest haem is an important trigger of the canonical inflammasome pathway [8,73,74], its functioning via non-canonical NLRP3 inflammasome activation in renal cells has not been explored.

4. Myoglobin-Mediated Pigment Nephropathy

Rhabdomyolysis is a clinical syndrome following physical, thermal, toxic, metabolic, ischaemic, infective and inflammatory insults to muscles [13]. The final step of the skeletal muscle breakdown is the release of toxic intracellular components, such as the hemoprotein myoglobin, into the circulation [10,75].

Myoglobinuric AKI is the most severe complication of rhabdomyolysis [76]. Myoglobin is one of the pathogenic drivers of renal injury following rhabdomyolysis. Myoglobin is cytotoxic, activating both pro-oxidant and inflammatory pathways. Cytotoxicity is augmented in the presence of volume depletion and aciduria, common features of AKI [77,78]. Renal vasoconstriction, tubular obstruction and apoptosis are additional pathological processes in myoglobin toxicity, see Figure 3 [10,12,79].

There is a large volume of published studies describing oxidative stress in myoglobinuric AKI [10,12,13,80]. As for other hemoproteins, myoglobin possesses a haem centre that can catalyse the production of ROS within the kidneys. The haem group within myoglobin is capable of cycling between various oxidative states (ferrous = Fe^{2+}; ferric = Fe^{3+}; and ferryl = Fe^{4+}) that may lead to lipid peroxidation independently of the Fenton reaction and iron release, see Figure 3 [12,13,80].

Most studies of the inflammatory pathogenic processes in myoglobinuric AKI are derived from experimental animal models and transformed cell lines. In a rat model of glycerol-induced rhabdomyolysis, macrophage infiltration was evident in the renal cortex as early as six hours following glycerol injection [79]. In vitro evidence suggests myoglobin polarizes macrophages toward both M1 (pro-inflammatory) and M2 (anti-inflammatory/pro-fibrotic) phenotypes, whilst in vivo research indicates that a reduction in oxidative stress may facilitate kidney tissue repair via a skewing of macrophages toward an M2 subtype [10,81].

Indeed, inflammation is involved in the pathogenesis of rhabdomyolysis-induced AKI, with emerging evidence of a functional role for the NLRP3 inflammasome in this disease process. Komada, et al. [17] reported greater expression of inflammasome-related molecules (NLRP3, ASC, caspase-1 and IL-1β) in the renal parenchyma following glycerol-induced myoglobinuric AKI [17]. Furthermore, activation of the inflammasome pathway correlated with leukocyte infiltration, tubular injury and dysfunction in the diseased kidney. Notably, these endpoints were markedly attenuated in *Nlrp3*^{-/-}, *Asc*^{-/-} and *Casp1*^{-/-} knockout mice [17].

At present, many questions regarding the potential triggers of the inflammasome cascade in myoglobinuric AKI remain unanswered. Komada, et al. [17] carried out in vitro experiments using renal tubular epithelial cells incubated with hemin (the oxidised form of haem), ferrous and ferric myoglobin, all potential stimuli of the NLRP3 inflammasome in myoglobinuric AKI. Although these experimental data were not published, the authors reported that these stimuli were insufficient to activate NLRP3 [17]. Although innate immune cells (DC, macrophages) have the required components for canonical inflammasome activation [74,82], the ability of tubular epithelial cells to secrete mature IL-1β via this two-step process remains uncertain [58,74,82]. Therefore, the absence of inflammatory cells in the in vitro experiments of Komada et al. may explain why they failed to demonstrate triggering of canonical inflammasome activation.

Finally, as the pathogenesis of rhabdomyolysis is multifactorial, the role of other concomitant factors, acting either as priming stimuli or directly activating the NLRP3 inflammasome, should not be ignored. For instance, data from several studies suggest that different types of crystals, such as calcium oxalate, monosodium urate and cholesterol, can function as DAMPs to trigger NLRP3 inflammasome activation [22,25,83]. Recently, we highlighted a potential role for urate crystals in generating oxidative stress and activating the NLRP3 inflammasome in an animal model of rhabdomyolysis-associated AKI [10]. Thus, additional research is required to validate this hypothesis as well as to further elucidate the mechanisms underlying inflammation in human myoglobinuric AKI.

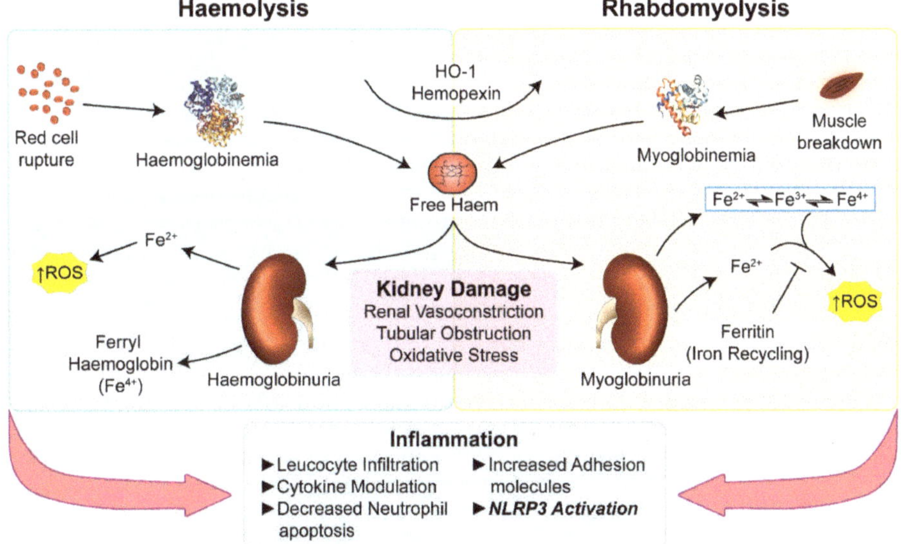

Figure 3. Potential pathways underlying haem-associated kidney injury. Free haem generated by rhabdomyolysis and haemolysis are effectively removed by HO-1 and hemopexin. The binding capacity of these proteins is saturated in pathological conditions and free haem continues to be present. Haemoglobin, myoglobin and plasma free-haem are freely filtered by the glomerulus and can be deposited within the tubules. Oxidative stress, renal vasoconstriction, tubular obstruction by casts, iron-mediated tubular toxicity and inflammation play an important role in acute pigment nephropathy. Myoglobin (PBD ID: 1MBN) and haemoglobin (PBD ID: 1BIJ) structures generated using the RCSB PDB NGL viewer [67]. NLRP3: nucleotide-binding domain-like receptor protein 3; HO-1: Haem Oxygenase-1; ROS: Reactive Oxygen Species.

5. Haemoglobin-Mediated Pigment Nephropathy

Haemolysis is defined as the rupture of red blood cells (RBC) as a result of intrinsic or extrinsic stresses, leading to the release of their intracellular contents, including hemoprotein haemoglobin [84]. Massive intravascular haemolysis is uncommon but occurs in life-threatening conditions such as poisoning, snake and insect envenomation, idiosyncratic drug reactions, haemolytic uraemic syndrome, paroxysmal nocturnal hemoglobinuria, malaria, haemorrhagic fevers, leptospirosis and septic shock [85–91].

In the event of haemolysis, plasma proteins such as haemoglobin-binding haptoglobin and haem-binding hemopexin effectively remove intravascular-produced haemoglobin/haem, thus mitigating haem-mediated deleterious effects [69]. However, under pathological conditions, the binding capacity of these plasma proteins is saturated, resulting in excess free haemoglobin in circulating blood [69]. Haemoglobulin and haem are filtered by the glomerulus, and free haemoglobin in the resultant ultrafiltrate is reabsorbed by the proximal tubules in an endocytic process involving the megalin-cubilin receptor system [65]. However, this absorption transport pathway is also concentration-dependent and large quantities of haemoglobin in the proximal tubules will saturate it, with free haemoglobulin/haem retained in the proximal tubules, leading to nephrotoxicity.

Many diseases featuring massive or recurrent haemolysis are complicated by AKI [9,64,84]. Prior to modern transfusion practices, ABO incompatibility was the most common cause of hemolysis-associated AKI [9]. With the exception of ABO-incompatible blood transfusions, haemolysis is now considered a contributing, rather than sole, trigger in the pathogenesis of haemoglobinuria-related AKI [9]. In fact, some conditions such as poisoning, envenomation and leptospirosis, may present with both haemolysis and rhabdomyolysis [85,92–95]. Furthermore, in malaria-associated AKI, other mechanisms play a greater pathogenic role than haemolysis, including mechanic obstruction by parasitized RBCs, the pro-inflammatory cytokine storm and immune-complex deposition [9,96].

The pathogenesis of haemoglobinuric AKI is multi-factorial, with aciduria, dehydration and renal ischaemia being the established contributing factors in the pathobiological processes [61,62]. These concomitant conditions are thought to enhance haem toxicity by favouring iron release and thus, pro-oxidant cytotoxic conditions [61].

As in myoglobin-derived PN, haemoglobin-derived free haem can drive oxidative stress, increased expression of adhesion molecules and elevated leukocyte infiltration into the diseased kidney [66,72]. Haemolysis also generates DAMP activity that triggers sterile inflammatory responses via the NLRP3 inflammasome [97]. In addition to haem, ruptured RBCs release heat shock proteins, ATP, IL-33 and mtDNA that are recognized triggers of the inflammasome cascade [97]. A correlate is found in humans with the disease of sickle cell, where patients commonly present with a state of chronic low-grade inflammation [69,98].

Intravascular hemolysis may also lead to haemoglobin in different oxidative states, i.e., hemoglobin (Fe^{2+}), methemoglobin (Fe^{3+}), and ferryl haemoglobin (Fe^{4+}) [99]. Nyakundi, et al. [99] demonstrated both haem and ferryl haemoglobin stimulated LPS-primed macrophages to upregulate IL-1β mRNA and induce active IL-1β secretion. Further experiments conducted by Dutra et al. showed that the iron present within the haem molecule, not free iron, was the most important stimulus triggering the NLRP3 inflammasome and IL-1β secretion in macrophages and ultimately contributed to hemolysis-associated lethality [8]. Understanding these molecular pathways triggered by distinct haem motifs may prove useful in identifying novel therapeutic targets for haemoglobin/myoglobin-mediated pigment nephropathies.

6. Inflammasome Inhibition as a Potential Therapeutic Target

The significant pathological role of inflammasome activation in several chronic inflammatory diseases has made it an attractive target for therapeutic intervention. There are two approaches in current strategies inhibiting the inflammasome: (1) Targeting inflammasome activation directly and/or (2) targeting down-stream effects of IL-1β. Here, we review several compounds that could be repurposed, in combination with existing therapies, to ameliorate inflammatory immune responses in PN.

6.1. NLRP3 Inflammasome Inhibitors

Several compounds have been identified and developed for therapeutic inhibition of NLRP3 inflammasome activation. These established inflammasome-inhibiting compounds have been extensively reviewed by Lopez-Castejon and Pelegrin [100] and, more recently, by Baldwin, et al. [101]. Several preclinical studies have already investigated the use of these inflammasome inhibitors in AKI and CKD nephropathies, but their therapeutic efficacy has not been tested in PN.

The second-generation sulfonylurea drug, glyburide (also glibenclamide), is an established compound for the treatment of human type II diabetes mellitus [100,101]. Glyburide blocks K_{ATP} channels, depolarizing the cell membrane, triggering the release of insulin from pancreatic β-cells [100,101]. Glyburide's actions were originally thought to be mediated via its role as a K_{ATP} channel blocker, but emerging evidence suggests that it, in fact, prevents the formation of ASC specks [101]. However, the specific mechanism of the interactions of glyburide and NLRP3 remain poorly understood.

Glyburide has been used in an adenine-rich diet rat model of CKD. In this study, glyburide treatment attenuated NLRP3 expression, improved renal function and ameliorated the CKD histopathology [102]. Unfortunately, glyburide is generally not a recommended treatment in CKD patients due to the increased risk of hypoglycemia [103]. In addition, patients with glucose-6-phosphate dehydrogenase deficiency are susceptible to developing haemolytic anemia following glyburide treatment [104,105].

A novel subclass of sulfonylurea containing compounds, derived from glyburide, was identified by Perregaux, et al. [106]. These compounds inhibited post-translational processing of IL-1β, resulting in little-to-no maturation or extracellular release of the cytokine. One of these compounds, MCC950 (also CP-456,773), was reported by Coll, et al. [107] as a potent, specific inhibitor of the NLRP3 inflammasome. Whilst the mechanism of MCC950-mediated NLRP3 inhibition is still poorly understood, MCC950 has been studied in several disease models, including colitis [108], Parkinson's disease [109], diabetic encephalopathy [110] and non-alcoholic steatohepatitis [111]. Recent studies also evaluated MCC950 in pre-clinical models of AKI and CKD. MCC950 treatment attenuated kidney fibrosis in a murine model of diet-induced oxalate crystal-nephropathy [20]. Furthermore, MCC950 treatment abrogated kidney damage and ameliorated systemic blood pressure in a murine model of hypertension, induced by both surgery (uninephrectomy) and treatment with deoxycorticosterone [60]. MCC950's relatively short half-life and its specificity for the NLRP3 inflammasome [107] make it, and its derivatives, ideal candidates for further investigations in PN.

6.2. Anti-IL-1β and IL-1 Receptor Antagonists

Inhibition of the down-stream IL-1β-signalling pathways has been widely adopted in rheumatology for treatment of auto-inflammatory diseases [112]. Strategies for these therapies involve: (1) Reducing the amount of IL-1β available for activating the endogenous IL-1 receptor (IL-1R) or (2) inhibiting the endogenous receptor directly.

Canakinumab is a potent monoclonal antibody specific for IL-1β [113,114] and an established therapeutic in the treatment of rheumatoid arthritis [112]. Canakinumab has been evaluated in patients with CKD, reducing the risk of major adverse cardiovascular event rates among high-risk atherosclerosis patients [115]. However, no differences in kidney function (as measured by the estimated Glomerulus Filtration Rate) were reported between placebo and Canakinumab-treated CKD patients [115]. A common CKD co-morbidity is gout, which arises as a consequence of increased uric acid. Inflammasome activation is imputed to be the prime mechanism of this auto-inflammatory condition [25]. A clinical trial using Canakinumab showed significantly reduced rates of gout attacks in patients, although no changes in serum uric acid concentrations were observed [116]. Studies such as these provide important foundational evidence for further pre-clinical studies of Canakinumab for the treatment of PN.

Therapeutic strategies targeting the IL-1 receptor (IL-1R) are also used in current clinical practice. Anakinra is a recombinant human IL-1R antagonist, competing with IL-1β for binding with the IL-1R [117]. Anakinra is another established therapeutic in the treatment of auto-inflammatory diseases in rheumatology. Notably, it has been successfully used in patients with Familial Mediterranean Fever (FMF) [118,119], an auto-inflammatory disease associated with mutations in the inflammasome component pyrin that results in triggering inflammasome activation [120,121]. The therapeutic use of anakinra for treating acute gout attacks in CKD patients is currently in clinical trials (ASGARD study), with the results yet to be published [117]. Interestingly, anakinra is being investigated as a third-line therapy in this ASGARD study, following non-response to second-line therapy, where the development of rhabdomyolysis was a reported side-effect [117,122].

Although these IL-1β- and IL-1R-targeting drugs are proving to be effective inflammasome inhibitors, pre-clinical studies investigating their efficacy for the treatment of PN are yet to be performed. These studies need to include in vivo and in vitro models of PN to not only establish therapeutic efficacy but also any unforeseen off-target effects.

7. Concluding Remarks

The release of haem by myoglobin and haemoglobin catabolism is pivotal in the pathogenesis of PN. Whilst haem toxicity is clinically recognized as important, the role of haem in the mechanism of the associated kidney inflammation may be overlooked. Irrespective of its source, haem triggers NLRP3 inflammasome activation, but this mechanistic pathway of disease in PN is still poorly understood. Contemporary studies have shifted to the role of haem driving kidney inflammation via NLRP3 inflammasome activation. The research is focused on the canonical activation of the inflammasome within immune cell populations by haem. The non-canonical activation of the inflammasome in immune cell populations by haem has not been investigated. Furthermore, neither canonical nor non-canonical mechanisms of inflammasome activation within kidney parenchymal cells are fully understood. Well-designed studies are required to address both, focusing on haemolytic driven AKI for which there is currently a lack of information.

The aim of future PN research is to provide evidence to move to pre-clinical studies of potential treatments for both myoglobinuric and haemolytic AKI. Non-renal studies with IL-1R antagonists and direct NLRP3 inflammasome inhibitors are advanced, with small molecules in clinical use for auto-immune rheumatological diseases. Several pre-clinical studies have investigated their therapeutic role in different patterns of kidney disease, but not PN. These studies provide the rationale for translation into clinical trials for the prevention and treatment of PN.

Author Contributions: P.H.F.G, A.J.K, H.H., and K.G. conceptualized the review article. P.H.F.G, K.T.K.G, A.J.K and H.H. contributed in writing, review and editing of the original draft. K.T.K.G. compiled the manuscript and P.H.F.G. supervised the study.

Funding: This research was supported by funds from Pathology Queensland, a Royal Brisbane and Women's Hospital Research Grant, the Kidney Research Foundation, a National Health and Medical Research Council Project Grant (GNT1099222). K.T.K.G. is supported by an Australian Government Research Training Program (RTP) Scholarship.

Acknowledgments: The authors wish to thank Madeleine Kersting-Flynn for her advice and assistance with the illustrations presented in this document. The authors also would like to express our profound thanks for the continued support from the staff and patients at the Royal Brisbane and Women's Hospital and Pathology Queensland.

Abbreviations

AKI	Acute Kidney Injury
ASC	Apoptosis-associated speck-like protein containing a CARD domain
ATP	Adenosine Triphosphate
CARD	Caspase activation and recruitment domain
CD	Cluster of differentiation
CKD	Chronic Kidney Disease
DAMPs	Damage-associated molecular patterns
DC	Dendritic cells
DKD	Diabetic kidney disease
ESCRT	Endosomal sorting complexes required for transport
FMF	Familial Mediterranean Fever

GSDMD	Gasdermin-D
HAMPs	Homeostasis-altering molecular processes
HO	Haem Oxygenase
HO-1	Haem Oxygenase-1
ICAM-l	Intercellular Adhesion Molecule-1
IL	Interleukin
IL-1R	IL-1 receptor
LPS	Lipopolysaccharide
MAVS	Mitochondrial antiviral signal
mtDNA	Mitochondrial DNA
NADPH	Dihydronicotinamide-adenine dinucleotide phosphate
NLRP3	Nucleotide-binding domain-like receptor protein 3
PAMPs	Pathogen-associated molecular patterns
PN	Pigment Nephropathy
PRRs	Pattern recognition receptors
PTEC	Proximal Tubule Epithelial Cells
RBC	Red Blood Cells
ROS	Reactive Oxygen Species
TLRs	Toll-like receptors
UUO	Unilateral ureteral obstruction
VCAM-l	Vascular Adhesion Molecule-1
XO	Xanthine Oxidase

References

1. Sikorski, Z.E. *Chemical and Functional Properties of Food Components*; CRC Press: Boc Raton, FL, USA, 2007.
2. Paoli, M.; Marles-Wright, J.; Smith, A. Structure–Function Relationships in Heme-Proteins. *DNA Cell Biol.* **2002**, *21*, 271–280. [CrossRef] [PubMed]
3. Larsen, R.; Gouveia, Z.; Soares, M.P.; Gozzelino, R.; Kapitulnik, J.; Hebrew, T.; Ryter, S.W.; Immenschuh, S. Heme cytotoxicity and the pathogenesis of immune-mediated inflammatory diseases. *Front. Pharmacol.* **2012**. [CrossRef] [PubMed]
4. Smith, L.J.; Kahraman, A.; Thornton, J.M. Heme proteins-Diversity in structural characteristics, function, and folding. *Proteins Struct. Function Bioinform.* **2010**, *78*, 2349–2368. [CrossRef] [PubMed]
5. Mense, S.M.; Zhang, L. Heme: A versatile signaling molecule controlling the activities of diverse regulators ranging from transcription factors to MAP kinases. *Cell Res.* **2006**, *16*, 681–692. [CrossRef] [PubMed]
6. Immenschuh, S.; Vijayan, V.; Janciauskiene, S.; Gueler, F. Heme as a Target for Therapeutic Interventions. *Front Pharmacol.* **2017**, *8*, 146. [CrossRef]
7. Nangaku, M. Hypoxia and Tubulointerstitial Injury: A Final Common Pathway to End-Stage Renal Failure. *Nephron Exp. Nephrol.* **2004**, *98*, e8–e12. [CrossRef] [PubMed]
8. Dutra, F.F.; Alves, L.S.; Rodrigues, D.; Fernandez, P.L.; de Oliveira, R.B.; Golenbock, D.T.; Zamboni, D.S.; Bozza, M.T. Hemolysis-induced lethality involves inflammasome activation by heme. *Proc. Natl. Acad. Sci. USA* **2014**. [CrossRef]
9. Perazella, M.A.; Rosner, M.H. Clinical features and diagnosis of heme pigment-induced acute kidney injury. Available online: https://www.uptodate.com/contents/clinical-features-and-diagnosis-of-heme-pigment-induced-acute-kidney-injury (accessed on 7 February 2019).
10. Gois, P.H.F.; Canale, D.; Volpini, R.A.; Ferreira, D.; Veras, M.M.; Andrade-Oliveira, V.; Câmara, N.O.S.; Shimizu, M.H.M.; Seguro, A.C. Allopurinol attenuates rhabdomyolysis-associated acute kidney injury: Renal and muscular protection. *Free Radic. Biol. Med.* **2016**, *101*, 176–189. [CrossRef] [PubMed]
11. Heyman, S.N.; Rosen, S.; Fuchs, S.; Epstein, F.H.; Brezis, M. Myoglobinuric acute renal failure in the rat: a role for medullary hypoperfusion, hypoxia, and tubular obstruction. *J. Am. Soc. Nephrol.* **1996**, *7*, 1066–1074.
12. Moore, K.P.; Holt, S.G.; Patel, R.P.; Svistunenko, D.A.; Zackert, W.; Goodier, D.; Reeder, B.J.; Clozel, M.; Anand, R.; Cooper, C.E.; et al. A causative role for redox cycling of myoglobin and its inhibition by alkalinization in the pathogenesis and treatment of rhabdomyolysis-induced renal failure. *J. Biol. Chem.* **1998**, *273*, 31731–31737. [CrossRef] [PubMed]

13. Zager, R.A.; Burkhart, K. Myoglobin toxicity in proximal human kidney cells: Roles of Fe, Ca2+, H2O2, and terminal mitochondrial electron transport. *Kidney Int.* **1997**, *51*, 728–738. [CrossRef] [PubMed]

14. Guo, H.; Callaway, J.B.; Ting, J.P.Y. Inflammasomes: Mechanism of action, role in disease, and therapeutics. *Nat. Med.* **2015**, *21*, 677–687. [CrossRef] [PubMed]

15. Dutra, F.F.; Bozza, M.T. Heme on innate immunity and inflammation. *Front. Pharmacol.* **2014**, *5*, 115. [CrossRef]

16. Erdei, J.; Tóth, A.; Balogh, E.; Nyakundi, B.B.; Bányai, E.; Ryffel, B.; Paragh, G.; Cordero, M.D.; Jeney, V. Induction of NLRP3 Inflammasome Activation by Heme in Human Endothelial Cells. *Oxid. Med. Cell. Longev.* **2018**. [CrossRef] [PubMed]

17. Komada, T.; Usui, F.; Kawashima, A.; Kimura, H.; Karasawa, T.; Inoue, Y.; Kobayashi, M.; Mizushina, Y.; Kasahara, T.; Taniguchi, S.I.; et al. Role of NLRP3 inflammasomes for rhabdomyolysis-induced acute kidney injury. *Sci. Rep.* **2015**. [CrossRef]

18. Schroder, K.; Tschopp, J. The Inflammasomes. *Cell* **2010**, *140*, 821–832. [CrossRef]

19. Brähler, S.; Zinselmeyer, B.H.; Raju, S.; Nitschke, M.; Suleiman, H.; Saunders, B.T.; Johnson, M.W.; Böhner, A.M.C.; Viehmann, S.F.; Theisen, D.J.; et al. Opposing Roles of Dendritic Cell Subsets in Experimental GN. *J. Am. Soc. Nephrol.* **2017**. [CrossRef]

20. Ludwig-Portugall, I.; Bartok, E.; Dhana, E.; Evers, B.D.G.; Primiano, M.J.; Hall, J.P.; Franklin, B.S.; Knolle, P.A.; Hornung, V.; Hartmann, G.; et al. An NLRP3-specific inflammasome inhibitor attenuates crystal-induced kidney fibrosis in mice. *Kidney Int.* **2016**, *90*, 525–539. [CrossRef]

21. Anders, H.J.; Muruve, D.A. The Inflammasomes in Kidney Disease. *J. Am. Soc. Nephrol.* **2011**, *22*, 1007–1018. [CrossRef]

22. Wilson, G.J.; Gois, P.H.F.; Zhang, A.; Wang, X.; Law, B.M.P.; Kassianos, A.J.; Healy, H.G. The Role of Oxidative Stress and Inflammation in Acute Oxalate Nephropathy Associated with Ethylene Glycol Intoxication. *Kidney Int. Rep.* **2018**, *3*, 1217–1221. [CrossRef]

23. Knauf, F.; Asplin, J.R.; Granja, I.; Schmidt, I.M.; Moeckel, G.W.; David, R.J.; Flavell, R.A.; Aronson, P.S. NALP3-mediated inflammation is a principal cause of progressive renal failure in oxalate nephropathy. *Kidney Int.* **2013**, *84*, 895–901. [CrossRef] [PubMed]

24. Yaribeygi, H.; Katsiki, N.; Butler, A.E.; Sahebkar, A. Effects of antidiabetic drugs on NLRP3 inflammasome activity, with a focus on diabetic kidneys. *Drug Discov. Today* **2018**. [CrossRef]

25. Martinon, F.; Pétrilli, V.; Mayor, A.; Tardivel, A.; Tschopp, J. Gout-associated uric acid crystals activate the NALP3 inflammasome. *Nature* **2006**, *440*, 237. [CrossRef] [PubMed]

26. Mulay, S.R.; Kulkarni, O.P.; Rupanagudi, K.V.; Migliorini, A.; Darisipudi, M.N.; Vilaysane, A.; Muruve, D.; Shi, Y.; Munro, F.; Liapis, H.; et al. Calcium oxalate crystals induce renal inflammation by NLRP3-mediated IL-1β secretion. *J. Clin. Investig.* **2013**, *123*, 236–246. [CrossRef]

27. Rajamäki, K.; Lappalainen, J.; Öörni, K.; Välimäki, E.; Matikainen, S.; Kovanen, P.T.; Eklund, K.K. Cholesterol Crystals Activate the NLRP3 Inflammasome in Human Macrophages: A Novel Link between Cholesterol Metabolism and Inflammation. *PLoS ONE* **2010**, *5*, e11765. [CrossRef]

28. Duewell, P.; Kono, H.; Rayner, K.J.; Sirois, C.M.; Vladimer, G.; Bauernfeind, F.G.; Abela, G.S.; Franchi, L.; Nuñez, G.; Schnurr, M.; et al. NLRP3 inflammasomes are required for atherogenesis and activated by cholesterol crystals. *Nature* **2010**, *464*, 1357. [CrossRef] [PubMed]

29. Liston, A.; Masters, S.L. Homeostasis-altering molecular processes as mechanisms of inflammasome activation. *Nat. Rev. Immunol.* **2017**, *17*, 208. [CrossRef] [PubMed]

30. He, Y.; Zeng, M.Y.; Yang, D.; Motro, B.; Núñez, G. NEK7 is an essential mediator of NLRP3 activation downstream of potassium efflux. *Nature* **2016**, *530*, 354–357. [CrossRef]

31. Amores-Iniesta, J.; Barberà-Cremades, M.; Martínez, C.M.; Pons, J.A.; Revilla-Nuin, B.; Martínez-Alarcón, L.; Di Virgilio, F.; Parrilla, P.; Baroja-Mazo, A.; Pelegrín, P. Extracellular ATP Activates the NLRP3 Inflammasome and Is an Early Danger Signal of Skin Allograft Rejection. *Cell Rep.* **2017**, *21*, 3414–3426. [CrossRef] [PubMed]

32. Chen, K.; Zhang, J.; Zhang, W.; Zhang, J.; Yang, J.; Li, K.; He, Y. ATP-P2X4 signaling mediates NLRP3 inflammasome activation: A novel pathway of diabetic nephropathy. *Int. J. Biochem. Cell Biol.* **2013**, *45*, 932–943. [CrossRef]

33. Sadatomi, D.; Nakashioya, K.; Mamiya, S.; Honda, S.; Tanimura, S.; Yamamura, Y.; Kameyama, Y.; Takeda, K. Mitochondrial function is required for extracellular ATP-induced NLRP3 inflammasome activation. *J. Biochem.* **2017**, *161*, 503–512. [CrossRef]

34. Elliott, E.I.; Miller, A.N.; Banoth, B.; Iyer, S.S.; Stotland, A.; Weiss, J.P.; Gottlieb, R.A.; Sutterwala, F.S.; Cassel, S.L. Cutting Edge: Mitochondrial Assembly of the NLRP3 Inflammasome Complex Is Initiated at Priming. *J. Immunol.* **2018**, *200*, 3047. [CrossRef] [PubMed]

35. Zhou, R.; Tardivel, A.; Thorens, B.; Choi, I.; Tschopp, J. Thioredoxin-interacting protein links oxidative stress to inflammasome activation. *Nat. Immunol.* **2010**, *11*, 136–140. [CrossRef] [PubMed]

36. Zhong, Z.; Liang, S.; Sanchez-Lopez, E.; He, F.; Shalapour, S.; Lin, X.j.; Wong, J.; Ding, S.; Seki, E.; Schnabl, B.; et al. New mitochondrial DNA synthesis enables NLRP3 inflammasome activation. *Nature* **2018**. [CrossRef] [PubMed]

37. Lin, K.-M.; Hu, W.; Troutman, T.D.; Jennings, M.; Brewer, T.; Li, X.; Nanda, S.; Cohen, P.; Thomas, J.A.; Pasare, C. IRAK-1 bypasses priming and directly links TLRs to rapid NLRP3 inflammasome activation. *Proc. Natl. Acad. Sci. USA* **2014**, *111*, 775–780. [CrossRef]

38. Liu, T.; Zhang, L.; Joo, D.; Sun, S.-C. NF-κB signaling in inflammation. *Signal Transduct. Target. Ther.* **2017**, *2*, 17023. [CrossRef]

39. Hari, A.; Zhang, Y.; Tu, Z.; Detampel, P.; Stenner, M.; Ganguly, A.; Shi, Y. Activation of NLRP3 inflammasome by crystalline structures via cell surface contact. *Sci. Rep.* **2014**, *4*, 7281. [CrossRef] [PubMed]

40. He, Y.; Hara, H.; Núñez, G. Mechanism and Regulation of NLRP3 Inflammasome Activation. *Trends Biochem. Sci.* **2016**, *41*, 1012–1021. [CrossRef]

41. Hornung, V.; Bauernfeind, F.; Halle, A.; Samstad, E.O.; Kono, H.; Rock, K.L.; Fitzgerald, K.A.; Latz, E. Silica crystals and aluminum salts activate the NALP3 inflammasome through phagosomal destabilization. *Nat. Immunol.* **2008**, *9*, 847. [CrossRef] [PubMed]

42. Bronner, D.N.; Abuaita, B.H.; Chen, X.; Fitzgerald, K.A.; Nuñez, G.; He, Y.; Yin, X.-M.; O'Riordan, M.X.D. Endoplasmic Reticulum Stress Activates the Inflammasome via NLRP3- and Caspase-2-Driven Mitochondrial Damage. *Immunity* **2015**, *43*, 451–462. [CrossRef]

43. Boucher, D.; Monteleone, M.; Coll, R.C.; Chen, K.W.; Ross, C.M.; Teo, J.L.; Gomez, G.A.; Holley, C.L.; Bierschenk, D.; Stacey, K.J.; et al. Caspase-1 self-cleavage is an intrinsic mechanism to terminate inflammasome activity. *J. Exp. Med.* **2018**. [CrossRef]

44. Monteleone, M.; Stanley, A.C.; Chen, K.W.; Brown, D.L.; Bezbradica, J.S.; von Pein, J.B.; Holley, C.L.; Boucher, D.; Shakespear, M.R.; Kapetanovic, R.; et al. Interleukin-1β Maturation Triggers Its Relocation to the Plasma Membrane for Gasdermin-D-Dependent and -Independent Secretion. *Cell Rep.* **2018**, *24*, 1425–1433. [CrossRef] [PubMed]

45. Sborgi, L.; Rühl, S.; Mulvihill, E.; Pipercevic, J.; Heilig, R.; Stahlberg, H.; Farady, C.J.; Müller, D.J.; Broz, P.; Hiller, S. GSDMD membrane pore formation constitutes the mechanism of pyroptotic cell death. *EMBO J.* **2016**, *35*, 1766–1778. [CrossRef] [PubMed]

46. Liu, X.; Zhang, Z.; Ruan, J.; Pan, Y.; Magupalli, V.G.; Wu, H.; Lieberman, J. Inflammasome-activated gasdermin D causes pyroptosis by forming membrane pores. *Nature* **2016**, *535*, 153–158. [CrossRef] [PubMed]

47. Rühl, S.; Shkarina, K.; Demarco, B.; Heilig, R.; Santos, J.C.; Broz, P. ESCRT-dependent membrane repair negatively regulates pyroptosis downstream of GSDMD activation. *Science* **2018**, *362*, 956–960. [CrossRef]

48. Sun, G.; Guzman, E.; Balasanyan, V.; Conner, C.M.; Wong, K.; Zhou, H.R.; Kosik, K.S.; Montell, D.J. A molecular signature for anastasis, recovery from the brink of apoptotic cell death. *J. Cell Biol.* **2017**, *216*, 3355–3368. [CrossRef]

49. Pellegrini, C.; Antonioli, L.; Lopez-Castejon, G.; Blandizzi, C.; Fornai, M. Canonical and non-canonical activation of NLRP3 inflammasome at the crossroad between immune tolerance and intestinal inflammation. *Front. Immunol.* **2017**, *8*, 36. [CrossRef]

50. Kayagaki, N.; Stowe, I.B.; Lee, B.L.; O'Rourke, K.; Anderson, K.; Warming, S.; Cuellar, T.; Haley, B.; Roose-Girma, M.; Phung, Q.T.; et al. Caspase-11 cleaves gasdermin D for non-canonical inflammasome signalling. *Nature* **2015**, *526*, 666–671. [CrossRef]

51. Knodler, L.A.; Crowley, S.M.; Sham, H.P.; Yang, H.; Wrande, M.; Ma, C.; Ernst, R.K.; Steele-Mortimer, O.; Celli, J.; Vallance, B.A. Noncanonical Inflammasome Activation of Caspase-4/Caspase-11 Mediates Epithelial Defenses against Enteric Bacterial Pathogens. *Cell Host Microbe* **2014**, *16*, 249–256. [CrossRef]

52. Vilaysane, A.; Chun, J.; Seamone, M.E.; Wang, W.; Chin, R.; Hirota, S.; Li, Y.; Clark, S.A.; Tschopp, J.; Trpkov, K.; et al. The NLRP3 Inflammasome Promotes Renal Inflammation and Contributes to CKD. *J. Am. Soc. Nephrol.* **2010**, *21*, 1732–1744. [CrossRef]

53. Braga, T.T.; Forni, M.F.; Correa-Costa, M.; Ramos, R.N.; Barbuto, J.A.; Branco, P.; Castoldi, A.; Hiyane, M.I.; Davanso, M.R.; Latz, E.; et al. Soluble Uric Acid Activates the NLRP3 Inflammasome. *Sci. Rep.* **2017**, *7*, 39884. [CrossRef]

54. Shahzad, K.; Bock, F.; Dong, W.; Wang, H.; Kopf, S.; Kohli, S.; Al-Dabet, M.D.M.; Ranjan, S.; Wolter, J.; Wacker, C.; et al. Nlrp3-inflammasome activation in non-myeloid-derived cells aggravates diabetic nephropathy. *Kidney Int.* **2015**, *87*, 74–84. [CrossRef] [PubMed]

55. Gersch, M.S.; Johnson, R.J. Uric acid and the immune response. *Nephrol. Dial. Transplant.* **2006**, *21*, 3046–3047. [CrossRef] [PubMed]

56. Ives, A.; Nomura, J.; Martinon, F.; Roger, T.; LeRoy, D.; Miner, J.N.; Simon, G.; Busso, N.; So, A. Xanthine oxidoreductase regulates macrophage IL1β secretion upon NLRP3 inflammasome activation. *Nat. Commun.* **2015**, *6*, 6555. [CrossRef] [PubMed]

57. Garlanda, C.; Dinarello, C.A.; Mantovani, A. The Interleukin-1 Family: Back to the Future. *Immunity* **2013**, *39*, 1003–1018. [CrossRef]

58. Kim, S.M.; Kim, Y.G.; Kim, D.J.; Park, S.H.; Jeong, K.H.; Lee, Y.H.; Lim, S.J.; Lee, S.H.; Moon, J.Y. Inflammasome-Independent Role of NLRP3 Mediates Mitochondrial Regulation in Renal Injury. *Front. Immunol.* **2018**, *9*, 2563. [CrossRef] [PubMed]

59. Kassianos, A.J.; Wang, X.; Sampangi, S.; Muczynski, K.; Healy, H.; Wilkinson, R. Increased tubulointerstitial recruitment of human CD141hi CLEC9A+ and CD1c+ myeloid dendritic cell subsets in renal fibrosis and chronic kidney disease. *AJP Renal Physiol.* **2013**, *305*, F1391–F1401. [CrossRef] [PubMed]

60. Krishnan, S.M.; Ling, Y.H.; Huuskes, B.M.; Ferens, D.M.; Saini, N.; Chan, C.T.; Diep, H.; Kett, M.M.; Samuel, C.S.; Kemp-Harper, B.K.; et al. Pharmacological inhibition of the NLRP3 inflammasome reduces blood pressure, renal damage, and dysfunction in salt-sensitive hypertension. *Cardiovasc. Res.* **2019**, *115*, 776–787. [CrossRef]

61. Paller, M.S. Hemoglobin- and myoglobin-induced acute renal failure in rats: Role of iron in nephrotoxicity. *Am. J. Physiol.* **1988**, *255*, F539–F544. [CrossRef]

62. Zager, R.A.; Gamelin, L.M. Pathogenetic mechanisms in experimental hemoglobinuric acute renal failure. *Am. J. Physiol.* **1989**, *256*, F446–F455. [CrossRef]

63. Biswas, S.K. Does the Interdependence between Oxidative Stress and Inflammation Explain the Antioxidant Paradox? *Oxid. Med. Cell. Longev.* **2016**. [CrossRef]

64. Qian, Q.; Nath, K.A.; Wu, Y.; Daoud, T.M.; Sethi, S. Hemolysis and acute kidney failure. *Am. J. Kidney Dis.* **2010**. [CrossRef] [PubMed]

65. Tracz, M.J.; Alam, J.; Nath, K.A. Physiology and Pathophysiology of Heme: Implications for Kidney Disease. *J. Am. Soc. Nephrol.* **2007**. [CrossRef]

66. Wagener, F.A.D.T.G.; Eggert, A.; Boerman, O.C.; Oyen, W.J.G.; Verhofstad, A.; Abraham, N.G.; Adema, G.; Van Kooyk, Y.; De Witte, T.; Figdor, C.G. Heme is a potent inducer of inflammation in mice and is counteracted by heme oxygenase. *Blood* **2001**. [CrossRef]

67. Rose, A.S.; Bradley, A.R.; Valasatava, Y.; Duarte, J.M.; Prlić, A.; Rose, P.W. NGL viewer: Web-based molecular graphics for large complexes. *Bioinformatics* **2018**, *34*, 3755–3758. [CrossRef] [PubMed]

68. Porto, B.N.; Alves, L.S.; Fernández, P.L.; Dutra, T.P.; Figueiredo, R.T.; Graça-Souza, A.V.; Bozza, M.T. Heme induces neutrophil migration and reactive oxygen species generation through signaling pathways characteristic of chemotactic receptors. *J. Biol. Chem.* **2007**. [CrossRef]

69. Graça-Souza, A.V.; Arruda, M.A.B.; De Freitas, M.S.; Barja-Fidalgo, C.; Oliveira, P.L. Neutrophil activation by heme: Implications for inflammatory processes. *Blood* **2002**. [CrossRef]

70. Arruda, M.A.; Rossi, A.G.; de Freitas, M.S.; Barja-Fidalgo, C.; Graça-Souza, A.V. Heme inhibits human neutrophil apoptosis: Involvement of phosphoinositide 3-kinase, MAPK, and NF-κB. *J. Immunol.* **2004**, *173*, 2023–2030. [CrossRef]

71. Figueiredo, R.T.; Fernandez, P.L.; Mourao-Sa, D.S.; Porto, B.N.; Dutra, F.F.; Alves, L.S.; Oliveira, M.F.; Oliveira, P.L.; Graça-Souza, A.V.; Bozza, M.T. Characterization of heme as activator of toll-like receptor 4. *J. Biolog. Chem.* **2007**. [CrossRef]

72. Wagener, F.A.; Feldman, E.; de Witte, T.; Abraham, N.G. Heme induces the expression of adhesion molecules ICAM-1, VCAM-1, and E selectin in vascular endothelial cells. *Proc. Soc. Exp. Biol. Med. Soc. Exp. Biol. Med.* **1997**, *216*, 456–463. [CrossRef]

73. Lv, J.; Su, W.; Yu, Q.; Zhang, M.; Di, C.; Lin, X.; Wu, M.; Xia, Z. Heme oxygenase-1 protects airway epithelium against apoptosis by targeting the proinflammatory NLRP3–RXR axis in asthma. *J. Biol. Chem.* **2018**, *293*, 18454–18465. [CrossRef]

74. Lorenz, G.; Darisipudi, M.N.; Anders, H.J. Canonical and non-canonical effects of the NLRP3 inflammasome in kidney inflammation and fibrosis. *Nephrol. Dial. Transplant.* **2014**, *29*, 41–48. [CrossRef]

75. Bosch, X.; Poch, E.; Grau, J.M. Rhabdomyolysis and Acute Kidney Injury. *N. Engl. J. Med.* **2009**, *361*, 62–72. [CrossRef]

76. Korrapati, M.C.; Shaner, B.E.; Schnellmann, R.G. Recovery from Glycerol-Induced Acute Kidney Injury Is Accelerated by Suramin. *J. Pharmacol. Exp. Ther.* **2012**. [CrossRef]

77. Desforges, J.F.; Better, O.S.; Stein, J.H. Early Management of Shock and Prophylaxis of Acute Renal Failure in Traumatic Rhabdomyolysis. *N. Engl. J. Med.* **1990**, *322*, 825–829. [CrossRef]

78. Zager, R.A. Rhabdomyolysis and myohemoglobinuric acute renal failure. *Kidney Int* **1996**, *49*, 314–326. [CrossRef] [PubMed]

79. Homsi, E.; Janino, P.; De Faria, J.B.L. Role of caspases on cell death, inflammation, and cell cycle in glycerol-induced acute renal failure. *Kidney Int.* **2006**, *69*, 1385–1392. [CrossRef]

80. Zager, R.A.; Foerder, C.A. Effects of inorganic iron and myoglobin on in vitro proximal tubular lipid peroxidation and cytotoxicity. *J. Clin. Investig.* **1992**, *89*, 989–995. [CrossRef] [PubMed]

81. Belliere, J.; Casemayou, A.; Ducasse, L.; Zakaroff-Girard, A.; Martins, F.; Iacovoni, J.S.; Guilbeau-Frugier, C.; Buffin-Meyer, B.; Pipy, B.; Chauveau, D.; et al. Specific macrophage subtypes influence the progression of rhabdomyolysis-induced kidney injury. *J. Am. Soc. Nephrol.* **2015**, *26*, 1363–1377. [CrossRef]

82. Lichtnekert, J.; Kulkarni, O.P.; Mulay, S.R.; Rupanagudi, K.V.; Ryu, M.; Allam, R.; Vielhauer, V.; Muruve, D.; Lindenmeyer, M.T.; Cohen, C.D.; et al. Anti-GBM Glomerulonephritis Involves IL-1 but Is Independent of NLRP3/ASC Inflammasome-Mediated Activation of Caspase-1. *PLoS ONE* **2011**, *6*, e26778. [CrossRef] [PubMed]

83. Karasawa, T.; Takahashi, M. The crystal-induced activation of NLRP3 inflammasomes in atherosclerosis. *Inflamm. Regen.* **2017**, *37*, 18. [CrossRef] [PubMed]

84. Nath, K.A.; Murali, N.S. *Myoglobinuric and Hemoglobinuric Acute Kidney Injury*, 5th ed.; Saunders Elsevier: Philadelphia, PA, USA, 2009; pp. 298–304.

85. Anuradha, S.; Arora, S.; Mehrotra, S.; Arora, A.; Kar, P. Acute renal failure following para-phenylenediamine (PPD) poisoning: A case report and review. *Renal Fail.* **2004**, *26*, 329–332. [CrossRef]

86. Fernandez, P.L.; Dutra, F.F.; Alves, L.; Figueiredo, R.T.; Mourão-Sa, D.; Fortes, G.B.; Bergstrand, S.; Lönn, D.; Cevallos, R.R.; Pereira, R.M.S.; et al. Heme Amplifies the Innate Immune Response to Microbial Molecules through Spleen Tyrosine Kinase (Syk)-dependent Reactive Oxygen Species Generation. *J. Biol. Chem.* **2010**, *285*, 32844–32851. [CrossRef]

87. Gois, P.H.F.; Martines, M.S.; Ferreira, D.; Volpini, R.; Canale, D.; Malaque, C.; Crajoinas, R.; Girardi, A.C.C.; Massola Shimizu, M.H.; Seguro, A.C. Allopurinol attenuates acute kidney injury following Bothrops jararaca envenomation. *PLoS Negl. Trop. Dis.* **2017**, *11*, e0006024. [CrossRef]

88. Mate-Kole, M.O.; Yeboah, E.D.; Affram, R.K.; Adu, D. Blackwater fever and acute renal failure in expatriates in Africa. *Renal Fail.* **1996**, *18*, 525–531. [CrossRef]

89. Schrier, S.L. Diagnosis of Hemolytic Anemia in the Adult. Available online: https://www.uptodate.com/contents/diagnosis-of-hemolytic-anemia-in-the-adult (accessed on 12 March 2019).

90. Viraraghavan, R.; Chakravarty, A.G.; Soreth, J. Cefotetan-induced haemolytic anaemia: A review of 85 cases. *Adverse Drug React. Toxicol. Rev.* **2002**, *21*, 101–107. [CrossRef]

91. Chapman, A.B.; Rahbari-Oskoui, F.F.; Bennett, W.M. Acquired cystic disease of the kidney in adults. Available online: https://www.uptodate.com/contents/acquired-cystic-disease-of-the-kidney-in-adults (accessed on 11 March 2019).

92. Abreu, P.A.E.; Seguro, A.C.; Canale, D.; Silva, A.M.G.d.; Matos, L.d.R.B.; Gotti, T.B.; Monaris, D.; Jesus, D.A.d.; Vasconcellos, S.A.; de Brito, T.; et al. Lp25 membrane protein from pathogenic Leptospira spp. is associated with rhabdomyolysis and oliguric acute kidney injury in a guinea pig model of leptospirosis. *PLoS Negl. Trop. Dis.* **2017**, *11*, e0005615. [CrossRef] [PubMed]

93. Albuquerque, P.L.; Jacinto, C.N.; Silva Junior, G.B.; Lima, J.B.; Veras, M.d.S.B.; Daher, E.F.; Daher, E.F. Acute kidney injury caused by Crotalus and Bothrops snake venom: A review of epidemiology, clinical manifestations and treatment. *Rev. Inst. Med. Trop. Sao Paulo* **2013**, *55*, 295–301. [CrossRef]

94. De Bragança, A.C.; Moreau, R.L.M.; De Brito, T.; Shimizu, M.H.M.; Canale, D.; De Jesus, D.A.; Silva, A.M.G.; Gois, P.H.; Seguro, A.C.; Magaldi, A.J. Ecstasy induces reactive oxygen species, kidney water absorption and rhabdomyolysis in normal rats. Effect of N-acetylcysteine and Allopurinol in oxidative stress and muscle fiber damage. *PLoS ONE* **2017**, *12*, e0179199. [CrossRef]

95. Trowbridge, A.A.; Green, J.B.; Bonnett, J.D.; Shohet, S.B.; Ponnappa, B.D.; McCombs, W.B. Hemolytic anemia associated with leptospirosis. Morphologic and lipid studies. *Am. J. Clin. Pathol.* **1981**, *76*, 493–498. [CrossRef]

96. Da Silva Junior, G.B.; Pinto, J.R.; Barros, E.J.G.; Farias, G.M.N.; Daher, E.D.F. Kidney involvement in malaria: An update. *Rev. Inst. Med. Trop. Sao Paulo* **2017**. [CrossRef]

97. Mendonça, R.; Silveira, A.A.A.; Conran, N. Red cell DAMPs and inflammation. *Inflamm. Res.* **2016**. [CrossRef]

98. Wagener, F.A.; Abraham, N.G.; Van Kooyk, Y.; De Witte, T.; Figdor, C.G. Heme-induced cell adhesion in the pathogenesis of sickle-cell disease and inflammation. *Trends Pharmacol. Sci.* **2001**. [CrossRef]

99. Nyakundi, B.B.; Tóth, A.; Balogh, E.; Nagy, B.; Erdei, J.; Ryffel, B.; Paragh, G.; Cordero, M.D.; Jeney, V. Oxidized hemoglobin forms contribute to NLRP3 inflammasome-driven IL-1β production upon intravascular hemolysis. *Biochim. Biophys. Acta Mol. Basis Dis.* **2019**. [CrossRef]

100. López-Castejón, G.; Pelegrín, P. Current status of inflammasome blockers as anti-inflammatory drugs. *Expert Opin. Investig. Drugs* **2012**, *21*, 995–1007. [CrossRef] [PubMed]

101. Baldwin, A.G.; Brough, D.; Freeman, S. Inhibiting the Inflammasome: A Chemical Perspective. *J. Med. Chem.* **2016**, *59*, 1691–1710. [CrossRef] [PubMed]

102. Diwan, V.; Gobe, G.; Brown, L. Glibenclamide improves kidney and heart structure and function in the adenine-diet model of chronic kidney disease. *Pharmacol. Res.* **2014**, *79*, 104–110. [CrossRef] [PubMed]

103. Berns, J.S.; Glickman, J.D. Management of Hyperglycemia in Patients with Type 2 Diabetes and Pre-Dialysis Chronic Kidney Disease or End-Stage Renal Disease. Available online: https://www.uptodate.com/contents/management-of-hyperglycemia-in-patients-with-type-2-diabetes-and-pre-dialysis-chronic-kidney-disease-or-end-stage-renal-disease (accessed on 15 March 2019).

104. Meloni, G.; Meloni, T. Glyburide-induced acute haemolysis in a G6PD-deficient patient with NIDDM. *Br. J. Haematol.* **1996**, *92*, 159–160. [CrossRef] [PubMed]

105. Vinzio, S.; Andrès, E.; Perrin, A.-E.; Schlienger, J.-L.; Goichot, B. Glibenclamide-induced acute haemolytic anaemia revealing a G6PD-deficiency. *Diabetes Res. Clin. Pract.* **2004**, *64*, 181–183. [CrossRef]

106. Perregaux, D.G.; McNiff, P.; Laliberte, R.; Hawryluk, N.; Peurano, H.; Stam, E.; Eggler, J.; Griffiths, R.; Dombroski, M.A.; Gabel, C.A. Identification and characterization of a novel class of interleukin-1 post-translational processing inhibitors. *J. Pharmacol. Exp. Ther.* **2001**, *299*, 187–197. [PubMed]

107. Coll, R.C.; Robertson, A.A.B.; Chae, J.J.; Higgins, S.C.; Muñoz-Planillo, R.; Inserra, M.C.; Vetter, I.; Dungan, L.S.; Monks, B.G.; Stutz, A.; et al. A small-molecule inhibitor of the NLRP3 inflammasome for the treatment of inflammatory diseases. *Nat. Med.* **2015**, *21*, 248–255. [CrossRef] [PubMed]

108. Perera, A.P.; Fernando, R.; Shinde, T.; Gundamaraju, R.; Southam, B.; Sohal, S.S.; Robertson, A.A.B.; Schroder, K.; Kunde, D.; Eri, R. MCC950, a specific small molecule inhibitor of NLRP3 inflammasome attenuates colonic inflammation in spontaneous colitis mice. *Sci. Rep.* **2018**, *8*, 8618. [CrossRef] [PubMed]

109. Gordon, R.; Albornoz, E.A.; Christie, D.C.; Langley, M.R.; Kumar, V.; Mantovani, S.; Robertson, A.A.B.; Butler, M.S.; Rowe, D.B.; O'Neill, L.A.; et al. Inflammasome inhibition prevents α-synuclein pathology and dopaminergic neurodegeneration in mice. *Sci. Transl. Med.* **2018**, *10*, eaah4066. [CrossRef]

110. Zhai, Y.; Meng, X.; Ye, T.; Xie, W.; Sun, G.; Sun, X. Inhibiting the NLRP3 Inflammasome Activation with MCC950 Ameliorates Diabetic Encephalopathy in db/db Mice. *Molecules* **2018**, *23*, 1–14. [CrossRef]

111. Mridha, A.R.; Wree, A.; Robertson, A.A.B.; Yeh, M.M.; Johnson, C.D.; Van Rooyen, D.M.; Haczeyni, F.; Teoh, N.C.H.; Savard, C.; Ioannou, G.N.; et al. NLRP3 inflammasome blockade reduces liver inflammation and fibrosis in experimental NASH in mice. *J. Hepatol.* **2017**, *66*, 1037–1046. [CrossRef]

112. Vitale, A.; Insalaco, A.; Sfriso, P.; Lopalco, G.; Emmi, G.; Cattalini, M.; Manna, R.; Cimaz, R.; Priori, R.; Talarico, R.; et al. A Snapshot on the On-Label and Off-Label Use of the Interleukin-1 Inhibitors in Italy among Rheumatologists and Pediatric Rheumatologists: A Nationwide Multi-Center Retrospective Observational Study. *Front. Pharmacol.* **2016**, *7*, 380. [CrossRef]

113. Alten, R.; Gram, H.; Joosten, L.A.; Berg, W.B.v.d.; Sieper, J.; Wassenberg, S.; Burmester, G.; van Riel, P.; Diaz-Lorente, M.; Bruin, G.J.M.; et al. The human anti-IL-1β monoclonal antibody ACZ885 is effective in joint inflammation models in mice and in a proof-of-concept study in patients with rheumatoid arthritis. *Arthritis Res. Ther.* **2008**, *10*, R67. [CrossRef]

114. Rondeau, J.-M.; Ramage, P.; Zurini, M.; Gram, H. The molecular mode of action and species specificity of canakinumab, a human monoclonal antibody neutralizing IL-1β. *mAbs* **2015**, *7*, 1151–1160. [CrossRef]

115. Ridker, P.M.; MacFadyen, J.G.; Glynn, R.J.; Koenig, W.; Libby, P.; Everett, B.M.; Lefkowitz, M.; Thuren, T.; Cornel, J.H. Inhibition of Interleukin-1beta by Canakinumab and Cardiovascular Outcomes in Patients With Chronic Kidney Disease. *J. Am. Coll. Cardiol.* **2018**, *71*, 2405–2414. [CrossRef] [PubMed]

116. Solomon, D.H.; Glynn, R.J.; MacFadyen, J.G.; Libby, P.; Thuren, T.; Everett, B.M.; Ridker, P.M. Relationship of Interleukin-1β Blockade With Incident Gout and Serum Uric Acid Levels: Exploratory Analysis of a Randomized Controlled TrialInterleukin-1β Blockade, Incident Gout, and Serum Uric Acid Levels. *Ann. Intern. Med.* **2018**, *169*, 535–542. [CrossRef] [PubMed]

117. Balasubramaniam, G.; Parker, T.; Turner, D.; Parker, M.; Scales, J.; Harnett, P.; Harrison, M.; Ahmed, K.; Bhagat, S.; Marianayagam, T.; et al. Feasibility randomised multicentre, double-blind, double-dummy controlled trial of anakinra, an interleukin-1 receptor antagonist versus intramuscular methylprednisolone for acute gout attacks in patients with chronic kidney disease (ASGARD): Protocol study. *BMJ Open* **2017**, *7*, e017121. [PubMed]

118. Ben-Zvi, I.; Kukuy, O.; Giat, E.; Pras, E.; Feld, O.; Kivity, S.; Perski, O.; Bornstein, G.; Grossman, C.; Harari, G.; et al. Anakinra for Colchicine-Resistant Familial Mediterranean Fever: A Randomized, Double-Blind, Placebo-Controlled Trial. *Arthritis Rheumatol.* **2017**, *69*, 854–862. [CrossRef] [PubMed]

119. Ugurlu, S.; Ergezen, B.; Ozdogan, H. Anakinra treatment in patients with Familial Mediterranean Fever: A single-center experience. *Pediatr. Rheumatol.* **2015**, *13*, P123. [CrossRef]

120. Moghaddas, F.; Llamas, R.; De Nardo, D.; Martinez-Banaclocha, H.; Martinez-Garcia, J.J.; Mesa-del-Castillo, P.; Baker, P.J.; Gargallo, V.; Mensa-Vilaro, A.; Canna, S.; et al. A novel Pyrin-Associated Autoinflammation with Neutrophilic Dermatosis mutation further defines 14-3-3 binding of pyrin and distinction to Familial Mediterranean Fever. *Ann. Rheum. Dis.* **2017**, *76*, 2085–2094. [CrossRef] [PubMed]

121. Masters, S.L.; Lagou, V.; Jéru, I.; Baker, P.J.; Van Eyck, L.; Parry, D.A.; Lawless, D.; De Nardo, D.; Garcia-Perez, J.E.; Dagley, L.F.; et al. Familial autoinflammation with neutrophilic dermatosis reveals a regulatory mechanism of pyrin activation. *Sci. Transl. Med.* **2016**, *8*, 332–345. [CrossRef] [PubMed]

122. Curiel, R.V.; Guzman, N.J. Challenges Associated with the Management of Gouty Arthritis in Patients with Chronic Kidney Disease: A Systematic Review. *Semin. Arthritis Rheum.* **2012**, *42*, 166–178. [CrossRef] [PubMed]

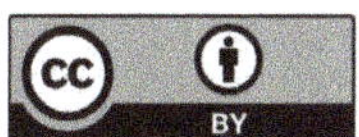

International Journal of
Molecular Sciences

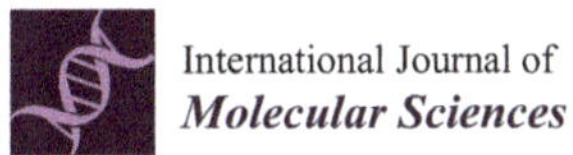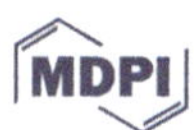

Review

Glomerular Hematuria: Cause or Consequence of Renal Inflammation?

Juan Antonio Moreno [1,2,*], Ángel Sevillano [3], Eduardo Gutiérrez [3], Melania Guerrero-Hue [1,2], Cristina Vázquez-Carballo [1], Claudia Yuste [3], Carmen Herencia [1], Cristina García-Caballero [1], Manuel Praga [3] and Jesús Egido [1,4,*]

[1]   Renal, Vascular and Diabetes Research Laboratory. Fundacion Jimenez Diaz University Hospital-Health Research Institute (FIIS-FJD), Autonoma University of Madrid (UAM), 28040 Madrid, Spain; mel10anie@gmail.com (M.G.-H.); cvazqu01@ucm.es (C.V.-C.); carmen_herencia@hotmail.com (C.H.); crisgcomplutense@gmail.com (C.G.-C.)
[2]   Department of Cell Biology, Physiology, and Immunology, Maimonides Biomedical Research Institute of Cordoba (IMIBIC), University of Cordoba, 14014 Cordoba, Spain
[3]   Department of Nephrology, Hospital 12 de Octubre, 28040 Madrid, Spain; sevillano.am@gmail.com (Á.S.); eduardogutmat90@hotmail.com (E.G.); claudiayustelozano@yahoo.es (C.Y.); mpragat@senefro.org (M.P.)
[4]   Spanish Biomedical Research Centre in Diabetes and Associated Metabolic Disorders (CIBERDEM), 28040 Madrid, Spain
*   Correspondence: juan.moreno@uco.es (J.A.M.); jegido@quironsalud.es (J.E.)

Received: 29 March 2019; Accepted: 28 April 2019; Published: 5 May 2019

Abstract: Glomerular hematuria is a cardinal symptom of renal disease. Glomerular hematuria may be classified as microhematuria or macrohematuria according to the number of red blood cells in urine. Recent evidence suggests a pathological role of persistent glomerular microhematuria in the progression of renal disease. Moreover, gross hematuria, or macrohematuria, promotes acute kidney injury (AKI), with subsequent impairment of renal function in a high proportion of patients. In this pathological context, hemoglobin, heme, or iron released from red blood cells in the urinary space may cause direct tubular cell injury, oxidative stress, pro-inflammatory cytokine production, and further monocyte/macrophage recruitment. The aim of this manuscript is to review the role of glomerular hematuria in kidney injury, the role of inflammation as cause and consequence of glomerular hematuria, and to discuss novel therapies to combat hematuria.

Keywords: hematuria; inflammation; oxidative stress; tubular injury; AKI; chronic kidney disease (CKD)

---

1. Introduction

Hematuria is described as the presence of red blood cells (RBCs) in the urine. Dysmorphic (abnormally shaped) RBCs in the urine are the consequence of RBC egression through the glomerular filtration barrier, and indicate hematuria of glomerular origin. Glomerular hematuria is a frequent manifestation of many renal diseases, and may be classified as microscopic or macroscopic according to its intensity. Recent evidence suggests a negative repercussion of glomerular hematuria on kidney function. In addition, gross hematuria promotes acute kidney injury (AKI), with a subsequent impairment of renal function by different pathological mechanisms, including an exacerbated inflammatory response. In the next sections, we will fully address the role of glomerular hematuria on kidney injury, emphasizing the causes as well as the pathophysiological consequences.

2. Glomerular Hematuria: An Important and Often-Neglected Clinical Sign

2.1. Prevalence of Glomerular Hematuria

The prevalence of hematuria in the general population is certainly unsettled. Screening programs show hematuria in 0.18–16.1% of healthy adults [1–5] and in between 0.03% and 3.9% of children [6–9]. This broad range reflects a relative lack of interest in hematuria, based in its traditionally benign consideration, the absence of standardized methods to detect and quantify hematuria [10,11], or even the difficulties in distinguishing non-glomerular from glomerular hematuria. Moreover, there is striking limited data on the prevalence and severity of glomerular hematuria in renal biopsy registries [12–16]. In these studies, the occurrence of glomerular hematuria ranged between 63.7% and 75.8% of cases. Glomerular hematuria seems to be more frequent in males than in females, regardless of age [17]. Children present more frequent macroscopic hematuria bouts than adults, whereas microhematuria is more common in adults [12,17].

2.2. Common Causes of Glomerular Hematuria

IgA nephropathy (IgAN), the commonest primary glomerulonephritis (GN), is the most frequent cause of glomerular hematuria (Table 1) [12,17]. Approximately half of patients can present with outbreaks of macroscopic gross hematuria (MGH), while the other half can do so with microhematuria. Macroscopic bouts of hematuria are more common in the early stages of IgAN and in children, concomitant with mucosal infections, usually in the respiratory tract and occasionally in the gastrointestinal tract [18].

Table 1. Significance of hematuria in glomerular disease.

Disease	Significance
Lupus nephritis	Classical symptom Marker of activity [19]
ANCA-associated vasculitis	Classical symptom Marker of activity Marker of risk to relapse after response to therapy [20]
Disorders of collagen IV α345	Classical symptom
IgAN	Classical symptom Marker of activity Probable implicated in progression of the disease Implicated in AKI associated to gross hematuria [21] Probable risk factor to progression to ESRD [22]
Other primary glomerulopathies	Classical symptom Marker of activity [19]

Rapidly progressive glomerulonephritis (RPGN), vasculitis, and acute glomerular inflammation, as observed in postinfectious GN or lupus, may also be associated with glomerular hematuria. Although hematuria is a usual urinalysis feature in endocapillary GN [23], extracapillary GN [12], and membranoproliferative GN [24], the real prevalence of hematuria in these diseases is mainly based in observational cohorts [25–27]. Data from the Spanish renal biopsy registry [17] reported an unexpectedly high rate of hematuria (50%) among patients that were traditionally considered as not hematuric GN, including minimal change disease, membranous GN, or focal and segmental glomerulosclerosis. In the recently characterized C3 glomerulonephritis (C3GN), hematuria—mainly microhematuria—was also present in 87% of the patients [28]. Interestingly, macrohematuria bouts have been also described in C3GN concurrently with upper respiratory tract infections, mimicking IgAN [29].

Current advances in genetic testing have allowed the condition previously known "benign familial hematuria" to be split into several type-IV collagen-associated diseases, such as Alport syndrome, thin basement membrane disease (TBMN), and the hereditary angiopathy, nephropathy, aneurysms and muscle cramps syndrome (HANAC) [30]. These type IV collagen-related disorders show persistent microscopic hematuria in the early stages, which progress over the years to proteinuria and chronic kidney disease (CKD), dependent on individual genetic background [31]. Further, infections have been reported as a trigger of macroscopic bouts of hematuria in collagen-associated disorders [32,33]. Finally, anticoagulant-related nephropathy (ARN) is a recently described entity characterized by gross glomerular hematuria and AKI in patients receiving warfarin [34] or other types of anticoagulant therapy [35,36]. ARN is secondary to a profuse glomerular hemorrhage as a consequence of over-anticoagulation (INR > 3) [37]. ARN shows a disease rate of 2–26 cases per year of follow-up [38–40] and a prevalence of the entity of 20% in over-coagulated patients (INR > 3) [41]. Unpublished data from our group shows that anticoagulant therapy is associated with AKI related to hematuria bouts in patients with IgAN. This could be a link between ARN and IgAN.

3. Hematuria and Renal Damage: Cause or Consequence?

3.1. Hematuria as a Sign of Glomerular Inflammation and Disease Progression

Although hematuria is a cardinal symptom of renal disease, it has occupied very little relevance as a negative prognostic factor, unlike proteinuria that continues to play a central role in the diagnosis and treatment of kidney diseases. This lack of interest in hematuria is surprising because it is a defining symptom of IgAN and other pathologies. New evidence suggests a link between inflammation and the genesis of glomerular hematuria. In an experimental model of IgAN, treatment with an IgA1 protease decreased IgA1 deposition—a fact that correlated with a decrease in inflammation, mesangial expansion, and from a clinical point of view, with a very significant reduction in hematuria without a significant influence on proteinuria [42]. In IgAN patients, macroscopic hematuria coincides with aero-digestive infections [43], indicating that dysregulation of the mucosal immune system may play an important role in the pathogenesis of hematuria through a mucosa–kidney axis [44]. In fact, the activation of Toll-like receptors (TLRs) by bacterial or viral antigens causes polyclonal lymphocyte proliferation [45,46] and the formation of circulating immune complex [43,47]. Another possible mechanism involved in the exacerbation of macrohematuria by inflammation includes the CX3CL1/CX3CR1 axis. The peripheral mononuclear cells of patients with IgAN have a higher expression of CX3CR1 during the episode of macrohematuria, as well as increased serum and urinary levels of CX3CL1, the unique ligand of CX3CR1 [48]. The CX3CL1/CX3CR1 axis may play a primordial role through its chemotactic activity to recruit infiltrating cells that can modify the glomerular filtration barrier. Increased CXC3CL1 expression is not exclusive to IgAN, and can be increased in other glomerular diseases associated with hematuria, such as lupus nephritis [49].

Recent data have shown the value of hematuria as a possible marker of relapse in antineutrophil cytoplasmic antibody (ANCA)-associated vasculitis. The authors found a significant positive association between the persistence of hematuria and subsequent nephritis relapse, although this association was not significant with the persistence of proteinuria [20]. One of the great future challenges is the establishment of a clear association between the glomerular damage and its potential utility to decide if it is necessary to increase the immunosuppressive treatment. Following these studies, the question arises as to whether hematuria is a simple marker of major renal damage. Hematuria could be an early indicator of recurrence, particularly if we consider that this is the first study examining the value of the level of hematuria in the relapse of vasculitis. Hematuria was previously demonstrated as a marker of flare in patients with systematic lupus erythematosus (SLE). Ding et al. suggested that alterations in the sediment, either in the form of isolated microhematuria or associated with sterile pyuria, were associated with the activity of the SLE, being able to serve as a marker of activity phase [19]. This hypothesis was confirmed in an analysis based on a prospective study of urine sediment changes in the Ohio SLE study [50].

3.2. Pathophysiological Consequences of Hematuria (AKI and CKD)

3.2.1. Hematuria and AKI

Renal findings in pathologies related to glomerular hematuria usually include tubules filled with RBC casts and acute tubular necrosis, mainly during the gross hematuria bouts. Massive hematuria of glomerular origin produces AKI and damage in tubular cells through different mechanisms: (a) direct tubular damage due to intratubular obstruction of the blood casts, (b) direct tubular toxic effect of hemoglobin (Hb) and heme produced after rupture of the erythrocytes in the tubular lumen, and (c) processes of erythrophagocytosis by the renal tubular cells. Taking all these aspects into account, the duration of macrohematuria bouts becomes a crucial phenomenon for the recovery of renal function. This may be especially relevant in elderly patients and patients with previous chronic renal failure, who may not be able to recover their full functional capacity, especially if the insult is prolonged [21,51].

From a physiopathological point of view, red blood cells in the urine in patients with hematuria release Hb and heme-related products, which are further taken up by tubular cells (Figure 1). Once inside the cell, Hb dissociates, releasing the globins and the heme group, which induces several pathological effects, including oxidative stress, cell death, inflammation, and fibrosis [51,52]. Recent data from our group show that, in addition to the tubular cells, podocytes may be the cellular target of Hb-mediated kidney damage. Thus, Hb induces oxidative damage, podocyte dysfunction, and finally apoptosis, with the detachment of the podocyte from the glomerular capillary [53]. The traffic of Hb through the capillary wall can damage the podocyte, and consequently originate an alteration of the glomerular filtration barrier in patients with glomerular diseases with outbreaks of macroscopic hematuria, such as IgAN. This could explain, at least in part, the deterioration of renal function suffered by those patients after a hematuria bout, especially in elderly patients [21]. However, this hypothesis has not yet been tested. The injury suffered by erythrocytes during their pass throughout the glomerular filtration barrier may promote the release of microvesicles containing microRNA (miRNA). miRNA can be swallowed by nearly all cells, playing an important role in the regulation of oxidative stress and intercellular communication by regulating gene expression. The more prevalent miRNA present in the urinary sediment of IgAN patients with hematuria were mainly derived from urinary erythrocytes, such as miR-25-3p, miR-144-3p, and miR-486-5p [54]. That implies that miRNA delivered by hematuria could act over renal parenchymal cells, changing their gene expression, and could be involved in the pathogenesis and evolution of kidney disease [55]. In other words, the presence of specific miRNA in the sediment could be a marker of the activity of hematuric disease, and may be a useful diagnostic tool. Thus, miR-215-5p and miR-378i appear more frequently in IgAN patients [54,56].

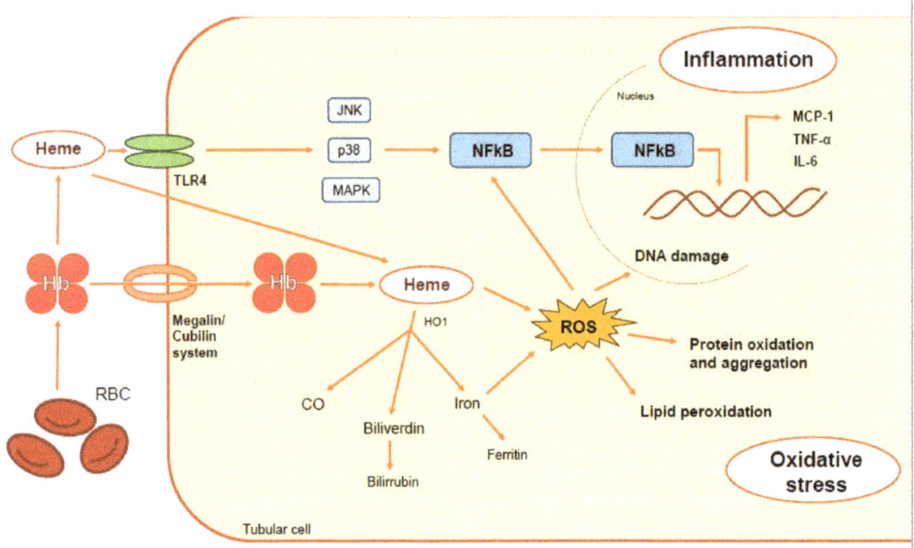

Figure 1. Pathophysiological mechanisms involved in renal damage associated with hematuria. Hemoglobin released by intratubular degradation of erythrocytes may be incorporated into proximal tubules through the megalin-cubilin receptor system or degraded in the tubular lumen, releasing heme. Hb, heme and iron accumulation within tubular cells triggers oxidative stress (lipid peroxidation, protein oxidation and aggregation and DNA damage) and inflammatory cytokine secretion (MCP-1 (monocyte chemoattractant protein 1), TNF-alpha (tumor necrosis factor-alpha), and interleukin 6 (IL-6)) throughout NF-κB transcription factor activation. The heme group may be recognized by the Toll-Like Receptor 4 (TLR4), resulting in the activation of the pro-inflammatory downstream signaling pathways like c-Jun kinases, p38, MAPK and NF-κB.

3.2.2. Hematuria as a Risk Factor for CKD

For many years, hematuria has been considered as only a symptom of some renal disorders. However, multiple studies have challenged this concept, pointing out that the presence of hematuria is associated with an increased risk of developing end-stage renal disease (ESRD). Glomerular diseases, specially IgAN, constitute the scenario where the association between hematuria and long-term renal dysfunction have been best analyzed. In this way, the persistence of hematuria in IgAN has been related to a greater probability of developing ESRD compared to patients with minimal or negative hematuria [22]. In fact, in that disease mild hematuria is associated with an increased risk of ESRD after 10 years of follow-up [57].

In an epidemiological study, the presence of isolated microhematuria significantly increased the risk for ESRD after 22 years of follow-up in a young Israeli population [6]. The presence of hematuria was also associated with a faster decline in renal function in advanced CKD patients compared with those without hematuria [58]. Similar findings emerged from the Chronic Renal Insufficiency Cohort (CRIC) Study [59] and the EPPIC (Evaluating Prevention of Progression In Chronic kidney disease) trials [60]. These studies evidenced an increase of the risk of ESRD after two years of follow-up among patients with baseline hematuria and a decrease of the risk to develop ESRD in those without hematuria. Finally, a recent report showed a significant association of hematuria with an increased risk of ESDR in a group of patients with diabetic nephropathy—the first cause of CKD in developed countries [61]. Based on these pieces of evidence, we consider that hematuria should be added to the traditional risk factor of CKD progression.

4. Should Hematuria be Included as a Surrogate Marker in Clinical Trials of Renal Diseases?

The search for adequate surrogate markers of disease progression, including the progression of renal diseases, is a key issue in many clinical conditions. However, the doubling of serum creatinine is currently the only validated marker associated with renal outcome [62]. Some evidence indicates that proteinuria disappearance could also be a good candidate as a surrogate marker, but further studies are necessary before its acceptance [62]. Hematuria is considered a marker of activity in ANCA vasculitis, lupus nephritis, or IgAN [19,20,63], and recent data indicate that the persistence of hematuria in IgAN is associated with increased risk of the development of ESRD [21,64,65]. For that reason, hematuria disappearance could be a surrogate marker of renal outcome in different diseases, such as vasculitis or glomerulonephritis. However, additional studies are necessary to validate this hypothesis.

5. Hematuria at the Crossroads of Inflammation and Oxidative Stress

The lysis of RBC in the urinary space releases Hb and heme-related products. Hb is incorporated into the kidney through the megalin/cubilin system, and after their oxidation and intracellular destabilization, heme is released and exerts its cytotoxic effect on the renal cells (particularly on the renal tubular epithelium) [66]. Heme consists of a tetrapyrrole ring with an iron atom bound in the center, coordinated to four pyrrole rings [67]. Heme released from the RBC generates oxidative stress, promoting the oxidation of proteins and lipids [68,69], altering the integrity of the cells, and damaging the DNA [70]. The structural instability of heme is essential for the induction of oxidative stress and inflammatory response [71]. Because of its structural properties, especially the hydrophobicity of the porphyrin ring, heme can be incorporated in the lipid bilayer that constitutes cell membranes, where it increases cellular susceptibility to oxidative damage [72]. Additionally, free iron is a potent oxidant and can generate free radicals through the Fenton reaction.

Heme has proinflammatory properties, including leukocyte activation and migration, increased expression of adhesion molecules, and the induction of acute-phase proteins. Thus, heme promotes endothelial activation and elicits the expression of adhesion molecules such as ICAM-1, VCAM-1, E-selectin, P-selectin, and von Willebrand factor [73–75], which facilitates the recruitment and migration of leukocytes [73,76].

Heme also promotes direct pro-inflammatory effects, for example, by activating the production of leukotriene B4 in tissue macrophages, which acts as a chemotactic agent of neutrophils [77]. Additionally, heme can act directly on neutrophils by delaying their apoptosis [78], enhancing their harmful effect on tissue [78]. Heme has been identified as a damage-associated molecular pattern (DAMP), a group of endogenous molecules derived from damaged cells capable of promoting and exacerbating the immune response. These DAMPs are recognized by pattern-recognition receptors (PRRs), within the family of TLRs. Specifically, heme is a ligand of a member of this family—the TLR4 receptor [79]. The activation of TLR4 by heme induces an inflammatory response through the activation of the transcription factor NF-kB [75,80]. As a ligand of TLR4, heme promotes the activation of several downstream signaling pathways, such as c-Jun kinases, p38, and MAPK [81], thus inducing an inflammatory response throughout MCP-1 production [82]. The TLR4 antagonist TAK-242 reduced these heme side effects, suggesting a direct relationship between inflammation and heme through TLR4 in renal tubular cells. Another pathway involved in the inflammation induced by heme is the activation of the NLRP3 (nitrogen permease regulator-like 3) inflammasome, leading to the release of different cytokines and chemokines involved in the recruitment of monocytes/macrophages [83].

6. Can We Envision a Therapeutic Approach for Hematuria-Associated Diseases?

There are no specific therapies to decrease adverse effects associated with hematuria in glomerular diseases. However, the more plausible therapeutic option would be oriented towards the prevention of hematuria bouts and treatment of the nephrotoxic effect of hematuria on renal cells.

6.1. Treatment for the Prevention of Gross Hematuria Bouts

Since hematuria was considered as just a benign symptom for decades, no significant effort has been made to treat macrohematuria. Indeed, the Kidney Disease: Improving Global Outcomes (KDIGO) guidelines only recommend supportive treatment for IgAN patients in this context, although this population is at high risk of developing acute or chronic kidney failure [21]. Immunosuppressor therapy, and most specifically corticosteroids, seems a logical option to treat macrohematuria episodes because inflammation is implicated in this phenomenon and because patients with IgAN, ANCA-vasculitis, or lupus nephritis that respond to this therapy usually experience hematuria disappearance. However, to date, there is no evidence to support this hypothesis.

The introduction of budesonide—a new oral corticosteroid with fewer systemic adverse events—provides opportunities to further explore therapeutic approaches for patients with persistent episodes of macroscopic hematuria [84]. Interestingly, budesonide treatment reduced hematuria in IgAN patients from the NEFIGAN clinical trial [85]. Since macrohematuria bouts are usually preceded by upper respiratory infection, tonsillectomy may be considered as another approach in IgAN patients with recurrent tonsillitis, though the results are contradictory [86].

6.2. Treatment of the Nephrotoxic Effect of Hematuria

No drug therapy has yet been tested in the management of nephrotoxicity induced by glomerular hematuria. However, based on the actual knowledge of pathogenesis of the damage, some therapeutic options could be effective: (1) alkalinization of the urine to reduce the dissociation of iron from the Hb, (2) diuretics to tubular obstruction by RBC casts, (3) iron chelators (deferiprone or deferoxamine) to decrease iron-nephrotoxicity, and (4) anti-oxidant and anti-inflammatory drugs, such as N-acetylcysteine or Nrf2 inducers. Although there are no current studies reporting beneficial effects on hematuria, a recent paper showed that the administration of N-acetylcysteine prevented Scr increase in 5/6 nephrectomized rats with warfarin-induced AKI [87].

7. Conclusions

Hematuria is a common urinary finding present in several glomerular diseases and patients with bad control of coagulation, among other conditions. Recent studies indicate a pathological role of hematuria in renal damage by promoting AKI and progression to CKD. The renal damage mediated by hematuria is related to nephrotoxic actions of Hb and heme on tubular cells, although data from our studies may suggest that the podocyte may be another cellular target of these molecules. Inflammation and oxidative stress are key processes involved in hematuria-related diseases, and may be plausible targets to develop novel therapeutic approaches.

Funding: Supported by FIS/FEDER CP14/00008, CP16/00017, PI15/00448, PI16/00735, PI16/02057, PI17/00130, PI17/01495, ISCIII-RETIC REDinREN RD012/0021, RD016/0009 FEDER funds, Spanish Ministry of Economy and Competitiveness (RYC-2017-22369), Sociedad Española de Nefrología, Fundacion Renal Iñigo Álvarez de Toledo (FRIAT), Comunidad de Madrid CIFRA2 B2017/BMD-3686 and Spanish Biomedical Research Centre in Diabetes and Associated Metabolic Disorders (CIBERDEM).

Conflicts of Interest: The authors declare no conflict of interest.

References

1. Woolhandler, S.; Pels, R.J.; Bor, D.H.; Himmelstein, D.U.; Lawrence, R.S. Dipstick urinalysis screening of asymptomatic adults for urinary tract disorders. I. Hematuria and proteinuria. *JAMA* **1989**, *262*, 1214–1219. [CrossRef] [PubMed]
2. Hiatt, R.A.; Ordoñez, J.D. Dipstick urinalysis screening, asymptomatic microhematuria, and subsequent urological cancers in a population-based sample. *Cancer Epidemiol. Biomarkers Prev.* **1994**, *3*, 439–443.

3. Ramirez, S.P.B.; Kapke, A.; Port, F.K.; Wolfe, R.A.; Saran, R.; Pearson, J.; Hirth, R.A.; Messana, J.M.; Daugirdas, J.T. Dialysis Dose Scaled to Body Surface Area and Size-Adjusted, Sex-Specific Patient Mortality. *Clin. J. Am. Soc. Nephrol.* **2012**, *7*, 1977–1987. [CrossRef] [PubMed]

4. Chadban, S.J.; Briganti, E.M.; Kerr, P.G.; Dunstan, D.W.; Welborn, T.A.; Zimmet, P.Z.; Atkins, R.C. Prevalence of kidney damage in Australian adults: The AusDiab kidney study. *J. Am. Soc. Nephrol.* **2003**, *14*, S131–S138. [CrossRef] [PubMed]

5. Ong, L.M.; Punithavathi, N.; Thurairatnam, D.; Zainal, H.; Beh, M.L.; Morad, Z.; Lee, S.Y.; Bavanandan, S.; Kok, L.S. Prevalence and risk factors for proteinuria: The National Kidney Foundation of Malaysia Lifecheck Health Screening programme. *Nephrology* **2013**, *18*, 569–575. [CrossRef]

6. Vivante, A.; Afek, A.; Frenkel-Nir, Y.; Tzur, D.; Farfel, A.; Golan, E.; Chaiter, Y.; Shohat, T.; Skorecki, K.; Calderon-Margalit, R. Persistent asymptomatic isolated microscopic hematuria in Israeli adolescents and young adults and risk for end-stage renal disease. *JAMA* **2011**, *306*, 729–736. [CrossRef] [PubMed]

7. Hajar, F.; Taleb, M.; Aoun, B.; Shatila, A. Dipstick urine analysis screening among asymptomatic school children. *N. Am. J. Med. Sci.* **2011**, 179–184. [CrossRef] [PubMed]

8. Chen, W.; Liu, Q.; Wang, H.; Chen, W.; Johnson, R.J.; Dong, X.; Li, H.; Ba, S.; Tan, J.; Luo, N.; et al. Prevalence and risk factors of chronic kidney disease: A population study in the Tibetan population. *Nephrol. Dial. Trans.* **2011**, *26*, 1592–1599. [CrossRef] [PubMed]

9. Murakami, M.; Hayakawa, M.; Yanagihara, T.; Hukunaga, Y. Proteinuria screening for children. *Kidney Int. Suppl.* **2005**, S23–S27. [CrossRef]

10. Cohen, R.A.; Brown, R.S. Clinical practice. Microscopic hematuria. *N. Engl. J. Med.* **2003**, *348*, 2330–2338. [CrossRef] [PubMed]

11. Moreno, J.A.; Martin-Cleary, C.; Gutierrez, E.; Rubio-Navarro, A.; Ortiz, A.; Praga, M.; Egido, J. Haematuria: The forgotten CKD factor? *Nephrol. Dial. Trans.* **2012**, *27*, 28–34. [CrossRef] [PubMed]

12. Rychlik, I.; Jancova, E.; Tesar, V.; Kolsky, A.; Lacha, J.; Stejskal, J.; Stejskalova, A.; Dusek, J.; Herout, V. The Czech registry of renal biopsies. Occurrence of renal diseases in the years 1994-2000. *Nephrol. Dial. Trans.* **2004**, *19*, 3040–3049. [CrossRef]

13. Maixnerova, D.; Jancova, E.; Skibova, J.; Rysava, R.; Rychlik, I.; Viklicky, O.; Merta, M.; Kolsky, A.; Reiterova, J.; Neprasova, M.; et al. Nationwide biopsy survey of renal diseases in the Czech Republic during the years 1994–2011. *J. Nephrol.* **2015**, *28*, 39–49. [CrossRef]

14. Schena, F.P. Survey of the Italian Registry of Renal Biopsies. Frequency of the renal diseases for 7 consecutive years. The Italian Group of Renal Immunopathology. *Nephrol. Dial. Trans.* **1997**, *12*, 418–426. [CrossRef]

15. Paripović, D.; Kostić, M.; Kruščić, D.; Spasojević, B.; Lomić, G.; Marković-Lipkovski, J.; Basta-Jovanović, G.; Smoljanić, Ž.; Peco-Antić, A. Indications and results of renal biopsy in children: A 10-year review from a single center in Serbia. *J. Nephrol.* **2012**, *25*, 1054–1059. [CrossRef] [PubMed]

16. Polito, M.G.; de Moura, L.A.R.; Kirsztajn, G.M. An overview on frequency of renal biopsy diagnosis in Brazil: Clinical and pathological patterns based on 9617 native kidney biopsies. *Nephrol. Dial. Trans.* **2010**, *25*, 490–496. [CrossRef] [PubMed]

17. Yuste, C.; Rivera, F.; Moreno, J.A.; López-Gómez, J.M. Haematuria on the Spanish Registry of Glomerulonephritis. *Sci. Rep.* **2016**, *6*, 19732. [CrossRef] [PubMed]

18. Haas, M.; Racusen, L.C.; Bagnasco, S.M. IgA-dominant postinfectious glomerulonephritis: A report of 13 cases with common ultrastructural features. *Hum. Pathol.* **2008**, *39*, 1309–1316. [CrossRef] [PubMed]

19. Ding, J.Y.C.; Ibañez, D.; Gladman, D.D.; Urowitz, M.B. Isolated Hematuria and Sterile Pyuria May Indicate Systemic Lupus Erythematosus Activity. *J. Rheumatol.* **2015**, *42*, 437–440. [CrossRef] [PubMed]

20. Rhee, R.L.; Davis, J.C.; Ding, L.; Fervenza, F.C.; Hoffman, G.S.; Kallenberg, C.G.M.; Langford, C.A.; McCune, W.J.; Monach, P.A.; Seo, P.; et al. The Utility of Urinalysis in Determining the Risk of Renal Relapse in ANCA-Associated Vasculitis. *Clin. J. Am. Soc. Nephrol.* **2018**, *13*, 251–257. [CrossRef]

21. Gutiérrez, E.; González, E.; Hernández, E.; Morales, E.; Martínez, M.A.; Usera, G.; Praga, M. Factors that determine an incomplete recovery of renal function in macrohematuria-induced acute renal failure of IgA nephropathy. *Clin. J. Am. Soc. Nephrol.* **2007**, *2*, 51–57. [CrossRef] [PubMed]

22. Sevillano, A.M.; Gutiérrez, E.; Yuste, C.; Cavero, T.; Mérida, E.; Rodríguez, P.; García, A.; Morales, E.; Fernández, C.; Martínez, M.A.; et al. Remission of Hematuria Improves Renal Survival in IgA Nephropathy. *J. Am. Soc. Nephrol.* **2017**, *28*, 3089–3099. [CrossRef]

23. Moroni, G.; Pozzi, C.; Quaglini, S.; Segagni, S.; Banfi, G.; Baroli, A.; Picardi, L.; Colzani, S.; Simonini, P.; Mihatsch, M.J.; et al. Long-term prognosis of diffuse proliferative glomerulonephritis associated with infection in adults. *Nephrol. Dial. Trans.* **2002**, *17*, 1204–1211. [CrossRef]

24. Sethi, S.; Fervenza, F.C. Membranoproliferative Glomerulonephritis—A New Look at an Old Entity. *N. Engl. J. Med.* **2012**, *366*, 1119–1131. [CrossRef]

25. Wyatt, R.J.; Julian, B.A. IgA Nephropathy. *N. Engl. J. Med.* **2013**, *368*, 2402–2414. [CrossRef]

26. D'Agati, V.D.; Kaskel, F.J.; Falk, R.J. Focal Segmental Glomerulosclerosis. *N. Engl. J. Med.* **2011**, *365*, 2398–2411. [CrossRef]

27. Sethi, S.; Zand, L.; Nasr, S.H.; Glassock, R.J.; Fervenza, F.C. Focal and segmental glomerulosclerosis: Clinical and kidney biopsy correlations. *Clin. Kidney J.* **2014**, *7*, 531–537. [CrossRef]

28. Medjeral-Thomas, N.R.; O'Shaughnessy, M.M.; O'Regan, J.A.; Traynor, C.; Flanagan, M.; Wong, L.; Teoh, C.W.; Awan, A.; Waldron, M.; Cairns, T.; et al. C3 glomerulopathy: Clinicopathologic features and predictors of outcome. *Clin. J. Am. Soc. Nephrol.* **2014**, *9*, 46–53. [CrossRef]

29. Pickering, M.C.; D'Agati, V.D.; Nester, C.M.; Smith, R.J.; Haas, M.; Appel, G.B.; Alpers, C.E.; Bajema, I.M.; Bedrosian, C.; Braun, M.; et al. C3 glomerulopathy: Consensus report. *Kidney Int.* **2013**, *84*, 1079–1089. [CrossRef]

30. Kovačević, Z.; Jovanović, D.; Rabrenović, V.; Dimitrijević, J.; Djukanović, J. Asymptomatic microscopic haematuria in young males. *Int. J. Clin. Pract.* **2008**, *62*, 406–412. [CrossRef] [PubMed]

31. Deltas, C.; Pierides, A.; Voskarides, K. The role of molecular genetics in diagnosing familial hematuria(s). *Pediatr. Nephrol.* **2012**, *27*, 1221–1231. [CrossRef]

32. Deltas, C.; Pierides, A.; Voskarides, K. Molecular genetics of familial hematuric diseases. *Nephrol. Dial. Trans.* **2013**, *28*, 2946–2960. [CrossRef]

33. Kashtan, C.E. Familial hematuria. *Pediatr. Nephrol.* **2009**, *24*, 1951–1958. [CrossRef] [PubMed]

34. Brodsky, S.V.; Satoskar, A.; Chen, J.; Nadasdy, G.; Eagen, J.W.; Hamirani, M.; Hebert, L.; Calomeni, E.; Nadasdy, T. Acute Kidney Injury During Warfarin Therapy Associated With Obstructive Tubular Red Blood Cell Casts: A Report of 9 Cases. *Am. J. Kidney Dis.* **2009**, *54*, 1121–1126. [CrossRef] [PubMed]

35. Escoli, R.; Santos, P.; Andrade, S.; Carvalho, F. Dabigatran-Related Nephropathy in a Patient with Undiagnosed IgA Nephropathy. *Case Rep. Nephrol.* **2015**, *2015*, 298261. [CrossRef]

36. Brodsky, S.V.; Mhaskar, N.S.; Thiruveedi, S.; Dhingra, R.; Reuben, S.C.; Calomeni, E.; Ivanov, I.; Satoskar, A.; Hemminger, J.; Nadasdy, G.; et al. Acute kidney injury aggravated by treatment initiation with apixaban: Another twist of anticoagulant-related nephropathy. *Kidney Res. Clin. Pract.* **2017**, *36*, 387–392. [CrossRef]

37. Brodsky, S.; Eikelboom, J.; Hebert, L.A. Anticoagulant-Related Nephropathy. *J. Am. Soc. Nephrol.* **2018**, *29*, 2787–2793. [CrossRef] [PubMed]

38. Shin, J.-I.; Luo, S.; Alexander, G.C.; Inker, L.A.; Coresh, J.; Chang, A.R.; Grams, M.E. Direct Oral Anticoagulants and Risk of Acute Kidney Injury in Patients With Atrial Fibrillation. *J. Am. Coll. Cardiol.* **2018**, *71*, 251–252. [CrossRef]

39. Chan, Y.-H.; Yeh, Y.-H.; See, L.-C.; Wang, C.-L.; Chang, S.-H.; Lee, H.-F.; Wu, L.-S.; Tu, H.-T.; Kuo, C.-T. Acute Kidney Injury in Asians With Atrial Fibrillation Treated With Dabigatran or Warfarin. *J. Am. Coll. Cardiol.* **2016**, *68*, 2272–2283. [CrossRef]

40. Yao, X.; Tangri, N.; Gersh, B.J.; Sangaralingham, L.R.; Shah, N.D.; Nath, K.A.; Noseworthy, P.A. Renal Outcomes in Anticoagulated Patients With Atrial Fibrillation. *J. Am. Coll. Cardiol.* **2017**, *70*, 2621–2632. [CrossRef] [PubMed]

41. Brodsky, S.V.; Nadasdy, T.; Rovin, B.H.; Satoskar, A.A.; Nadasdy, G.M.; Wu, H.M.; Bhatt, U.Y.; Hebert, L.A. Warfarin-related nephropathy occurs in patients with and without chronic kidney disease and is associated with an increased mortality rate. *Kidney Int.* **2011**, *80*, 181–189. [CrossRef]

42. Lechner, S.M.; Abbad, L.; Boedec, E.; Papista, C.; Le Stang, M.-B.; Moal, C.; Maillard, J.; Jamin, A.; Bex-Coudrat, J.; Wang, Y.; et al. IgA1 Protease Treatment Reverses Mesangial Deposits and Hematuria in a Model of IgA Nephropathy. *J. Am. Soc. Nephrol.* **2016**, *27*, 2622–2629. [CrossRef]

43. Robert, T.; Berthelot, L.; Cambier, A.; Rondeau, E.; Monteiro, R.C. Molecular Insights into the Pathogenesis of IgA Nephropathy. *Trends Mol. Med.* **2015**, *21*, 762–775. [CrossRef]

44. Suzuki, Y.; Suzuki, H.; Nakata, J.; Sato, D.; Kajiyama, T.; Watanabe, T.; Tomino, Y. Pathological role of tonsillar B cells in IgA nephropathy. *Clin. Dev. Immunol.* **2011**, *2011*, 639074. [CrossRef]

45. Meng, T.; Li, X.; Ao, X.; Zhong, Y.; Tang, R.; Peng, W.; Yang, J.; Zou, M.; Zhou, Q. Hemolytic Streptococcus may exacerbate kidney damage in IgA nephropathy through CCL20 response to the effect of Th17 cells. *PLoS ONE* **2014**, *9*, e108723. [CrossRef]

46. Nishikawa, Y.; Shibata, R.; Ozono, Y.; Ichinose, H.; Miyazaki, M.; Harada, T.; Kohno, S. Streptococcal M protein enhances TGF-beta production and increases surface IgA-positive B cells in vitro in IgA nephropathy. *Nephrol. Dial. Trans.* **2000**, *15*, 772–777. [CrossRef]

47. Barratt, J.; Smith, A.C.; Feehally, J. The pathogenic role of IgA1 O-linked glycosylation in the pathogenesis of IgA nephropathy. *Nephrology (Carlton)* **2007**, *12*, 275–284. [CrossRef]

48. Cox, S.N.; Sallustio, F.; Serino, G.; Loverre, A.; Pesce, F.; Gigante, M.; Zaza, G.; Stifanelli, P.F.; Ancona, N.; Schena, F.P. Activated innate immunity and the involvement of CX3CR1-fractalkine in promoting hematuria in patients with IgA nephropathy. *Kidney Int.* **2012**, *82*, 548–560. [CrossRef]

49. Nakatani, K.; Yoshimoto, S.; Iwano, M.; Asai, O.; Samejima, K.; Sakan, H.; Terada, M.; Hasegawa, H.; Nose, M.; Saito, Y. Fractalkine expression and CD16+ monocyte accumulation in glomerular lesions: Association with their severity and diversity in lupus models. *Am. J. Physiol. Renal Physiol.* **2010**, *299*, F207–16. [CrossRef]

50. Ayoub, I.; Birmingham, D.; Rovin, B.; Hebert, L. Commentary on the Current Guidelines for the Diagnosis of Lupus Nephritis Flare. *Curr. Rheumatol. Rep.* **2019**, *21*, 12. [CrossRef]

51. Moreno, J.A.; Martin-Cleary, C.; Gutierrez, E.; Toldos, O.; Blanco-Colio, L.M.; Praga, M.; Ortiz, A.; Egido, J. AKI Associated with Macroscopic Glomerular Hematuria: Clinical and Pathophysiologic Consequences. *Clin. J. Am. Soc. Nephrol.* **2012**, *7*, 175–184. [CrossRef] [PubMed]

52. Gutiérrez, E.; Egido, J.; Rubio-Navarro, A.; Buendía, I.; Blanco Colio, L.M.; Toldos, O.; Manzarbeitia, F.; de Lorenzo, A.; Sanchez, R.; Ortiz, A.; et al. Oxidative stress, macrophage infiltration and CD163 expression are determinants of long-term renal outcome in macrohematuria-induced acute kidney injury of IgA nephropathy. *Nephron. Clin. Pract.* **2012**, *121*, c42–53. [CrossRef]

53. Rubio-Navarro, A.; Sanchez-Niño, M.D.; Guerrero-Hue, M.; García-Caballero, C.; Gutiérrez, E.; Yuste, C.; Sevillano, Á.; Praga, M.; Egea, J.; Román, E.; et al. Podocytes are new cellular targets of haemoglobin-mediated renal damage. *J. Pathol.* **2018**, *244*. [CrossRef]

54. Duan, Z.-Y.; Cai, G.-Y.; Bu, R.; Lu, Y.; Hou, K.; Chen, X.-M. Selection of urinary sediment miRNAs as specific biomarkers of IgA nephropathy. *Sci. Rep.* **2016**, *6*, 23498. [CrossRef] [PubMed]

55. Duan, Z.-Y.; Cai, G.-Y.; Li, J.-J.; Bu, R.; Chen, X.-M. Urinary Erythrocyte-Derived miRNAs: Emerging Role in IgA Nephropathy. *Kidney Blood Press. Res.* **2017**, *42*, 738–748. [CrossRef]

56. Tan, K.; Chen, J.; Li, W.; Chen, Y.; Sui, W.; Zhang, Y.; Dai, Y. Genome-wide analysis of microRNAs expression profiling in patients with primary IgA nephropathy. *Genome* **2013**, *56*, 161–169. [CrossRef]

57. Goto, M.; Wakai, K.; Kawamura, T.; Ando, M.; Endoh, M.; Tomino, Y. A scoring system to predict renal outcome in IgA nephropathy: A nationwide 10-year prospective cohort study. *Nephrol. Dial. Trans.* **2009**, *24*, 3068–3074. [CrossRef]

58. Barraca, D.; Moreno, J.A.; Aragoncillo, I.; Praga, M.; Gutiérrez, E.; Vega, A.; Egido, J.; Rubio-Navarro, A.; Mahillo, I.; Santos, A.; et al. Haematuria Increases Progression of Advanced Proteinuric Kidney Disease. *PLoS ONE* **2015**, *10*, e0128575.

59. Orlandi, P.F.; Fujii, N.; Roy, J.; Chen, H.Y.; Lee Hamm, L.; Sondheimer, J.H.; He, J.; Fischer, M.J.; Rincon-Choles, H.; Krishnan, G.; et al. Hematuria as a risk factor for progression of chronic kidney disease and death: Findings from the Chronic Renal Insufficiency Cohort (CRIC) Study. *BMC Nephrol.* **2018**, *19*, 1–11. [CrossRef] [PubMed]

60. Schulman, G.; Berl, T.; Beck, G.J.; Remuzzi, G.; Ritz, E.; Shimizu, M.; Kikuchi, M.; Shobu, Y. Risk factors for progression of chronic kidney disease in the EPPIC trials and the effect of AST-120. *Clin. Exp. Nephrol.* **2018**, *22*, 299–308. [CrossRef] [PubMed]

61. Lin, H.Y.H.; Niu, S.W.; Kuo, I.C.; Lim, L.M.; Hwang, D.Y.; Lee, J.J.; Hwang, S.J.; Chen, H.C.; Hung, C.C. Hematuria and Renal Outcomes in Patients With Diabetic Chronic Kidney Disease. *Am. J. Med. Sci.* **2018**, *356*, 268–276. [CrossRef]

62. Levey, A.S.; Cattran, D.; Friedman, A.; Miller, W.G.; Sedor, J.; Tuttle, K.; Kasiske, B.; Hostetter, T. Proteinuria as a surrogate outcome in CKD: report of a scientific workshop sponsored by the National Kidney Foundation and the US Food and Drug Administration. *Am. J. Kidney Dis.* **2009**, *54*, 205–226. [CrossRef] [PubMed]

63. Berthoux, F.; Mohey, H.; Laurent, B.; Mariat, C.; Afiani, A.; Thibaudin, L. Predicting the Risk for Dialysis or Death in IgA Nephropathy. *J. Am. Soc. Nephrol.* **2011**, *22*, 752–761. [CrossRef]

64. Le, W.; Liang, S.; Hu, Y.; Deng, K.; Bao, H.; Zeng, C.; Liu, Z. Long-term renal survival and related risk factors in patients with IgA nephropathy: Results from a cohort of 1155 cases in a Chinese adult population. *Nephrol. Dial. Trans.* **2012**, *27*, 1479–1485. [CrossRef] [PubMed]

65. Coppo, R.; Fervenza, F.C. Persistent Microscopic Hematuria as a Risk Factor for Progression of IgA Nephropathy: New Floodlight on a Nearly Forgotten Biomarker. *J. Am. Soc. Nephrol.* **2017**, *28*, 2831–2834. [CrossRef] [PubMed]

66. Tracz, M.J.; Alam, J.; Nath, K.A. Physiology and Pathophysiology of Heme: Implications for Kidney Disease. *J. Am. Soc. Nephrol.* **2007**, *18*, 414–420. [CrossRef]

67. Kumar, S.; Bandyopadhyay, U. Free heme toxicity and its detoxification systems in human. *Toxicol. Lett.* **2005**, *157*, 175–188. [CrossRef]

68. Vincent, S.H. Oxidative effects of heme and porphyrins on proteins and lipids. *Semin. Hematol.* **1989**, *26*, 105–113. [PubMed]

69. TAPPEL, A.L. The mechanism of the oxidation of unsaturated fatty acids catalyzed by hematin compounds. *Arch. Biochem. Biophys.* **1953**, *44*, 378–395. [CrossRef]

70. Aft, R.L.; Mueller, G.C. Hemin-mediated DNA strand scission. *J. Biol. Chem.* **1983**, *258*, 12069–12072.

71. Dutra, F.F.; Bozza, M.T. Heme on innate immunity and inflammation. *Front. Pharmacol.* **2014**, *5*, 115. [CrossRef]

72. Balla, G.; Jacob, H.S.; Eaton, J.W.; Belcher, J.D.; Vercellotti, G.M. Hemin: A possible physiological mediator of low density lipoprotein oxidation and endothelial injury. *Arterioscler. Thromb. J. Vasc. Biol.* **1991**, *11*, 1700–1711. [CrossRef]

73. Wagener, F.A.; Feldman, E.; de Witte, T.; Abraham, N.G. Heme induces the expression of adhesion molecules ICAM-1, VCAM-1, and E selectin in vascular endothelial cells. *Proc. Soc. Exp. Biol. Med.* **1997**, *216*, 456–463. [CrossRef]

74. Immenschuh, S.; Vijayan, V.; Janciauskiene, S.; Gueler, F. Heme as a Target for Therapeutic Interventions. *Front. Pharmacol.* **2017**, *8*, 146. [CrossRef]

75. Belcher, J.D.; Chen, C.; Nguyen, J.; Milbauer, L.; Abdulla, F.; Alayash, A.I.; Smith, A.; Nath, K.A.; Hebbel, R.P.; Vercellotti, G.M. Heme triggers TLR4 signaling leading to endothelial cell activation and vaso-occlusion in murine sickle cell disease. *Blood* **2014**, *123*, 377–390. [CrossRef]

76. Graça-Souza, A.V.; Arruda, M.A.B.; de Freitas, M.S.; Barja-Fidalgo, C.; Oliveira, P.L. Neutrophil activation by heme: Implications for inflammatory processes. *Blood* **2002**, *99*, 4160–4165. [CrossRef] [PubMed]

77. Monteiro, A.P.T.; Pinheiro, C.S.; Luna-Gomes, T.; Alves, L.R.; Maya-Monteiro, C.M.; Porto, B.N.; Barja-Fidalgo, C.; Benjamim, C.F.; Peters-Golden, M.; Bandeira-Melo, C.; et al. Leukotriene B4 mediates neutrophil migration induced by heme. *J. Immunol.* **2011**, *186*, 6562–6567. [CrossRef]

78. Arruda, M.A.; Rossi, A.G.; de Freitas, M.S.; Barja-Fidalgo, C.; Graça-Souza, A. V Heme inhibits human neutrophil apoptosis: Involvement of phosphoinositide 3-kinase, MAPK, and NF-kappaB. *J. Immunol.* **2004**, *173*, 2023–2030. [CrossRef]

79. Figueiredo, R.T.; Fernandez, P.L.; Mourao-Sa, D.S.; Porto, B.N.; Dutra, F.F.; Alves, L.S.; Oliveira, M.F.; Oliveira, P.L.; Graça-Souza, A.V.; Bozza, M.T. Characterization of heme as activator of Toll-like receptor 4. *J. Biol. Chem.* **2007**, *282*, 20221–20229. [CrossRef]

80. Lin, T.; Sammy, F.; Yang, H.; Thundivalappil, S.; Hellman, J.; Tracey, K.J.; Warren, H.S. Identification of hemopexin as an anti-inflammatory factor that inhibits synergy of hemoglobin with HMGB1 in sterile and infectious inflammation. *J. Immunol.* **2012**, *189*, 2017–2022. [CrossRef] [PubMed]

81. Medzhitov, R. Origin and physiological roles of inflammation. *Nature* **2008**, *454*, 428–435. [CrossRef]

82. Nath, K.A.; Belcher, J.D.; Nath, M.C.; Grande, J.P.; Croatt, A.J.; Ackerman, A.W.; Katusic, Z.S.; Vercellotti, G.M. Role of TLR4 signaling in the nephrotoxicity of heme and heme proteins. *Am. J. Physiol. Renal Physiol.* **2018**, *314*, F906–F914. [CrossRef]

83. Komada, T.; Usui, F.; Kawashima, A.; Kimura, H.; Karasawa, T.; Inoue, Y.; Kobayashi, M.; Mizushina, Y.; Kasahara, T.; Taniguchi, S.; et al. Role of NLRP3 Inflammasomes for Rhabdomyolysis-induced Acute Kidney Injury. *Sci. Rep.* **2015**, *5*, 10901. [CrossRef]

84. Lee, C.M.; Hardy, C.M. Cocoa feeding and human lactose intolerance. *Am. J. Clin. Nutr.* **1989**, *49*, 840–844. [CrossRef]

85. Fellström, B.C.; Barratt, J.; Cook, H.; Coppo, R.; Feehally, J.; de Fijter, J.W.; Floege, J.; Hetzel, G.; Jardine, A.G.; Locatelli, F.; et al. Targeted-release budesonide versus placebo in patients with IgA nephropathy (NEFIGAN): A double-blind, randomised, placebo-controlled phase 2b trial. *Lancet* **2017**, *389*, 2117–2127. [CrossRef]
86. Floege, J.; Barbour, S.J.; Cattran, D.C.; Hogan, J.J.; Nachman, P.H.; Tang, S.C.W.; Wetzels, J.F.M.; Cheung, M.; Wheeler, D.C.; Winkelmayer, W.C.; et al. Management and treatment of glomerular diseases (part 1): Conclusions from a Kidney Disease: Improving Global Outcomes (KDIGO) Controversies Conference. *Kidney Int.* **2019**, *95*, 268–280. [CrossRef]
87. Ware, K.; Qamri, Z.; Ozcan, A.; Satoskar, A.A.; Nadasdy, G.; Rovin, B.H.; Hebert, L.A.; Nadasdy, T.; Brodsky, S. V N-acetylcysteine ameliorates acute kidney injury but not glomerular hemorrhage in an animal model of warfarin-related nephropathy. *Am. J. Physiol. Renal Physiol.* **2013**, *304*, F1421–F1427. [CrossRef] [PubMed]

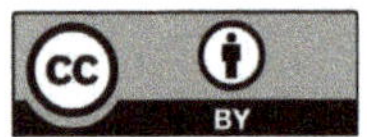

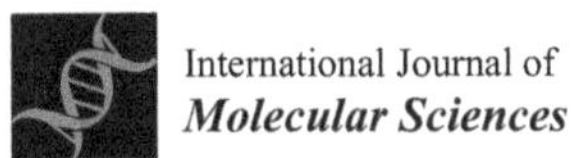

International Journal of
Molecular Sciences

MDPI

Review

Arachidonic Acid Metabolism and Kidney Inflammation

Tianqi Wang [1,2,†], Xianjun Fu [2,3,†], Qingfa Chen [4], Jayanta Kumar Patra [5], Dongdong Wang [6,7], Zhenguo Wang [2,*] and Zhibo Gai [3,*]

[1] Traditional Chinese Medicine History and Literature, Institute for Literature and Culture of Chinese Medicine, Shandong University of Traditional Chinese Medicine, Jinan 250355, China
[2] Institute for Literature and Culture of Chinese Medicine, Shandong University of Traditional Chinese Medicine, Jinan 250355, China
[3] Key Laboratory of Traditional Chinese Medicine for Classical Theory, Ministry of Education, Shandong University of Traditional Chinese Medicine, Jinan 250355, China
[4] The Institute for Tissue Engineering and Regenerative Medicine, The Liaocheng University, Liaocheng 252000, China
[5] Research Institute of Biotechnology & Medical Converged Science, Dongguk University-Seoul, Goyangsi 10326, Korea
[6] Institute of Clinical Chemistry, University Hospital Zurich, University of Zurich, Wagistrasse 14, 8952 Schlieren, Switzerland
[7] Guizhou University of Traditional Chinese Medicine, Fei Shan Jie 32, Guiyang 550003, China
[*] Correspondence: zhenguow@126.com (Z.W.); zhibo.gai@usz.ch (Z.G.); Tel.: +86-13505312372 (Z.W.); +41-43-253-2068 (Z.G.)
[†] These authors contributed equally to this work.

Received: 8 July 2019; Accepted: 20 July 2019; Published: 27 July 2019

Abstract: As a major component of cell membrane lipids, Arachidonic acid (AA), being a major component of the cell membrane lipid content, is mainly metabolized by three kinds of enzymes: cyclooxygenase (COX), lipoxygenase (LOX), and cytochrome P450 (CYP450) enzymes. Based on these three metabolic pathways, AA could be converted into various metabolites that trigger different inflammatory responses. In the kidney, prostaglandins (PG), thromboxane (Tx), leukotrienes (LTs) and hydroxyeicosatetraenoic acids (HETEs) are the major metabolites generated from AA. An increased level of prostaglandins (PGs), TxA_2 and leukotriene B4 (LTB_4) results in inflammatory damage to the kidney. Moreover, the LTB_4-leukotriene B4 receptor 1 (BLT1) axis participates in the acute kidney injury via mediating the recruitment of renal neutrophils. In addition, AA can regulate renal ion transport through 19-hydroxystilbenetetraenoic acid (19-HETE) and 20-HETE, both of which are produced by cytochrome P450 monooxygenase. Epoxyeicosatrienoic acids (EETs) generated by the CYP450 enzyme also plays a paramount role in the kidney damage during the inflammation process. For example, 14 and 15-EET mitigated ischemia/reperfusion-caused renal tubular epithelial cell damage. Many drug candidates that target the AA metabolism pathways are being developed to treat kidney inflammation. These observations support an extraordinary interest in a wide range of studies on drug interventions aiming to control AA metabolism and kidney inflammation.

Keywords: arachidonic acid; cyclooxygenase; lipoxygenase; cytochrome P450; kidney inflammation; therapeutic target

---

1. Introduction

Arachidonic acid (AA), also named eicosa-5,8,11,14-tetraenoic acid, is a ω-6 polyunsaturated fatty acid (PFA) and is mainly present in the form of phospholipids in the cell membrane. When cells are under stress, AA is released from the phospholipids by phospholipase A_2 (PLA_2) and phospholipase

C (PLC) as free arachidonic acids [1–3], which become the precursor of proinflammatory bioactive mediators through three metabolic pathways. Through the cyclooxygenase (COX) pathway, AA can be metabolized into prostaglandins (PGs) and thromboxanes (TXs). AA can also be converted into leukotrienes (LTs) and lipoxins (LXs) by the lipoxygenase (LOX) pathway [4–6]. Moreover, AA also generates epoxyeicosatrienoic acids (EETs) or hydroxyeicosatetraenoic acids (HETEs) through the cytochrome P450 (CYP450) pathway. Together, these AA metabolites are referred as eicosanoids, which are effective autocrine and paracrine bioactive mediators, and are widely involved in a variety of physiological and pathological processes [7–10].

Kidney inflammation, characterized by hematuria, proteinuria, edema, hypertension, etc., is caused by immune-mediated inflammatory mediators (such as complement, cytokines, reactive oxygen species, etc.), resulting in a group of kidney diseases with a varying degree of renal dysfunction. Without prompt treatment, it will lead to thromboembolism, acute renal failure (and even chronic nephritis), chronic renal failure and finally uremia [11].

The relationship between AA and inflammation attracts our interest in the effect of AA metabolism on kidney inflammation. Therefore, we systematically summarized the effect of AA-derived bioactive mediators on kidney inflammation by discussing the regulatory mechanism of AA metabolism in the kidney, followed by the mechanism of AA-induced renal inflammation and a potential treatment targeting the AA metabolism.

2. Regulation of the AA Metabolism in the Kidney

2.1. The Release of AA

Normally, AA exists in the cell membrane in the form of phospholipids. When the cell membrane is subjected to stimuli, especially the inflammatory reaction, the phospholipids are released from the cell membrane. Through the hydrolysis of phospholipids by PLA_2 and PLC [1,3,12], AA is released and then transformed into a bioactive metabolite with the help of different enzymes, thus promoting inflammatory cascades. At present, it is well known that at least three metabolic pathways (the COX pathway, LOX pathway and CYP450 pathway) are involved in the metabolism of AA, which are closely related to the occurrence, development, and regression of renal inflammation (Figure 1) [1].

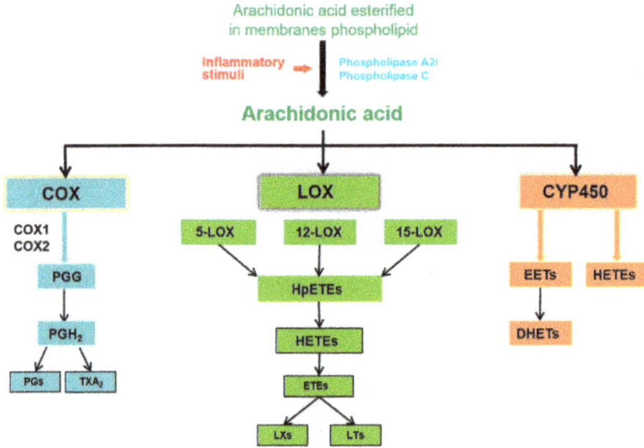

Figure 1. Scheme of eicosanoids biosynthesis pathways from arachidonic acid.

2.2. COX Pathway

COX-1/2, also called prostaglandin H synthase (PGHS), is one of the key enzymes involved in the AA metabolism [13]. The constitutive enzyme COX-1 is responsible for the expression of prostaglandin E_2 (PGE_2) at the background level or the expression of PG under hypotonic swelling stimulation [14]. COX-2 is almost not expressed at normal physiological conditions; however, it is highly expressed when the kidney is under the influence of stimuli, such as chronic sodium deficiency and ultrafiltration [15]. It is important to note that COX-2 is the dominating source of prostacyclin [16]. Once AA is released, it can be metabolized by two isozymes of PGHS, PGHS-1 and PGHS-2 [17]. PGHSs have two different but complementary enzyme activities, one is cyclooxygenase (dioxygenase) activity, which catalyzes the production of PGG_2 from arachidonic acid, and the other is peroxidase activity, which promotes the reduction of PGG_2 to PGH_2 [18]. In general, the COX protein contains a cyclooxygenase site and a peroxidase site. AA is converted to the endogenous hydrogen peroxide PGG_2 by the cyclooxygenase site, and the peroxidase site is responsible for reducing PGG_2 to PGH_2 [19]. COXs initially metabolize AA to unstable PGG_2 by their COX function and then convert it to PGH_2 by their peroxidase function. PGH_2, like cell-and tissue-selective prostanoid synthases and isomerases, is not stable, and can easily generate many bioactive prostaglandins, such as prostaglandins D2, E2, F2α, and I_2, and TXA_2, depending on the differential expression of these synthetases in different tissues [20–23]. PGH_2 can also be decomposed into malonaldehyde (MDA) and 12L-hydroxy-5,8,10-heptadecatrienoic acid (HHT) by thromboxane synthase [24]. The process of converting PGH_2 to PGD requires two PGD synthetases, namely hematopoietic PGD synthase (H-PGDS) and lipocalin-type PGD synthase (L-PGDS). Then the PGD_2 is metabolized to 15-deoxy-Δ 12,14-prostaglandin J 2 (15d-PGJ 2) [25]. PGI_2 is extremely unstable, with a half-life of only two to three minutes, and is easily converted to 6-keto-prostaglandin F1α spontaneously [26,27]. In particular, PGH_2 is produced in most cells by the action of microsomal PGE_2 synthase (mPGES). PGE_2 is synthesized in almost all human cells and exerts extremely complex physiological effects in the inflammatory response through the signaling pathway which is composed of four G protein-coupled receptors: E-type prostanoid receptors (EP)1, EP2, EP3 and EP4 [28–30]. As for TXA_2, AA can generate TXA_2 via the action of thromboxane synthase [31], which has a half-life of only about 30 s and is then spontaneously converted to thromboxane B_2 (TXB_2) [32,33]. Three things that need to be especially pointed out are that platelets mainly form TXA_2, endothelial cells mainly form PGI_2, and PGE_2 is the main prostatic body produced by renal collecting tubule cells [34]. In recent years, another variant of the COX family, COX-3 (or CX-1b), which is an allosteric splice variant of COX-1, has been discovered, and its gene sequence differs from COX-2 in such a way that the COX-3 retains the intron 1 sequences [35]. COX-3 also catalyzes the production of PGH_2, its activity can be inhibited by crude aminophenol, and it is mainly expressed in the microvessels of the brain and heart [36–38]. Hence, its role in AA metabolism and kidney inflammation needs to be further explored.

2.3. LOX Pathway

Under the catalysis of lipoxygenase, AA is metabolized into hydroperoxyeicosatetraenoic acid (HpETE). Current research suggests that at least four enzymes, namely 5-LOX, 8-LOX, 12-LOX, and 15-LOX are involved in the metabolism of AA in the LOX pathway. However, the 5-, 12-, and 15-positions are the main oxidation sites of AA, leading to oxidation reactions that are based on the catalysis of 5-LOX, 12-LOX, and 15-LOX enzymes. In this review, we focus on the 5-LOX, 12-LOX and 15-LOX pathways (Figure 2).

Human 5-LOX holds a major function in kidney inflammation, ranging from kidney tubules to glomeruli. In this pathway, AA forms 5-hydroperoxyeicosatetraenoic acid (5-HpETE) by dioxygenase [39], and then 95% is generated into 5-hydroxyeicosatetraenoic acid (5-hydroxy-6,8,11,15-eicosatetraenoic acid, 5-HETE) at C7 and 5% is generated into 8-HETE at C10, which are the first two steps during the conversion process of AA to proinflammatory LTs [40]. Besides, Oxo-ETE is generated via the LOX product, HETEs by the microsomal dehydrogenase in the human polymorphonuclear leukocytes (PMNLs) [39,41]. Then, oxo-ETEs are formed through the oxidation of HETEs [42,43], which is the strongest eosinophil chemoattractant among bioactive mediators. From here, AA metabolites are further converted to LTA_4 and LXs via 5-LOX activator protein (5-FLAP) and dehydrase [44]. Basically, the catalytic function of the 5-LOX enzyme is mainly manifested in the following two aspects: one is the insertion of molecular oxygen by dioxygenase activity and the other is the formation of epoxide by LTA_4 synthase activity. Regarding 5-HpETE, it is generated from AA through homolytic cleavage and removal of hydrogen on the pro-S hydrogen at carbon-7 [39]. 5-LOX can generate LTA$_4$ by removing the C10 hydrogen atom from 5-HpETE [45]. LTA$_4$ is unstable and can be hydrolyzed or combined with glutathione or transcellularly transferred to generate bioactive eicosanoids. In neutrophils and other inflammatory cells of kidney tissue, LTA$_4$ is catalyzed by epoxide hydrolase to form LTB$_4$ [46]. LTA$_4$ and glutathione (GSH) catalyze the production of LTC$_4$ using glutathione S-transferase (GST) and then remove glutamic acid to form LTD$_4$ via γ-glutamyl transferase, which is further metabolized by dipeptidase to form LTE$_4$. Then, LTF$_4$ is synthesized from LTE$_4$ by γ-glutamyl transferase [47].

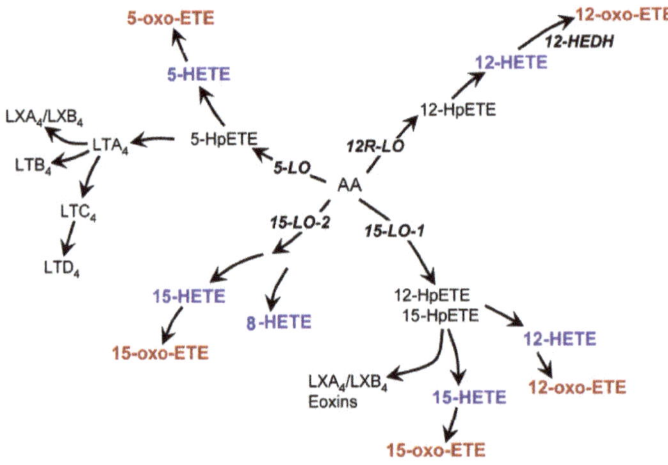

Figure 2. Lipoxygenase, and dehydrogenase pathways for the formation of HETEs, oxo-ETEs, and related eicosanoids.

The roles of the 12-LOX and 15-LOX pathways are mainly in the production of HETEs and LXs. The 12-LOX pathway is similar to the 5-LOX pathway. AA first generates 12-HpETE and 12-hydroxyeicosatetraenoic acid (12-HETE) via 12-LOX [48,49]. But there is a difference between them, as in addition to the conversion of AA to 12-HETE, 12-LOX can also convert 5(S)-HETE to 5(S),12(S)-dihydroxyeicosatetraenoic acid (-diHETE) as well as metabolize 15(S)-HETE to 14(R),15(S)-diHETE in the leukocytes. These products ultimately convert into extra-platelet LTA$_4$ [50,51]. Another biosynthetic pathway for LXs involves 5-LOX in neutrophils and 12-LOX in the platelets. 5-LOX generates LTA$_4$ in the neutrophil, which is then transferred to the platelet, where 12-LOX subsequently generates either LXA$_4$ or LXB$_4$ [45,52,53]. Same as the 12-LOX pathway, the principal effect of the 15-LOX pathway is to ultimately generate HETEs, ETEs and LXs. There are two isoforms in mammalian cells: 15-LOX-1 and 15-LOX-2. 15-LOX-1 (12/15-LOX), which is encoded by the arachidonate 15-lipoxygenase (ALOX15) gene, could metabolize AA into LXA$_4$, LXB$_4$ and 15-oxo-ETEs [43,45], while 15-LOX-2 will metabolize AA into 15-oxo-ETE and 8SHETE. HpETEs. In particular, when using 5, 15-diHpETE as a substrate, the primary product catalyzed by 12-LOX and 15-LOX-1 is LXB$_4$, and the efficiency of 15-LOX-1 is 20 times higher than that of 12-LOX [45]. In humans, 15-LOX-1 and leukocyte 12-LOX have high homology and can form 12(S)-HETE and 15(S)-HETE simultaneously, so these two pathways can be collectively called 12/15-LOX (12/15-LOX). When 15-LOX-2 metabolizes AA to produce only 15-HETE, 15-LOX-1 also metabolizes linoleic acid to synthesize hydroxyoctadecadienoic acid [54]. Then, 15-HETE is rapidly converted into LXA$_4$ or LXB$_4$ by hydrolase [55].

2.4. Cytochrome P450 (CYP450) Pathway

The CYP450 pathway is the major metabolic pathway of AA in the kidney [56]. CYP450 can be detected in the endoplasmic reticulum, mitochondria and nuclear membrane of the kidney [57,58]. In general, AA produces corresponding metabolites mainly through three kinds of reduced triphosphopyridine nucleotide (NADPH, or reduced coenzyme II)-dependent oxidation in the CYP450 pathway. The first is the formation of 5,6-; 8,9-; 11,12-; and 14,15-epoxyeicosatrienoic acids (EETs) through surface oxidation [59–63]. The kidney is an organ with high expoxygenase activity, which, like the liver, also produces enantioselective EETs. In the case of lipoxygenase and cyclooxygenase, AA is first converted to hydrogen peroxide (HpETEs) [43], and then through CYP450 isozymes, oxo-ETEs can also be formed directly from HpETEs (just like the common process of forming HETEs via enzymatic oxidation) [42]. 14,15-EET is the main epoxy compound formed by kidney, and most of the isomers in this region are in (R,S) configuration. CYP2 is the main CYP450 epoxygenase family, and more importantly, CYP2C8 is the most paramount and plays a central epoxygenase role in the metabolism of AA to biologically active EETs in human kidney [64,65]. In addition, the CYP2J family also contributes to the formation of EETs in human and mouse kidneys [64,65]. Early research of CYP2C epoxygenases suggested that CYP2C29 and CYP2C39 produced 14,15-EET, and the CYP2C38 produced 11,12-EET [66]. In particularly, human CYP2J2 isoforms are extremely efficient at epoxidation of AA at the 14,15-position [67]. CYP2J5 is an epoxygenase enzyme that is confined in tubular cells and metabolizes AA to 8,9-EET; 11,12-EET; and 14,15-EET in the mouse kidney [68]. Therefore, different vascular smooth muscle cells and epithelial transport processes controlled by EETs have led to the differential localization and regulation of renal vascular and tubular CYP450 cyclooxygenase, and these conclusions are consistent throughout [69]. Then, EETs are mainly hydrolyzed by soluble epoxide hydrolase (sEH) to form 5,6-; 8,9-; 11,12-; and 14,15-dihydroxyepoxyeicosatrienoic acids (DHETs), which possess weak biological activity [70]. Recent research has confirmed that sEH is one of the key enzymes in the metabolism of EETs, and the regulation of sEH activity and can change the level of EETs in vivo [70].

The other two CYP450 pathways ultimately produce HETEs. One is the formation of 5-, 8-, 9-, 11-, 12-, or 15-HETEs by propylene oxidation. HpETEs produced by lipoxygenase and cyclooxygenase can be reduced to monohydroxy fatty acids (HETEs) by peroxidase [43], which means the hydroxyl group is adjacent to a conjugated diene system. CYP2J5 can also facilitate the process, which has been confirmed in tubular cells, and metabolizes AA to 11-HETE and 15-HETE in mouse kidney [68]. The other is the formation of 19- and 20-Hydroxyeicosatetraenoic (19- and 20-HETE) by ω-1 hydroxylation. The CYP ω-hydroxylase that has been discovered so far is mainly in the CYP4 family. In kidney, proximal straight tubules are capable of converting AA to 20-HETE and 19(S)-HETE by ω-hydroxylase [71]. What's more, 20-HETE is the main product of AA catalyzed by CYP ω-hydroxylase, and in the human kidney, 20-HETE formation is mediated by both CYP4F2 and CYP4A11 [56,72]. Then, 20-HETE can be further oxidized to 20-carboxy arachidonic acid (20-COOH-AA) by alcohol dehydrogenase [73]. It is now well established from a few studies that, CYP4A1, CYP4A2, and CYP4A3 have remarkable AA ω-hydroxylase activity [74]. Moreover, CYP4A1 as an arachidonate ω-hydroxylase has a higher catalytic efficiency, with a turnover rate 20 times higher than that of CYP4A2 or CYP4A3 [74]. Besides, CYP4A1 can also convert AA to 11,12-EET in the mouse kidney [74].

3. Mechanism of AA-induced Renal Inflammation

3.1. PGs and Renal Inflammation

PGs produced by the COX pathway, function differently in case of renal vascular disease. The impact of PGs on renal inflammation is mainly focused in the field of lupus nephritis (LN). In mice and humans, urinary prostaglandin D synthase (uPGDS) is considered as a biomarker of LN, which makes the role of PGD_2 important in the development of LN [75]. PGD_2 are considered as an inflammatory marker, while lipocalin-like-prostaglandin-D synthase (L-PGDS) is considered as a urinary biomarker for human active lupus nephritis [76]. One study of 184 longitudinal observations in 80 patients showed that lipocalin-like-prostaglandin-D synthase could predict the onset/remission of LN [77]. In patients with systemic lupus erythematosus (SLE), increased expression of PGD_2 receptors (PTGDRs) in blood basophils causes an increase of PGD_2 metabolites in the plasma [78]. PGD_2 regulates the inflammatory response through two receptors, PTGDR-1 and PTGDR-2, which are also called D prostanoid receptor-1 (DP-1) and D prostanoid receptor-2 (DP-2). DP-2 also functions as the chemo-attractant receptor-homologous molecule, which is expressed on the T helper type 2 (TH2) cells (CRTH2) [79,80]. Under in vivo condition, the targeted cells of PGD_2 are mainly basophils, and the two PTGDRs are expressed at the highest level in the peripheral blood leukocytes. Interestingly, PTGDR-1 is ubiquitously expressed in the leukocytes, whereas PTGDR-2 only mediates the activation and chemotaxis of basophils, eosinophils, and $CD4^+$ TH2 cells [81]. PGD_2 and PTGDR induce the activation and infiltration of basophils in the kidneys of patients with SLE via mediating C-X-C motif ligand 12 (CXCL12) [78]. CXCL12 plays a biological role mainly through the chemokine receptor CXCR4, and regulates the physiological distribution of neutrophils in the kidney [82,83]. Inflammatory tissues and secondary lymphoid organs (SLOs) are associated with high levels of CXCL12, and CXCL12 mediates immune cell recruitment, which are the factors associated with the pathogenesis of SLE [78]. More importantly, basophil autocrine PGD_2 is the main factor of PGD2-induced CXCR4 epoxidation. In humans and mice, the CXCL12-CXCR4 axis promotes the accumulation of basophils in SLOs during lupus through its mediating effect on the PGD_2-PTGDR axis [78]. At the same time, we also can't deny the bad consequence caused by PGE_2 and TXB_2 in the LN. High levels of PGE_2 and TXB_2 promoted the activation of T cells and the production of IL-4 and IL-10 cytokines, which in turn leads to glomerulosclerosis in LN [84].

In addition, a potential link between PGs and tubulointerstitial lesions and glomerulonephritis was well studied. In the kidney with unilateral ureteral obstruction (UUO), PGD_2 has penetrated all the sides of tubulointerstitial lesions by DP-2 expressed on CD4-positive T cells to activate Th2 lymphocytes. High levels of L-PGDS increased the degree of tubular fibrosis, while L-PGDS-knockout mice and prostaglandin D2 receptor CRTH2-knockout mice revealed a reduction in renal fibrosis, which may be related to the reduced infiltration of Th2 lymphocytes as well as reduced generation of the Th2 cytokines IL-4 and IL-13 [85]. In contrast, the PGD_2 metabolite, 15d-PGJ2, can activate PPARγ and modulate the adhesion process via inhibiting the TNFα-triggered IKK-NFκB pathway, which eventually suppresses inflammation in mouse renal tubular epithelial cells [86]. Moreover, PGs are also regulators of renal ischemia and vasoconstriction. Conversely, PGl_2 and PGE_1 have the effect of relaxing blood vessels and preventing hypoxia-mediated renal tissue damage. More importantly, in the case of renal artery stenosis, PGl_2 and PGE_1 selectively prevent tissue contraction and inhibit the decline of GFR [87,88].

It is well known that PGE_2 is the major product of the COX-2 pathway in the kidneys, which mediates kidney damage [89]. PGE2 play a crucial role in renal hemodynamics, renin release, and renal tubular sodium/water resorption [90,91]. In pathological environments such as diabetic nephropathy, PGE2 synthesis is increased, which may affect cell proliferation, differentiation or apoptosis [92,93]. Current studies indicate that four different EP receptors for PGE_2 are closely associated with rapidly progressive glomerulonephritis (RPGN) [94]. In humans, EP1 receptor mRNA is predominantly expressed in the glomerulus [95]. In diabetic mouse models, activation of EP1 promotes the progression of diabetic nephropathy [96]. On the other hand, deletion of EP1 inhibited the down-regulation of nephrin, and improved glomerular basement membrane thickening and foot process regression [96]. In contrast, a few studies have shown that EP1 deficiency caused severe renal impairment in mice with glomerulonephritis, and the cause of this difference has not yet been discovered [97]. Interestingly, PGE_2 has both vasodilation and vasoconstriction effects on renal afferent arterioles. Treatment with high concentrations of PGE_2 (between 1 and 10 nmol/L) caused arterial vasodilation, and at lower concentrations (0.100 nmol/L), PGE_2 leads to vasoconstriction and aggravates hydronephrosis, which may be due to the binding of the EP3 receptor to the pertussis toxin (PTX)-sensitive G protein $Gα_i$. [98]. Glomerular hypertrophy caused by unilateral nephrectomy in mice may be associated with increased expression of EP2 [99]. In netrin-1-deficient mice, proximal tubular injury can be attributed to the COX-2-PGE_2-mediated inflammatory response [100]. Further studies have confirmed that activation of the COX-2-PGE_2-EP2 axis may be a specific response of podocytes to fluid flow shear stress. This appears to provide a mechanistic basis for changes in podocyte structure and glomerular filtration barrier, leading to proteinuria in high filtration-mediated renal injury [99]. EP3 also plays a paramount role in the progression of renal diseases. $Ep3^{-/-}$ -STZ mice have less volume of urine and higher urine osmotic pressure compared with wild-type STZ (WT-STZ) mice, indicating enhanced water reabsorption. In parallel, the expressions of aquaporin-1, aquaporin-2, and urea transporter A1 in $Ep3^{-/-}$ -STZ mice were increased, so the presence of EP3 was an important promoting factor in the progression of renal disease [101]. EP4 is abundant in almost all types of kidney cells [95], and plays different roles at the glomeruli [102] and tubules [103]. The $G\alpha_s$-conjugated EP4 receptor directly activates adenylate cyclase, increases cAMP, and also activates phosphoinositide kinase 3 [94,104]. In addition, EP4 also stimulates AMP-activated protein kinase and COX2 in mouse podocytes in a p38-dependent manner [105]. When the rats were treated with a low-salt diet, EP4 transcripts in the glomeruli increased significantly, which in turn mediated PGE_2-induced renin secretion and maintained renal blood flow [106]. More importantly, the overexpression of EP4 contributed to podocyte injury and compromised the glomerular filtration barrier in podocyte-specific EP4 receptor transgenic (EP4^{pod+}) mice after 5/6 nephrectomy [107]. On the other hand, in a rat model of cisplatin-induced renal failure, the COX1-PGE2-EP4 axis plays more important roles than dose COX-2 in regulating renal epithelial regeneration [108]. The endogenous PGE_2-EP4 system is involved in tubule-interstitial fibrosis in a mouse UUO model. EP4 knockout significantly augmented obstruction-induced histological alterations. The effects of EP4 agonist are controversial. Use of EP4-sepicific agonist down-regulated the expression of renal macrophage chemokines and pro-fibrinogen growth factors, and inhibited the progression of renal inflammation [103]. In the rat model of acute renal failure, EP4 agonist reduces serum creatinine level and improve survival rate [109]. Moreover, in chronic kidney failure both EP2 and EP4 receptors are shown to be equally important in preserving the progression of chronic kidney disease [109]. In addition, PGE2 can alter renal cell growth, matrix transformation, fibrosis, and apoptosis by activating the EP4 receptor [89]. However, in a STZ-induced diabetic mouse model, the level of cytokines (TNFα and IL-6) and chemokines (MCP-1 and IP-10) in urine of EP4 agonist-treated mice were remarkably higher than those of vehicle-treated diabetes mice, which aggravated glomerular sclerosis and renal tubular interstitial fibrosis [110]. The exact mechanisms of EP4 agonists for the treatment of different kidney diseases need to be further studied.

3.2. HETEs and Renal Inflammation

It has been argued that the regulatory effects of HETEs on platelet function by autocrine or paracrine play a crucial role in the renal inflammation. In view of renal inflammation, which is often associated with renal vascular disease, HETEs have a dual role of anti-thrombotic and pro-thrombotic effects. 5-HETE, 12-HETE and 15-HETE inhibited platelet PLA_2 activity [111]. Platelets are more sensitive to ADP-induced aggregation, and mouse platelets disrupted by gene targeting 12-lipoxygenase (P-12LO$^{-/-}$) of the 12-LOX gene exhibit selective hypersensitivity to ADP [112]. Current study found that in patients with type 2 diabetes, exogenous 12-HpETE activates platelet p38 mitogen-activated protein kinase (p38 MAPK), which in turn promotes the platelet activation in the oxidative stress-related pathophysiological states [113]. Under oxidative stress, a decrease in the glutathione peroxidase activity promotes the formation of 12-HpETE and further causes an increase in the phosphorylation level of p38 MAPK, which further activates platelets [113], exacerbating the kidney damage [114]. Therefore, HETE-induced renal inflammation can be achieved through the regulation of platelets.

In recent years, increasing literatures reveal the activation of peroxisome proliferator-activated receptors (PPARs) by HETEs. PPARs, with three isotypes (PPARα, PPARδ, and PPARγ), are all transcriptional factors for lipogenesis and mainly expressed in the adipocytes and immune cells that regulate the expression of a quantity of genes associated with renal inflammation [115–117]. In macrophages, high concentrations of HETEs activate PPARγ [118,119], the latter gives rise to the increasing expression of CD36, which induces the apoptosis of tubule-interstitial cells, and ultimately leads to the inflammation and fibrosis of renal tubules [120]. In addition, HETEs can also activate PPARα [121], which has an important effect on renal inflammation by participating in the regulation of lipid metabolism [122,123]. Moreover, the metabolite of 20-HETE, 20-COOH-AA, is an endogenous dual activator of PPARα and PPARγ, and its efficiency to activate PPARγ is twice than that of 20-HETE, revealing the potential modulatory effects of 20-COOH-AA on renal inflammation via activation of PPARs.

The roles of HETEs are also of interest in regulating the renal ion transport during renal inflammation. 20-HETE has a wide range of biological effects, including cell proliferation and angiogenesis, and is a relevant factor that regulates the renal function [124]. 20-HETE is widely synthesized in the renal tubules, including proximal tubules, thick ascending rings, small arteries of the renal cortex and the outer medulla. 20-HETE can fully bind to major vasoconstrictors, such as angiotensin II [125], adrenaline, and endothelin [126]. As early as 1991, Escalante had pointed out that both 20-HETE and 20-COOH-AA, acting similarly to furosemide, reduce the Na^+ and K^+ concentrations of medullary thick ascending limb of Henle (mTALH) cells, suggesting the potential impact of HETEs on renal blood flow, GFR and urinary sodium excretion rates [127]. CYP4A11 is a key enzyme in the synthesis of 20-HETE. Both CYP4A and CYP4F belong to the CYP4 gene family, which catalyzes the conversion of arachidonic acid to 20-HETE [128]. The expression of CYP4A protein and the production of 20-HETE were significantly higher in the renal cortex and outer medulla of Dahl S salt-sensitive rats that fed either a low-salt or high-salt diet, indicating that the increased levels of renal 20-HETE in Dahl S rats promoted sodium retention and the development of salt sensitive hypertension [129]. Normalization of the 20-HETE levels with fibrates or transfer of wild-type CYP4A genes in congenic Dahl S strains is of great significance for inhibiting the progression of proteinuria and renal injury [129–131]. In the kidney, especially in the renal cortex, CYP4A also increases pressure natriuresis in the Dahl salt-sensitive rat [132]. The amount of 20-HETE metabolites in the CYP450 pathway produced by the extra renal medullary microsomes of salt-sensitive (SS/Jr) rats was significantly lower than that of salt-resistant (SR/Jr) rats [133].

In contrast, pharmacological inhibition of 20-HETE production in the outer medulla of the kidney in Lewis rats renders salt-sensitive [134], which means 20-HETE is a powerful vasoconstrictor in the kidney [135,136]. In renal microvessels, 20-HETE can strongly inhibit the activity of Na^+/K^+-ATPase and is a highly effective vasoconstrictor [137]. Increased production of 20-HETE in the renal microcirculation will decrease glomerular capillary pressure and GFR [124,138]. More importantly, 20-HETE can also reduce the pressure of post-glomerular circulation and ultimately promote the development of hypertension [138]. Interestingly though, 20-HETE-mediated increases in renal vascular resistance also reduce stress during glomerular circulation, thereby preventing the occurrence of glomerular damage caused by hypertension [139]. Therefore, when the synthesis of 20-HETE in the kidney is disturbed, the self-regulation of renal blood flow and the renal tubule-glomerular feedback system will be affected, resulting in reduced ion transport, increasing the difficulty of blood pressure control, and eventually aggravating glomerulonephritis and renal tubular interstitial nephritis [124]. The effect of 20-HETE on vascular function causes an ischemia-reperfusion injury (IRI) change that prolongs vasoconstriction after reperfusion and increased I/R injury [140]. It is well known that IRI is the most common cause of AKI, and 20-HETE production is elevated after renal ischemia (I/R) [141–143]. Use of 20-HETE analogues at a lower dosage can reduce the elevated plasma creatinine levels after I/R injury. In addition, 20-HETE analogues preconditioning reduced the area of tubular epithelial necrosis after I/R injury [143]. Moreover, 20-HETE can also be used to attenuate IRI by increasing medullary oxygen cooperation because it increases medullary blood flow and inhibits the renal tubular sodium transport [143,144]. On the other hand, in the kidney, 20-HETE overexpression significantly aggravated cell damage caused by I/R damage, which was mediated by the activation of caspase-3 and partly by enhanced CYP4A-producing free radicals [140]. Thus, the relationship between 20-HETE and AKI may be further clarified. 20-HETE may also promote the progression of renal inflammation by mediating apoptosis [145,146]. Studies have proved that CYP4A and NADPH oxidase expression was up-regulated in glomeruli of diabetic OVE26 mice [145]. And hyperglycemia increases 20-HETE production and enhances 20-HETE-dependent ROS formation and apoptosis in the mouse podocytes and rat tubuli epithelial cells, while 20-HETE blockade reduces ROS and improves apoptosis and albuminuria [145,146]. Recent research indicated that 20-HETE can increase the TRPC6 activity in podocytes, secondary to podocytes and activate ROS production [147]. Activation of TRPC6 results in the disappearance of the foot processes, but eliminates the detachment of podocyte [148]. Similar to 20-HETE, the correlation between 19-HETE and renal inflammation is mainly achieved through its effects on renal hemodynamics and blood pressure, which will not be repeated here [149].

3.3. LTs/LXs and Renal Inflammation

As the major metabolite of the LOX pathway, LTs and LXs both play considerable roles in kidney inflammation. LTs are a class of powerful chemotactic molecules that regulate leukocyte migration and activation [150]. Current studies have confirmed increases of LTs and LXs in the kidneys after ischemia, which further mediates a series of inflammatory reactions leading to the kidney damage [151]. More importantly, studies have shown that renal tissue can produce LTs without relying on circulating inflammatory cells [152]. The action of LTB_4 on neutrophil aggregation and infiltration and kidney tissue damage in the rat iARF model was first reported. In the rat kidney ischemia-reperfusion (I/R) model, LTB_4 played a leading role in the polymorphonuclear neutrophils (PMNs) [153]. LTB_4-dependent cells migrate to ischemic renal parenchyma and activate neutrophils, which can rapidly up-regulate leukocyte adhesion molecules, and then promote the initial infiltration of PMNs. Activated neutrophils induce endothelial cell injury, and vasodilation is blocked, further aggravating ischemic tubulointerstitial damage and causing a vicious circle of renal tissue damage [153]. A recent study by Landgraf on LTB_4-mediated renal tissue inflammation has found that LTB_4 and LTD_4 inhibited the endocytosis of albumin in LLC-PK1 cells (pig kidney cells), attenuating the activation of protein kinase C (PKC) and protein kinase B (PKB) and thereby reducing the absorption of albumin. Meanwhile, in mice models, LTs inhibited the secretion of the anti-inflammatory cytokine IL-10, hindered the PI-3K/PKB pathway, and caused albumin overload that finally gave rise to tubule-interstitial damage [154,155]. After a few minutes of reperfusion, PMNs were recruited and LTA_4 was immediately transformed into LTB_4 in the kidney. Once PMNs entered the interstitial space, the above mechanism will be performed at high speed, thus accelerating the extensive migration of PMNs and forming a vicious cycle of tissue damage [153]. The role of LTs in glomerular injury has also been demonstrated in the nephrotoxic serum-induced glomerular injury model, due to increased recruitment/activation of polymorphonuclear cells and increased LTB_4 production in the kidney, which eventually amplifies the reduction of glomerular filtration rate [156]. Moreover, LTB_4 and $LTC_4/D_4/E_4$ levels are both increased in patients with nephrotic syndrome (NS), and this may be the reason why the serum creatinine, diastolic blood pressure, and protein/creatinine ratio of patients are significantly reduced [157].

As another major metabolite of the LOX pathway, LXs are important endogenous anti-inflammatory lipid transmitters that have been discovered earlier and can act on a variety of cells, including neutrophils, mononuclear macrophages, mesangial cells etc., to exert complex anti-inflammatory effects [158–160]. In glomerulonephritis, LXA_4 inhibits LTs and reduces further infiltration of leukocytes [161,162]. In acute poststreptococcal glomerulonephritis (APSGN), one of the crucial pathological effects is the infiltration of neutrophils and monocytes in the glomeruli during the acute phase [163]. In vitro experiments with human mesangial cells showed that very low concentrations of LXA_4 (1–10 nmol/L) inhibited the expression of cell fibrosis-related genes induced by platelet-derived growth factor and connective tissue growth factor [164]. Leukocytes infiltrate and LTB_4 synthesis increases in rat kidneys at the early stage after nephrotoxic serum injection. At the same time, IL-4 and IL-13 produced by Th2 cells stimulate glomerular expression of LOX and synthesis of 15S-HETE and LXA_4. The later inhibits LTB_4 signaling, reduces leukocyte chemotaxis and transforms neutrophil infiltration into mononuclear macrophage infiltration, resulting in removal of apoptotic neutrophils and repairmen of tissue damage [165,166]. Another nephritis involving LXs is Henoch-Schonlein purpura nephritis (HSPN), which is a common secondary glomerulonephritis in pediatrics [167]. In HSPN, both plasma and urinary levels of LTB_4 and LTE_4 increase, while LXA_4 levels decrease, indicating that endogenous LXA_4 deficiency may be one of the causes of HSPN (which provides a basis for exploring new methods for the treatment of HSPN) [167]. Recent studies have shown that LXs inhibited the increase of renal/body weight ratio in diabetic animals and also reduced the glomerular dilatation and mesangial matrix deposition, in both high-fat diet-induced diabetes mouse model and unilateral ureteral obstruction (UUO) mouse model [168,169]. In addition, LXs can significantly reduce proteinuria and play an important role in reversing the CKD induced in diabetic *ApoE*$^{-/-}$ male mice [170]. In cultured human renal epithelial cells, treatment with LXs reduced TNF-α-driven Egr-1 activation, which may regulate the inflammation of kidney disease [170] [171,172]. As Egr-1 activity is elevated in renal tubular cells in patients with renal failure [173], this may be related to Egr-1, which mediates the TGF-β signaling pathway in the kidney, immune cell infiltration, and regulates the NF-κB activity and cytokine/chemokine expression in the kidney [173]. Brennan et al. had identified that Egr-1 as a downstream target for LXs, besides, they also confirmed the interaction between LXs and Egr-1 in studies of human renal tubular epithelial cells [170]. In summary, LXs have a significant positive effect on inhibiting kidney inflammation.

3.4. EETs and Renal Inflammation

It has been reported that 14,15-EET can alleviate the proteinuria and renal dysfunction caused by cyclosporine, which may be related to the inhibition of inflammatory cells infiltration into the kidney and reduction of renal fibrosis [174]. In the rat model of renal tubule-interstitial inflammation induced by unilateral ureteral obstruction (UUO), sEH deficiency has a beneficial effect on renal fibrosis and interstitial inflammation. The molecular mechanism may be associated with lack of sEH and the reduction of EETs degradation, which inhibited the transforming growth factor (TGF)-1/Smad3 signaling, diminished infiltration of neutrophils and macrophages, prevented expression levels of NF-κB target gene proteins (TNF-α and ICAM-1), decrease cell death caused by ROS, and causes PPAR inactivation [175]. Manhiani proved that soluble epoxide hydrolase gene deletion attenuated renal injury and inflammation with DOCA-salt hypertension [176]. In the kidney, EET has anti-inflammatory effects by blocking the activation of NF-kB and inhibiting the progression of renal inflammation by reducing renal macrophage infiltration [176]. Research also showed that, increased production of EET prevented microalbuminuria and kidney inflammation in the hyperglycemic overweight mice [177]. However, in the kidney, EET/DHET-ratios were increased in sEH knockout mice, but surprisingly, plasma creatinine concentration and IRI were higher than in the control group, which may be due to the formation of 20-HETE that eliminates the potentially beneficial effects of EET degradation [178]. In an I/R-induced AKI mouse model, the administration of 14,15-EET alleviated the dilated renal tubules, leading to an obvious reduction in plasma Cr, TNF-α and IL-6 [179]. These effects, discovered in I/R-caused AKI mice, may be due to the 14,15-EET reversing the I/R-induced declination of p-GSK3β expression, which induced the ratio of p-GSK3β/GSK3β back to a normal level [180]. In addition, the CYP450-derived eicosanoids could activate the eNOS and NO release. 14,15-EET can activate the endothelial cell NO synthase (eNOS) and NO release by blocking the Ca^{2+}-activated K$^+$, which eventually caused afferent arteries dilatation and reduces renal inflammation [181]. 5,6-EET, found in the kidneys of rabbits, is involved in the metabolism of two types of vasodilators, one being PGE$_2$/PGI$_2$ and the other being the adenosine analogue 5,6-epoxy-PGE [182]. In contrast, in the rat I/R kidney model, 5,6-EET caused COX-dependent renal vasoconstriction, whereas in isolated rat kidneys, 5,6-EET dilated blood vessels. In spontaneously hypertensive rats, 5,6-EET and 11,12-EET induced renal vasodilation more than 2 times greater than in Wistar Kyoto rats [183]. Stimulation of EETs activating adenosine 2A (A2A) may be an important mechanism for regulating microvascular tension in glomeruli [184]. It has been reported that 11,12-EET may represent an A2A-mediated mediator of glomerular microvascular expansion in rats. In rat glomerular pre-microvasculature, EET release was an important step in the activation of A2A receptors and adenylyl cyclase activation, and EETs mediated the activation of the Gs alpha protein by stimulating mono-ADP-ribosyltransferase [185]. The mechanism by which 11,12-EET dilates the afferent arterioles is possibly due to the phosphorylation of protein phosphatase 2A activity and Ca^{2+}-activated K$^+$ channels [186]. Recent research has proven that 11,12-EET is a major product of Cyp2c44 in mice, which is involved in regulating the excretion of epithelial sodium in the collecting duct. Cyp2c44 in the collecting duct can promote the excretion of Na^+ in the kidney under high salt or high K^+ environment by inhibiting epithelial Na^+ channel (ENaC), thus preventing excessive Na^+ absorption, suggesting that 11,12-EET may indirectly affect the renal inflammation through its role in regulation of blood pressure [187]. It is worth mentioning that 8,9-EET has a unique protective effect on the glomerulus [188]. Exogenous 8,9-EET (1–1000 nM) dose-dependently prevented a circulating permeability factor (FSPF)-induced increase in the glomerular albumin permeability [188]. The other three EET regioisomers, 8,9-EET metabolite, 8,9-dihydroxyeicosatrienoic acid and unrelated 11,14-eicosadienoic acid were ineffective, indicating the specificity of 8,9-EET for glomerular protection [188]. More importantly, a synthetic analog of 8,9-EET containing a double bond antagonized the effect of 8,9-EET on FSPF-induced increase in glomerular albumin permeability. These results indicate that the development of stable analogs of 8,9-EET may make sense to the effective management of glomerular dysfunction [188].

4. Treatments

A number of drugs for kidney inflammation based on the AA metabolic pathway are in the early stages of development for human disease treatment, and their study output is limited. The treatment of kidney disease based on AA is varied and many factors are involved, so here we only introduce strategies that are relevant to humans (Table 1).

Table 1. Drugs related to AA metabolism for kidney inflammation.

Compounds	Species	Targets	Kidney Disease	Outcome	Reference
Cyclosporine+ methylprednisolone	Human	Calcineurin and corticosteroid hormone receptor	IMN	Proteinuria ↓ PLA2R Ab ↓ Infiltration of defense cells ↓	[189]
Tacrolimus+corticosteroids, corticosteroids+cyclophosphamide, or corticosteroids alone.	Human	Peptidyl-prolyl isomerase and glucocorticoid receptors	IMN	Proteinuria ↓ Serum albumin ↑ Glomerular PLA2R ↓ Serum PLA2R-Ab ↓ Infiltration of defense cells ↑	[190]
Rituximab	Human	Pan-B-cell marker CD20	IMN/IgA Nephritis	Proteinuria ↓ GFR ↑ Serum albumin ↑ PLA2R Ab ↓ Infiltration of defense cells ↓	[191–193]
Prednisolone	Human	glucocorticoid receptors	IMN	GFR ↑ Proteinuria ↓ Serum albumin ↑ PLA2R Ab ↓ Infiltration of defense cells ↓	[194]
Cyclophosphamide or +corticosteroids	Human	glucocorticoid receptors (for corticosteroids)	IMN/IgA Nephritis	GFR ↑ Proteinuria ↓ Serum albumin ↑ PLA2R Ab ↓ Infiltration of defense cells ↓	[193,194]
Aspirin	Mouse and Human	COX-1/COX-2	AKI	GFR ↑ Serum creatinine ↓ Urinary output ↑ Proteinuria ↓	[195,196]
Ibuprofen	Human	COX-1/COX-2	ATIN	Pain control ↓	[197,198]
Nimesulide	Rats and Human	COX-1/COX-2	ATIN	Plasma renin activity ↓ Aldosterone level ↓ Urinary PTE2 level ↓	[199]
Indomethacin	Human	COX-1/COX-2	Renal failure	IL-6 ↓ IL-10 ↓	[199]
Carprofen	Human	COX-2	Renal failure	IL-1β ↓	[199]

Table 1. *Cont.*

Compounds	Species	Targets	Kidney Disease	Outcome	Reference
Diclofenac acid	Rats and Human	COX1/COX2	Renal cancer	PGE2 level ↓	[200]
Zileuton	Human Mesangial Cells	LOX/COX-2	Renal cancer	Serum creatinine ↓ Interstitial fibrosis ↓	[201]
Licofelone	Mouse and Human	5-LOX/COX	Glomerulonephritis	IL-18 ↓ PGE2 ↓	[201]
Baicalein	Mouse	12/15-LOX	Diabetic nephropathy	12-HETE ↓ IL-6 ↓ Proteinuria ↓	[202]
PVPA	Rats	CYP450	Acute and chronic glomerulonephritis	Proteinuria ↓ Apoptosis in tubular epithelial cells ↓ Generation of reactive oxygen species ↓	[174]

4.1. Phospholipase-Associated Therapy

Current research has suggested that the M-type phospholipase A2 receptor (PLA$_2$R) is sensitive and specific for idiopathic membranous nephropathy (MN). Serum phospholipase A$_2$ receptor antibody (PLA$_2$R Ab) and circulating anti-phospholipase A$_2$ receptor antibodies (anti-PLA2R Abs) are now regarded as a valuable indicator of prognosis for patients with nephritis, especially in patients with idiopathic membranous nephropathy (IMN) [203,204]. IMN is one of the most common causes of adult primary NS. The KDIGO guidelines have recommend treatment with glucocorticoids and immunosuppressive agents for IMN [191,194]. Beck et al. reported that 35 patients with IMN were treated with rituximab (the anti- autoimmune disease drug), within whom 71% of patients were serum anti-PLA$_2$R -positive. After 12 months of rituximab therapy, serum anti-PLA$_2$R decreased or disappeared in 17 (68%) of these patients. After 12 months and 24 months of therapy, the rates of complete remission (CR) and partial response (PR) were 59% and 88%, respectively, and the decrease in antibody titer was earlier than the remission of proteinuria [189]. An earlier study of 37 biopsy confirmed IMN patients indicated that, after receiving standard immunosuppressive therapy (cyclosporine combined with methylprednisolone), the titer of PLA$_2$R-Ab positive patients gradually decreased with an ameliorated proteinuria [190]. A retrospective study that includes 113 IMN patients showed that, the tacrolimus (TAC) and corticosteroids, corticosteroids and cyclophosphamide (CYC) and corticosteroids alone respectively can decrease the serum PLA$_2$R-Ab titer and proteinuria in IMN patients [192]. As a conventional anti-tumor drug, rituximab seems to have a favorable result on MN [205]. 8 months after receiving rituximab, 22 patients with PLA$_2$R-related MN showed a decrease of proteinuria and PLA$_2$R Ab titer. At the meantime, renal function remained stable, and serum albumin increased [205]. Similar results were obtained in Beck's study, which suggested that rituximab can inhibit the progression of IMN by lowering the PLA$_2$R Ab titer [189]. Lowered PLA$_2$R Ab titer could also be achieved by oral administration of prednisolone or cyclical cyclophosphamide (CTX) or cyclophosphamide or mycophenolate mofetil (MMF) in combination with steroids in IMN patients, showing a beneficial result with elevated glomerular filtration rate (eGFR) [191,193]. A recent study showed that combination with corticosteroids and rituximab also decreases the serum creatinine and PLA$_2$R-Ab level [206]. However, one cannot ignore the fact that steroid treatment aggravated tubule-interstitial fibrosis in patients with acute interstitial nephritis [207]. A recent study also reported that corticosteroid treatment seems to increase the recurrence rate of TIN [208], suggesting that the PLA$_2$R-Ab therapy may only work in IMN patients. The data from this research seems contradictory, especially the small sample size, which makes it difficult to draw firm conclusions regarding their outcomes. Therefore, the prospect of corticosteroids for the anti- PLA$_2$R-Ab therapy needs more research and exploration.

4.2. COX-Associated Therapy

Nonsteroidal anti-inflammatory drugs (NSAIDs) are the main COX inhibitors. Their common mechanism of action is the inhibition of COX, and the most important result of this inhibition is the reduction of the production of PGs, thus playing anti-inflammatory, pain relieving and antipyretic roles [209]. COX inhibitors fall into two broad categories: non-specific COX inhibitors and specific COX-2 inhibitors. Among them, aspirin, ibuprofen, naproxen, etc. are usually used as non-specific COX inhibitors in the treatment of nephritis. Certain functional groups of COX-2 inhibitors (coxibs) can insert into the hydrophobic cavity formed by some amino acid residues of COX-2, causing the loss of their catalytic function [18]. In this case, AA cannot perform biological transformations under the catalysis of COX-2, thus blocking the synthesis of PGs as well as the inflammatory process [58]. Aspirin, also known as acetylsalicylic acid, is a well-known antipyretic analgesic that inhibits platelet aggregation and prevents thrombosis, which could also be used in kidney inflammatory diseases [210]. Aspirin is a non-specific COX inhibitor that inhibits both COX-1 and COX-2, which has a good effect on the prevention of primary and secondary thrombosis [211–213]. Aspirin treatment in MRL/MpJ-*Fas^{lpr}*/J (MRL/lpr) mouse could alleviate LN [195] and reduce the risk of platelet aggregation and micro-embolization, which may improve the GFR during renal perfusion, thereby improving kidney function [196]. At the same time, perioperative aspirin can reduce the thromboxane level in the urine, which is a powerful vasoconstrictor, and improve renal function [196]. A large prospective cohort study of more than 5000 patients undergoing cardiac surgery indicated that patients taking aspirin had a lower incidence of AKI than patients who did not take aspirin ($P < 0.001$) [214]. Above all, the incidence of renal failure was reduced by 74% in those who were taking aspirin [214]. However, according to a recent study, low-dose aspirin oral intake was shown to have no significant effect on kidney function during the 15 years after kidney transplantation [215]. This may be because aspirin can be rapidly hydrolyzed to salicylate immediately, a product that has an almost negligible effect on COX [210]. Further, the results found that aspirin increased the risk of massive hemorrhage and further increased the risk of subsequent AKI [197]. Since the findings in numerous studies are contradictory, additional research on the value of aspirin for kidney inflammation is essential.

As the most widely used NSAID, ibuprofen is the first choice for the treatment of inflammatory pain [198]. Compared with other NSAIDs and coxibs, ibuprofen has fewer side effects on the gastrointestinal tract and a relatively low incidence of liver and kidney damage [216]. However, the amount of urine was obviously reduced after the first day of treatment with ibuprofen in premature infants, and the serum creatinine concentration was significantly increased on the third day of treatment [217]. There seems to be a latent relationship between ibuprofen and acute tubule-interstitial nephritis (ATIN), which is a major factor contributing to the acute renal insufficiency that must be kept in mind when it is used for treatment [199,218,219].

Nimesulide, another NSAID, has selective inhibition of COX-2 and qualitative inhibition of COX-1, and the principal effect of nimesulide on kidney inflammation mainly involves renal hemodynamics and electrolyte excretion. The use of nimesulide in healthy volunteers during long-term use of furosemide causes a brief and acute decline in renal hemodynamics and attenuated the natriuretic, kaliuretic and diuretic effects of furosemide [220]. Nimesulide reduced the plasma renin activity, aldosterone levels, and urinary PTE_2 levels [220]. Meanwhile, diuretic-induced renin activity was attenuated by nimesulide. This suggests that nimesulide protects kidney function by allowing sodium and potassium retention [220]. However, it is interesting to remark that there was no significant change in serum creatinine and Tamm-Horsfall glycoprotein (THG) concentrations as well as no significant effect on GFR after nimesulide in 16 healthy human volunteers [221]. The weak effect of nimesulide on renal toxicity may suggest that it has no strong inhibitory effect on renal COX at the therapeutic dose, which is similar to the results from Ceserani et al., who showed that nimesulide did not dramatically reduced urinary PTE_2 excretion in rats [222].

Several other NSAIDs also plays active role in the treatment of nephritis. Carprofen, an inhibitor of COX-mediated PG synthesis, increased the thick ascending limb of the loop of Henle at the tubular level and increased resorption of solute in the medullary segment of the upper extremity, thereby reducing sodium and chlorine excretion and potentially improving GFR or overall excretion of solute in the human kidney [200]. Diclofenac acid can reduce the recurrence survival rate and improve the survival rate of patients with renal cancer after surgery, which may be related to the fact that diclofenac acid inhibits the production of PGE_2, which in turn inhibited the process by which PGE_2 alters intracellular cyclic adenosine monophosphate levels to reduce the number and activity of natural killer cells [223–225].

However, as a COX-2 inhibitor, rofecoxib increases the risk of major cardiovascular events during treatment [226]. In addition, naproxen and celecoxib were related to the occurrence of AKI [227]. Studies have associated people who take naproxen, regardless of the dosage, with a higher risk of nephrotic syndrome and AIN [228]. Other NSAIDs may also have potential adverse effects on renal function [229], such as indomethacin, which can cause acute sodium retention in healthy adults and reduce GFR levels by inhibiting COX [230]. Studies have shown that live-donor nephrectomy patients that were treated with ketolic acid had significant increases of urinary albumin/creatinine ratio after 1 year and is an independent risk factor for reducing GFR (odds ratio 1.38) [231]. A study from *Lancet* indicated that NSAIDs, such as rofecoxib, celecoxib, ibuprofen, naproxen, and diclofenac, increase the risk of vascular events during treatment [232]. However, it has also been pointed out that all COX-2 inhibitors did not significantly promote renal events and arrhythmia events [233]. These findings provide insight for future research, and prospective clinical trials are needed to assess the curative effect and safety of NSAIDs for the treatment of renal inflammation.

4.3. LOX-Associated Therapy

The research related to LOX-associated therapy is mostly studied on experimental animals, and when it comes to human studies, zileuton is often mentioned. Zileuton blocks the conversion of AA to LTB_4 by inhibiting the 5-LOX activity and is often used for the prevention of inflammation-related diseases and for cancer treatment [234]. However, whether zileuton could be used to treat renal inflammation in humans still needs to be further confirmed by clinical trials. Licofelone is a novel dual anti-inflammatory drug that inhibits both COX and 5-LOX. A study has indicated that licofelone improved inflammation in human mesangial cells (HMCs) exposed to IL-18 in a dose-dependent manner, through inhibiting COX-2 enzyme activity and reducing PGE_2 release in HMCs [201]. Similarly, licofelone inhibited IL-18-induced 5-LOX enzyme activity and thereby reduces leukotriene release. In addition, licofelone blocked IL-18-induced phosphorylation of p38 proliferation protein kinase, inhibited the expression of monocyte chemoattractant protein 1 and interferon-γ. Licofelone also suppressed mesangial cell proliferation caused by IL-18 [201]. These results indicate that licofelone alleviates human glomerular inflammation by inhibiting IL-18-induced proinflammatory cytokine release and cell proliferation. A more exciting result was that licofelone inhibited IL-18-induced mesangial cell proliferation, and the results indicated that licofelone might be effective for the treatment of glomerulonephritis in children [201]. 2,3-diarylxanthones, dual inhibitors of COX and 5-LOX, are capable of preventing the production of LTB_4 in human neutrophils as well as decreasing PGE_2 production in human whole blood in a concentration-dependent manner [235]. According to the current results, the effect of lox-related drugs in regulating inflammation is still in the experimental study stage. Baicalein, a 12/15-LOX inhibitor, was demonstrated to prevent the elevation in renal 12-HETE production and reduce renal inflammation in strptozotocin-induced diabetic mice [202].

4.4. CYP450/sEH-Associated Therapy

There are two pharmacological approaches that have been used to chronically elevate endogenous levels of EETs in order to evaluate their renal and vascular protective effects in vivo. One approach is to increase the levels of EETs by inducing epoxygenases with fibric acid derivatives such as clofibrate, fenofibrate, and bezafibrate [236]. Fenofibrate has been shown to strongly induce renal protein expression of CYP2C23, a major CYP epoxygenase in the rat kidney, and increase the renal epoxygenase activity [236]. We have previously reported that a CYP450 inducer, gemfibrozil, has shown positive effects on CYP2C-related non-alcoholic steatotic hepatitis [237]. More importantly, the potential link between dyslipidemia and renal inflammation also reveals the potential values of fibric acid derivatives for the treatment of renal inflammation [238,239] among diabetic dyslipidemia patients [240–242]. However, some reports suggested that, the combined action of metamizole and gemfibrozil could synergistically affect the proximal tubule and increase the chances of renal damage [243]. Some studies have shown that the epoxyeicosatrienoic acid analog can effectively slow down the kidney damage associated with oxidative stress, inflammation, and endoplasmic reticulum stress [244,245]. For example, a new oral drug, PVPA, reduces the proteinuria and renal dysfunction caused by cyclosporine, inhibits the inflammatory cell infiltration in the kidney, and reduces the renal fibrosis [174]. Warfarin, an anticoagulant, is mainly metabolized by CYP2C [246–248], which can inhibit the proliferation of mesangial cells by interfering with the activation of Gas6, and plays an important role in the treatment of various human kidney diseases, such as acute and chronic glomerulonephritis and diabetic nephropathy [249].

Another approach to elevate EETs is to inhibit the conversion of EETs to their less active metabolites by soluble epoxide hydrolase (sEH) [250]. sEH plays a major role in several diseases, including hypertension, cardiac hypertrophy, arteriosclerosis [251]. Because of its possible role in cardiovascular and other diseases, sEH is being pursued as a pharmacological target, and potent small molecule inhibitors are available [252]. Such inhibitors, like UC1153 (AR9281) and GSK2256294, were taken to clinical trials for treatment of hypertension and chronic obstructive pulmonary disease respectively [252]. However, even with the promise of epoxygenase metabolites to protect the kidney and vasculature, further research in this area is necessary in view of the small number of trials on humans.

5. Conclusions

The present review aims to discuss the effect of AA metabolism on kidney inflammation, as well as to provide a theoretical basis for the treatment of kidney inflammation. AA metabolism and kidney inflammation are closely linked in multiple ways. Through a summary of previous studies, our conclusions help us to understand the effects of AA metabolism on the kidney in several ways and provide the therapeutical treatment for renal inflammation. However, the studies on the treatment of kidney inflammation based on AA metabolism require a large sample of randomized controlled trails to elucidate their efficacy.

Author Contributions: Z.W., and Z.G. conceived and designed the article; T.W., X.F., Z.G., Z.W., Q.C. and D.W. wrote the paper. J.K.P and D.W. edited the manuscript. All authors read and approved the manuscript.

Funding: This work was funded by the National Key Research and Development Program of China, grant number [2017YFC1702703], the Key R&D programs in Shandong, grant number [2016CYJS08A01-1], and the National Science Foundation of China, grant number [81473369].

Conflicts of Interest: The authors declare no conflict of interest.

References

1. Van Dorp, D.A. Essential fatty acid metabolism. *Proc. Nutr. Soc.* **1975**, *34*, 279–286. [CrossRef] [PubMed]
2. Sperling, R.I.; Benincaso, A.I.; Knoell, C.T.; Larkin, J.K.; Austen, K.F.; Robinson, D.R. Dietary omega-3 polyunsaturated fatty acids inhibit phosphoinositide formation and chemotaxis in neutrophils. *J. Clin. Investig.* **1993**, *91*, 651–660. [CrossRef] [PubMed]
3. De Jonge, H.W.; Dekkers, D.H.; Lamers, J.M. Polyunsaturated fatty acids and signalling via phospholipase C-beta and A2 in myocardium. *Mol. Cell. Biochem.* **1996**, *157*, 199–210. [CrossRef] [PubMed]
4. Calder, P.C. Marine omega-3 fatty acids and inflammatory processes: Effects, mechanisms and clinical relevance. *Biochim. Biophys. Acta* **2015**, *1851*, 469–484. [CrossRef] [PubMed]

5. Yates, C.M.; Calder, P.C.; Ed Rainger, G. Pharmacology and therapeutics of omega-3 polyunsaturated fatty acids in chronic inflammatory disease. *Pharmacol. Ther.* **2014**, *141*, 272–282. [CrossRef] [PubMed]

6. Rae, S.A.; Davidson, E.M.; Smith, M.J. Leukotriene B4, an inflammatory mediator in gout. *Lancet* **1982**, *2*, 1122–1124. [CrossRef]

7. Arachidonic acid, analgesics, and asthma. *Lancet* **1981**, *2*, 1266–1267.

8. Rand, A.A.; Barnych, B.; Morisseau, C.; Cajka, T.; Lee, K.S.S.; Panigrahy, D.; Hammock, B.D. Cyclooxygenase-derived proangiogenic metabolites of epoxyeicosatrienoic acids. *Proc. Natl. Acad. Sci. USA* **2017**, *114*, 4370–4375. [CrossRef]

9. Kopp, B.T.; Thompson, R.; Kim, J.; Konstan, R.; Diaz, A.; Smith, B.; Shrestha, C.; Rogers, L.K.; Hayes, D., Jr.; Tumin, D.; et al. Secondhand smoke alters arachidonic acid metabolism and inflammation in infants and children with cystic fibrosis. *Thorax* **2019**, *74*, 237–246. [CrossRef]

10. Chauhan, G.; Roy, K.; Kumar, G.; Kumari, P.; Alam, S.; Kishore, K.; Panjwani, U.; Ray, K. Distinct influence of COX-1 and COX-2 on neuroinflammatory response and associated cognitive deficits during high altitude hypoxia. *Neuropharmacology* **2019**, *146*, 138–148. [CrossRef]

11. Goldstein, A.R.; White, R.H.; Akuse, R.; Chantler, C. Long-term follow-up of childhood Henoch-Schonlein nephritis. *Lancet* **1992**, *339*, 280–282. [CrossRef]

12. Murakami, M.; Nakatani, Y.; Kuwata, H.; Kudo, I. Cellular components that functionally interact with signaling phospholipase A(2)s. *Biochim. Biophys. Acta* **2000**, *1488*, 159–166. [CrossRef]

13. Dubois, R.N.; Abramson, S.B.; Crofford, L.; Gupta, R.A.; Simon, L.S.; Van De Putte, L.B.; Lipsky, P.E. Cyclooxygenase in biology and disease. *FASEB J.* **1998**, *12*, 1063–1073. [CrossRef] [PubMed]

14. Lambert, I.H.; Hoffmann, E.K.; Christensen, P. Role of prostaglandins and leukotrienes in volume regulation by Ehrlich ascites tumor cells. *J. Membr. Biol.* **1987**, *98*, 247–256. [CrossRef] [PubMed]

15. Lipsky, P.E.; Brooks, P.; Crofford, L.J.; DuBois, R.; Graham, D.; Simon, L.S.; van de Putte, L.B.; Abramson, S.B. Unresolved issues in the role of cyclooxygenase-2 in normal physiologic processes and disease. *Arch. Intern. Med.* **2000**, *160*, 913–920. [CrossRef] [PubMed]

16. Ricciotti, E.; Yu, Y.; Grosser, T.; Fitzgerald, G.A. COX-2, the dominant source of prostacyclin. *Proc. Natl. Acad. Sci. USA* **2013**, *110*, E183. [CrossRef] [PubMed]

17. Thuresson, E.D.; Lakkides, K.M.; Rieke, C.J.; Sun, Y.; Wingerd, B.A.; Micielli, R.; Mulichak, A.M.; Malkowski, M.G.; Garavito, R.M.; Smith, W.L. Prostaglandin endoperoxide H synthase-1: The functions of cyclooxygenase active site residues in the binding, positioning, and oxygenation of arachidonic acid. *J. Biol. Chem.* **2001**, *276*, 10347–10357. [CrossRef]

18. Hawkey, C.J. COX-2 inhibitors. *Lancet* **1999**, *353*, 307–314. [CrossRef]

19. Kawahara, K.; Hohjoh, H.; Inazumi, T.; Tsuchiya, S.; Sugimoto, Y. Prostaglandin E2-induced inflammation: Relevance of prostaglandin E receptors. *Biochim. Biophys. Acta* **2015**, *1851*, 414–421. [CrossRef]

20. Smith, W.L.; Garavito, R.M.; DeWitt, D.L. Prostaglandin endoperoxide H synthases (cyclooxygenases)-1 and -2. *J. Biol. Chem.* **1996**, *271*, 33157–33160. [CrossRef]

21. Naraba, H.; Murakami, M.; Matsumoto, H.; Shimbara, S.; Ueno, A.; Kudo, I.; Oh-ishi, S. Segregated coupling of phospholipases A2, cyclooxygenases, and terminal prostanoid synthases in different phases of prostanoid biosynthesis in rat peritoneal macrophages. *J. Immunol.* **1998**, *160*, 2974–2982. [PubMed]

22. Smith, W.L.; Song, I. The enzymology of prostaglandin endoperoxide H synthases-1 and -2. *Prostaglandins Other Lipid Mediat.* **2002**, *68–69*, 115–128. [CrossRef]

23. Bahia, M.S.; Katare, Y.K.; Silakari, O.; Vyas, B.; Silakari, P. Inhibitors of microsomal prostaglandin E2 synthase-1 enzyme as emerging anti-inflammatory candidates. *Med. Res. Rev.* **2014**, *34*, 825–855. [CrossRef] [PubMed]

24. Hecker, M.; Haurand, M.; Ullrich, V.; Diczfalusy, U.; Hammarstrom, S. Products, kinetics, and substrate specificity of homogeneous thromboxane synthase from human platelets: Development of a novel enzyme assay. *Arch. Biochem. Biophys.* **1987**, *254*, 124–135. [CrossRef]

25. Goetzl, E.J.; An, S.; Smith, W.L. Specificity of expression and effects of eicosanoid mediators in normal physiology and human diseases. *FASEB J.* **1995**, *9*, 1051–1058. [CrossRef] [PubMed]

26. Stenson, W.F. The universe of arachidonic acid metabolites in inflammatory bowel disease: Can we tell the good from the bad? *Curr. Opin. Gastroenterol.* **2014**, *30*, 347–351. [CrossRef] [PubMed]

27. Alhouayek, M.; Muccioli, G.G. COX-2-derived endocannabinoid metabolites as novel inflammatory mediators. *Trends Pharmacol. Sci.* **2014**, *35*, 284–292. [CrossRef]

28. Li, H.S.; Hebda, P.A.; Kelly, L.A.; Ehrlich, G.D.; Whitcomb, D.C.; Dohar, J.E. Up-regulation of prostaglandin EP4 receptor messenger RNA in fetal rabbit skin wound. *Arch. Otolaryngol. Head Neck Surg.* **2000**, *126*, 1337–1343. [CrossRef]

29. Breyer, R.M.; Bagdassarian, C.K.; Myers, S.A.; Breyer, M.D. Prostanoid receptors: Subtypes and signaling. *Annu. Rev. Pharmacol. Toxicol.* **2001**, *41*, 661–690. [CrossRef]

30. Sandulache, V.C.; Chafin, J.B.; Li-Korotky, H.S.; Otteson, T.D.; Dohar, J.E.; Hebda, P.A. Elucidating the role of interleukin 1beta and prostaglandin E2 in upper airway mucosal wound healing. *Arch. Otolaryngol. Head Neck Surg.* **2007**, *133*, 365–374. [CrossRef]

31. Bauer, J.; Ripperger, A.; Frantz, S.; Ergun, S.; Schwedhelm, E.; Benndorf, R.A. Pathophysiology of isoprostanes in the cardiovascular system: Implications of isoprostane-mediated thromboxane A2 receptor activation. *Br. J. Pharmacol.* **2014**, *171*, 3115–3131. [CrossRef] [PubMed]

32. Ekambaram, P.; Lambiv, W.; Cazzolli, R.; Ashton, A.W.; Honn, K.V. The thromboxane synthase and receptor signaling pathway in cancer: An emerging paradigm in cancer progression and metastasis. *Cancer Metast. Rev.* **2011**, *30*, 397–408. [CrossRef] [PubMed]

33. Zhou, Z.; Sun, C.; Tilley, S.L.; Mustafa, S.J. Mechanisms underlying uridine adenosine tetraphosphate-induced vascular contraction in mouse aorta: Role of thromboxane and purinergic receptors. *Vasc. Pharmacol.* **2015**, *73*, 78–85. [CrossRef] [PubMed]

34. Smith, W.L.; DeWitt, D.L.; Garavito, R.M. Cyclooxygenases: Structural, cellular, and molecular biology. *Annu. Rev. Biochem.* **2000**, *69*, 145–182. [CrossRef] [PubMed]

35. Davies, N.M.; Good, R.L.; Roupe, K.A.; Yanez, J.A. Cyclooxygenase-3: Axiom, dogma, anomaly, enigma or splice error?—Not as easy as 1, 2, 3. *J. Pharm. Pharm. Sci.* **2004**, *7*, 217–226. [PubMed]

36. Chandrasekharan, N.V.; Dai, H.; Roos, K.L.; Evanson, N.K.; Tomsik, J.; Elton, T.S.; Simmons, D.L. COX-3, a cyclooxygenase-1 variant inhibited by acetaminophen and other analgesic/antipyretic drugs: Cloning, structure, and expression. *Proc. Natl. Acad. Sci. USA* **2002**, *99*, 13926–13931. [CrossRef] [PubMed]

37. Schwab, J.M.; Beiter, T.; Linder, J.U.; Laufer, S.; Schulz, J.E.; Meyermann, R.; Schluesener, H.J. COX-3—A virtual pain target in humans? *FASEB J.* **2003**, *17*, 2174–2175. [CrossRef] [PubMed]

38. Willoughby, D.A.; Moore, A.R.; Colville-Nash, P.R. COX-1, COX-2, and COX-3 and the future treatment of chronic inflammatory disease. *Lancet* **2000**, *355*, 646–648. [CrossRef]

39. Radmark, O.; Werz, O.; Steinhilber, D.; Samuelsson, B. 5-Lipoxygenase, a key enzyme for leukotriene biosynthesis in health and disease. *Biochim. Biophys. Acta* **2015**, *1851*, 331–339. [CrossRef]

40. Mittal, M.; Kumar, R.B.; Balagunaseelan, N.; Hamberg, M.; Jegerschold, C.; Radmark, O.; Haeggstrom, J.Z.; Rinaldo-Matthis, A. Kinetic investigation of human 5-lipoxygenase with arachidonic acid. *Bioorganic Med. Chem. Lett.* **2016**, *26*, 3547–3551. [CrossRef]

41. Powell, W.S.; Gravelle, F.; Gravel, S. Metabolism of 5(S)-hydroxy-6,8,11,14-eicosatetraenoic acid and other 5(S)-hydroxyeicosanoids by a specific dehydrogenase in human polymorphonuclear leukocytes. *J. Biol. Chem.* **1992**, *267*, 19233–19241. [PubMed]

42. Mastyugin, V.; Aversa, E.; Bonazzi, A.; Vafaes, C.; Mieyal, P.; Schwartzman, M.L. Hypoxia-induced production of 12-hydroxyeicosanoids in the corneal epithelium: Involvement of a cytochrome P-4504B1 isoform. *J. Pharmacol. Exp. Ther.* **1999**, *289*, 1611–1619. [PubMed]

43. Powell, W.S.; Rokach, J. Biosynthesis, biological effects, and receptors of hydroxyeicosatetraenoic acids (HETEs) and oxoeicosatetraenoic acids (oxo-ETEs) derived from arachidonic acid. *Biochim. Biophys. Acta* **2015**, *1851*, 340–355. [CrossRef] [PubMed]

44. Shimizu, T.; Radmark, O.; Samuelsson, B. Enzyme with dual lipoxygenase activities catalyzes leukotriene A4 synthesis from arachidonic acid. *Proc. Natl. Acad. Sci. USA* **1984**, *81*, 689–693. [CrossRef] [PubMed]

45. Green, A.R.; Freedman, C.; Tena, J.; Tourdot, B.E.; Liu, B.; Holinstat, M.; Holman, T.R. 5 S,15 S-Dihydroperoxyeicosatetraenoic Acid (5,15-diHpETE) as a Lipoxin Intermediate: Reactivity and Kinetics with Human Leukocyte 5-Lipoxygenase, Platelet 12-Lipoxygenase, and Reticulocyte 15-Lipoxygenase-1. *Biochemistry* **2018**, *57*, 6726–6734. [CrossRef] [PubMed]

46. Nakao, A.; Watanabe, T.; Ohishi, N.; Toda, A.; Asano, K.; Taniguchi, S.; Nosaka, K.; Noiri, E.; Suzuki, T.; Sakai, T.; et al. Ubiquitous localization of leukotriene A4 hydrolase in the rat nephron. *Kidney Int.* **1999**, *55*, 100–108. [CrossRef] [PubMed]

47. Baba, T.; Black, K.L.; Ikezaki, K.; Chen, K.N.; Becker, D.P. Intracarotid infusion of leukotriene C4 selectively increases blood-brain barrier permeability after focal ischemia in rats. *J. Cereb. Blood Flow Metab.* **1991**, *11*, 638–643. [CrossRef] [PubMed]
48. Porro, B.; Songia, P.; Squellerio, I.; Tremoli, E.; Cavalca, V. Analysis, physiological and clinical significance of 12-HETE: A neglected platelet-derived 12-lipoxygenase product. *J. Chromatogr. B* **2014**, *964*, 26–40. [CrossRef] [PubMed]
49. Witola, W.H.; Liu, S.R.; Montpetit, A.; Welti, R.; Hypolite, M.; Roth, M.; Zhou, Y.; Mui, E.; Cesbron-Delauw, M.F.; Fournie, G.J.; et al. ALOX12 in human toxoplasmosis. *Infect. Immun.* **2014**, *82*, 2670–2679. [CrossRef]
50. Serhan, C.N.; Sheppard, K.A. Lipoxin formation during human neutrophil-platelet interactions. Evidence for the transformation of leukotriene A4 by platelet 12-lipoxygenase in vitro. *J. Clin. Investig.* **1990**, *85*, 772–780. [CrossRef]
51. Fiore, S.; Ryeom, S.W.; Weller, P.F.; Serhan, C.N. Lipoxin recognition sites. Specific binding of labeled lipoxin A4 with human neutrophils. *J. Biol. Chem.* **1992**, *267*, 16168–16176. [PubMed]
52. Edenius, C.; Haeggstrom, J.; Lindgren, J.A. Transcellular conversion of endogenous arachidonic acid to lipoxins in mixed human platelet-granulocyte suspensions. *Biochem. Biophys. Res. Commun.* **1988**, *157*, 801–807. [CrossRef]
53. Sheppard, K.A.; Greenberg, S.M.; Funk, C.D.; Romano, M.; Serhan, C.N. Lipoxin generation by human megakaryocyte-induced 12-lipoxygenase. *Biochim. Biophys. Acta* **1992**, *1133*, 223–234. [CrossRef]
54. Moreno, J.J. New aspects of the role of hydroxyeicosatetraenoic acids in cell growth and cancer development. *Biochem. Pharmacol.* **2009**, *77*, 1–10. [CrossRef] [PubMed]
55. Medzhitov, R. Origin and physiological roles of inflammation. *Nature* **2008**, *454*, 428–435. [CrossRef] [PubMed]
56. Lasker, J.M.; Chen, W.B.; Wolf, I.; Bloswick, B.P.; Wilson, P.D.; Powell, P.K. Formation of 20-hydroxyeicosatetraenoic acid, a vasoactive and natriuretic eicosanoid, in human kidney. Role of Cyp4F2 and Cyp4A11. *J. Biol. Chem.* **2000**, *275*, 4118–4126. [CrossRef] [PubMed]
57. Wang, J.F.; Zhang, C.C.; Chou, K.C.; Wei, D.Q. Structure of cytochrome p450s and personalized drug. *Curr. Med. Chem.* **2009**, *16*, 232–244. [CrossRef]
58. Nebert, D.W.; Russell, D.W. Clinical importance of the cytochromes P450. *Lancet* **2002**, *360*, 1155–1162. [CrossRef]
59. Tacconelli, S.; Patrignani, P. Inside epoxyeicosatrienoic acids and cardiovascular disease. *Front. Pharmacol.* **2014**, *5*, 239. [CrossRef]
60. Aspromonte, N.; Monitillo, F.; Puzzovivo, A.; Valle, R.; Caldarola, P.; Iacoviello, M. Modulation of cardiac cytochrome P450 in patients with heart failure. *Expert Opin. Drug Metab. Toxicol.* **2014**, *10*, 327–339. [CrossRef]
61. Shahabi, P.; Siest, G.; Visvikis-siest, S. Influence of inflammation on cardiovascular protective effects of cytochrome P450 epoxygenase-derived epoxyeicosatrienoic acids. *Drug Metab. Rev.* **2014**, *46*, 33–56. [CrossRef]
62. Alsaad, A.M.; Zordoky, B.N.; Tse, M.M.; El-Kadi, A.O. Role of cytochrome P450-mediated arachidonic acid metabolites in the pathogenesis of cardiac hypertrophy. *Drug Metab. Rev.* **2013**, *45*, 173–195. [CrossRef]
63. Bellien, J.; Joannides, R. Epoxyeicosatrienoic acid pathway in human health and diseases. *J. Cardiovasc. Pharmacol.* **2013**, *61*, 188–196. [CrossRef] [PubMed]
64. Makita, K.; Falck, J.R.; Capdevila, J.H. Cytochrome P450, the arachidonic acid cascade, and hypertension: New vistas for an old enzyme system. *FASEB J.* **1996**, *10*, 1456–1463. [CrossRef] [PubMed]
65. Zeldin, D.C.; DuBois, R.N.; Falck, J.R.; Capdevila, J.H. Molecular cloning, expression and characterization of an endogenous human cytochrome P450 arachidonic acid epoxygenase isoform. *Arch. Biochem. Biophys.* **1995**, *322*, 76–86. [CrossRef] [PubMed]
66. Luo, G.; Zeldin, D.C.; Blaisdell, J.A.; Hodgson, E.; Goldstein, J.A. Cloning and expression of murine CYP2Cs and their ability to metabolize arachidonic acid. *Arch. Biochem. Biophys.* **1998**, *357*, 45–57. [CrossRef]
67. Wu, S.; Moomaw, C.R.; Tomer, K.B.; Falck, J.R.; Zeldin, D.C. Molecular cloning and expression of CYP2J2, a human cytochrome P450 arachidonic acid epoxygenase highly expressed in heart. *J. Biol. Chem.* **1996**, *271*, 3460–3468. [CrossRef]

68. Ma, J.; Qu, W.; Scarborough, P.E.; Tomer, K.B.; Moomaw, C.R.; Maronpot, R.; Davis, L.S.; Breyer, M.D.; Zeldin, D.C. Molecular cloning, enzymatic characterization, developmental expression, and cellular localization of a mouse cytochrome P450 highly expressed in kidney. *J. Biol. Chem.* **1999**, *274*, 17777–17788. [CrossRef]

69. Zhao, X.; Imig, J.D. Kidney CYP450 enzymes: Biological actions beyond drug metabolism. *Curr. Drug Metab.* **2003**, *4*, 73–84. [CrossRef]

70. Yu, Z.; Xu, F.; Huse, L.M.; Morisseau, C.; Draper, A.J.; Newman, J.W.; Parker, C.; Graham, L.; Engler, M.M.; Hammock, B.D.; et al. Soluble epoxide hydrolase regulates hydrolysis of vasoactive epoxyeicosatrienoic acids. *Circ. Res.* **2000**, *87*, 992–998. [CrossRef]

71. Quigley, R.; Baum, M.; Reddy, K.M.; Griener, J.C.; Falck, J.R. Effects of 20-HETE and 19(S)-HETE on rabbit proximal straight tubule volume transport. *Am. J. Physiol. Ren. Physiol.* **2000**, *278*, F949–F953. [CrossRef] [PubMed]

72. Snider, N.T.; Kornilov, A.M.; Kent, U.M.; Hollenberg, P.F. Anandamide metabolism by human liver and kidney microsomal cytochrome p450 enzymes to form hydroxyeicosatetraenoic and epoxyeicosatrienoic acid ethanolamides. *J. Pharmacol. Exp. Ther.* **2007**, *321*, 590–597. [CrossRef] [PubMed]

73. Collins, X.H.; Harmon, S.D.; Kaduce, T.L.; Berst, K.B.; Fang, X.; Moore, S.A.; Raju, T.V.; Falck, J.R.; Weintraub, N.L.; Duester, G.; et al. Omega-oxidation of 20-hydroxyeicosatetraenoic acid (20-HETE) in cerebral microvascular smooth muscle and endothelium by alcohol dehydrogenase 4. *J. Biol. Chem.* **2005**, *280*, 33157–33164. [CrossRef] [PubMed]

74. Nguyen, X.; Wang, M.H.; Reddy, K.M.; Falck, J.R.; Schwartzman, M.L. Kinetic profile of the rat CYP4A isoforms: Arachidonic acid metabolism and isoform-specific inhibitors. *Am. J. Physiol.* **1999**, *276*, R1691–R1700. [CrossRef] [PubMed]

75. Gupta, R.; Yadav, A.; Misra, R.; Aggarwal, A. Urinary prostaglandin D synthase as biomarker in lupus nephritis: A longitudinal study. *Clin. Exp. Rheumatol.* **2015**, *33*, 694–698. [PubMed]

76. Somparn, P.; Hirankarn, N.; Leelahavanichkul, A.; Khovidhunkit, W.; Thongboonkerd, V.; Avihingsanon, Y. Urinary proteomics revealed prostaglandin H(2)D-isomerase, not Zn-alpha2-glycoprotein, as a biomarker for active lupus nephritis. *J. Proteom.* **2012**, *75*, 3240–3247. [CrossRef] [PubMed]

77. Smith, E.M.D.; Eleuteri, A.; Goilav, B.; Lewandowski, L.; Phuti, A.; Rubinstein, T.; Wahezi, D.; Jones, C.A.; Marks, S.D.; Corkhill, R.; et al. A Markov Multi-State model of lupus nephritis urine biomarker panel dynamics in children: Predicting changes in disease activity. *Clin. Immunol.* **2019**, *198*, 71–78. [CrossRef] [PubMed]

78. Pellefigues, C.; Dema, B.; Lamri, Y.; Saidoune, F.; Chavarot, N.; Loheac, C.; Pacreau, E.; Dussiot, M.; Bidault, C.; Marquet, F.; et al. Prostaglandin D2 amplifies lupus disease through basophil accumulation in lymphoid organs. *Nat. Commun.* **2018**, *9*, 725. [CrossRef]

79. Pettipher, R.; Hansel, T.T.; Armer, R. Antagonism of the prostaglandin D2 receptors DP1 and CRTH2 as an approach to treat allergic diseases. *Nat. Rev. Drug Discov.* **2007**, *6*, 313–325. [CrossRef]

80. Rajakariar, R.; Hilliard, M.; Lawrence, T.; Trivedi, S.; Colville-Nash, P.; Bellingan, G.; Fitzgerald, D.; Yaqoob, M.M.; Gilroy, D.W. Hematopoietic prostaglandin D2 synthase controls the onset and resolution of acute inflammation through PGD2 and 15-deoxyDelta12 14 PGJ2. *Proc. Natl. Acad. Sci. USA* **2007**, *104*, 20979–20984. [CrossRef]

81. Hirai, H.; Tanaka, K.; Yoshie, O.; Ogawa, K.; Kenmotsu, K.; Takamori, Y.; Ichimasa, M.; Sugamura, K.; Nakamura, M.; Takano, S.; et al. Prostaglandin D2 selectively induces chemotaxis in T helper type 2 cells, eosinophils, and basophils via seven-transmembrane receptor CRTH2. *J. Exp. Med.* **2001**, *193*, 255–261. [CrossRef] [PubMed]

82. Togel, F.; Isaac, J.; Hu, Z.; Weiss, K.; Westenfelder, C. Renal SDF-1 signals mobilization and homing of CXCR4-positive cells to the kidney after ischemic injury. *Kidney Int.* **2005**, *67*, 1772–1784. [CrossRef] [PubMed]

83. Devi, S.; Wang, Y.; Chew, W.K.; Lima, R.; Gonzalez, N.A.; Mattar, C.N.; Chong, S.Z.; Schlitzer, A.; Bakocevic, N.; Chew, S.; et al. Neutrophil mobilization via plerixafor-mediated CXCR4 inhibition arises from lung demargination and blockade of neutrophil homing to the bone marrow. *J. Exp. Med.* **2013**, *210*, 2321–2336. [CrossRef] [PubMed]

84. Daza, L.; Kornhauser, C.; Zamora, L.; Flores, J. Captopril effect on prostaglandin E2, thromboxane B2 and proteinuria in lupus nephritis patients. *Prostaglandins Other Lipid Mediat.* **2005**, *78*, 194–201. [CrossRef] [PubMed]

85. Ito, H.; Yan, X.; Nagata, N.; Aritake, K.; Katsumata, Y.; Matsuhashi, T.; Nakamura, M.; Hirai, H.; Urade, Y.; Asano, K.; et al. PGD2-CRTH2 pathway promotes tubulointerstitial fibrosis. *J. Am. Soc. Nephrol.* **2012**, *23*, 1797–1809. [CrossRef] [PubMed]

86. Lu, Y.; Zhou, Q.; Zhong, F.; Guo, S.; Hao, X.; Li, C.; Wang, W.; Chen, N. 15-Deoxy-Delta(12,14)-prostaglandin J(2) modulates lipopolysaccharide-induced chemokine expression by blocking nuclear factor-kappaB activation via peroxisome proliferator activated receptor-gamma-independent mechanism in renal tubular epithelial cells. *Nephron Exp. Nephrol.* **2013**, *123*, 1–10. [CrossRef] [PubMed]

87. Hart, D.; Lifschitz, M.D. Renal physiology of the prostaglandins and the effects of nonsteroidal anti-inflammatory agents on the kidney. *Am. J. Nephrol.* **1987**, *7*, 408–418. [CrossRef]

88. Dunn, M.J.; Hood, V.L. Prostaglandins and the kidney. *Am. J. Physiol.* **1977**, *233*, 169–184. [CrossRef]

89. Nasrallah, R.; Hassouneh, R.; Hebert, R.L. Chronic kidney disease: Targeting prostaglandin E2 receptors. *Am. J. Physiol. Ren. Physiol.* **2014**, *307*, F243–F250. [CrossRef]

90. Breyer, M.D.; Breyer, R.M. Prostaglandin E receptors and the kidney. *Am. J. Physiol. Ren. Physiol.* **2000**, *279*, F12–F23. [CrossRef]

91. Kotnik, P.; Nielsen, J.; Kwon, T.H.; Krzisnik, C.; Frokiaer, J.; Nielsen, S. Altered expression of COX-1, COX-2, and mPGES in rats with nephrogenic and central diabetes insipidus. *Am. J. Physiol. Ren. Physiol.* **2005**, *288*, F1053–F1068. [CrossRef] [PubMed]

92. Sanchez, T.; Moreno, J.J. Role of EP(1) and EP(4) PGE(2) subtype receptors in serum-induced 3T6 fibroblast cycle progression and proliferation. *Am. J. Physiol. Cell Physiol.* **2002**, *282*, C280–C288. [CrossRef] [PubMed]

93. Moore, B.B.; Ballinger, M.N.; White, E.S.; Green, M.E.; Herrygers, A.B.; Wilke, C.A.; Toews, G.B.; Peters-Golden, M. Bleomycin-induced E prostanoid receptor changes alter fibroblast responses to prostaglandin E2. *J. Immunol.* **2005**, *174*, 5644–5649. [CrossRef] [PubMed]

94. Yokoyama, U.; Iwatsubo, K.; Umemura, M.; Fujita, T.; Ishikawa, Y. The prostanoid EP4 receptor and its signaling pathway. *Pharmacol. Rev.* **2013**, *65*, 1010–1052. [CrossRef] [PubMed]

95. Breyer, M.D.; Davis, L.; Jacobson, H.R.; Breyer, R.M. Differential localization of prostaglandin E receptor subtypes in human kidney. *Am. J. Physiol.* **1996**, *270*, F912–F918. [CrossRef] [PubMed]

96. Thibodeau, J.F.; Nasrallah, R.; Carter, A.; He, Y.; Touyz, R.; Hebert, R.L.; Kennedy, C.R.J. PTGER1 deletion attenuates renal injury in diabetic mouse models. *Am. J. Pathol.* **2013**, *183*, 1789–1802. [CrossRef]

97. Rahal, S.; McVeigh, L.I.; Zhang, Y.; Guan, Y.; Breyer, M.D.; Kennedy, C.R. Increased severity of renal impairment in nephritic mice lacking the EP1 receptor. *Can. J. Physiol. Pharmacol.* **2006**, *84*, 877–885. [CrossRef]

98. Tang, L.; Loutzenhiser, K.; Loutzenhiser, R. Biphasic actions of prostaglandin E(2) on the renal afferent arteriole: Role of EP(3) and EP(4) receptors. *Circ. Res.* **2000**, *86*, 663–670. [CrossRef]

99. Srivastava, T.; Alon, U.S.; Cudmore, P.A.; Tarakji, B.; Kats, A.; Garola, R.E.; Duncan, R.S.; McCarthy, E.T.; Sharma, R.; Johnson, M.L.; et al. Cyclooxygenase-2, prostaglandin E2, and prostanoid receptor EP2 in fluid flow shear stress-mediated injury in the solitary kidney. *Am. J. Physiol. Ren. Physiol.* **2014**, *307*, F1323–F1333. [CrossRef]

100. Mohamed, R.; Jayakumar, C.; Ranganathan, P.V.; Ganapathy, V.; Ramesh, G. Kidney proximal tubular epithelial-specific overexpression of netrin-1 suppresses inflammation and albuminuria through suppression of COX-2-mediated PGE2 production in streptozotocin-induced diabetic mice. *Am. J. Pathol.* **2012**, *181*, 1991–2002. [CrossRef]

101. Hassouneh, R.; Nasrallah, R.; Zimpelmann, J.; Gutsol, A.; Eckert, D.; Ghossein, J.; Burns, K.D.; Hebert, R.L. PGE2 receptor EP3 inhibits water reabsorption and contributes to polyuria and kidney injury in a streptozotocin-induced mouse model of diabetes. *Diabetologia* **2016**, *59*, 1318–1328. [CrossRef] [PubMed]

102. Frolich, S.; Olliges, A.; Kern, N.; Schreiber, Y.; Narumiya, S.; Nusing, R.M. Temporal expression of the PGE2 synthetic system in the kidney is associated with the time frame of renal developmental vulnerability to cyclooxygenase-2 inhibition. *Am. J. Physiol. Ren. Physiol.* **2012**, *303*, F209–F219. [CrossRef] [PubMed]

103. Nakagawa, N.; Yuhki, K.; Kawabe, J.; Fujino, T.; Takahata, O.; Kabara, M.; Abe, K.; Kojima, F.; Kashiwagi, H.; Hasebe, N.; et al. The intrinsic prostaglandin E2-EP4 system of the renal tubular epithelium limits the development of tubulointerstitial fibrosis in mice. *Kidney Int.* **2012**, *82*, 158–171. [CrossRef] [PubMed]

104. Fujino, H.; Xu, W.; Regan, J.W. Prostaglandin E2 induced functional expression of early growth response factor-1 by EP4, but not EP2, prostanoid receptors via the phosphatidylinositol 3-kinase and extracellular signal-regulated kinases. *J. Biol. Chem.* **2003**, *278*, 12151–12156. [CrossRef] [PubMed]

105. Faour, W.H.; Gomi, K.; Kennedy, C.R. PGE(2) induces COX-2 expression in podocytes via the EP(4) receptor through a PKA-independent mechanism. *Cell Signal.* **2008**, *20*, 2156–2164. [CrossRef] [PubMed]

106. Jensen, B.L.; Mann, B.; Skott, O.; Kurtz, A. Differential regulation of renal prostaglandin receptor mRNAs by dietary salt intake in the rat. *Kidney Int.* **1999**, *56*, 528–537. [CrossRef] [PubMed]

107. Stitt-Cavanagh, E.M.; Faour, W.H.; Takami, K.; Carter, A.; Vanderhyden, B.; Guan, Y.; Schneider, A.; Breyer, M.D.; Kennedy, C.R. A maladaptive role for EP4 receptors in podocytes. *J. Am. Soc. Nephrol.* **2010**, *21*, 1678–1690. [CrossRef] [PubMed]

108. Yamamoto, E.; Izawa, T.; Juniantito, V.; Kuwamura, M.; Sugiura, K.; Takeuchi, T.; Yamate, J. Involvement of endogenous prostaglandin E2 in tubular epithelial regeneration through inhibition of apoptosis and epithelial-mesenchymal transition in cisplatin-induced rat renal lesions. *Histol. Histopathol.* **2010**, *25*, 995–1007. [CrossRef]

109. Vukicevic, S.; Simic, P.; Borovecki, F.; Grgurevic, L.; Rogic, D.; Orlic, I.; Grasser, W.A.; Thompson, D.D.; Paralkar, V.M. Role of EP2 and EP4 receptor-selective agonists of prostaglandin E(2) in acute and chronic kidney failure. *Kidney Int.* **2006**, *70*, 1099–1106. [CrossRef]

110. Mohamed, R.; Jayakumar, C.; Ramesh, G. Chronic administration of EP4-selective agonist exacerbates albuminuria and fibrosis of the kidney in streptozotocin-induced diabetic mice through IL-6. *Lab. Investig.* **2013**, *93*, 933–945. [CrossRef]

111. Chang, J.; Blazek, E.; Kreft, A.F.; Lewis, A.J. Inhibition of platelet and neutrophil phospholipase A2 by hydroxyeicosatetraenoic acids (HETES). A novel pharmacological mechanism for regulating free fatty acid release. *Biochem. Pharmacol.* **1985**, *34*, 1571–1575. [CrossRef]

112. Johnson, E.N.; Brass, L.F.; Funk, C.D. Increased platelet sensitivity to ADP in mice lacking platelet-type 12-lipoxygenase. *Proc. Natl. Acad. Sci. USA* **1998**, *95*, 3100–3105. [CrossRef] [PubMed]

113. Coulon, L.; Calzada, C.; Moulin, P.; Vericel, E.; Lagarde, M. Activation of p38 mitogen-activated protein kinase/cytosolic phospholipase A2 cascade in hydroperoxide-stressed platelets. *Free Radic. Biol. Med.* **2003**, *35*, 616–625. [CrossRef]

114. Jansen, M.P.; Emal, D.; Teske, G.J.; Dessing, M.C.; Florquin, S.; Roelofs, J.J. Release of extracellular DNA influences renal ischemia reperfusion injury by platelet activation and formation of neutrophil extracellular traps. *Kidney Int.* **2017**, *91*, 352–364. [CrossRef] [PubMed]

115. Fajas, L.; Auboeuf, D.; Raspe, E.; Schoonjans, K.; Lefebvre, A.M.; Saladin, R.; Najib, J.; Laville, M.; Fruchart, J.C.; Deeb, S.; et al. The organization, promoter analysis, and expression of the human PPARgamma gene. *J. Biol. Chem.* **1997**, *272*, 18779–18789. [CrossRef] [PubMed]

116. Berger, J.P.; Akiyama, T.E.; Meinke, P.T. PPARs: Therapeutic targets for metabolic disease. *Trends Pharmacol. Sci.* **2005**, *26*, 244–251. [CrossRef] [PubMed]

117. Platt, C.; Coward, R.J. Peroxisome proliferator activating receptor-gamma and the podocyte. *Nephrol. Dial. Transplant.* **2017**, *32*, 423–433. [CrossRef]

118. Nagy, L.; Tontonoz, P.; Alvarez, J.G.; Chen, H.; Evans, R.M. Oxidized LDL regulates macrophage gene expression through ligand activation of PPARgamma. *Cell* **1998**, *93*, 229–240. [CrossRef]

119. Huang, J.T.; Welch, J.S.; Ricote, M.; Binder, C.J.; Willson, T.M.; Kelly, C.; Witztum, J.L.; Funk, C.D.; Conrad, D.; Glass, C.K. Interleukin-4-dependent production of PPAR-gamma ligands in macrophages by 12/15-lipoxygenase. *Nature* **1999**, *400*, 378–382. [CrossRef]

120. Okamura, D.M.; Lopez-Guisa, J.M.; Koelsch, K.; Collins, S.; Eddy, A.A. Atherogenic scavenger receptor modulation in the tubulointerstitium in response to chronic renal injury. *Am. J. Physiol. Ren. Physiol.* **2007**, *293*, F575–F585. [CrossRef]

121. Fruchart, J.C. Peroxisome proliferator-activated receptor-alpha (PPARalpha): At the crossroads of obesity, diabetes and cardiovascular disease. *Atherosclerosis* **2009**, *205*, 1–8. [CrossRef] [PubMed]

122. Tanaka, Y.; Kume, S.; Araki, S.; Isshiki, K.; Chin-Kanasaki, M.; Sakaguchi, M.; Sugimoto, T.; Koya, D.; Haneda, M.; Kashiwagi, A.; et al. Fenofibrate, a PPARalpha agonist, has renoprotective effects in mice by enhancing renal lipolysis. *Kidney Int.* **2011**, *79*, 871–882. [CrossRef] [PubMed]

123. Stadler, K.; Goldberg, I.J.; Susztak, K. The evolving understanding of the contribution of lipid metabolism to diabetic kidney disease. *Curr. Diabetes Rep.* **2015**, *15*, 40. [CrossRef] [PubMed]

124. Fan, F.; Muroya, Y.; Roman, R.J. Cytochrome P450 eicosanoids in hypertension and renal disease. *Curr. Opin. Nephrol. Hypertens.* **2015**, *24*, 37–46. [CrossRef] [PubMed]

125. Croft, K.D.; McGiff, J.C.; Sanchez-Mendoza, A.; Carroll, M.A. Angiotensin II releases 20-HETE from rat renal microvessels. *Am. J. Physiol. Ren. Physiol.* **2000**, *279*, F544–F551. [CrossRef] [PubMed]

126. Parmentier, J.H.; Muthalif, M.M.; Saeed, A.E.; Malik, K.U. Phospholipase D activation by norepinephrine is mediated by 12(s)-, 15(s)-, and 20-hydroxyeicosatetraenoic acids generated by stimulation of cytosolic phospholipase a2. Tyrosine phosphorylation of phospholipase d2 in response to norepinephrine. *J. Biol. Chem.* **2001**, *276*, 15704–15711. [CrossRef] [PubMed]

127. Escalante, B.; Erlij, D.; Falck, J.R.; McGiff, J.C. Effect of cytochrome P450 arachidonate metabolites on ion transport in rabbit kidney loop of Henle. *Science* **1991**, *251*, 799–802. [CrossRef]

128. Capdevila, J.H.; Falck, J.R. The CYP P450 arachidonic acid monooxygenases: From cell signaling to blood pressure regulation. *Biochem. Biophys. Res. Commun.* **2001**, *285*, 571–576. [CrossRef]

129. Williams, J.M.; Fan, F.; Murphy, S.; Schreck, C.; Lazar, J.; Jacob, H.J.; Roman, R.J. Role of 20-HETE in the antihypertensive effect of transfer of chromosome 5 from Brown Norway to Dahl salt-sensitive rats. *Am. J. Physiol. Regul. Integr. Comp. Physiol.* **2012**, *302*, R1209–R1218. [CrossRef]

130. Williams, J.M.; Sarkis, A.; Hoagland, K.M.; Fredrich, K.; Ryan, R.P.; Moreno, C.; Lopez, B.; Lazar, J.; Fenoy, F.J.; Sharma, M.; et al. Transfer of the CYP4A region of chromosome 5 from Lewis to Dahl S rats attenuates renal injury. *Am. J. Physiol. Ren. Physiol.* **2008**, *295*, F1764–F1777. [CrossRef]

131. Dahly-Vernon, A.J.; Sharma, M.; McCarthy, E.T.; Savin, V.J.; Ledbetter, S.R.; Roman, R.J. Transforming growth factor-beta, 20-HETE interaction, and glomerular injury in Dahl salt-sensitive rats. *Hypertension* **2005**, *45*, 643–648. [CrossRef] [PubMed]

132. Roman, R.J.; Ma, Y.H.; Frohlich, B.; Markham, B. Clofibrate prevents the development of hypertension in Dahl salt-sensitive rats. *Hypertension* **1993**, *21*, 985–988. [CrossRef] [PubMed]

133. Ma, Y.H.; Schwartzman, M.L.; Roman, R.J. Altered renal P-450 metabolism of arachidonic acid in Dahl salt-sensitive rats. *Am. J. Physiol.* **1994**, *267*, R579–R589. [CrossRef] [PubMed]

134. Moreno, C.; Maier, K.G.; Hoagland, K.M.; Yu, M.; Roman, R.J. Abnormal pressure-natriuresis in hypertension: Role of cytochrome P450 metabolites of arachidonic acid. *Am. J. Hypertens.* **2001**, *14*, 90S–97S. [CrossRef]

135. Alonso-Galicia, M.; Maier, K.G.; Greene, A.S.; Cowley, A.W., Jr.; Roman, R.J. Role of 20-hydroxyeicosatetraenoic acid in the renal and vasoconstrictor actions of angiotensin II. *Am. J. Physiol. Regul. Integr. Comp. Physiol.* **2002**, *283*, R60–R68. [CrossRef] [PubMed]

136. McGiff, J.C.; Quilley, J. 20-HETE and the kidney: Resolution of old problems and new beginnings. *Am. J. Physiol.* **1999**, *277*, R607–R623. [CrossRef] [PubMed]

137. Roman, R.J. P-450 metabolites of arachidonic acid in the control of cardiovascular function. *Physiol. Rev.* **2002**, *82*, 131–185. [CrossRef]

138. Williams, J.M.; Sarkis, A.; Lopez, B.; Ryan, R.P.; Flasch, A.K.; Roman, R.J. Elevations in renal interstitial hydrostatic pressure and 20-hydroxyeicosatetraenoic acid contribute to pressure natriuresis. *Hypertension* **2007**, *49*, 687–694. [CrossRef]

139. Williams, J.M.; Murphy, S.; Burke, M.; Roman, R.J. 20-hydroxyeicosatetraeonic acid: A new target for the treatment of hypertension. *J. Cardiovasc. Pharmacol.* **2010**, *56*, 336–344. [CrossRef]

140. Nilakantan, V.; Maenpaa, C.; Jia, G.; Roman, R.J.; Park, F. 20-HETE-mediated cytotoxicity and apoptosis in ischemic kidney epithelial cells. *Am. J. Physiol. Ren. Physiol.* **2008**, *294*, F562–F570. [CrossRef]

141. Lameire, N.; Vanholder, R. Pathophysiologic features and prevention of human and experimental acute tubular necrosis. *J. Am. Soc. Nephrol.* **2001**, *12* (Suppl. 17), S20–S32.

142. Fan, F.; Ge, Y.; Lv, W.; Elliott, M.R.; Muroya, Y.; Hirata, T.; Booz, G.W.; Roman, R.J. Molecular mechanisms and cell signaling of 20-hydroxyeicosatetraenoic acid in vascular pathophysiology. *Front. Biosci.* **2016**, *21*, 1427–1463.

143. Regner, K.R.; Zuk, A.; Van Why, S.K.; Shames, B.D.; Ryan, R.P.; Falck, J.R.; Manthati, V.L.; McMullen, M.E.; Ledbetter, S.R.; Roman, R.J. Protective effect of 20-HETE analogues in experimental renal ischemia reperfusion injury. *Kidney Int.* **2009**, *75*, 511–517. [CrossRef] [PubMed]

144. Roman, R.J.; Akbulut, T.; Park, F.; Regner, K.R. 20-HETE in acute kidney injury. *Kidney Int.* **2011**, *79*, 10–13. [CrossRef]

145. Eid, A.A.; Gorin, Y.; Fagg, B.M.; Maalouf, R.; Barnes, J.L.; Block, K.; Abboud, H.E. Mechanisms of podocyte injury in diabetes: Role of cytochrome P450 and NADPH oxidases. *Diabetes* **2009**, *58*, 1201–1211. [CrossRef] [PubMed]

146. Eid, S.; Maalouf, R.; Jaffa, A.A.; Nassif, J.; Hamdy, A.; Rashid, A.; Ziyadeh, F.N.; Eid, A.A. 20-HETE and EETs in diabetic nephropathy: A novel mechanistic pathway. *PLoS ONE* **2013**, *8*, e70029. [CrossRef] [PubMed]

147. Roshanravan, H.; Kim, E.Y.; Dryer, S.E. 20-Hydroxyeicosatetraenoic Acid (20-HETE) Modulates Canonical Transient Receptor Potential-6 (TRPC6) Channels in Podocytes. *Front. Physiol.* **2016**, *7*, 351. [CrossRef]

148. Kriz, W.; Lemley, K.V. A potential role for mechanical forces in the detachment of podocytes and the progression of CKD. *J. Am. Soc. Nephrol.* **2015**, *26*, 258–269. [CrossRef]

149. Omata, K.; Tsutsumi, E.; Sheu, H.L.; Utsumi, Y.; Abe, K. Effect of aging on renal cytochrome P450-dependent arachidonic acid metabolism in Dahl rats. *J. Lipid Mediat.* **1993**, *6*, 369–373. [PubMed]

150. Moore, K.P.; Wood, J.; Gove, C.; Tan, K.C.; Eason, J.; Taylor, G.W.; Williams, R. Synthesis and metabolism of cysteinyl leukotrienes by the isolated pig kidney. *Adv. Prostaglandin Thromboxane Leukot. Res.* **1991**, *21B*, 697–700. [CrossRef] [PubMed]

151. Klausner, J.M.; Paterson, I.S.; Goldman, G.; Kobzik, L.; Rodzen, C.; Lawrence, R.; Valeri, C.R.; Shepro, D.; Hechtman, H.B. Postischemic renal injury is mediated by neutrophils and leukotrienes. *Am. J. Physiol.* **1989**, *256*, F794–F802. [CrossRef] [PubMed]

152. Sener, G.; Sakarcan, A.; Sehirli, O.; Eksioglu-Demiralp, E.; Sener, E.; Ercan, F.; Gedik, N.; Yegen, B.C. Chronic renal failure-induced multiple-organ injury in rats is alleviated by the selective CysLT1 receptor antagonist montelukast. *Prostaglandins Other Lipid Mediat.* **2007**, *83*, 257–267. [CrossRef] [PubMed]

153. Noiri, E.; Yokomizo, T.; Nakao, A.; Izumi, T.; Fujita, T.; Kimura, S.; Shimizu, T. An in vivo approach showing the chemotactic activity of leukotriene B(4) in acute renal ischemic-reperfusion injury. *Proc. Natl. Acad. Sci. USA* **2000**, *97*, 823–828. [CrossRef] [PubMed]

154. Landgraf, S.S.; Silva, L.S.; Peruchetti, D.B.; Sirtoli, G.M.; Moraes-Santos, F.; Portella, V.G.; Silva-Filho, J.L.; Pinheiro, C.S.; Abreu, T.P.; Takiya, C.M.; et al. 5-Lypoxygenase products are involved in renal tubulointerstitial injury induced by albumin overload in proximal tubules in mice. *PLoS ONE* **2014**, *9*, e107549. [CrossRef] [PubMed]

155. Zimmerman, G.A.; McIntyre, T.M. Neutrophil adherence to human endothelium in vitro occurs by CDw18 (Mo1, MAC-1/LFA-1/GP 150,95) glycoprotein-dependent and -independent mechanisms. *J. Clin. Investig.* **1988**, *81*, 531–537. [CrossRef] [PubMed]

156. Yared, A.; Albrightson-Winslow, C.; Griswold, D.; Takahashi, K.; Fogo, A.; Badr, K.F. Functional significance of leukotriene B4 in normal and glomerulonephritic kidneys. *J. Am. Soc. Nephrol.* **1991**, *2*, 45–56. [PubMed]

157. Zedan, M.M.; El-Refaey, A.; Zaghloul, H.; Abdelrahim, M.E.; Osman, A.; Zedan, M.M.; Eltantawy, N. Montelukast as an add-on treatment in steroid dependant nephrotic syndrome, randomised-controlled trial. *J. Nephrol.* **2016**, *29*, 585–592. [CrossRef]

158. Planaguma, A.; Kazani, S.; Marigowda, G.; Haworth, O.; Mariani, T.J.; Israel, E.; Bleecker, E.R.; Curran-Everett, D.; Erzurum, S.C.; Calhoun, W.J.; et al. Airway lipoxin A4 generation and lipoxin A4 receptor expression are decreased in severe asthma. *Am. J. Respir. Crit. Care Med.* **2008**, *178*, 574–582. [CrossRef]

159. Cheng, X.; He, S.; Yuan, J.; Miao, S.; Gao, H.; Zhang, J.; Li, Y.; Peng, W.; Wu, P. Lipoxin A4 attenuates LPS-induced mouse acute lung injury via Nrf2-mediated E-cadherin expression in airway epithelial cells. *Free Radic. Biol. Med.* **2016**, *93*, 52–66. [CrossRef]

160. Kieran, N.E.; Maderna, P.; Godson, C. Lipoxins: Potential anti-inflammatory, proresolution, and antifibrotic mediators in renal disease. *Kidney Int.* **2004**, *65*, 1145–1154. [CrossRef]

161. Christie, P.E.; Spur, B.W.; Lee, T.H. The effects of lipoxin A4 on airway responses in asthmatic subjects. *Am. Rev. Respir. Dis.* **1992**, *145*, 1281–1284. [CrossRef] [PubMed]

162. Dahlen, S.E.; Franzen, L.; Raud, J.; Serhan, C.N.; Westlund, P.; Wikstrom, E.; Bjorck, T.; Matsuda, H.; Webber, S.E.; Veale, C.A.; et al. Actions of lipoxin A4 and related compounds in smooth muscle preparations and on the microcirculation in vivo. *Adv. Exp. Med. Biol.* **1988**, *229*, 107–130. [PubMed]

163. Wu, S.H.; Liao, P.Y.; Yin, P.L.; Zhang, Y.M.; Dong, L. Elevated expressions of 15-lipoxygenase and lipoxin A4 in children with acute poststreptococcal glomerulonephritis. *Am. J. Pathol.* **2009**, *174*, 115–122. [CrossRef] [PubMed]

164. Rodgers, K.; McMahon, B.; Mitchell, D.; Sadlier, D.; Godson, C. Lipoxin A4 modifies platelet-derived growth factor-induced pro-fibrotic gene expression in human renal mesangial cells. *Am. J. Pathol.* **2005**, *167*, 683–694. [CrossRef]

165. O'Meara, Y.M.; Brady, H.R. Lipoxins, leukocyte recruitment and the resolution phase of acute glomerulonephritis. *Kidney Int. Suppl.* **1997**, *58*, S56–S61. [PubMed]

166. Munger, K.A.; Montero, A.; Fukunaga, M.; Uda, S.; Yura, T.; Imai, E.; Kaneda, Y.; Valdivielso, J.M.; Badr, K.F. Transfection of rat kidney with human 15-lipoxygenase suppresses inflammation and preserves function in experimental glomerulonephritis. *Proc. Natl. Acad. Sci. USA* **1999**, *96*, 13375–13380. [CrossRef] [PubMed]

167. Davin, J.C.; Coppo, R. Henoch-Schonlein purpura nephritis in children. *Nat. Rev. Nephrol.* **2014**, *10*, 563–573. [CrossRef] [PubMed]

168. Borgeson, E.; Docherty, N.G.; Murphy, M.; Rodgers, K.; Ryan, A.; O'Sullivan, T.P.; Guiry, P.J.; Goldschmeding, R.; Higgins, D.F.; Godson, C. Lipoxin A(4) and benzo-lipoxin A(4) attenuate experimental renal fibrosis. *FASEB J.* **2011**, *25*, 2967–2979. [CrossRef]

169. Borgeson, E.; Johnson, A.M.; Lee, Y.S.; Till, A.; Syed, G.H.; Ali-Shah, S.T.; Guiry, P.J.; Dalli, J.; Colas, R.A.; Serhan, C.N.; et al. Lipoxin A4 Attenuates Obesity-Induced Adipose Inflammation and Associated Liver and Kidney Disease. *Cell Metab.* **2015**, *22*, 125–137. [CrossRef]

170. Brennan, E.P.; Mohan, M.; McClelland, A.; Tikellis, C.; Ziemann, M.; Kaspi, A.; Gray, S.P.; Pickering, R.; Tan, S.M.; Ali-Shah, S.T.; et al. Lipoxins Regulate the Early Growth Response-1 Network and Reverse Diabetic Kidney Disease. *J. Am. Soc. Nephrol.* **2018**, *29*, 1437–1448. [CrossRef]

171. Sun, S.; Ning, X.; Zhai, Y.; Du, R.; Lu, Y.; He, L.; Li, R.; Wu, W.; Sun, W.; Wang, H. Egr-1 mediates chronic hypoxia-induced renal interstitial fibrosis via the PKC/ERK pathway. *Am. J. Nephrol.* **2014**, *39*, 436–448. [CrossRef] [PubMed]

172. McMahon, B.; Stenson, C.; McPhillips, F.; Fanning, A.; Brady, H.R.; Godson, C. Lipoxin A4 antagonizes the mitogenic effects of leukotriene D4 in human renal mesangial cells. Differential activation of MAP kinases through distinct receptors. *J. Biol. Chem.* **2000**, *275*, 27566–27575. [CrossRef] [PubMed]

173. Ho, L.C.; Sung, J.M.; Shen, Y.T.; Jheng, H.F.; Chen, S.H.; Tsai, P.J.; Tsai, Y.S. Egr-1 deficiency protects from renal inflammation and fibrosis. *J. Mol. Med.* **2016**, *94*, 933–942. [CrossRef] [PubMed]

174. Yeboah, M.M.; Hye Khan, M.A.; Chesnik, M.A.; Sharma, A.; Paudyal, M.P.; Falck, J.R.; Imig, J.D. The epoxyeicosatrienoic acid analog PVPA ameliorates cyclosporine-induced hypertension and renal injury in rats. *Am. J. Physiol. Ren. Physiol.* **2016**, *311*, F576–F585. [CrossRef] [PubMed]

175. Kim, J.; Imig, J.D.; Yang, J.; Hammock, B.D.; Padanilam, B.J. Inhibition of soluble epoxide hydrolase prevents renal interstitial fibrosis and inflammation. *Am. J. Physiol. Ren. Physiol.* **2014**, *307*, F971–F980. [CrossRef]

176. Manhiani, M.; Quigley, J.E.; Knight, S.F.; Tasoobshirazi, S.; Moore, T.; Brands, M.W.; Hammock, B.D.; Imig, J.D. Soluble epoxide hydrolase gene deletion attenuates renal injury and inflammation with DOCA-salt hypertension. *Am. J. Physiol. Ren. Physiol.* **2009**, *297*, F740–F748. [CrossRef] [PubMed]

177. Roche, C.; Guerrot, D.; Harouki, N.; Duflot, T.; Besnier, M.; Remy-Jouet, I.; Renet, S.; Dumesnil, A.; Lejeune, A.; Morisseau, C.; et al. Impact of soluble epoxide hydrolase inhibition on early kidney damage in hyperglycemic overweight mice. *Prostaglandins Other Lipid Mediat.* **2015**, *120*, 148–154. [CrossRef]

178. Zhu, Y.; Blum, M.; Hoff, U.; Wesser, T.; Fechner, M.; Westphal, C.; Gurgen, D.; Catar, R.A.; Philippe, A.; Wu, K.; et al. Renal Ischemia/Reperfusion Injury in Soluble Epoxide Hydrolase-Deficient Mice. *PLoS ONE* **2016**, *11*, e0145645. [CrossRef]

179. Hercule, H.C.; Schunck, W.H.; Gross, V.; Seringer, J.; Leung, F.P.; Weldon, S.M.; da Costa Goncalves, A.; Huang, Y.; Luft, F.C.; Gollasch, M. Interaction between P450 eicosanoids and nitric oxide in the control of arterial tone in mice. *Arterioscler. Thromb. Vasc. Biol.* **2009**, *29*, 54–60. [CrossRef]

180. Deng, B.Q.; Luo, Y.; Kang, X.; Li, C.B.; Morisseau, C.; Yang, J.; Lee, K.S.S.; Huang, J.; Hu, D.Y.; Wu, M.Y.; et al. Epoxide metabolites of arachidonate and docosahexaenoate function conversely in acute kidney injury involved in GSK3beta signaling. *Proc. Natl. Acad. Sci. USA* **2017**, *114*, 12608–12613. [CrossRef]

181. Wang, D.; Borrego-Conde, L.J.; Falck, J.R.; Sharma, K.K.; Wilcox, C.S.; Umans, J.G. Contributions of nitric oxide, EDHF, and EETs to endothelium-dependent relaxation in renal afferent arterioles. *Kidney Int.* **2003**, *63*, 2187–2193. [CrossRef] [PubMed]

182. Ma, S.K.; Wang, Y.; Chen, J.; Zhang, M.Z.; Harris, R.C.; Chen, J.K. Overexpression of G-protein-coupled receptor 40 enhances the mitogenic response to epoxyeicosatrienoic acids. *PLoS ONE* **2015**, *10*, e0113130. [CrossRef] [PubMed]

183. Pomposiello, S.I.; Quilley, J.; Carroll, M.A.; Falck, J.R.; McGiff, J.C. 5,6-epoxyeicosatrienoic acid mediates the enhanced renal vasodilation to arachidonic acid in the SHR. *Hypertension* **2003**, *42*, 548–554. [CrossRef] [PubMed]

184. Cheng, M.K.; Doumad, A.B.; Jiang, H.; Falck, J.R.; McGiff, J.C.; Carroll, M.A. Epoxyeicosatrienoic acids mediate adenosine-induced vasodilation in rat preglomerular microvessels (PGMV) via A2A receptors. *Br. J. Pharmacol.* **2004**, *141*, 441–448. [CrossRef] [PubMed]

185. Carroll, M.A.; Doumad, A.B.; Li, J.; Cheng, M.K.; Falck, J.R.; McGiff, J.C. Adenosine2A receptor vasodilation of rat preglomerular microvessels is mediated by EETs that activate the cAMP/PKA pathway. *Am. J. Physiol. Ren. Physiol.* **2006**, *291*, F155–F161. [CrossRef] [PubMed]

186. Imig, J.D.; Dimitropoulou, C.; Reddy, D.S.; White, R.E.; Falck, J.R. Afferent arteriolar dilation to 11, 12-EET analogs involves PP2A activity and Ca2+-activated K+ Channels. *Microcirculation* **2008**, *15*, 137–150. [CrossRef] [PubMed]

187. Wang, W.H.; Zhang, C.; Lin, D.H.; Wang, L.; Graves, J.P.; Zeldin, D.C.; Capdevila, J.H. Cyp2c44 epoxygenase in the collecting duct is essential for the high K+ intake-induced antihypertensive effect. *Am. J. Physiol. Ren. Physiol.* **2014**, *307*, F453–F460. [CrossRef]

188. Sharma, M.; McCarthy, E.T.; Reddy, D.S.; Patel, P.K.; Savin, V.J.; Medhora, M.; Falck, J.R. 8,9-Epoxyeicosatrienoic acid protects the glomerular filtration barrier. *Prostaglandins Other Lipid Mediat.* **2009**, *89*, 43–51. [CrossRef]

189. Beck, L.H., Jr.; Fervenza, F.C.; Beck, D.M.; Bonegio, R.G.; Malik, F.A.; Erickson, S.B.; Cosio, F.G.; Cattran, D.C.; Salant, D.J. Rituximab-induced depletion of anti-PLA2R autoantibodies predicts response in membranous nephropathy. *J. Am. Soc. Nephrol.* **2011**, *22*, 1543–1550. [CrossRef]

190. Thokhonelidze, I.; Maglakelidze, N.; Sarishvili, N.; Kasradze, T.; Dalakishvili, K. Association of anti-phospholipasea2-receptor antibodies with clinical course of idiopathic membranous nephropathy. *Georgian Med News* **2015**, 49–53.

191. Ramachandran, R.; Hn, H.K.; Kumar, V.; Nada, R.; Yadav, A.K.; Goyal, A.; Kumar, V.; Rathi, M.; Jha, V.; Gupta, K.L.; et al. Tacrolimus combined with corticosteroids versus Modified Ponticelli regimen in treatment of idiopathic membranous nephropathy: Randomized control trial. *Nephrology* **2016**, *21*, 139–146. [CrossRef] [PubMed]

192. Wei, S.Y.; Wang, Y.X.; Li, J.S.; Zhao, S.L.; Diao, T.T.; Wang, Y.; Wang, C.; Qin, Y.; Cao, Y.; Wei, Q.; et al. Serum Anti-PLA2R Antibody Predicts Treatment Outcome in Idiopathic Membranous Nephropathy. *Am. J. Nephrol.* **2016**, *43*, 129–140. [CrossRef] [PubMed]

193. Bech, A.P.; Hofstra, J.M.; Brenchley, P.E.; Wetzels, J.F. Association of anti-PLA(2)R antibodies with outcomes after immunosuppressive therapy in idiopathic membranous nephropathy. *Clin. J. Am. Soc. Nephrol.* **2014**, *9*, 1386–1392. [CrossRef] [PubMed]

194. Radhakrishnan, J.; Cattran, D.C. The KDIGO practice guideline on glomerulonephritis: Reading between the (guide)lines–application to the individual patient. *Kidney Int.* **2012**, *82*, 840–856. [CrossRef] [PubMed]

195. Gonzalo-Gil, E.; Garcia-Herrero, C.; Toldos, O.; Usategui, A.; Criado, G.; Perez-Yague, S.; Barber, D.F.; Pablos, J.L.; Galindo, M. Microthrombotic Renal Vascular Lesions Are Associated to Increased Renal Inflammatory Infiltration in Murine Lupus Nephritis. *Front. Immunol.* **2018**, *9*, 1948. [CrossRef] [PubMed]

196. Gerrah, R.; Ehrlich, S.; Tshori, S.; Sahar, G. Beneficial effect of aspirin on renal function in patients with renal insufficiency postcardiac surgery. *J. Cardiovasc. Surg.* **2004**, *45*, 545–550.

197. Garg, A.X.; Kurz, A.; Sessler, D.I.; Cuerden, M.; Robinson, A.; Mrkobrada, M.; Parikh, C.R.; Mizera, R.; Jones, P.M.; Tiboni, M.; et al. Perioperative aspirin and clonidine and risk of acute kidney injury: A randomized clinical trial. *JAMA* **2014**, *312*, 2254–2264. [CrossRef] [PubMed]

198. De Martino, M.; Chiarugi, A.; Boner, A.; Montini, G.; De' Angelis, G.L. Working towards an Appropriate Use of Ibuprofen in Children: An Evidence-Based Appraisal. *Drugs* **2017**, *77*, 1295–1311. [CrossRef]

199. Lipman, G.S.; Shea, K.; Christensen, M.; Phillips, C.; Burns, P.; Higbee, R.; Koskenoja, V.; Eifling, K.; Krabak, B.J. Ibuprofen versus placebo effect on acute kidney injury in ultramarathons: A randomised controlled trial. *Emerg. Med. J.* **2017**, *34*, 637–642. [CrossRef] [PubMed]

200. Kaojarern, S.; Chennavasin, P.; Anderson, S.; Brater, D.C. Nephron site of effect of nonsteroidal anti-inflammatory drugs on solute excretion in humans. *Am. J. Physiol.* **1983**, *244*, F134–F139. [CrossRef]

201. Wu, Y.J.; Xue, M.; Chen, H. Licofelone inhibits interleukin-18-induced pro-inflammatory cytokine release and cellular proliferation in human mesangial cells. *Basic Clin. Pharmacol. Toxicol.* **2012**, *111*, 166–172. [CrossRef] [PubMed]

202. Faulkner, J.; Pye, C.; Al-Shabrawey, M.; Elmarakby, A.A. Inhibition of 12/15-Lipoxygenase Reduces Renal Inflammation and Injury in Streptozotocin-Induced Diabetic Mice. *J. Diabetes Metab.* **2015**, *6*. [CrossRef]

203. Hofstra, J.M.; Beck, L.H., Jr.; Beck, D.M.; Wetzels, J.F.; Salant, D.J. Anti-phospholipase A(2) receptor antibodies correlate with clinical status in idiopathic membranous nephropathy. *Clin. J. Am. Soc. Nephrol.* **2011**, *6*, 1286–1291. [CrossRef] [PubMed]

204. Debiec, H.; Ronco, P. PLA2R autoantibodies and PLA2R glomerular deposits in membranous nephropathy. *N. Engl. J. Med.* **2011**, *364*, 689–690. [CrossRef] [PubMed]

205. Pourcine, F.; Dahan, K.; Mihout, F.; Cachanado, M.; Brocheriou, I.; Debiec, H.; Ronco, P. Prognostic value of PLA2R autoimmunity detected by measurement of anti-PLA2R antibodies combined with detection of PLA2R antigen in membranous nephropathy: A single-centre study over 14 years. *PLoS ONE* **2017**, *12*, e0173201. [CrossRef] [PubMed]

206. Jullien, P.; Seitz Polski, B.; Maillard, N.; Thibaudin, D.; Laurent, B.; Ollier, E.; Alamartine, E.; Lambeau, G.; Mariat, C. Anti-phospholipase A2 receptor antibody levels at diagnosis predicts spontaneous remission of idiopathic membranous nephropathy. *Clin. Kidney J.* **2017**, *10*, 209–214. [CrossRef] [PubMed]

207. Buysen, J.G.; Houthoff, H.J.; Krediet, R.T.; Arisz, L. Acute interstitial nephritis: A clinical and morphological study in 27 patients. *Nephrol. Dial. Transplant.* **1990**, *5*, 94–99. [CrossRef] [PubMed]

208. Eddy, A.A. Drug-induced tubulointerstitial nephritis: Hypersensitivity and necroinflammatory pathways. *Pediatric Nephrol.* **2019**, 1–8. [CrossRef] [PubMed]

209. Di Rosa, M.; Giroud, J.P.; Willoughby, D.A. Studies on the mediators of the acute inflammatory response induced in rats in different sites by carrageenan and turpentine. *J. Pathol.* **1971**, *104*, 15–29. [CrossRef] [PubMed]

210. De Gaetano, G.; Bucchi, F.; Gambino, M.C.; Cerletti, C. Does oral aspirin spare the kidney? *Lancet* **1986**, *1*, 736. [CrossRef]

211. Berger, J.S.; Brown, D.L.; Becker, R.C. Low-dose aspirin in patients with stable cardiovascular disease: A meta-analysis. *Am. J. Med.* **2008**, *121*, 43–49. [CrossRef] [PubMed]

212. Antithrombotic Trialists, C.; Baigent, C.; Blackwell, L.; Collins, R.; Emberson, J.; Godwin, J.; Peto, R.; Buring, J.; Hennekens, C.; Kearney, P.; et al. Aspirin in the primary and secondary prevention of vascular disease: Collaborative meta-analysis of individual participant data from randomised trials. *Lancet* **2009**, *373*, 1849–1860. [CrossRef]

213. Vandvik, P.O.; Lincoff, A.M.; Gore, J.M.; Gutterman, D.D.; Sonnenberg, F.A.; Alonso-Coello, P.; Akl, E.A.; Lansberg, M.G.; Guyatt, G.H.; Spencer, F.A. Primary and secondary prevention of cardiovascular disease: Antithrombotic Therapy and Prevention of Thrombosis, 9th ed: American College of Chest Physicians Evidence-Based Clinical Practice Guidelines. *Chest* **2012**, *141*, e637S–e668S. [CrossRef] [PubMed]

214. Karzai, W.; Priebe, H.J. Aspirin and mortality from coronary bypass surgery. *N. Engl. J. Med.* **2003**, *348*, 1057–1059. [PubMed]

215. Ali, H.; Shaaban, A.; Murtaza, A.; Howell, L.E.; Ahmed, A. Effect of Long-Term, Low-Dose Aspirin Therapy on Renal Graft Function. *Exp. Clin. Transplant.* **2017**, *15*, 400–404. [CrossRef] [PubMed]

216. Rainsford, K.D. Ibuprofen: Pharmacology, efficacy and safety. *Inflammopharmacology* **2009**, *17*, 275–342. [CrossRef] [PubMed]

217. Van Overmeire, B.; Allegaert, K.; Casaer, A.; Debauche, C.; Decaluwe, W.; Jespers, A.; Weyler, J.; Harrewijn, I.; Langhendries, J.P. Prophylactic ibuprofen in premature infants: A multicentre, randomised, double-blind, placebo-controlled trial. *Lancet* **2004**, *364*, 1945–1949. [CrossRef]

218. Haas, M.; Spargo, B.H.; Wit, E.J.; Meehan, S.M. Etiologies and outcome of acute renal insufficiency in older adults: A renal biopsy study of 259 cases. *Am. J. Kidney Dis.* **2000**, *35*, 433–447. [CrossRef]

219. Martinez Lopez, A.B.; Alvarez Blanco, O.; De Pablos, A.L.; San-Jose, M.D.M.; De La Blanca, A.R.S. Ibuprofen-induced acute interstitial nephritis in the paediatric population. *Nefrologia* **2016**, *36*, 69–71. [CrossRef]

220. Steinhauslin, F.; Munafo, A.; Buclin, T.; Macciocchi, A.; Biollaz, J. Renal effects of nimesulide in furosemide-treated subjects. *Drugs* **1993**, *46* (Suppl. 1), 257–262. [CrossRef]

221. Warrington, S.J.; Ravic, M.; Dawnay, A. Renal and general tolerability of repeated doses of nimesulide in normal subjects. *Drugs* **1993**, *46* (Suppl. 1), 263–269. [CrossRef]

222. Ceserani, R.; Casciarri, I.; Cavalletti, E.; Cazzulani, P. Action of Nimesulide on Rat Gastric Prostaglandins and Renal Function. *Drug Investig.* **1991**, *3*, 14–21. [CrossRef]

223. Forget, P.; Machiels, J.P.; Coulie, P.G.; Berliere, M.; Poncelet, A.J.; Tombal, B.; Stainier, A.; Legrand, C.; Canon, J.L.; Kremer, Y.; et al. Neutrophil: Lymphocyte ratio and intraoperative use of ketorolac or diclofenac are prognostic factors in different cohorts of patients undergoing breast, lung, and kidney cancer surgery. *Ann. Surg. Oncol.* **2013**, *20* (Suppl. 3), S650–S660. [CrossRef]

224. Yakar, I.; Melamed, R.; Shakhar, G.; Shakhar, K.; Rosenne, E.; Abudarham, N.; Page, G.G.; Ben-Eliyahu, S. Prostaglandin e(2) suppresses NK activity in vivo and promotes postoperative tumor metastasis in rats. *Ann. Surg. Oncol.* **2003**, *10*, 469–479. [CrossRef] [PubMed]

225. Ostrand-Rosenberg, S.; Sinha, P. Myeloid-derived suppressor cells: Linking inflammation and cancer. *J. Immunol.* **2009**, *182*, 4499–4506. [CrossRef] [PubMed]

226. Bombardier, C.; Laine, L.; Reicin, A.; Shapiro, D.; Burgos-Vargas, R.; Davis, B.; Day, R.; Ferraz, M.B.; Hawkey, C.J.; Hochberg, M.C.; et al. Comparison of upper gastrointestinal toxicity of rofecoxib and naproxen in patients with rheumatoid arthritis. VIGOR Study Group. *N. Engl. J. Med.* **2000**, *343*, 1520–1528. [CrossRef]

227. Ungprasert, P.; Cheungpasitporn, W.; Crowson, C.S.; Matteson, E.L. Individual non-steroidal anti-inflammatory drugs and risk of acute kidney injury: A systematic review and meta-analysis of observational studies. *Eur. J. Intern. Med.* **2015**, *26*, 285–291. [CrossRef] [PubMed]

228. Colebatch, A.N.; Marks, J.L.; van der Heijde, D.M.; Edwards, C.J. Safety of nonsteroidal antiinflammatory drugs and/or paracetamol in people receiving methotrexate for inflammatory arthritis: A Cochrane systematic review. *J. Rheumatol. Suppl.* **2012**, *90*, 62–73. [CrossRef] [PubMed]

229. Nawaz, F.A.; Larsen, C.P.; Troxell, M.L. Membranous nephropathy and nonsteroidal anti-inflammatory agents. *Am. J. Kidney Dis.* **2013**, *62*, 1012–1017. [CrossRef] [PubMed]

230. Catella-Lawson, F.; McAdam, B.; Morrison, B.W.; Kapoor, S.; Kujubu, D.; Antes, L.; Lasseter, K.C.; Quan, H.; Gertz, B.J.; FitzGerald, G.A. Effects of specific inhibition of cyclooxygenase-2 on sodium balance, hemodynamics, and vasoactive eicosanoids. *J. Pharmacol. Exp. Ther.* **1999**, *289*, 735–741. [PubMed]

231. Takahashi, K.; Patel, A.K.; Nagai, S.; Safwan, M.; Putchakayala, K.G.; Kane, W.J.; Malinzak, L.E.; Denny, J.E.; Yoshida, A.; Kim, D.Y. Perioperative Ketorolac Use: A Potential Risk Factor for Renal Dysfunction After Live-Donor Nephrectomy. *Ann. Transplant.* **2017**, *22*, 563–569. [CrossRef] [PubMed]

232. Griffin, M.R. High-dose non-steroidal anti-inflammatories: Painful choices. *Lancet* **2013**, *382*, 746–748. [CrossRef]

233. Zhang, J.; Ding, E.L.; Song, Y. Adverse effects of cyclooxygenase 2 inhibitors on renal and arrhythmia events: Meta-analysis of randomized trials. *JAMA* **2006**, *296*, 1619–1632. [CrossRef] [PubMed]

234. Gounaris, E.; Heiferman, M.J.; Heiferman, J.R.; Shrivastav, M.; Vitello, D.; Blatner, N.R.; Knab, L.M.; Phillips, J.D.; Cheon, E.C.; Grippo, P.J.; et al. Zileuton, 5-lipoxygenase inhibitor, acts as a chemopreventive agent in intestinal polyposis, by modulating polyp and systemic inflammation. *PLoS ONE* **2015**, *10*, e0121402. [CrossRef] [PubMed]

235. Santos, C.M.M.; Ribeiro, D.; Silva, A.M.S.; Fernandes, E. 2,3-Diarylxanthones as Potential Inhibitors of Arachidonic Acid Metabolic Pathways. *Inflammation* **2017**, *40*, 956–964. [CrossRef] [PubMed]

236. Muller, D.N.; Theuer, J.; Shagdarsuren, E.; Kaergel, E.; Honeck, H.; Park, J.K.; Markovic, M.; Barbosa-Sicard, E.; Dechend, R.; Wellner, M.; et al. A peroxisome proliferator-activated receptor-alpha activator induces renal CYP2C23 activity and protects from angiotensin II-induced renal injury. *Am. J. Pathol.* **2004**, *164*, 521–532. [CrossRef]

237. Gai, Z.; Visentin, M.; Gui, T.; Zhao, L.; Thasler, W.E.; Hausler, S.; Hartling, I.; Cremonesi, A.; Hiller, C.; Kullak-Ublick, G.A. Effects of Farnesoid X Receptor Activation on Arachidonic Acid Metabolism, NF-kB Signaling, and Hepatic Inflammation. *Mol. Pharmacol.* **2018**, *94*, 802–811. [CrossRef]

238. Shlipak, M.G.; Fried, L.F.; Cushman, M.; Manolio, T.A.; Peterson, D.; Stehman-Breen, C.; Bleyer, A.; Newman, A.; Siscovick, D.; Psaty, B. Cardiovascular mortality risk in chronic kidney disease: Comparison of traditional and novel risk factors. *JAMA* **2005**, *293*, 1737–1745. [CrossRef]

239. Muntner, P.; He, J.; Astor, B.C.; Folsom, A.R.; Coresh, J. Traditional and nontraditional risk factors predict coronary heart disease in chronic kidney disease: Results from the atherosclerosis risk in communities study. *J. Am. Soc. Nephrol.* **2005**, *16*, 529–538. [CrossRef]

240. Garg, A.; Grundy, S.M. Management of dyslipidemia in NIDDM. *Diabetes Care* **1990**, *13*, 153–169. [CrossRef]
241. Garg, A.; Grundy, S.M. Gemfibrozil alone and in combination with lovastatin for treatment of hypertriglyceridemia in NIDDM. *Diabetes* **1989**, *38*, 364–372. [CrossRef] [PubMed]
242. Siavash, M.; Amini, M. Vitamin C may have similar beneficial effects to Gemfibrozil on serum high-density lipoprotein-cholesterol in type 2 diabetic patients. *J. Res. Pharm. Pract.* **2014**, *3*, 77–82. [CrossRef] [PubMed]
243. Martin-Navarro, J.A.; Petkov-Stoyanov, V.; Gutierrez-Sanchez, M.J.; Pedraza-Cezon, L. Acute renal failure secondary to interstitial acute nephritis and Fanconi syndrome for metamizole and gemfibrozil. *Nefrologia* **2016**, *36*, 321–323. [CrossRef] [PubMed]
244. Khan, M.A.; Liu, J.; Kumar, G.; Skapek, S.X.; Falck, J.R.; Imig, J.D. Novel orally active epoxyeicosatrienoic acid (EET) analogs attenuate cisplatin nephrotoxicity. *FASEB J.* **2013**, *27*, 2946–2956. [CrossRef] [PubMed]
245. Node, K.; Huo, Y.; Ruan, X.; Yang, B.; Spiecker, M.; Ley, K.; Zeldin, D.C.; Liao, J.K. Anti-inflammatory properties of cytochrome P450 epoxygenase-derived eicosanoids. *Science* **1999**, *285*, 1276–1279. [CrossRef] [PubMed]
246. Farzamikia, N.; Sakhinia, E.; Afrasiabirad, A. Pharmacogenetics-Based Warfarin Dosing in Patients with Cardiac Valve Replacement: The Effects of CYP2C9 and VKORC1 Gene Polymorphisms. *Lab. Med.* **2017**, *49*, 25–34. [CrossRef]
247. Pei, L.; Tian, X.; Long, Y.; Nan, W.; Jia, M.; Qiao, R.; Zhang, J. Establishment of a Han Chinese-specific pharmacogenetic-guided warfarin dosing algorithm. *Medicine* **2018**, *97*, e12178. [CrossRef]
248. Spatzenegger, M.; Jaeger, W. Clinical importance of hepatic cytochrome P450 in drug metabolism. *Drug Metab. Rev.* **1995**, *27*, 397–417. [CrossRef]
249. Yanagita, M. Gas6, warfarin, and kidney diseases. *Clin. Exp. Nephrol.* **2004**, *8*, 304–309. [CrossRef]
250. Zeldin, D.C.; Wei, S.; Falck, J.R.; Hammock, B.D.; Snapper, J.R.; Capdevila, J.H. Metabolism of epoxyeicosatrienoic acids by cytosolic epoxide hydrolase: Substrate structural determinants of asymmetric catalysis. *Arch. Biochem. Biophys.* **1995**, *316*, 443–451. [CrossRef]
251. Imig, J.D.; Hammock, B.D. Soluble epoxide hydrolase as a therapeutic target for cardiovascular diseases. *Nat. Rev. Drug Discov.* **2009**, *8*, 794–805. [CrossRef] [PubMed]
252. Shen, H.C.; Hammock, B.D. Discovery of inhibitors of soluble epoxide hydrolase: A target with multiple potential therapeutic indications. *J. Med. Chem.* **2012**, *55*, 1789–1808. [CrossRef] [PubMed]

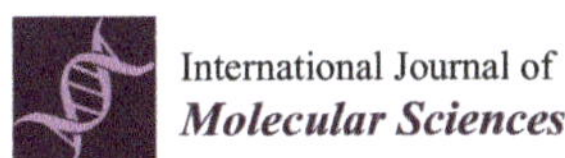

International Journal of
Molecular Sciences

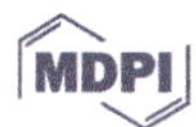

Review

Efficacy of Polyunsaturated Fatty Acids on Inflammatory Markers in Patients Undergoing Dialysis: A Systematic Review with Network Meta-Analysis of Randomized Clinical Trials

Po-Kuan Wu [1], Shu-Ching Yeh [2], Shan-Jen Li [3,*] and Yi-No Kang [4,*]

[1] School of Medicine, College of Medicine, Taipei Medical University, Taipei 11042, Taiwan
[2] Division of Nephrology, Department of Internal Medicine, Taipei Medical University Hospital, Taipei 11042, Taiwan
[3] Department of Emergency Medicine, Taipei Medical University Hospital, Taipei 11042, Taiwan
[4] Evidence-Based Medicine Center, Wan Fang Hospital, Taipei Medical University, Taipei 11696, Taiwan
* Correspondence: b8401121@gmail.com (S.-J.L.); academicnono@gmail.com (Y.-N.K.);
   Tel.: +886-2-27372181 (ext. 3759) (S.-J.L.); +886-2-27372181 (ext. 3759) (Y.-N.K.)

Received: 28 May 2019; Accepted: 19 July 2019; Published: 25 July 2019

Abstract: The effects of polyunsaturated fatty acids (PUFAs) on inflammatory markers among patients receiving dialysis have been discussed for a long time, but previous syntheses made controversial conclusion because of highly conceptual heterogeneity in their synthesis. Thus, to further understanding of this topic, we comprehensively gathered relevant randomized clinical trials (RCTs) before April 2019, and two authors independently extracted data of C-reactive protein (CRP), high-sensitivity C-reactive protein (hs-CRP), and interleukin-6 (IL-6) for conducting network meta-analysis. Eighteen eligible RCTs with 962 patients undergoing dialysis were included in our study. The result showed that with placebo as the reference, PUFAs was the only treatment showing significantly lower CRP (weighted mean difference (WMD): −0.37, 95% confidence interval (CI): −0.07 to −0.68), but the CRP in PUFAs group was not significantly lower than vitamin E, PUFAs plus vitamin E, or medium-chain triglyceride. Although no significant changes were noted for hs-CRP and IL-6 levels, PUFAs showed the best ranking among treatments according to surface under the cumulative ranking. Therefore, PUFAs could be a protective option for patients receiving dialysis in clinical practice.

Keywords: polyunsaturated fatty acids; omega-3 fatty acid; inflammatory maker; C-reactive protein; interleukin-6

---

1. Introduction

Patients with end-stage renal disease around the world suffer from chronic inflammation caused by dialysis, especially hemodialysis. For instance, vascular access of hemodialysis [1], filter membrane of hemodialysis machine [2], and endotoxin from the dialysate [3] all cause chronic inflammation. Chronic inflammation not only reduces the quality-of-life among patients with chronic kidney disease, but also increases the mortality rate of these populations [4,5]. Previous reports have noted about 30% to 50% of patients undergoing hemodialysis have activated inflammatory response [6]. Chronic inflammation is related to pathogenesis of atherosclerosis [7], and cardiovascular disease accounts for the largest proportion of mortality in patients with chronic kidney disease [8]. As a result, detecting Interleukin-6 (IL-6), C-reactive protein (CRP), and high-sensitivity C-reactive protein (hs-CRP) are imperative for understanding and managing inflammatory conditions among these patients [4,5]. The association between IL-6, CRP, and cardiovascular disease is well known. Also, hs-CRP is another important marker manifesting inflammation and endothelial damage; it is also an indicator of defective coronary artery blood flow [9].

To improve the outcomes among patients with hemodialysis, controlling their inflammatory status is an important aspect in clinical practice. In the past decade, many trials have tried to control these inflammations among this group of patients through nutrient supplements [10–30]. Commonly-used nutrient supplements such as polyunsaturated fatty acids (PUFAs), vitamin D, antioxidants, polyphenol-rich foods, fibers, and probiotics to modulate patient's immune response are becoming more and more popular [31]. Unlike consuming drugs, nutrient supplements are usually free from increment of patients' physical stress. PUFAs are the top two popular nutrient supplements with many trials and Omega-3 fatty acids are the main nutrients as trials used PUFAs for reducing inflammatory among patients with chronic kidney disease [31]. The association of PUFA and inflammatory processes has been widely discussed in the past decade [32–40]. With regard to Omega-3 fatty acids, it commonly involves eicosapentaenoic acid, docosahexaenoic acid, and alpha-linolenic acid. Eicosapentaenoic acid and docosahexaenoic acid upregulate peroxisome proliferators' active receptors, and decrease CRP and IL-6. The peroxisome proliferators' active receptors also decrease CRP and IL-6 through downregulation of nuclear factor kappa B (NF-κB) [41,42].

A good synthesis for the topic of nutrients on inflammatory markers among patients with hemodialysis in 2018, yet there is a very high heterogeneity (I-square = 84.3%) existing in the result of CRP mean changes after Omega-3 fatty acids supplementation [31]. Therefore, this topic needs further analysis to provide a clearer picture for the effects of PUFAs on inflammatory markers among patients undergoing hemodialysis. Moreover, there is another meta-analysis in 2018 showing that alpha-linolenic acid cannot affect relevant inflammatory markers [43]. Therefore, our study aimed to clarify whether using PUFAs can reduce inflammatory cytokines (CRP, IL-6, hs-CRP) among patients undergoing dialysis through systematic review and meta-analysis of randomized clinical trials.

2. Results

Through comprehensive search, this systematic review identified 1485 references from the EMBASE (*n* = 656), PubMed (*n* = 388), and Web of Science (*n* = 441). Three records were found from hand search of reference lists. After the exclusion of 437 duplications, 1051 references were reviewed for eligibility. Then, two systematic reviews and 25 randomized clinical trials without relevant outcomes were excluded [31,44–69]. There were 21 references from 18 RCTs meeting the eligibility criteria (Figure 1) [10–30].

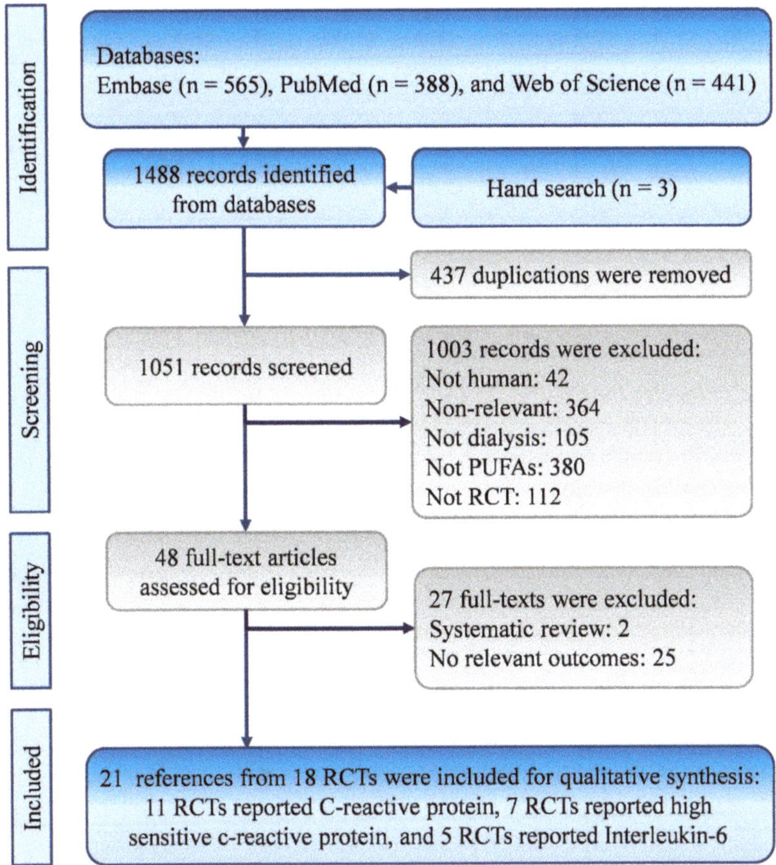

Figure 1. Flowchart of the systematic review and meta-analysis according to PRISMA guidelines.

2.1. Characteristics and Quality of Included Studies

The 18 trials recruited 962 patient undergoing dialysis from Brazil [24], Denmark [13,18], Greece [27], Egypt [30], Iran [10,14,21,22,25,26], Korea [23], United States [11,12,19,20,29], and Sweden [28]. The treatments in the 18 trials could be categorized into five treating strategies including placebo, PUFAs, vitamin E, medium chain triglyceride (MCT), and PUFAs plus vitamin E. The available data in each study showed mean ages from 46.4 to 68 years old, and a total of 598 (62.2%) men were included in the studies. Other information about trial location, inclusion years, treatments, number of patients, and dialysis period are shown in Table 1. Overall, the quality of the studies is presented in Table 2.

Table 1. Characteristics of the included randomized clinical trials.

Author	Location	Inclusion Year	Treatments	Patients	Mean Age	Sex (M/F)	Dialysis Period
Asemi [10]	Iran	2014	1. ω-3	30	55.2	20/10	3.6
			2. αT	30	61.2	20/10	3.5
			3. ω-3 + αT	30	54.9	20/10	3.4
			4. Placebo	30	59.9	20/10	3.4
Bowden [11]	USA	NR	1. ω-3	18	57.2	11/7	1.5
			2. corn oil	15	64.3	8/7	2.8
Daud [12]	USA	NR	1. ω-3	28	59	20/11	3.6
			2. placebo	27	58	12/20	3.3
Ewers [13]	Denmark	2007	1. ω-3	14	64.6	30/10	NR
			2. No supplement	14	64.6	30/10	NR
Gharekhani [14–17]	Iran	NR	1. ω-3	25	56.8	12/13	5
			2. paraffin (placebo)	20	57.2	8/12	6
Harving [18]	Denmark	NR	1. ω-3	83	65.5	55/28	4
			2. Olive oil	79	68	51/28	3.6
Himmelifarb [19]	USA	2008 to 2011	1. ω-3	31	58	23/8	2.1
			2. placebo	32	61.2	17/15	2.6
Hung [20]	USA	2008 to 2011	1. ω-3	17	50	14/3	4.2
			2. placebo	17	53	13/4	3.6
Khalatbari Soltani [21]	Iran	NR	1. ground flaxseed	15	54	10/5	2.6
			2. Usual diet	15	54.5	6/9	2.8
Kooshki [22]	Iran	NR	1. ω-3	17	50	10/7	1.75
			2. placebo	17	50	11/6	2.3
Lemos [24]	Brazil	NR	1. flaxseed oil + αT	70	55.7	39/31	2.4
			2. mineral oil + αT	75	58.3	46/29	2.9
Lee [23]	Korea	2012	1. ω-3	8	60	2/6	NR
			2. Olive oil	7	64	3/4	NR
Mirfatahi [25]	Iran	NR	1. flaxseed oil	17	68	12/5	4.4
			2. medium-chain triglycerides oil	17	59	10/7	4.6
Naini [26]	Iran	NR	1. ω-3	20	57.7	11/9	NR
			2. placebo	20	59.3	12/8	NR
Poulia [27]	Greece	NR	1. ω-3 + αT	22	51	16/9	9.4
			2. αT	23	51	16/9	
Rodhe [28]	Sweden	NR	1. sea buckthorn + vit-E	24	62	29/16	NR
			2. Coconut oil	21	62	29/16	NR
Saifullah [29]	USA	NR	1. ω-3	15	58	11/4	NR
			2. placebo	8	57	7/1	NR
Zakaria [30]	Egypt	NR	1. ω-3 + vit-E	20	50.2	12/8	4
			2. Placebo	20	46.4	11/9	4.5

CRP, C-reactive protein; hs-CRP, high-sensitivity C-reactive protein; IL-6, interleukin-6; NR, no report; vit-E, vitamin E; αT, alpha-tocopherol; ω-3, omega-3 fatty acids.

Table 2. Quality of the included randomized clinical trials.

Study	Randomization	Concealment	Blinding	Follow-Up Duration	Loss Follow-Up	Type of Analysis	Relevant Outcomes	Quality Judgement
Asemi	Computer generated	Yes	Double-blind	12 weeks	0	ITT	hs-CRP	Low risk
Bowden	4-block permuted randomization	No	Double-blind	26 weeks	7	PP	hs-CRP	High risk
Daud	NR	NR	Triple-blind	26 weeks	2	ITT	CRP	Moderate
Ewers	Computer generated	NR	Single-blind	6 weeks	10	PP	CRP	High risk
Gharekhani	Blocked randomization	NR	Single-blind	16 weeks	9	PP	CRP, IL-6	High risk
Harving	NR	NR	NR	12 weeks	44	PP	hs-CRP	High risk
Himmelifarb	4-block permuted randomization	NR	Double-blind	8 weeks	0	ITT	CRP, IL-6	Moderate
Hung	Randomized in 1:1 ratio	NR	Double-blind	12 weeks	4	PP	hs-CRP, IL-6	Moderate
KhalatbariSoltani	NR	NR	Unblind	8 weeks	8	PP	CRP	High risk
Kooshki	Blocked randomization	Yes	Double-blind	10 weeks	0	ITT	CRP, IL-6	Low risk
Lee	Random number table	NR	Double-blind	12 weeks	0	PP	CRP	Moderate
Lemos	NR	Yes	Double-blind	7 weeks	22	ITT	CRP	High risk
Mirfatahi	Blocked randomization	NR	Double-blind	8 weeks	0	PP	hs-CRP	Moderate
Naini	NR	Yes	Double-blind	8 weeks	0	ITT	CRP, IL-6	Moderate
Poulia	Flip coin	NR	Single-blind	4 weeks	8	PP	CRP	High risk
Rodhe	NR	Yes	Double-blind	8 weeks	21	PP	hs-CRP	High risk
Saifullah	Computer generated	Yes	Double-blind	12 weeks	3	PP	CRP	Moderate
Zakaria	Flip coin	NR	Double-blind	16 weeks	0	PP	hs-CRP	Moderate

CRP, C-reactive protein; hs-CRP, high-sensitivity C-reactive protein; IL-6, interleukin-6; ITT, intention to treat; NR, no report; PP, per protocol.

2.2. C-Reactive Protein

A total of 11 RCTs with 632 cases in five treatments were included in the network meta-analysis of CRP (Figure 2A) [12–14,18,21–24,26,27,29]. The result showed that with placebo as the reference, PUFAs was the only one treatment showing significantly lower CRP (WMD: −0.37, 95% CI: −0.07 to −0.68), but the CRP in PUFAs group was not significantly lower than vitamin E, PUFAs plus vitamin E, and MCT (Figure 3A; Supplementary File 1). Similarly, in SUCRA, PUFAs also had the highest value (Mean rank = 2.1; SUCRA = 72.7) and placebo had the lowest value (Mean rank = 4.3; SUCRA = 16.3; Supplementary File 2). Because placebo, PUFA, vitamin E, PUFAs plus vitamin E, and MCT did not form any loop in the network meta-analysis of CRP, it is not required to test inconsistency in this consistency model. Moreover, no evidence detected serious small study effects (*t* = 0.49, 95% CI: −1.27 to 1.98; Supplementary File 3).

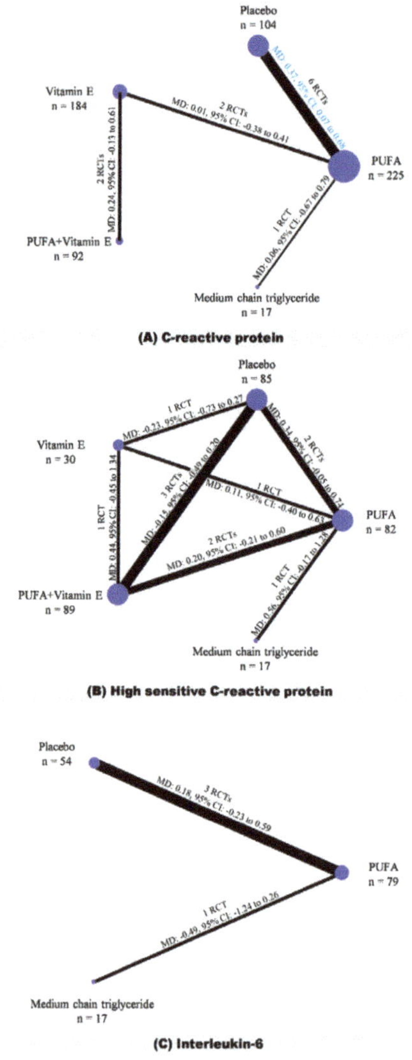

Figure 2. Network plots of (**A**) CRP, (**B**) high sensitivity CRP, and (**C**) IL-6.

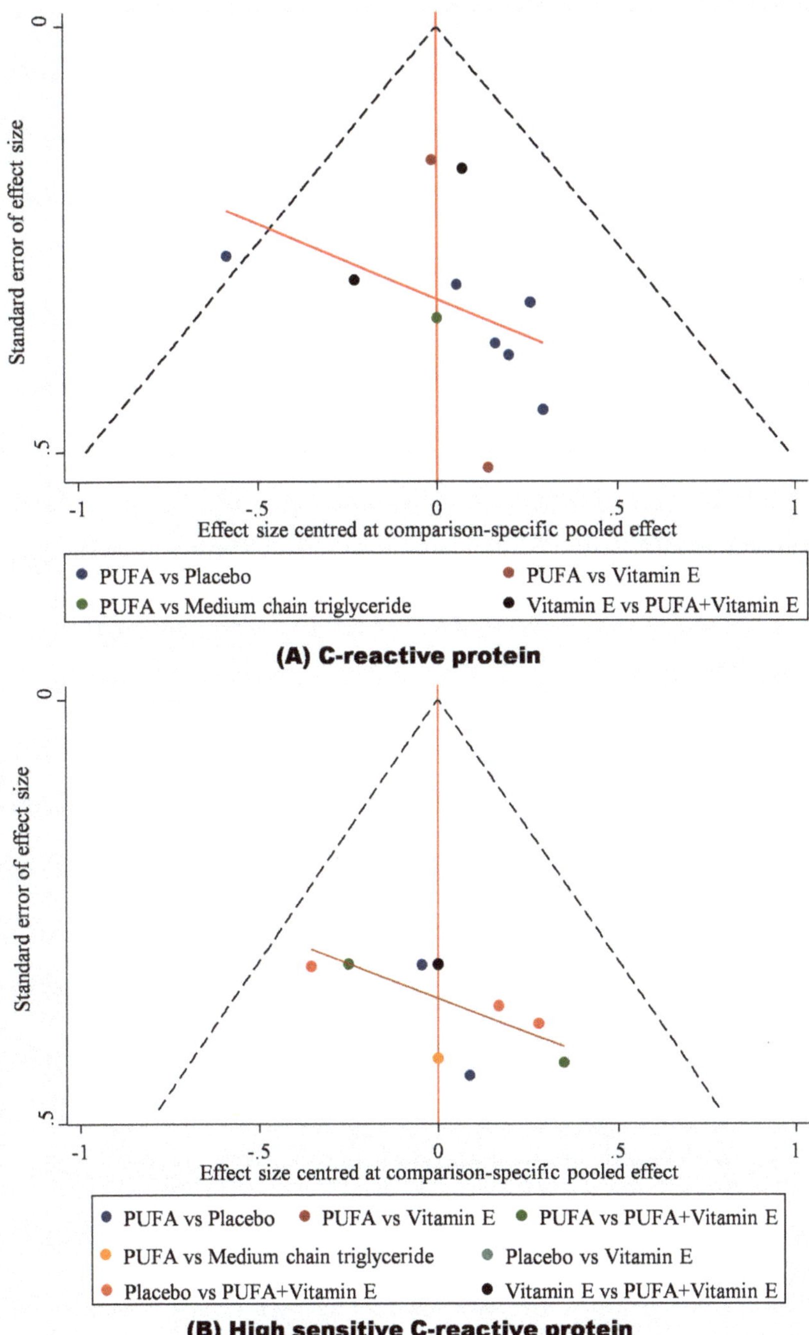

Figure 3. Funnel plots of (**A**) CRP and (**B**) high sensitivity CRP.

2.3. High-Sensitivity C-Reactive Protein

Six trials provided data on hs-CRP among the five treatments (n = 303) (Figure 2B) [10,11,20,25,28,30]. According to the available data, our network meta-analysis of hs-CRP showed no significant differences among placebo, PUFA, vitamin E, PUFAs plus vitamin E, and MCT (Supplementary File 4). There were some hints from ranking the best hs-CRP probability showing that PUFAs (54.7%) was the best choice, whereas placebo (1.2%) should be avoided. Similarly, in SUCRA, PUFAs had the highest value (Mean rank = 1.6; SUCRA = 84.6), whereas placebo (Mean rank = 3.9; SUCRA = 28.2) and MCT (Mean rank = 4.3; SUCRA = 18.4; Supplementary File 5) were the two treatments with lowest values. The loop inconsistency test for the network meta-analysis of hs-CRP showed insignificance (chi-square = 2.25, p < 0.13; Supplementary File 6), yet the Egger's test detected small study effects (t = 2.34, 95% CI: 0.10 to 6.06, p = 0.04; Supplementary File 7).

2.4. Interleukin-6

Four of the included trials provided data on IL-6 among placebo, PUFA, and MCT (n = 140) (Figure 2A) [14,20,22,26]. The network meta-analysis of IL-6 also showed no significant differences among placebo, PUFA, and MCT (Supplementary File 8). Interestingly, ranking the best IL-6 probability showing that MCT (88.8%) had the highest probability, whereas placebo (3.2%) and PUFAs (8.0%) were the two treatments with lowest probabilities. SUCRA also depicted similar phenomenon showing that MCT had the highest value (Mean rank = 1.2; SUCRA = 92.0), whereas placebo (Mean rank = 2.7; SUCRA = 12.7) and MCT (Mean rank = 2.1; SUCRA = 45.2) were the two treatments with lowest values. The loop inconsistency test for the network meta-analysis of hs-CRP showed no significance (chi-square = 1.64, p < 0.20; Supplementary File 9), and the Egger's test also detected no small study effects (t = 1.44, 95% CI: −14.26 to 28.63, p = 0.29; Supplementary File 10).

2.5. Further Analysis

We further examined albumin, a minor parameter of inflammatory, based on the included evidence, and we also detected the influences from regions because of lifestyle and dietary style. For albumin, A total of nine trials formed network for placebo, PUFA, vitamin E, and PUFAs plus vitamin E with 407 cases [10,12,13,15,20,23,27–29]. The pooled result also showed insignificant differences among those four treatments (Supplementary File 11). Yet, SUCRA indicated that PUFA had the highest value (Mean rank = 1.4, SUCRA = 86.9; Supplementary File 12). We did not observe significant inconsistency (chi-square = 5.38, p < 0.06; Supplementary File 13) and small study effects (t = 1.02, 95% CI: −1.69 to 4.65, p = 0.33; Supplementary File 14).

Moreover, we only found available and appropriate information for detecting region effects on the pooled results of CRP and hs-CRP. Then, the meta-regression did not show any significant findings. Current evidence is insufficient to prove that region plays an important role in the effects of PUFA on CRP (Supplementary File 15) and hs-CRP (Supplementary File 16).

A cluster plot for CRP and hs-CRP scores demonstrated that the best balance was achieved by PUFAs (Cophenetic Correlation Coefficient = 0.86; Supplementary File 17). Therefore, PUFAs may be recommended for treating patients undergoing dialysis. By contrast, placebo exhibited poor performance in the cluster plot.

3. Discussion

In our systematic review, we successfully identified 18 randomized clinical trials (n = 962) investigating the effect of PUFAs on inflammatory markers among patients undergoing dialysis. In our network meta-analysis, we depicted an overview of comparisons among placebo, PUFA, vitamin E, PUFAs plus vitamin E, and MCT. Then, the results showed that the current evidence only supports PUFAs group having significant lower CRP than placebo. Yet, other active treatments did not reach the statistical significance when they were compared to placebo. The results of hs-CRP and IL-6 failed to support PUFAs having more benefits than other treatment, even no significant benefit as it was compared to placebo. These results about limited anti-inflammatory effects from PUFAs are similar to a previous synthesis indicating that alpha-linolenic acid has no effects on blood inflammatory markers [43].

These insignificant results may relate to the complex comparators among trials. Some of the trials treated control group with vitamin E, and some of them used combined supplements of PUFAs and vitamin E. Apart from PUFA, antioxidants such as vitamin E can also reduce the inflammatory responses by decreasing reactive oxygen species and NF-κB [70]. Besides, combination of PUFAs and antioxidants can reduce the oxidative stress caused by PUFAs [1]. Thus, our synthesis separated PUFAs alone and combined supplements of PUFAs and vitamin E. Then, we found PUFAs alone having a significantly higher CRP level than placebo, whereas no significant difference in CRP level between combined supplements of PUFAs and vitamin E and placebo. The pooled result also did not support that combined supplements of PUFAs and vitamin E having significant benefits on hs-CRP.

We agree that Omega-3 fatty acids play some roles in anti-inflammatory among patients undergoing dialysis because eicosapentaenoic acid and docosahexaenoic acid have been well-known in anti-inflammatory action through regulating gene expression, lowering membrane content of arachidonic acid, inhibiting arachidonic acid metabolism, and competing with arachidonic acid [41,71]. To be more specific, eicosapentaenoic acid and docosahexaenoic acid affect cyclooxygenase and lipoxygenase pathway through being substrates for the key enzymes. The patients of chronic kidney disease have much higher systemic concentration of inflammatory cytokine because of the decrease renal clearance and the insufficiency of nutrient [72,73]. This situation will cause the destruction of endothelial cell and eventually lead to cardiovascular disease [72,74]. To control the chronic inflammation of these patients, dietary fat supplement has important biological effect. PUFA can clean up the reactive oxygen species and inhibit activation of NF-κB, which plays a significant role in regulating inflammatory response [31]. Furthermore, PUFA will compete with arachidonic acid for the substance in the cyclooxygenase pathway to produce less pro-inflammatory cytokine [41]. Collectively, PUFA can decrease the systemic inflammation and the cardiovascular disease mortality among patients with chronic kidney disease. Although our evidence did not show the significant benefit of Omega-3 fatty acids on hs-CRP among patients receiving dialysis, the pooled hs-CRP had similar trends with the pooled results of CRP. A potential reason for the insignificant difference in hs-CRP may be smaller sample size (n = 303). In addition, another important potential factor causing the insignificant finding is that hs-CRP detects inflammatory with better sensitivity than CRP, especially for those patients with cardiovascular problems. It is well-published that cardiovascular problems are common comorbidities of chronic kidney disease. Thus, the difference between hs-CRP and traditional CRP may be more obvious for patients undergoing dialysis than for healthy people.

3.1. Comparing to the Previous Syntheses

Besides the good systematic review and meta-analysis in 2018 we mentioned above [31], there is another important synthesis in 2016 on this topic [69]. These two systematic reviews concluded similarly by declaring that Omega-3 fatty acids are effective supplements for reducing CRP levels among patients undergoing dialysis. However, their meta-analyses of CRP reflected very high heterogeneities. They did not successfully explain the source of heterogeneities though the systematic review by Khor et al. in 2018 separated alpha-linolenic acid (I-square = 93.4%) from eicosapentaenoic acid and docosahexaenoic acid. As we know, the anti-inflammatory effects of alpha-linolenic acid share similar pathway with eicosapentaenoic acid and docosahexaenoic acid [31]. Thus, subgroup analysis for alpha-linolenic acid may be not the best way to explore the heterogeneity in the pooled result of CRP mean change.

To face the challenge of high heterogeneity in the pooled CRP reported by the previous syntheses, in our study, we carefully clarified comparators by mainly relevant nutrients and outcomes for giving fewer biased results because of conceptual heterogeneity according to methodological guidance [75]. These two conceptual heterogeneities may result in the statistical heterogeneity in the pooled CRP level. Our study not only distinguished placebo, PUFA, vitamin E, PUFAs plus vitamin E, and MCT for comparators, but also separated hs-CRP from CRP for outcome synthesis. For instance, four trials included in the previous synthesis used hs-CRP [10,11,20,25], and we pooled these four trials with the other two trials that were not included in the previous synthesis for hs-CRP [28,30]. As a result of reduction of conceptual heterogeneity, we successfully gave this topic reasonable results without inconsistency and highly statistical heterogeneity.

3.2. Limitations

Although our synthesis overcame some limitations in previous syntheses and clarified the effects of PUFAs on inflammatory markers among patients receiving dialysis, the present synthesis still has three limitations. Firstly, the use of PUFAs is not clear, though our study separated combined supplements of PUFAs and vitamin E from PUFAs alone. The separation resulted in lower heterogeneity than previous syntheses, but our study cannot make a practical suggestion with a specific dosage for the use of PUFAs. Secondly, interaction of PUFAs and vitamin E on the anti-inflammatory effects remains unclear. Our synthesis did not find better results as the trials treating patients with combined supplements of PUFAs and vitamin E. Thirdly, our synthesis showed some trends about the benefits of PUFAs on hs-CRP and IL-6, but the results may be under power because of small sample size. We suggest that future studies should use hs-CRP measurement to confirm whether using PUFAs can reduce inflammatory responses, especially among those patients undergoing dialysis.

4. Materials and Methods

This comprehensive review team consisting of nephrologists and an experienced researcher conducted this study according to the Cochrane handbook, and reported the systematic review and meta-analysis according to the PRISMA guidelines [76]. The experienced researcher previously participated in some studies about nutrient, internal medicine, and chronic kidney disease [77–80]. The researcher also has some experience in conducting network meta-analysis [81,82]. Because this meta-analysis uses published data, it was exempted from institutional review board approval.

4.1. Study Selection Criteria

According to our study purpose, this comprehensive review selected evidence if (1) the study recruited patients undergoing dialysis, (2) the intervention was PUFA, and (3) the study prospectively randomized patients into two or more groups. However, this comprehensive review removed studies when they met following exclusion criteria: (1) the reference was gray literature without detailed information or data, (2) the study did not separate outcome reporting as it concurrently recruited patients with and without dialysis, and (3) the article did not report any relevant outcomes (CRP, hs-CRP, and IL-6).

4.2. Search Strategy and Study Selection

Data sources were three important online databases including EMBASE, PubMed, and the Web of Science. PubMed was the platform for building search strategy with relevant terms of dialysis and PUFA, and the search strategy was adapted to the other two databases. The relevant terms involved free-text and medical subject heading. Boolean operator "OR" combined the relevant terms of dialysis, and we also used "OR" for combining relevant terms of PUFA. Then, Boolean operator "AND" connected both dialysis part and PUFAs part. This search strategy did not restrict language and publication date from database inception until April 2019. Supplemental Material 18 showed the detail of the searching strategy.

After relevant references were identified from online databases, two investigators excluded ineligible references according to criteria in two phases. The first phase was title and abstract screening, and the second phase was full-text review. Any references meeting exclusion criteria were removed.

4.3. Quality Assessment and Data Extraction

The two investigators independently identified relevant information, and extracted outcome data. They identified the data about the details of trial design, location, inclusion year, treatments, sample size, mean age, sex, and dialysis period. The outcome data included three inflammatory markers, namely CRP, hs-CRP, IL-6, and albumin at the end of treatment. Because these data were continuous, the investigators extracted them in mean and standard deviation (SD). This network meta-analysis estimated SD from standard error (SE) according to the formula $SE = SD/\sqrt{N}$ when the trial only provided SE. When the trial only presented interquartile range (IQR), this study estimated SD using formula IQR/1.35. Moreover, the network meta-analysis estimated SD from maximum and minimum according to Hozo's method [83].

Based on the identified information, the investigators completed the risk of bias in each trial. The assessment involved randomization, concealment, blinding, follow-up duration, loss follow-up, and analysis type. These items reflected selection bias, performance bias, detection bias, and attrition bias. In case of any disagreements on risk of bias between the two investigators, a third reviewer participated into discussion to resolve the disagreement.

4.4. Evidence Synthesis and Statistical Analysis

Evidence synthesis consisted of qualitative and quantitative parts. The quantitative synthesis was contrast-based network meta-analysis. Because of conceptual heterogeneity among trial design, the network meta-analysis should be in random-effects model. The main outcomes were CRP, hs-CRP, and IL-6 at the end of treatment. Thus, the analysis performed weighted mean difference (WMD) and 95% confidence interval (CI). Standardized mean difference was the solution for units of measurement including mg/L, mg/dL, ng/L, ng/mL, and pg/mL. To clarify the effects among active treatments, the quantitative synthesis also showed surface under the cumulative ranking (SUCRA). This statistical technique estimated the probability of each treatment among the most effective treatments, and formed a hierarchy through the treatment ranking of probability. We would like to foster the understanding on this topic, and therefore we further analyzed albumin and the influence from region. The influence from region was detected by using meta-regression in network meta-analysis model. For conducting meta-regression, we applied dummy variables for America, Asia, and Europe. To confirm the quality of the quantitative synthesis, the network meta-analysis detected both the small-study effect and inconsistency. The small-study effect in a network meta-analysis can be assessed by an adjusted funnel plot and Egger's regression intercept. Concerning inconsistency, the meta-analysis implemented Lu–Ades' loop inconsistency test. The analyses mentioned above were completed using STATA version 14 for Microsoft Windows. In all analysis, $p < 0.05$ was considered as statistically significant.

5. Conclusions

Based on available evidence, the very first network meta-analysis on this topic, PUFAs could be an option for controlling inflammatory to patients undergoing dialysis. However, the evidence is not strong enough, especially with regards to the results of hs-CRP and IL-6. For practical recommendation, we anticipate further studies investigating in this topic to further elucidate how PUFAs reduce inflammatory among patients receiving dialysis.

Supplementary Materials: Supplementary materials can be found at http://www.mdpi.com/1422-0067/20/15/3645/s1.

Author Contributions: P.-K.W.: Conception of the study, data acquisition, manuscript drafting, and final approval of the version to be published. S.-C.Y.: Critical revision of the draft for enhancing crucial intellectual content, and final approval of the version to be published. S.-J.L.: Interpretation of data, supervision of the study, critical revision of the draft for enhancing crucial intellectual content, and final approval of the version to be published. Y.-N.K.: Design of the study, formal analysis and interpretation of data, manuscript drafting, and final approval of the version to be published.

Funding: This research received no external funding.

Conflicts of Interest: The authors declare no conflict of interest.

Abbreviations

CI	confidence interval
CRP	C-reactive protein
hs-CRP	high-sensitivity C-reactive protein
IQR	interquartile range
IL-6	interleukin-6
MCT	medium chain triglyceride
NF-κB	nuclear factor kappa B
PUFA	polyunsaturated fatty acids
RCT	randomized clinical trial
SD	standard deviation.
SE	standard error
SUCRA	surface under the cumulative ranking curve
WMD	weighted mean difference

References

1. Sachdeva, M.; Hung, A.; Kovalchuk, O.; Bitzer, M.; Mokrzycki, M.H. The initial vascular access type contributes to inflammation in incident hemodialysis patients. *Int. J. Nephrol.* **2012**, *2012*, 917465. [CrossRef] [PubMed]
2. Caglar, K.; Peng, Y.; Pupim, L.B.; Flakoll, P.J.; Levenhagen, D.; Hakim, R.M.; Ikizler, T.A. Inflammatory signals associated with hemodialysis. *Kidney Int.* **2002**, *62*, 1408–1416. [CrossRef] [PubMed]
3. Carrero, J.J.; Stenvinkel, P. Inflammation in end-stage renal disease—What have we learned in 10 years? *Semin. Dial.* **2010**, *23*, 498–509. [CrossRef] [PubMed]
4. Bazeley, J.; Bieber, B.; Li, Y.; Morgenstern, H.; de Sequera, P.; Combe, C.; Yamamoto, H.; Gallagher, M.; Port, F.K.; Robinson, B.M. C-reactive protein and prediction of 1-year mortality in prevalent hemodialysis patients. *Clin. J. Am. Soc. Nephrol. CJASN* **2011**, *6*, 2452–2461. [CrossRef] [PubMed]
5. Panichi, V.; Maggiore, U.; Taccola, D.; Migliori, M.; Rizza, G.M.; Consani, C.; Bertini, A.; Sposini, S.; Perez-Garcia, R.; Rindi, P.; et al. Interleukin-6 is a stronger predictor of total and cardiovascular mortality than c-reactive protein in haemodialysis patients. *Nephrol. Dial. Transplant. Off. Publ. Eur. Dial. Transplant. Assoc. Eur. Ren. Assoc.* **2004**, *19*, 1154–1160. [CrossRef] [PubMed]
6. Stenvinkel, P. Inflammation in end-stage renal failure: Could it be treated? *Nephrol. Dial. Transplant. Off. Publ. Eur. Dial. Transplant. Assoc. Eur. Ren. Assoc.* **2002**, *17* (Suppl. 8), 33–38. [CrossRef] [PubMed]
7. Stenvinkel, P.; Alvestrand, A. Inflammation in end-stage renal disease: Sources, consequences, and therapy. *Semin. Dial.* **2002**, *15*, 329–337. [CrossRef]
8. Machowska, A.; Carrero, J.J.; Lindholm, B.; Stenvinkel, P. Therapeutics targeting persistent inflammation in chronic kidney disease. *Transl. Res. J. Lab. Clin. Med.* **2016**, *167*, 204–213. [CrossRef]
9. Barutcu, I.; Sezgin, A.T.; Sezgin, N.; Gullu, H.; Esen, A.M.; Topal, E.; Ozdemir, R.; Kosar, F.; Cehreli, S. Increased high sensitive crp level and its significance in pathogenesis of slow coronary flow. *Angiology* **2007**, *58*, 401–407. [CrossRef]
10. Asemi, Z.; Soleimani, A.; Shakeri, H.; Mazroii, N.; Esmaillzadeh, A. Effects of omega-3 fatty acid plus alpha-tocopherol supplementation on malnutrition-inflammation score, biomarkers of inflammation and oxidative stress in chronic hemodialysis patients. *Int. Urol. Nephrol.* **2016**, *48*, 1887–1895. [CrossRef]
11. Bowden, R.G.; Wilson, R.L.; Deike, E.; Gentile, M. Fish oil supplementation lowers c-reactive protein levels independent of triglyceride reduction in patients with end-stage renal disease. *Nutr. Clin. Pract.* **2009**, *24*, 508–512. [CrossRef] [PubMed]
12. Daud, Z.A.; Tubie, B.; Adams, J.; Quainton, T.; Osia, R.; Tubie, S.; Kaur, D.; Khosla, P.; Sheyman, M. Effects of protein and omega-3 supplementation, provided during regular dialysis sessions, on nutritional and inflammatory indices in hemodialysis patients. *Vasc. Health Risk Manag.* **2012**, *8*, 187–195. [PubMed]

13. Ewers, B.; Riserus, U.; Marckmann, P. Effects of unsaturated fat dietary supplements on blood lipids, and on markers of malnutrition and inflammation in hemodialysis patients. *J. Ren. Nutr.* **2009**, *19*, 401–411. [CrossRef] [PubMed]

14. Gharekhani, A.; Dashti-Khavidaki, S.; Lessan-Pezeshki, M.; Khatami, M.R. Potential effects of omega-3 fatty acids on insulin resistance and lipid profile in maintenance hemodialysis patients a randomized placebo-controlled trial. *Iran. J. Kidney Dis.* **2016**, *10*, 310–318. [PubMed]

15. Gharekhani, A.; Khatami, M.R.; Dashti-Khavidaki, S.; Razeghi, E.; Abdollahi, A.; Hashemi-Nazari, S.S.; Mansournia, M.A. Effects of oral supplementation with omega-3 fatty acids on nutritional state and inflammatory markers in maintenance hemodialysis patients. *J. Ren. Nutr.* **2014**, *24*, 177–185. [CrossRef] [PubMed]

16. Gharekhani, A.; Khatami, M.R.; Dashti-Khavidaki, S.; Razeghi, E.; Abdollahi, A.; Hashemi-Nazari, S.S.; Mansournia, M.A. Potential effects of omega-3 fatty acids on anemia and inflammatory markers in maintenance hemodialysis patients. *DARU* **2014**, *22*, 11. [CrossRef] [PubMed]

17. Gharekhani, A.; Khatami, M.R.; Dashti-Khavidaki, S.; Razeghi, E.; Noorbala, A.A.; Hashemi-Nazari, S.S.; Mansournia, M.A. The effect of omega-3 fatty acids on depressive symptoms and inflammatory markers in maintenance hemodialysis patients: A randomized, placebo-controlled clinical trial. *Eur. J. Clin. Pharmacol.* **2014**, *70*, 655–665. [CrossRef]

18. Harving, F.; Svensson, M.; Flyvbjerg, A.; Schmidt, E.B.; Jorgensen, K.A.; Eriksen, H.H.; Christensen, J.H. N-3 polyunsaturated fatty acids and adiponectin in patients with end-stage renal disease. *Clin. Nephrol.* **2015**, *83*, 279–285. [CrossRef]

19. Himmelifarb, J.; Phinney, S.; Ikizler, T.A.; Kane, J.; McMonagle, E.; Miller, G. Gamma-tocopherol and docosahexaenoic acid decrease inflammation in dialysis patients. *J. Ren. Nutr.* **2007**, *17*, 296–304. [CrossRef]

20. Hung, A.M.; Booker, C.; Ellis, C.D.; Siew, E.D.; Graves, A.J.; Shintani, A.; Abumrad, N.N.; Himmelfarb, J.; Ikizler, T.A. Omega-3 fatty acids inhibit the up-regulation of endothelial chemokines in maintenance hemodialysis patients. *Nephrol. Dial. Transplant.* **2015**, *30*, 266–274. [CrossRef]

21. Khalatbari Soltani, S.; Jamaluddin, R.; Tabibi, H.; Mohd Yusof, B.N.; Atabak, S.; Loh, S.P.; Rahmani, L. Effects of flaxseed consumption on systemic inflammation and serum lipid profile in hemodialysis patients with lipid abnormalities. *Hemodial. Int.* **2013**, *17*, 275–281. [CrossRef] [PubMed]

22. Kooshki, A.; Taleban, F.A.; Tabibi, H.; Hedayati, M. Effects of marine omega-3 fatty acids on serum systemic and vascular inflammation markers and oxidative stress in hemodialysis patients. *Ann. Nutr. Metab.* **2011**, *58*, 197–202. [CrossRef] [PubMed]

23. Lee, S.M.; Son, Y.K.; Kim, S.E.; An, W.S. The effects of omega-3 fatty acid on vitamin d activation in hemodialysis patients: A pilot study. *Mar. Drugs* **2015**, *13*, 741–755. [CrossRef] [PubMed]

24. Lemos, J.R.N.; de Alencastro, M.G.; Konrath, A.V.; Cargnin, M.; Manfro, R.C. Flaxseed oil supplementation decreases c-reactive protein levels in chronic hemodialysis patients. *Nutr. Res.* **2012**, *32*, 921–927. [CrossRef] [PubMed]

25. Mirfatahi, M.; Tabibi, H.; Nasrollahi, A.; Hedayati, M.; Taghizadeh, M. Effect of flaxseed oil on serum systemic and vascular inflammation markers and oxidative stress in hemodialysis patients: A randomized controlled trial. *Int. Urol. Nephrol.* **2016**, *48*, 1335–1341. [CrossRef]

26. Naini, A.E.; Asiabi, R.E.; Keivandarian, N.; Moeinzadeh, F. Effect of omega-3 supplementation on inflammatory parameters in patients on chronic ambulatory peritoneal dialysis. *Adv. Biomed. Res.* **2015**, *4*, 167. [PubMed]

27. Poulia, K.A.; Panagiotakos, D.B.; Tourlede, E.; Rezou, A.; Stamatiadis, D.; Boletis, J.; Zampelas, A. Omega-3 fatty acids supplementation does not affect serum lipids in chronic hemodialysis patients. *J. Ren. Nutr.* **2011**, *21*, 479–484. [CrossRef]

28. Rodhe, Y.; Woodhill, T.; Thorman, R.; Moller, L.; Hylander, B. The effect of sea buckthorn supplement on oral health, inflammation, and DNA damage in hemodialysis patients: A double-blinded, randomized crossover study. *J. Ren. Nutr.* **2013**, *23*, 172–179. [CrossRef]

29. Saifullah, A.; Watkins, B.A.; Saha, C.; Li, Y.; Moe, S.M.; Friedman, A.N. Oral fish oil supplementation raises blood omega-3 levels and lowers c-reactive protein in haemodialysis patients—A pilot study. *Nephrol. Dial. Transplant.* **2007**, *22*, 3561–3567. [CrossRef]

30. Zakaria, H.; Mostafa, T.M.; El-Azab, G.A.; Abd El Wahab, A.M.; Elshahawy, H.; Sayed-Ahmed, N.A.H. The impact of fish oil and wheat germ oil combination on mineral-bone and inflammatory markers in maintenance hemodialysis patients: A randomized, double-blind, placebo-controlled clinical trial. *Int. Urol. Nephrol.* **2017**, *49*, 1851–1858. [CrossRef]

31. Khor, B.H.; Narayanan, S.S.; Sahathevan, S.; Gafor, A.H.A.; Daud, Z.A.M.; Khosla, P.; Sabatino, A.; Fiaccadori, E.; Chinna, K.; Karupaiah, T. Efficacy of nutritional interventions on inflammatory markers in haemodialysis patients: A systematic review and limited meta-analysis. *Nutrients* **2018**, *10*, 397. [CrossRef] [PubMed]

32. Bersch-Ferreira, A.C.; Sampaio, G.R.; Gehringer, M.O.; Ross-Fernandes, M.B.; Kovacs, C.; Alves, R.; Pereira, J.L.; Magnoni, C.D.; Weber, B.; Rogero, M.M. Association between polyunsaturated fatty acids and inflammatory markers in patients in secondary prevention of cardiovascular disease. *Nutr.* **2017**, *37*, 30–36. [CrossRef] [PubMed]

33. Calder, P.C. N-3 polyunsaturated fatty acids, inflammation, and inflammatory diseases. *Am. J. Clin. Nutr.* **2006**, *83*, 1505s–1519s. [CrossRef] [PubMed]

34. Calder, P.C. Omega-3 polyunsaturated fatty acids and inflammatory processes: Nutrition or pharmacology? *Br. J. Clin. Pharmacol.* **2013**, *75*, 645–662. [CrossRef] [PubMed]

35. Calder, P.C. Omega-3 fatty acids and inflammatory processes: From molecules to man. *Biochem. Soc. Trans.* **2017**, *45*, 1105–1115. [CrossRef] [PubMed]

36. Laye, S.; Nadjar, A.; Joffre, C.; Bazinet, R.P. Anti-inflammatory effects of omega-3 fatty acids in the brain: Physiological mechanisms and relevance to pharmacology. *Pharmacol. Rev.* **2018**, *70*, 12–38. [CrossRef] [PubMed]

37. Scaioli, E.; Liverani, E.; Belluzzi, A. The imbalance between n-6/n-3 polyunsaturated fatty acids and inflammatory bowel disease: A comprehensive review and future therapeutic perspectives. *Int. J. Mol. Sci.* **2017**, *18*, 2619. [CrossRef]

38. Thomas, J.; Thomas, C.J.; Radcliffe, J.; Itsiopoulos, C. Omega-3 fatty acids in early prevention of inflammatory neurodegenerative disease: A focus on alzheimer's disease. *Biomed. Res. Int* **2015**, *2015*, 172801. [CrossRef]

39. Tortosa-Caparros, E.; Navas-Carrillo, D.; Marin, F.; Orenes-Pinero, E. Anti-inflammatory effects of omega 3 and omega 6 polyunsaturated fatty acids in cardiovascular disease and metabolic syndrome. *Crit. Rev. Food Sci. Nutr.* **2017**, *57*, 3421–3429. [CrossRef]

40. Yates, C.M.; Calder, P.C.; Ed Rainger, G. Pharmacology and therapeutics of omega-3 polyunsaturated fatty acids in chronic inflammatory disease. *Pharmacol. Ther.* **2014**, *141*, 272–282. [CrossRef]

41. Calder, P.C. Mechanisms of action of (n-3) fatty acids. *J. Nutr.* **2012**, *142*, 592s–599s. [CrossRef] [PubMed]

42. Reiter, E.; Jiang, Q.; Christen, S. Anti-inflammatory properties of alpha- and gamma-tocopherol. *Mol. Asp. Med.* **2007**, *28*, 668–691. [CrossRef] [PubMed]

43. Su, H.; Liu, R.J.; Chang, M.; Huang, J.H.; Jin, Q.Z.; Wang, X.G. Effect of dietary alpha-linolenic acid on blood inflammatory markers: A systematic review and meta-analysis of randomized controlled trials. *Eur. J. Nutr.* **2018**, *57*, 877–891. [CrossRef] [PubMed]

44. Yoshimoto-Furuie, K.; Yoshimoto, K.; Tanaka, T.; Saima, S.; Kikuchi, Y.; Shay, J.; Horrobin, D.F.; Echizen, H. Effects of oral supplementation with evening primrose oil for six weeks on plasma essential fatty acids and uremic skin symptoms in hemodialysis patients. *Nephron* **1999**, *81*, 151–159. [CrossRef] [PubMed]

45. Taziki, O.; Lessan-Pezeshki, M.; Akha, O.; Vasheghani, F. The effect of low dose omega-3 on plasma lipids in hemodialysis patients. *Saudi J. Kidney Dis. Transplant. Off. Publ. Saudi Cent. Organ. Transplant. Saudi Arab.* **2007**, *18*, 571–576.

46. Tabibi, H.; Mirfatahi, M.; Hedayati, M.; Nasrollahi, A. Effects of flaxseed oil on blood hepcidin and hematologic factors in hemodialysis patients. *Hemodial. Int.* **2017**, *21*, 549–556. [CrossRef] [PubMed]

47. Svensson, M.; Schrnidt, E.B.; Jorgense, K.A.; Christensen, J.H. The effect of n-3 fatty acids on lipids and lipoproteins in patients treated with chronic haemodialysis: A randomized placebo-controlled intervention study. *Nephrol. Dial. Transplant.* **2008**, *23*, 2918–2924. [CrossRef]

48. Svensson, M.; Schmidt, E.B.; Jorgensen, K.A.; Christensen, J.H. The effect of n-3 fatty acids on heart rate variability in patients treated with chronic hemodialysis. *J. Ren. Nutr.* **2007**, *17*, 243–249. [CrossRef]

49. Sorensen, G.V.B.; Svensson, M.; Strandhave, C.; Schmidt, E.B.; Jorgensen, K.A.; Christensen, J.H. The effect of n-3 fatty acids on small dense low-density lipoproteins in patients with end-stage renal disease: A randomized placebo-controlled intervention study. *J. Ren. Nutr.* **2015**, *25*, 376–380. [CrossRef]

50. Schmitz, P.G.; McCloud, L.K.; Reikes, S.T.; Leonard, C.L.; Gellens, M.E. Prophylaxis of hemodialysis graft thrombosis with fish oil: Double-blind, randomized, prospective trial. *J. Am. Soc. Nephrol.* **2002**, *13*, 184–190.

51. Rantanen, J.M.; Riahi, S.; Johansen, M.B.; Schmidt, E.B.; Christensen, J.H. Effects of marine n-3 polyunsaturated fatty acids on heart rate variability and heart rate in patients on chronic dialysis: A randomized controlled trial. *Nutrients* **2018**, *10*, 1313. [CrossRef] [PubMed]

52. Omrani, H.R.; Pasdar, Y.; Raisi, D.; Najafi, F.; Esfandiari, A. The effect of omega-3 on serum lipid profile in hemodialysis patients. *J. Ren. Inj. Prev.* **2015**, *4*, 68–72. [PubMed]

53. Madsen, T.; Hagstrup Christensen, J.; Toft, E.; Aardestrup, I.; Lundbye-Christensen, S.; Schmidt, E.B. Effect of intravenous ω-3 fatty acid infusion and hemodialysis on fatty acid composition of free fatty acids and phospholipids in patients with end-stage renal disease. *J. Parenter. Enter. Nutr.* **2011**, *35*, 97–106. [CrossRef] [PubMed]

54. Lok, C.E.; Moist, L.; Hemmelgarn, B.R.; Tonelli, M.; Vazquez, M.A.; Dorval, M.; Oliver, M.; Donnelly, S.; Allon, M.; Stanley, K. Effect of fish oil supplementation on graft patency and cardiovascular events among patients with new synthetic arteriovenous hemodialysis grafts a randomized controlled trial. *JAMA J. Am. Med. Assoc.* **2012**, *307*, 1809–1816. [CrossRef] [PubMed]

55. Khosroshahi, H.T.; Dehgan, R.; Asl, B.H.; Safaian, A.; Panahi, F.; Estakhri, R.; Purasgar, B. Effect of omega-3 supplementation on serum level of homocysteine in hemodialysis patients. *Iran. J. Kidney Dis.* **2013**, *7*, 479–484.

56. Khajehdehi, P. Lipid-lowering effect of polyunsaturated fatty acids in hemodialysis patients. *J. Ren. Nutr. Off. J. Counc. Ren. Nutr. Natl. Kidney Found.* **2000**, *10*, 191–195. [CrossRef]

57. Kajbaf, M.H.; Khorvash, F.; Mortazavi, M.; Shahidi, S.; Moeinzadeh, F.; Farajzadegan, Z.; Tirani, S.A. Does omega-3 supplementation decrease carotid intima-media thickening in hemodialysis patients? *J. Res. Pharm. Pract.* **2016**, *5*, 252–256.

58. Jabbari, M.; Khoshnevis, T.; Jenabi, A.; Yousefi, F. The effect of omega-3 supplement on serum lipid profile in patients undergoing hemodialysis: A randomized clinical trial. *Rom. J. Intern. Med. Rev. Roum. Med. Interne* **2016**, *54*, 222–227. [CrossRef]

59. Irish, A.B.; Viecelli, A.K.; Hawley, C.M.; Hooi, L.S.; Pascoe, E.M.; Paul-Brent, P.A.; Badve, S.V.; Mori, T.A.; Cass, A.; Kerr, P.G.; et al. Effect of fish oil supplementation and aspirin use on arteriovenous fistula failure in patients requiring hemodialysis a randomized clinical trial. *JAMA Intern. Med.* **2017**, *177*, 184–193. [CrossRef]

60. Ghanei, E.; Zeinali, J.; Borghei, M.; Homayouni, M. Efficacy of omega-3 fatty acids supplementation in treatment of uremic pruritus in hemodialysis patients: A double-blind randomized controlled trial. *Iran. Red Crescent Med. J.* **2012**, *14*, 515–522.

61. Deger, S.M.; Hung, A.M.; Ellis, C.D.; Booker, C.; Bian, A.H.; Chen, G.H.; Abumrad, N.N.; Ikizler, T.A. High dose omega-3 fatty acid administration and skeletal muscle protein turnover in maintenance hemodialysis patients. *Clin. J. Am. Soc. Nephrol.* **2016**, *11*, 1227–1235. [CrossRef] [PubMed]

62. De Mattos, A.M.; da Costa, J.A.C.; Jordao, A.A.; Chiarello, P.G. Omega-3 fatty acid supplementation is associated with oxidative stress and dyslipidemia, but does not contribute to better lipid and oxidative status on hemodialysis patients. *J. Ren. Nutr.* **2017**, *27*, 333–339. [CrossRef] [PubMed]

63. Dashti-Khavidaki, S.; Gharekhani, A.; Khatami, M.R.; Miri, E.S.; Khalili, H.; Razeghi, E.; Hashemi-Nazari, S.S.; Mansournia, M.A. Effects of omega-3 fatty acids on depression and quality of life in maintenance hemodialysis patients. *Am. J. Ther.* **2014**, *21*, 275–287. [CrossRef] [PubMed]

64. Begum, R.; Belury, M.A.; Burgess, J.R.; Peck, L.W. Supplementation with n-3 and n-6 polyunsaturated fatty acids: Effects on lipoxygenase activity and clinical symptoms of pruritus in hemodialysis patients. *J. Ren. Nutr.* **2004**, *14*, 233–241. [CrossRef]

65. Beavers, K.M.; Beavers, D.P.; Bowden, R.G.; Wilson, R.L.; Gentile, M. Effect of over-the-counter fish-oil administration on plasma lp(a) levels in an end-stage renal disease population. *J. Ren. Nutr.* **2009**, *19*, 443–449. [CrossRef] [PubMed]

66. Beavers, K.M.; Beavers, D.P.; Bowden, R.G.; Wilson, R.L.; Gentile, M. Omega-3 fatty acid supplementation and total homocysteine levels in end-stage renal disease patients. *Nephrology* **2008**, *13*, 284–288. [CrossRef]

67. Ateya, A.M.; Sabri, N.A.; El Hakim, I.; Shaheen, S.M. Effect of omega-3 fatty acids on serum lipid profile and oxidative stress in pediatric patients on regular hemodialysis: A randomized placebo-controlled study. *J. Ren. Nutr.* **2017**, *27*, 169–174. [CrossRef] [PubMed]

68. Allawi, A.A.D.; Wahab Alwardi, M.A.; Altemimi, H.M. Effects of omega-3 on vitamin d activation in iraqi patients with chronic kidney disease treated by maintenance hemodialysis. *J. Pharm. Sci. Res.* **2017**, *9*, 1812–1816.

69. Xu, T.H.; Sun, Y.T.; Sun, W.; Yao, L.; Sun, L.; Liu, L.L.; Ma, J.F.; Wang, L.N. Effect of omega-3 fatty acid supplementation on serum lipids and vascular inflammation in patients with end-stage renal disease: A meta-analysis. *Sci Rep.* **2016**, *6*, 39346. [CrossRef]

70. Khan, A.Q.; Khan, R.; Rehman, M.U.; Lateef, A.; Tahir, M.; Ali, F.; Sultana, S. Soy isoflavones (daidzein & genistein) inhibit 12-o-tetradecanoylphorbol-13-acetate (tpa)-induced cutaneous inflammation via modulation of cox-2 and nf-kappab in swiss albino mice. *Toxicology* **2012**, *302*, 266–274.

71. Mori, T.A.; Beilin, L.J. Omega-3 fatty acids and inflammation. *Curr. Atheroscler. Rep.* **2004**, *6*, 461–467. [CrossRef] [PubMed]

72. Carrero, J.J.; Stenvinkel, P. Persistent inflammation as a catalyst for other risk factors in chronic kidney disease: A hypothesis proposal. *Clin. J. Am. Soc. Nephrol. CJASN* **2009**, *4* (Suppl. 1), S49–S55. [CrossRef] [PubMed]

73. Huang, X.; Stenvinkel, P.; Qureshi, A.R.; Riserus, U.; Cederholm, T.; Barany, P.; Heimburger, O.; Lindholm, B.; Carrero, J.J. Essential polyunsaturated fatty acids, inflammation and mortality in dialysis patients. *Nephrol. Dial. Transplant. Off. Publ. Eur. Dial. Transplant. Assoc. Eur. Ren. Assoc.* **2012**, *27*, 3615–3620. [CrossRef]

74. Foley, R.N.; Parfrey, P.S.; Sarnak, M.J. Clinical epidemiology of cardiovascular disease in chronic renal disease. *Am. J. Kidney Dis. Off. J. Natl. Kidney Found.* **1998**, *32*, S112–S119. [CrossRef]

75. Mills, E.J.; Thorlund, K.; Ioannidis, J.P. Demystifying trial networks and network meta-analysis. *BMJ (Clin. Res. Ed.)* **2013**, *346*, f2914. [CrossRef] [PubMed]

76. Hutton, B.; Salanti, G.; Caldwell, D.M.; Chaimani, A.; Schmid, C.H.; Cameron, C.; Ioannidis, J.P.; Straus, S.; Thorlund, K.; Jansen, J.P.; et al. The prisma extension statement for reporting of systematic reviews incorporating network meta-analyses of health care interventions: Checklist and explanations. *Ann. Intern. Med.* **2015**, *162*, 777–784. [CrossRef] [PubMed]

77. Chi, S.C.; Tuan, H.I.; Kang, Y.N. Effects of polyunsaturated fatty acids on nonspecific typical dry eye disease: A systematic review and meta-analysis of randomized clinical trials. *Nutrients* **2019**, *11*, 942. [CrossRef] [PubMed]

78. Kang, Y.N.; Chi, S.C.; Wu, M.H.; Chiu, H.H. The effects of losartan versus beta-blockers on cardiovascular protection in marfan syndrome: A systematic review and meta-analysis. *J. Formos. Med Assoc. Taiwan Yi Zhi* **2019**, in press. [CrossRef]

79. Lin, T.M.; Chi, J.E.; Chang, C.C.; Kang, Y.N. Do etoricoxib and indometacin have similar effects and safety for gouty arthritis? A meta-analysis of randomized controlled trials. *J. Pain Res.* **2019**, *12*, 83–91. [CrossRef]

80. Lin, Y.C.; Lin, J.W.; Wu, M.S.; Chen, K.C.; Peng, C.C.; Kang, Y.N. Effects of calcium channel blockers comparing to angiotensin-converting enzyme inhibitors and angiotensin receptor blockers in patients with hypertension and chronic kidney disease stage 3 to 5 and dialysis: A systematic review and meta-analysis. *PLoS ONE* **2017**, *12*, e0188975. [CrossRef]

81. Kao, C.C.; Lin, Y.S.; Chu, H.C.; Fang, T.C.; Wu, M.S.; Kang, Y.N. Association of renal function and direct-acting antiviral agents for hcv: A network meta-analysis. *J. Clin. Med.* **2018**, *7*, 341. [CrossRef] [PubMed]

82. Lin, E.Y.; Kuo, Y.K.; Kang, Y.N. Effects of three common lumbar interbody fusion procedures for degenerative disc disease: A network meta-analysis of prospective studies. *Int. J. Surg.* **2018**, *60*, 224–230. [CrossRef] [PubMed]

83. Hozo, S.P.; Djulbegovic, B.; Hozo, I. Estimating the mean and variance from the median, range, and the size of a sample. *BMC Med Res. Methodol.* **2005**, *5*, 13. [CrossRef] [PubMed]

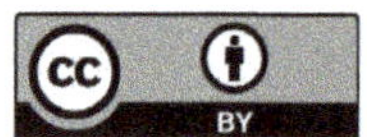

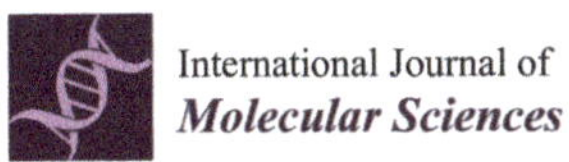 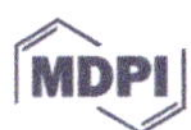

International Journal of
Molecular Sciences

Review

Molecular Mechanisms of the Acute Kidney Injury to Chronic Kidney Disease Transition: An Updated View

Francesco Guzzi [1,2,3,*], Luigi Cirillo [3], Rosa Maria Roperto [3], Paola Romagnani [1,2,3] and Elena Lazzeri [1,2]

1   Excellence Centre for Research, Transfer and High Education for the development of DE NOVO
     Therapies (DENOTHE), University of Florence, 50139 Florence, Italy; paola.romagnani@unifi.it (P.R.);
     elena.lazzeri@unifi.it (E.L.)
2   Department of Experimental and Clinical Biomedical Sciences "Mario Serio", University of Florence,
     50134 Florence, Italy
3   Nephrology and Dialysis Unit, Meyer Children's University Hospital, 50139 Florence, Italy;
     cirlui89@gmail.com (L.C.); rosa.roperto@meyer.it (R.M.R.)
*   Correspondence: francesco.guzzi@gmail.com

Received: 19 September 2019; Accepted: 4 October 2019; Published: 6 October 2019

Abstract: Increasing evidence has demonstrated the bidirectional link between acute kidney injury (AKI) and chronic kidney disease (CKD) such that, in the clinical setting, the new concept of a unified syndrome has been proposed. The pathophysiological reasons, along with the cellular and molecular mechanisms, behind the ability of a single, acute, apparently self-limiting event to drive chronic kidney disease progression are yet to be explained. This acute injury could promote progression to chronic disease through different pathways involving the endothelium, the inflammatory response and the development of fibrosis. The interplay among endothelial cells, macrophages and other immune cells, pericytes and fibroblasts often converge in the tubular epithelial cells that play a central role. Recent evidence has strengthened this concept by demonstrating that injured tubules respond to acute tubular necrosis through two main mechanisms: The polyploidization of tubular cells and the proliferation of a small population of self-renewing renal progenitors. This alternative pathophysiological interpretation could better characterize functional recovery after AKI.

Keywords: acute kidney injury; chronic kidney disease; renal progenitors; polyploidization

1. AKI Is Not a Self-Limiting Event

Despite the common belief of a generally benign nature, the profound, long-term implications of acute kidney injury (AKI) are appearing more and more evident. In particular, the emergent finding of a progression to various degrees of chronic kidney disease (CKD) after apparently self-limiting AKI episodes, independent from the etiology, has attracted great attention.

In the last decade, the assumption of an existing association between AKI and CKD has gradually spread in the nephrology and intensive care fields with evidence of a tight link between even mild serum creatinine elevation and long-term CKD [1–3]. The classic teaching case regarding acute renal failure, in particular acute tubular necrosis (ATN), has been that those patients generally achieve full or nearly full recovery [4,5]. The consensus on a new definition of AKI has helped to improve the understanding of its long-term clinical consequences and to demonstrate a clear link between AKI episodes, their severity, and their outcome [6]. With the help of standardized criteria for the definition of AKI and CKD, diverse observational studies collecting data from large administrative databases have increasingly showed a possible association between these two clinical entities [7–9]. Indeed, the more recent assumption is now to consider AKI and CKD as two interconnected syndromes where CKD is a risk factor for AKI and, in the meantime, AKI is a risk factor for the development and progression of CKD [3]. A recent systematic review and meta-analysis by See et al. [7] aimed to quantify the association between AKI and CKD by evaluating the results from 82 studies comprising more than 2 million patients experiencing AKI. The authors confirmed an increase in the risk of new or progressive CKD after AKI (HR 2.67, 95% CI 1.99–3.58) with a gradient of risk across AKI stages, an increased risk of end stage renal disease (ESRD) (HR 4.81, 95% CI 3.04–7.62), and an increased risk of death (HR 1.80, 95% CI 1.61–2.02) [7]. Moreover, previous studies have demonstrated that AKI severity [10], duration [11] and frequency [12] are associated with an increased risk of CKD progression. The AKI–CKD link has also been highlighted in pediatric studies [13–15].

Despite continuous progresses in the field and the recent ability to better identify the molecular signature of different renal cell types following acute injury, the mechanisms that drive the transition to chronic disease remain debated [16,17]. The traditional beliefs are now challenged by clinical observations and new advances in experimental transgenic models. Researchers have made significant effort trying to elucidate the pathophysiological link from AKI to CKD on cellular and molecular levels by using experimental models. CKD can occur through several pathologic mechanisms involving one or more of the kidney compartments: Vasculature, the tubule-interstitium or the glomerulus. Microvascular loss occurs along with increased fibrosis, worsening relative hypoxia within the kidney and in particular within the outer medulla. This is associated with changes in pericytes to adopt a pro-fibrotic myofibroblast phenotype. Moreover, consequent to altered oxygen availability, tubular injury and necrosis cause tubular dysfunction, oliguria and reduced glomerular filtration via tubulo-glomerular feedback. Thus, after an ischemic injury, the loss of nephronic mass, with remnant nephron hyperfiltration, renin-angiotensin system (RAS) activation, systemic hypertension and subsequent glomerulosclerosis have been described to pave the way from AKI to CKD [18–20]. Regardless of the initial insult, evidence of tubular cell loss and replacement by collagen scars and infiltrating macrophages are associated with further renal functional loss and progression towards end stage renal failure. Experimental models have shown that selective epithelial injury could drive capillary rarefaction, interstitial fibrosis, glomerulosclerosis and progression to CKD, substantiating a direct role for damaged tubular epithelial cells (TECs) [21]. Therefore, tubular epithelial cells have attracted increasing attention [22,23].

A new interpretation of this pathophysiology is that the epithelial tubular cell may allow for a better understanding of this somehow unexpected turn in the AKI natural history. Altogether, there is a need for the further investigation of the AKI-to-CKD transition as a public health priority.

2. Pathophysiology of the AKI-to-CKD Transition

From a pathophysiological point of view, microvascular integrity, changes in leukocyte and pericyte behavior, and tubular cell survival and function are all features of both AKI and CKD, and several cellular and molecular pathways have been considered to define the transition process. The main pathological mechanisms which concur to explain the AKI-to-CKD transition include: (i) Endothelial dysfunction, vasoconstriction and vascular congestion [24,25]; (ii) interstitial inflammation and the associated infiltration of monocytes/macrophages, neutrophils, T- and B-cells [26–30]; (iii) fibrosis via myofibroblasts recruitment and matrix deposition [31–33]; and (iv) tubular epithelial injury and dysregulated repair [23,34,35] (Figure 1). After a brief description of the main molecular pathways of the endothelial, inflammatory and fibrotic response to injury, we focus on the proximal tubular epithelial cell, the main player of the AKI-to-CKD transition [35].

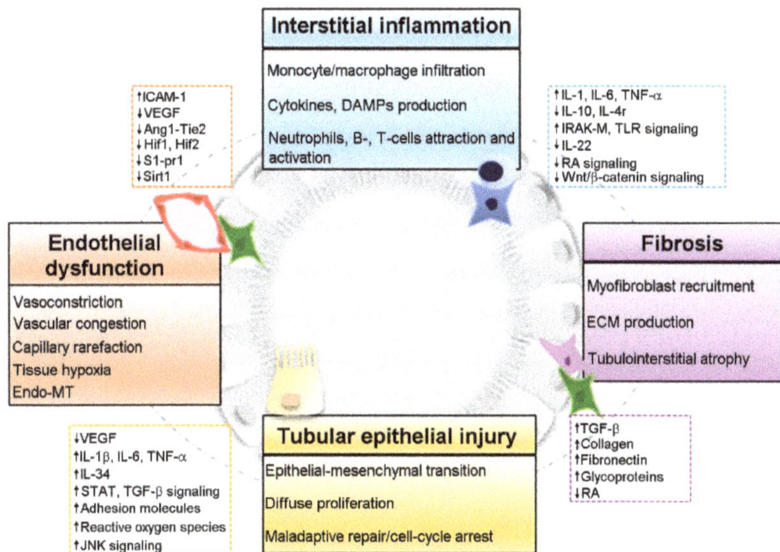

Figure 1. The interplay between endothelial dysfunction, interstitial inflammation, fibrosis and tubular epithelial injury concur to explain the acute kidney injury-to-chronic kidney disease (AKI-to-CKD) transition.

2.1. Endothelial Dysfunction

Capillary rarefaction has been extensively described as a consistent feature of the acutely injured nephron and has been linked to progression as a potential initiator of chronic nephropathy. A reduction in regional renal oxygen delivery leads to inflammation, ischemia, and necrosis, thus reflecting an imbalance between arterial pressure and vascular resistance, with a particularly vulnerable area in the outer stripe of the outer medulla. The existence of a putative bone marrow-derived endothelial progenitor cell (EPC) population has been hypothesized and linked to progression to chronic disease [36]. However, a recent study that combined bone marrow and kidney transplantation in a transgenic murine model demonstrated that no extra-renal cells substantially contribute to endothelial repair after selective injury [37].

Once capillary rarefaction is established, tissue hypoxia, mitochondrial dysfunction, inflammation and subsequent fibrosis occur [24]. The cellular and molecular pathways that underlie capillary rarefaction—in particular, the interplay between hypoxia, anti-angiogenic, and angiogenic factors—have yet to be explained [38]. Among angiogenic factors, vascular endothelial growth factor (VEGF), an endogenous cytokine produced by epithelial cells and directed to endothelial cells, is crucial for the preservation of vascular networks. Its reduced production could promote microvascular dysfunction and morphologic changes in the nephron [39,40]. The effects of its exogenous administration, with restoration of the microvascular density, improved renal blood flow, and reduced fibrogenic activity have been described in swine kidneys [41]. Similar effects, with improved endothelial cell survival and prevention of capillary leakage, resulted from the activation of the endothelium-specific receptor Tie2 through angiopoietin-1 (Ang-1)—a protein produced by vasculature support cells and specialized pericytes [42]. Moreover, the transgenic murine inactivation of endothelial hypoxia-inducible factors (Hif1-α and Hif2-α), as well as the deletion of endothelial sphingosine 1-phosphate receptor 1 (S1-pr1), resulted in increased acute and chronic inflammation and fibrosis after injury without affecting capillary permeability [43,44]. Therefore, there is considerable interest in the potential for Hif-stabilizing agents as therapeutic tools in renal injury [45]. In two models of folic acid-induced AKI and ureteral obstruction, Sirtuin 1 (Sirt 1) inactivation in endothelial cells caused impaired recovery, increased fibrosis, and disease progression [46,47].

Endothelial-to-mesenchymal transition (EndoMT) has been proposed as a contributor to capillary rarefaction, interstitial fibrosis, and, therefore, chronic damage [48]. Indeed, the reduction of EndoMT, obtained by reducing endothelium-specific transforming growth factor β (TGF-β) in a transgenic mouse model, was followed by the preservation of renal blood flow and microvasculature, less tissue hypoxia and tubulointerstitial fibrosis, thereby supporting the hypothesis of a link between EndoMT and chronic changes [49]. Moreover, the renal pericyte is now recognized as a key contributor to vascular stability in response to kidney injury [50].

Pericytes sit in close proximity to the endothelial cells within many organs, where they maintain vascular stability and release factors, including PDGF (platelet-derived growth factor) [51], angiopoietin [52], TGF-β [53], VEGF [54] and sphingosine-1-phosphate [55]. There is now an increasing understanding of the role played by these cells in acute and chronic kidney injury, where they leave their perivascular site in response to injury and differentiate to become myofibroblasts. Thus, either injuries or defects in pericyte function induce their detachment, contributing to both vascular rarefaction and increased fibrosis. In the end, recent advances have elucidated a contribution of endothelial cells and their products to capillary rarefaction, inflammation and tubulogenic pathways in a complex cellular interplay [43,44].

2.2. Interstitial Inflammation

Both resident and infiltrating immune cells participate in inflammation, injury and repair in the acute phase of kidney injury; through a tight cross-talk with endothelial cells, epithelial cells, and pericytes, they also contribute to disease progression [56]. The recent identification of a particular subset of renal resident macrophages, located at the abluminal side of the peritubular capillaries and capable of monitoring endothelial transport, has provided a perfect paradigm of the interplay between endothelium and immune system [57]. Resident macrophages seem to form a distinct anatomical and functional unit with the peritubular capillary endothelial cells that have the ability to detect and scavenge small immune complexes, possibly explaining the further recruitment of monocytes and neutrophils, as well as tissue injury in immune complex diseases [57]. This macrophage-endothelial functional unit, with a specific cross-talk at both the cellular and molecular levels, is also likely to be involved in the response to AKI [38].

The link between endothelial cells and inflammation is also suggested by CD169+ monocytes/macrophages that counteract the inflammatory response induced by intercellular adhesion molecule-1 (ICAM-1) expression after ischemic AKI [58]. Because they regulate inflammation, neutrophils infiltration, and because of their paracrine effects on tubular epithelial cells, macrophages can play an important role as determinants of AKI outcomes. Two populations of macrophages have been proposed by in vitro studies on behalf of their chemokine receptor repertoire: Pro-inflammatory or M1-subtype (interleukin (IL)-1, IL-6, and tumor necrosis factor-α (TNF-α)) and anti-inflammatory or M2-subtype (arginase, mannose receptor, IL-10, and IL-4 receptor-α), the first classically activated and the latter alternatively activated [59]. Despite being recently revised in regards to these two populations' in vivo behavior [60,61], this classification has been useful to identify different responses after acute injury in the kidney and a putative role for these cells in disease progression [28]. Macrophages have contrasting roles in renal injury and repair, first increasing the number of M1-polarized cells and then switching to an M2 phenotype supporting epithelial cell repair. Indeed, the depletion of M2 macrophages in mice with established AKI has resulted in prolongation of renal injury [62].

In a post-ischemic transgenic murine model, IL-1 receptor-associated kinase-M (IRAK-M), specifically expressed by monocyte/macrophages, has been demonstrated to influence the progression of AKI to CKD. IRAK-M expression induces the healing phase by inhibiting the toll-like receptor (TLR) and IL-1 receptor signaling, resolving TNF-α-dependent inflammation, and dampening the M1 pro-inflammatory response, all of which have been found to allow for improved functional recovery and structural regeneration [26]. Macrophages also participate in endogenous repair by secreting cytokines, such as IL-22, and providing ligands for retinoic acid (RA) and Wnt/β-catenin. In an ischemia-reperfusion injury (IRI) transgenic murine model, the administration or overexpression of IL-22 has been found to preserve renal function by increasing signal transducer and transcription factor 3 (STAT3) and protein kinase B (Akt) phosphorylation in proximal tubular epithelial cells, upregulating anti-apoptotic genes (e.g., *Bcl-2*), and downregulating pro-apoptotic genes (e.g., *Bad*) [63]. Retinoic acid (RA) signaling, activated in macrophages and tubular epithelial cells within hours of injury, has been found to reduce macrophage-dependent injury and fibrosis after AKI [64]. In zebrafish and murine models, the activation of RA signaling between epithelial cells and macrophages after AKI has been found to limit the injury extent by promoting the activation of M2 macrophages and tubular epithelial cell repair [64]. Wnt/β-catenin is another important pathway in recovery from AKI. Its activation by macrophages has been found to stimulate repair [65], and its early intervention is required to minimize renal damage after AKI in the initial phase [66]. However, its persistent activation and Wnt1 overexpression have been shown to play a role in progression to CKD through uncontrolled fibroblasts activation and inflammation [66,67]. Therefore, while important in facilitating repair after AKI, the presence of macrophages is also correlated with fibrosis and adverse outcomes. Moreover, the reciprocal expression of colony-stimulating factor-1 (CSF-1) and its receptor between macrophages and tubular epithelial cells could enhance cell proliferation and stimulate the anti-inflammatory M2 subtype [68]. Interestingly, to highlight the complexity of the interplay between these cells upon injury, IL-34 produced by injured TECs may have a pro-inflammatory ability despite sharing the same macrophage receptor of CSF-1 [69].

After the initial phase of injury, early inflammation is followed by the infiltration of circulating immune cells (T- and B-cells) attracted by cytokines and damage-associated molecular patterns (DAMPs) released by injured cells [27]. While interacting with activated monocytes/macrophages, injured TECs, and endothelial cells, DAMPs participate in the development of a pro-fibrotic milieu which activates pericytes to proliferate and evolve into myofibroblasts, thereby inducing matrix deposition, renal fibrosis, and CKD [70]. In contrast, a subset of regulatory T-cells (Treg) may act like self-tolerance inducers and suppress inflammation by enhancing immune homeostasis [71]. Together with their positive effects, Treg depletion has been shown to aggravate ischemic AKI [72]. Interestingly, the protective role of CD4+ and CD8+ T-cells in a murine model of toxic nephropathy (aristolochic acid nephropathy) has recently been described after treatment with selective monoclonal antibodies [73]. Concerning B-cells, immunoglobulins production, antigen presentation, and subsequent complement activation have been described as possible contributors to the progression from acute to chronic renal injury [74].

2.3. Fibrosis

Several obstructive, ischemia-reperfusion and nephrotoxic animal models have investigated the link between AKI and CKD by focusing on the development of interstitial fibrosis [31–33]. Myofibroblasts, whether derived from activated resident fibroblasts or from pericytes, are responsible for extracellular matrix (ECM) production, with the deposition of collagens, fibronectins and other glycoproteins, which, together with TGF-β, contribute to fibrosis [32,75]. The expression of α-smooth muscle actin (α-SMA), usually confined to the vascular compartment, and platelet-derived growth factor receptor-β (PDGFR-β), identifies these cells in the interstitium of injured kidneys [75]. A number of studies have consistently linked peritubular capillaries rarefaction, pericytes detachment, interstitial hypoxia and tubular epithelial injury as triggers of renal fibrosis [21,50]. In particular, whereas an ischemic injury could be responsible for capillary rarefaction and pericyte detachment, pericyte loss could be a trigger for endothelial damage and capillary rarefaction followed by tubular epithelial injury and fibrosis [50]. Though the severity of interstitial fibrosis in renal biopsies has been recognized as the major prognostic factor for CKD/ESRD, fibrosis has been considered a self-sustaining process [76], and a causal relationship between ECM deposition, fibrosis and chronic kidney injury has not yet been identified.

Recent studies have suggested that fibrosis could also be beneficial for the healing processes [34]. During repair from experimental AKI, tubules that fail to recover become atrophic, and fibrosis surrounds them in well-demarcated areas that separate the injured parenchyma from restored or not injured tubules [34]. In this view, fibrosis is itself essentially a self-limiting repair process that restricts injury, and it is not autonomously progressive. Indeed, many other experimental data do not support a major role of self-perpetuating tubulointerstitial fibrosis in the transition from AKI to CKD and highlight that progressive renal fibrosis requires additional injuries—unless primary interstitial disease is itself the triggering factor for fibrosis [23,77]. Recently, in a transgenic mouse model expressing diphtheria toxin receptor on renal fibroblasts, Nakamura et al. showed that fibroblasts depletion could worsen the expression of tubular injury markers, with a marked increase after unilateral ureteral obstruction [33]. While the transition of resident fibroblasts to myofibroblasts has been described to trigger fibrosis [78], myofibroblasts can also acquire retinoic acid-production ability—lost by the injured tubular epithelial cells—supporting epithelial integrity and repair [33] and dampening pro-inflammatory macrophages [64]. In the aged kidney, the ability of resident fibroblasts to support repair is less pronounced [79].

Altogether, a deeper understanding of the cellular and molecular pathways involving fibrosis in different types of acute kidney injury will be of great importance for the development of therapeutic strategies to halt the progression of AKI to CKD [80,81].

2.4. Tubular Epithelial Injury

The most sensitive cells to acute ischemic and nephrotoxic injury are the proximal S3 segment tubular epithelial cells of the outer stripe of the outer medulla due to their intense workload, high metabolic demand, and limited capacity for anaerobic energy production [82]. In fact, this region accounts for a unique microvascular environment which is extremely vulnerable to hypoperfusion, renal hypoxia, and mitochondrial damage [82,83]. Recently, a shift from a victim to the driving force of the AKI-to-CKD transition has been proposed for the tubular epithelial cell [35]. Indeed, injured TECs have been shown to act as drivers of both inflammation and fibrosis. They produce a large variety of cytokines (e.g., IL-6, IL-1β, and TNF-α), thereby gaining a pro-inflammatory phenotype and directly influencing macrophage behavior [84,85], and they are an important source of chemokines—via several pathways including STAT signaling and TGF-β signaling—adhesion molecules and reactive oxygen species [35]. Traditionally, injured TECs have been thought to undergo a process of dedifferentiation, a partial epithelial–mesenchymal transition (EMT) [86,87], i.e., the de novo expression of mesenchymal marker such as vimentin in TECs [88] induced by the injury-mediated reactivation of snail family zinc finger 1 (Snail1) [89,90]. This transient dedifferentiation is also characterized by the re-expression of developmental genes such as *Pax2* and cell cycle markers such as proliferating cell nuclear antigen (PCNA)—thus suggesting extensive proliferation—followed by a loss of mesenchymal markers, which has been interpreted as re-differentiation into fully viable epithelial cells [91,92]. This extensive proliferative ability could be responsible for rapid repair upon acute injury.

This proliferative capacity is thought to explain why young and mildly injured patients regain normal (or near-normal) renal function within days from acute injury, regardless of etiology. According to this view, the kidney's reparative potential is counterbalanced by maladaptive repair, as if they are on a balance pan. Shifting from proliferation to maladaptive repair would explain disease progression. In one toxic and one obstructive nephropathy models, Yang et al. demonstrated a causal association between cell cycle arrest and fibrosis [93]. Due to abnormal repair processes, TECs can become atrophic and gain a pro-fibrotic phenotype after AKI. G2/M-arrested TECs may activate the JNK signaling to induce the production of pro-fibrotic cytokines (e.g., TGF-β and connective tissue growth factor (CTGF)) [22]. Altogether, whereas favorable cell cycle events could be responsible for repair, cell cycle arrest could determine the progression of injury. Dysregulated and inefficient (i.e., maladaptive) tubular repair has been related to the persistence of an inflammatory milieu, ECM deposition and subsequent tubular cells convergence towards a pro-fibrotic and senescent phenotype [94]. Indeed, dedifferentiated TECs acquire pro-fibrotic characteristics that elicit CKD progression [23].

An alternative pathophysiological interpretation of cell cycle events after acute injury has recently been proposed [95,96]. Indeed, several studies have recently pointed toward the existence of a scattered population of undifferentiated, self-renewing, renal progenitors with the ability to regenerate fully differentiated TECs rather than acquire a dedifferentiation state [97–102]. After their identification in the human kidney, further studies were able to provide detailed characterization in both humans and mice [100] and to identify these cells as a source of tubular regeneration after AKI [103]. This strategy for kidney regeneration appears to be highly conserved across species [104] and involved in kidney development, maintenance, and regeneration [105]. New experimental evidence provided by lineage tracing studies has strengthened the concept that tubular epithelial cell regeneration is mostly due to a scattered progenitors' population rather than to the majority of remnant cells [95]. Renal progenitors are more numerous in the proximal tubule S3 segment, the segment which is more sensitive to ischemic and nephrotoxic injury and from where tubular cells detach in large numbers, thus explaining the high proliferation of tubular epithelial cells observed in this area (Figure 2) [95]. The intense immunoreactivity of nuclear proliferation markers (such as proliferating cell nuclear antigen-PCNA and Ki-67) has also been observed after acute injury in the proximal tubule S2 segment and other uninjured areas of the nephron [88,106]. Regardless, although such cell cycle markers confirm the cell's entry in the cell cycle, they do not entail its completion with the formation of two new differentiated daughter cells. Thanks to simultaneous cell cycle phase lineage tracing analysis and DNA content measurement with FUCCI (fluorescent ubiquitination-based cell cycle indicator) technology, it has been shown that the majority of remnant TECs do enter the cell cycle, but they undergo endoreplication-mediated hypertrophy (Figure 2). Endoreplication is an evolutionary conserved cell cycle program by which cells replicate their genome without division, resulting in polyploid cells (i.e., polyploidization). Polyploidization increases the gene copy number in response to the need to quickly support increased functional requests for a higher metabolic output while persistently maintaining differentiated and specialized cell functions. This permits hypertrophy and function recovery [95,96].

In mammals, endoreplication-induced polyploidy has been observed in multiple tissue and organs (including the skin, placenta, liver, and blood) during normal development and under stressful conditions [107]. In the kidney, tubular cell polyploidization has frequently been observed in the proximal convoluted tubule S2 segment that is not directly injured during ATN (Figure 2). Accordingly, a new interpretation could follow: i) AKI causes TEC loss; ii) a small subset of progenitor cells showing resistance to death and proliferative ability are responsible for parenchymal regeneration; and iii) remnant TECs enter the cell cycle but undergo endoreplication-mediated polyploidy rather than mitosis, thus rapidly compensating for function loss [95].

According to this new hypothesis, the physiological response to AKI could imply a limited regeneration mediated by scattered renal progenitors and a polyploidization response by remnant TECs [96]. Polyploid TECs do not truly reconstitute parenchymal loss; thus, they might be a marker of irreversible loss and elicit progression towards chronic disease. In this view, a response to AKI is a costly process which cannot endlessly repeat without any consequence; rather, the tubular epithelium is more susceptible to further damage after every hit, better mirroring the clinical spectrum of the AKI-to-CKD transition.

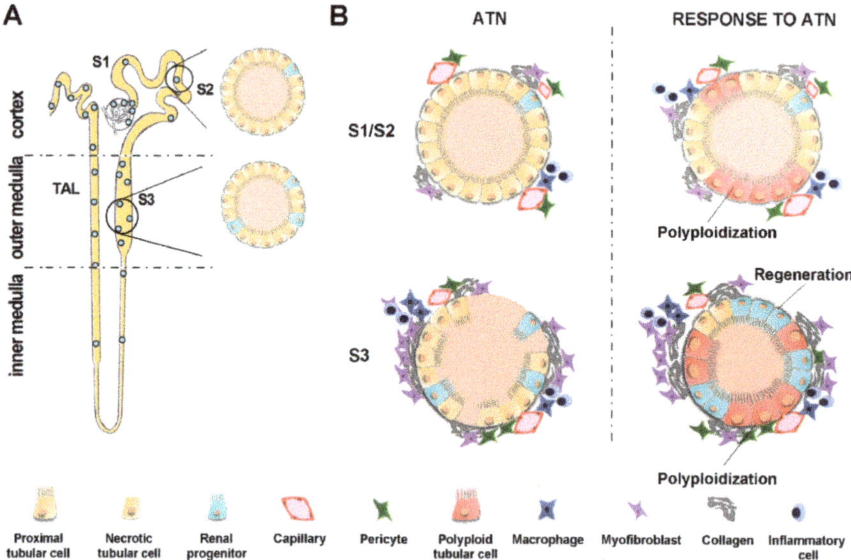

Figure 2. A new pathophysiological interpretation of tubular response to AKI leading towards CKD: The proliferation of renal progenitors and polyploidization of tubular cells. (**A**) Schematic localization of renal progenitors scattered along the S1–S2 segment, the S3 segment, and thick ascending limb (TAL) in the nephron. (Figure modified from Lazzeri et al., Trends Mol Med, 2019); (**B**) Top: In the uninjured proximal tubule S1–S2 segment, tubular epithelial cells enhance their working capacity by entering the cell cycle to increase their DNA content without division, resulting in polyploid tubular cells (i.e., polyploidization). Bottom: In the necrotic proximal tubule S3 segment, renal progenitors proliferate and complete cell division to drive regeneration, while the remnant tubular epithelial cells undergo polyploidization rather than mitosis. ATN: Acute tubular necrosis.

3. Conclusions

A tight link between AKI and CKD is now becoming evident, both in the clinical and experimental settings. AKI severity, duration and frequency are associated with the development of CKD, but even mild episodes are associated with an increased risk of disease progression. Recent experimental findings have provided new insight into the cellular and molecular mechanisms of the AKI-to-CKD transition; these experiments have been trying to unveil the relative contribution of endothelial dysfunction, immune cell response, pericytes and fibroblasts activation. Regardless of the AKI etiology, endothelial dysfunction and subsequent hypoxia (as well as death of tubular cells from a toxic injury) trigger a cascade of self-sustaining events involving myofibroblast activation derived from resident fibroblasts or pericytes, extracellular matrix deposition, and interstitial inflammation. The overall view has shown that all the molecular and cellular mechanisms converge to the tubular epithelial cell dysfunction. Indeed, the lack of recovery of the tubular structure's integrity sustains the above-mentioned events, thus promoting the progression of interstitial injury. The direct increase in the risk of CKD development and progression, which mirrors the severity of the acute episode, suggests a causative role of the final effector of acute function loss, i.e., epithelial cell injury. In several highly specialized organs, widespread parenchymal proliferation is likely to be a counterproductive strategy. Indeed, the mitosis and cytokinesis of highly specialized parenchymal cells determines a temporary loss of function that might become critical for the organ's survival. It is now becoming evident that, to minimize the mitotic ability of specialized parenchymal cells without losing their functional performance, evolution has selected an alternative type of response: Hypertrophy via polyploidization.

The biological rationale for increasing genome content through polyploidization could be to increase cell size and to facilitate amplified cell metabolism so that polyploid cells could sustain acute organ function recovery. Renal progenitor cells instead, thanks to their clonogenic ability, could be responsible for the true tissue regeneration and structural recovery of the necrotic S3 segment of the proximal tubule in affected nephrons, as highlighted by lineage tracing studies. Overall, these results suggest that injured tubules respond to ATN through two main mechanisms: The polyploidization of tubular cells and the proliferation of renal progenitors. New advances in the understanding of the biology and pathophysiology of epithelial tubular cells, renal progenitors, and their adaptation mechanisms will permit the better characterization of functional recovery after AKI and the tracing of the cascade of events leading towards CKD.

Author Contributions: F.G. and E.L. wrote the paper; F.G., L.C., R.M.R., P.R. and E.L. critically revised the manuscript.

Funding: This manuscript is supported by the European Research Council under the Consolidator Grant RENOIR to Paola Romagnani (ERC-2014-CoG), grant number 648274.

Conflicts of Interest: The authors declare no conflict of interest.

Abbreviations

AKI	Acute kidney injury
Akt	Protein kinase B
Ang-1	Angiopoietin-1
ATN	Acute tubular necrosis
CKD	Chronic kidney disease
CSF-1	Colony-stimulating factor-1
CTGF	Connective tissue growth factor
DAMPs	Damage-associated molecular patterns
ECM	Extracellular matrix
EMT	Epithelial-mesenchymal transition
EndoMT	Endothelial to mesenchymal transition
EPC	Endothelial progenitor cells
ESRD	End stage renal disease
FUCCI	Fluorescent ubiquitination-based cell cycle indicator
Hif	Hypoxia-inducible factor
ICAM-1	Intercellular adhesion molecule-1
IL	Interleukin
IRAK-M	IL-1 receptor-associated kinase-M
IRI	Ischemia-reperfusion injury
PCNA	Proliferating cell nuclear antigen
PDGF	Platelet-derived growth factor
PDGFR-β	Platelet-derived growth factor receptor-β
RA	Retinoic acid
RAS	Renin-angiotensin system
S1-pr1	Sphingosine 1-phosphate receptor 1
Sirt 1	Sirtuin 1
Snail1	Snail family zinc finger 1
STAT3	Signal transducer and transcription factor 3
TEC	Tubular epithelial cell
TGF-β	Transforming growth factor β
TLR	Toll-like receptor
TNF-α	Tumor necrosis factor-α
VEGF	Vascular endothelial growth factor
α-SMA	α-smooth muscle actin

References

1. Ponte, B.; Felipe, C.; Muriel, A.; Tenorio, M.T.; Liaño, F. Long-term functional evolution after an acute kidney injury: A 10-year study. *Nephrol. Dial. Transplant. Off. Publ. Eur. Dial. Transpl. Assoc.—Eur. Ren. Assoc.* **2008**, *23*, 3859–3866. [CrossRef] [PubMed]

2. Coca, S.G.; Singanamala, S.; Parikh, C.R. Chronic kidney disease after acute kidney injury: A systematic review and meta-analysis. *Kidney Int.* **2012**, *81*, 442–448. [CrossRef] [PubMed]

3. Chawla, L.S.; Eggers, P.W.; Star, R.A.; Kimmel, P.L. Acute kidney injury and chronic kidney disease as interconnected syndromes. *N. Engl. J. Med.* **2014**, *371*, 58–66. [CrossRef] [PubMed]

4. Lowe, K.G. The late prognosis in acute tubular necrosis. *Lancet* **1952**, *259*, 1086–1088. [CrossRef]

5. Liaño, F.; Felipe, C.; Tenorio, M.-T.; Rivera, M.; Abraira, V.; Sáez-de-Urturi, J.-M.; Ocaña, J.; Fuentes, C.; Severiano, S. Long-term outcome of acute tubular necrosis: A contribution to its natural history. *Kidney Int.* **2007**, *71*, 679–686. [CrossRef] [PubMed]

6. Ricci, Z.; Cruz, D.N.; Ronco, C. Classification and staging of acute kidney injury: Beyond the RIFLE and AKIN criteria. *Nat. Rev. Nephrol.* **2011**, *7*, 201–208. [CrossRef] [PubMed]

7. See, E.J.; Jayasinghe, K.; Glassford, N.; Bailey, M.; Johnson, D.W.; Polkinghorne, K.R.; Toussaint, N.D.; Bellomo, R. Long-term risk of adverse outcomes after acute kidney injury: A systematic review and meta-analysis of cohort studies using consensus definitions of exposure. *Kidney Int.* **2019**, *95*, 160–172. [CrossRef]

8. Ishani, A.; Xue, J.L.; Himmelfarb, J.; Eggers, P.W.; Kimmel, P.L.; Molitoris, B.A.; Collins, A.J. Acute kidney injury increases risk of ESRD among elderly. *J. Am. Soc. Nephrol.* **2009**, *20*, 223–228. [CrossRef]

9. Amdur, R.L.; Chawla, L.S.; Amodeo, S.; Kimmel, P.L.; Palant, C.E. Outcomes following diagnosis of acute renal failure in U.S. veterans: Focus on acute tubular necrosis. *Kidney Int.* **2009**, *76*, 1089–1097. [CrossRef]

10. Ishani, A.; Nelson, D.; Clothier, B.; Schult, T.; Nugent, S.; Greer, N.; Slinin, Y.; Ensrud, K.E. The Magnitude of Acute Serum Creatinine Increase After Cardiac Surgery and the Risk of Chronic Kidney Disease, Progression of Kidney Disease, and Death. *Arch. Intern. Med.* **2011**, *171*, 226–233. [CrossRef]

11. Mehta, S.; Chauhan, K.; Patel, A.; Patel, S.; Pinotti, R.; Nadkarni, G.N.; Parikh, C.R.; Coca, S.G. The prognostic importance of duration of AKI: A systematic review and meta-analysis. *BMC Nephrol.* **2018**, *19*, 91. [CrossRef] [PubMed]

12. Thakar, C.V.; Christianson, A.; Himmelfarb, J.; Leonard, A.C. Acute kidney injury episodes and chronic kidney disease risk in diabetes mellitus. *Clin. J. Am. Soc. Nephrol.* **2011**, *6*, 2567–2572. [CrossRef] [PubMed]

13. Devarajan, P.; Jefferies, J.L. Progression of chronic kidney disease after acute kidney injury. *Prog. Pediatr. Cardiol.* **2016**, *41*, 33–40. [CrossRef] [PubMed]

14. Uber, A.M.; Sutherland, S.M. Acute kidney injury in hospitalized children: Consequences and outcomes. *Pediatr. Nephrol. Berl. Ger.* **2018**, 1–8. [CrossRef] [PubMed]

15. Sigurjonsdottir, V.K.; Chaturvedi, S.; Mammen, C.; Sutherland, S.M. Pediatric acute kidney injury and the subsequent risk for chronic kidney disease: Is there cause for alarm? *Pediatr. Nephrol. Berl. Ger.* **2018**, *33*, 2047–2055. [CrossRef]

16. Basile, D.P.; Bonventre, J.V.; Mehta, R.; Nangaku, M.; Unwin, R.; Rosner, M.H.; Kellum, J.A.; Ronco, C.; ADQI XIII Work Group. Progression after AKI: Understanding Maladaptive Repair Processes to Predict and Identify Therapeutic Treatments. *J. Am. Soc. Nephrol.* **2016**, *27*, 687–697. [CrossRef]

17. Bellomo, R.; Kellum, J.A.; Ronco, C. Acute kidney injury. *Lancet* **2012**, *380*, 756–766. [CrossRef]

18. Venkatachalam, M.A.; Griffin, K.A.; Lan, R.; Geng, H.; Saikumar, P.; Bidani, A.K. Acute kidney injury: A springboard for progression in chronic kidney disease. *Am. J. Physiol. Renal Physiol.* **2010**, *298*, F1078–F1094. [CrossRef]

19. Rodriguez-Romo, R.; Benitez, K.; Barrera-Chimal, J.; Perez-Villalva, R.; Gomez, A.; Aguilar-Leon, D.; Rangel-Santiago, J.F.; Huerta, S.; Gamba, G.; Uribe, N.; et al. AT1 receptor antagonism before ischemia prevents the transition of acute kidney injury to chronic kidney disease. *Kidney Int.* **2016**, *89*, 363–373. [CrossRef]

20. Chou, Y.-H.; Chu, T.-S.; Lin, S.-L. Role of renin-angiotensin system in acute kidney injury-chronic kidney disease transition. *Nephrol. Carlton Vic* **2018**, *23*, 121–125. [CrossRef]

21. Grgic, I.; Campanholle, G.; Bijol, V.; Wang, C.; Sabbisetti, V.S.; Ichimura, T.; Humphreys, B.D.; Bonventre, J.V. Targeted proximal tubule injury triggers interstitial fibrosis and glomerulosclerosis. *Kidney Int.* **2012**, *82*, 172–183. [CrossRef] [PubMed]

22. Ferenbach, D.A.; Bonventre, J.V. Mechanisms of maladaptive repair after AKI leading to accelerated kidney ageing and CKD. *Nat. Rev. Nephrol.* **2015**, *11*, 264–276. [CrossRef] [PubMed]

23. Venkatachalam, M.A.; Weinberg, J.M.; Kriz, W.; Bidani, A.K. Failed Tubule Recovery, AKI-CKD Transition, and Kidney Disease Progression. *J. Am. Soc. Nephrol.* **2015**, *26*, 1765–1776. [CrossRef] [PubMed]

24. Basile, D.P. The endothelial cell in ischemic acute kidney injury: Implications for acute and chronic function. *Kidney Int.* **2007**, *72*, 151–156. [CrossRef] [PubMed]

25. Basile, D.P.; Collett, J.A.; Yoder, M.C. Endothelial colony-forming cells and pro-angiogenic cells: Clarifying definitions and their potential role in mitigating acute kidney injury. *Acta. Physiol. Oxf. Engl.* **2018**, *222*, e12914. [CrossRef] [PubMed]

26. Lech, M.; Gröbmayr, R.; Ryu, M.; Lorenz, G.; Hartter, I.; Mulay, S.R.; Susanti, H.E.; Kobayashi, K.S.; Flavell, R.A.; Anders, H.-J. Macrophage phenotype controls long-term AKI outcomes—Kidney regeneration versus atrophy. *J. Am. Soc. Nephrol.* **2014**, *25*, 292–304. [CrossRef] [PubMed]

27. Anders, H.-J.; Schaefer, L. Beyond Tissue Injury—Damage-Associated Molecular Patterns, Toll-Like Receptors, and Inflammasomes Also Drive Regeneration and Fibrosis. *J. Am. Soc. Nephrol.* **2014**, *25*, 1387–1400. [CrossRef]

28. Belliere, J.; Casemayou, A.; Ducasse, L.; Zakaroff-Girard, A.; Martins, F.; Iacovoni, J.S.; Guilbeau-Frugier, C.; Buffin-Meyer, B.; Pipy, B.; Chauveau, D.; et al. Specific Macrophage Subtypes Influence the Progression of Rhabdomyolysis-Induced Kidney Injury. *J. Am. Soc. Nephrol.* **2015**, *26*, 1363–1377. [CrossRef] [PubMed]

29. Jang, H.R.; Rabb, H. Immune cells in experimental acute kidney injury. *Nat. Rev. Nephrol.* **2015**, *11*, 88–101. [CrossRef]

30. Sato, Y.; Yanagita, M. Immune cells and inflammation in AKI to CKD progression. *Am. J. Physiol. Renal Physiol.* **2018**, *315*, 1501–1512. [CrossRef]

31. Gomez, I.G.; Duffield, J.S. The FOXD1 lineage of kidney perivascular cells and myofibroblasts: Functions and responses to injury. *Kidney Int. Suppl.* **2014**, *4*, 26–33. [CrossRef] [PubMed]

32. Mack, M.; Yanagita, M. Origin of myofibroblasts and cellular events triggering fibrosis. *Kidney Int.* **2015**, *87*, 297–307. [CrossRef] [PubMed]

33. Nakamura, J.; Sato, Y.; Kitai, Y.; Wajima, S.; Yamamoto, S.; Oguchi, A.; Yamada, R.; Kaneko, K.; Kondo, M.; Uchino, E.; et al. Myofibroblasts acquire retinoic acid–producing ability during fibroblast-to-myofibroblast transition following kidney injury. *Kidney Int.* **2019**, *95*, 526–539. [CrossRef] [PubMed]

34. Kaissling, B.; Lehir, M.; Kriz, W. Renal epithelial injury and fibrosis. *Biochim. Biophys. Acta* **2013**, *1832*, 931–939. [CrossRef] [PubMed]

35. Liu, B.-C.; Tang, T.-T.; Lv, L.-L.; Lan, H.-Y. Renal tubule injury: A driving force toward chronic kidney disease. *Kidney Int.* **2018**, *93*, 568–579. [CrossRef]

36. Patschan, D.; Kribben, A.; Müller, G.A. Postischemic microvasculopathy and endothelial progenitor cell-based therapy in ischemic AKI: Update and perspectives. *Am. J. Physiol.-Ren. Physiol.* **2016**, *311*, 382–394. [CrossRef]

37. Sradnick, J.; Rong, S.; Luedemann, A.; Parmentier, S.P.; Bartaun, C.; Todorov, V.T.; Gueler, F.; Hugo, C.P.; Hohenstein, B. Extrarenal Progenitor Cells Do Not Contribute to Renal Endothelial Repair. *J. Am. Soc. Nephrol.* **2016**, *27*, 1714–1726. [CrossRef]

38. Kumar, S. Cellular and molecular pathways of renal repair after acute kidney injury. *Kidney Int.* **2018**, *93*, 27–40. [CrossRef]

39. Tanaka, S.; Tanaka, T.; Nangaku, M. Hypoxia as a key player in the AKI-to-CKD transition. *Am. J. Physiol. Renal Physiol.* **2014**, *307*, 1187–1195. [CrossRef]

40. Chade, A.R. Vascular Endothelial Growth Factor Therapy for the Kidney: Are We There Yet? *J. Am. Soc. Nephrol.* **2016**, *27*, 1–3. [CrossRef]

41. Chade, A.R.; Tullos, N.A.; Harvey, T.W.; Mahdi, F.; Bidwell, G.L. Renal Therapeutic Angiogenesis Using a Bioengineered Polymer-Stabilized Vascular Endothelial Growth Factor Construct. *J. Am. Soc. Nephrol.* **2016**, *27*, 1741–1752. [CrossRef] [PubMed]

42. Hörbelt, M.; Lee, S.-Y.; Mang, H.E.; Knipe, N.L.; Sado, Y.; Kribben, A.; Sutton, T.A. Acute and chronic microvascular alterations in a mouse model of ischemic acute kidney injury. *Am. J. Physiol.-Ren. Physiol.* **2007**, *293*, 688–695. [CrossRef] [PubMed]

43. Kapitsinou, P.P.; Sano, H.; Michael, M.; Kobayashi, H.; Davidoff, O.; Bian, A.; Yao, B.; Zhang, M.-Z.; Harris, R.C.; Duffy, K.J.; et al. Endothelial HIF-2 mediates protection and recovery from ischemic kidney injury. *J. Clin. Invest.* **2014**, *124*, 2396–2409. [CrossRef] [PubMed]

44. Perry, H.M.; Huang, L.; Ye, H.; Liu, C.; Sung, S.J.; Lynch, K.R.; Rosin, D.L.; Bajwa, A.; Okusa, M.D. Endothelial Sphingosine 1-Phosphate Receptor-1 Mediates Protection and Recovery from Acute Kidney Injury. *J. Am. Soc. Nephrol.* **2016**, *27*, 3383–3393. [CrossRef] [PubMed]

45. Tanaka, T.; Wiesener, M.; Bernhardt, W.; Eckardt, K.-U.; Warnecke, C. The human *HIF* (hypoxia-inducible factor)-*3α* gene is a HIF-1 target gene and may modulate hypoxic gene induction. *Biochem. J.* **2009**, *424*, 143–151. [CrossRef] [PubMed]

46. Vasko, R.; Xavier, S.; Chen, J.; Lin, C.H.S.; Ratliff, B.; Rabadi, M.; Maizel, J.; Tanokuchi, R.; Zhang, F.; Cao, J.; et al. Endothelial Sirtuin 1 Deficiency Perpetrates Nephrosclerosis through Downregulation of Matrix Metalloproteinase-14: Relevance to Fibrosis of Vascular Senescence. *J. Am. Soc. Nephrol.* **2014**, *25*, 276–291. [CrossRef] [PubMed]

47. Kida, Y.; Zullo, J.A.; Goligorsky, M.S. Endothelial sirtuin 1 inactivation enhances capillary rarefaction and fibrosis following kidney injury through Notch activation. *Biochem. Biophys. Res. Commun.* **2016**, *478*, 1074–1079. [CrossRef] [PubMed]

48. Basile, D.P.; Friedrich, J.L.; Spahic, J.; Knipe, N.; Mang, H.; Leonard, E.C.; Changizi-Ashtiyani, S.; Bacallao, R.L.; Molitoris, B.A.; Sutton, T.A. Impaired endothelial proliferation and mesenchymal transition contribute to vascular rarefaction following acute kidney injury. *Am. J. Physiol.-Ren. Physiol.* **2011**, *300*, 721–733. [CrossRef]

49. Xavier, S.; Vasko, R.; Matsumoto, K.; Zullo, J.A.; Chen, R.; Maizel, J.; Chander, P.N.; Goligorsky, M.S. Curtailing Endothelial TGF-β Signaling Is Sufficient to Reduce Endothelial-Mesenchymal Transition and Fibrosis in CKD. *J. Am. Soc. Nephrol.* **2015**, *26*, 817–829. [CrossRef]

50. Kramann, R.; Wongboonsin, J.; Chang-Panesso, M.; Machado, F.G.; Humphreys, B.D. Gli1+ Pericyte Loss Induces Capillary Rarefaction and Proximal Tubular Injury. *J. Am. Soc. Nephrol.* **2017**, *28*, 776–784. [CrossRef]

51. Betsholtz, C. Insight into the physiological functions of PDGF through genetic studies in mice. *Cytokine Growth Factor Rev.* **2004**, *15*, 215–228. [CrossRef] [PubMed]

52. Sundberg, C.; Kowanetz, M.; Brown, L.F.; Detmar, M.; Dvorak, H.F. Stable expression of angiopoietin-1 and other markers by cultured pericytes: Phenotypic similarities to a subpopulation of cells in maturing vessels during later stages of angiogenesis in vivo. *Lab. Investig. J. Tech. Methods Pathol.* **2002**, *82*, 387–401. [CrossRef]

53. Carvalho, R.L.C. Defective paracrine signalling by TGF in yolk sac vasculature of endoglin mutant mice: A paradigm for hereditary haemorrhagic telangiectasia. *Development* **2004**, *131*, 6237–6247. [CrossRef] [PubMed]

54. Benjamin, L.E.; Hemo, I.; Keshet, E. A plasticity window for blood vessel remodelling is defined by pericyte coverage of the preformed endothelial network and is regulated by PDGF-B and VEGF. *Dev. Camb. Engl.* **1998**, *125*, 1591–1598.

55. Chae, S.-S.; Paik, J.-H.; Allende, M.L.; Proia, R.L.; Hla, T. Regulation of limb development by the sphingosine 1-phosphate receptor S1p1/EDG-1 occurs via the hypoxia/VEGF axis. *Dev. Biol.* **2004**, *268*, 441–447. [CrossRef] [PubMed]

56. Anders, H.-J. Immune system modulation of kidney regeneration—mechanisms and implications. *Nat. Rev. Nephrol.* **2014**, *10*, 347–358. [CrossRef]

57. Stamatiades, E.G.; Tremblay, M.-E.; Bohm, M.; Crozet, L.; Bisht, K.; Kao, D.; Coelho, C.; Fan, X.; Yewdell, W.T.; Davidson, A.; et al. Immune Monitoring of Trans-endothelial Transport by Kidney-Resident Macrophages. *Cell* **2016**, *166*, 991–1003. [CrossRef]

58. Karasawa, K.; Asano, K.; Moriyama, S.; Ushiki, M.; Monya, M.; Iida, M.; Kuboki, E.; Yagita, H.; Uchida, K.; Nitta, K.; et al. Vascular-Resident CD169-Positive Monocytes and Macrophages Control Neutrophil Accumulation in the Kidney with Ischemia-Reperfusion Injury. *J. Am. Soc. Nephrol.* **2015**, *26*, 896–906. [CrossRef]

59. Mantovani, A.; Sica, A.; Sozzani, S.; Allavena, P.; Vecchi, A.; Locati, M. The chemokine system in diverse forms of macrophage activation and polarization. *Trends Immunol.* **2004**, *25*, 677–686. [CrossRef]

60. Martinez, F.O.; Gordon, S. The M1 and M2 paradigm of macrophage activation: Time for reassessment. *F1000Prime Rep.* **2014**, *6*, 13. [CrossRef]

61. Clements, M.; Gershenovich, M.; Chaber, C.; Campos-Rivera, J.; Du, P.; Zhang, M.; Ledbetter, S.; Zuk, A. Differential Ly6C Expression after Renal Ischemia-Reperfusion Identifies Unique Macrophage Populations. *J. Am. Soc. Nephrol.* **2016**, *27*, 159–170. [CrossRef] [PubMed]

62. Jang, H.-S.; Kim, J.; Park, Y.-K.; Park, K.M. Infiltrated Macrophages Contribute to Recovery after Ischemic Injury But Not to Ischemic Preconditioning in Kidneys. *Transplantation* **2008**, *85*, 447–455. [CrossRef] [PubMed]

63. Xu, M.-J.; Feng, D.; Wang, H.; Guan, Y.; Yan, X.; Gao, B. IL-22 Ameliorates Renal Ischemia-Reperfusion Injury by Targeting Proximal Tubule Epithelium. *J. Am. Soc. Nephrol.* **2014**, *25*, 967–977. [CrossRef] [PubMed]

64. Chiba, T.; Skrypnyk, N.I.; Skvarca, L.B.; Penchev, R.; Zhang, K.X.; Rochon, E.R.; Fall, J.L.; Paueksakon, P.; Yang, H.; Alford, C.E.; et al. Retinoic Acid Signaling Coordinates Macrophage-Dependent Injury and Repair after AKI. *J. Am. Soc. Nephrol.* **2016**, *27*, 495–508. [CrossRef] [PubMed]

65. Lin, S.-L.; Li, B.; Rao, S.; Yeo, E.-J.; Hudson, T.E.; Nowlin, B.T.; Pei, H.; Chen, L.; Zheng, J.J.; Carroll, T.J.; et al. Macrophage Wnt7b is critical for kidney repair and regeneration. *Proc. Natl. Acad. Sci. USA* **2010**, *107*, 4194–4199. [CrossRef] [PubMed]

66. Zhou, D.; Tan, R.J.; Fu, H.; Liu, Y. Wnt/β-catenin signaling in kidney injury and repair: A double-edged sword. *Lab. Invest.* **2016**, *96*, 156–167. [CrossRef]

67. Tan, R.J.; Zhou, D.; Zhou, L.; Liu, Y. Wnt/β-catenin signaling and kidney fibrosis. *Kidney Int. Suppl.* **2014**, *4*, 84–90. [CrossRef] [PubMed]

68. Zhang, M.-Z.; Yao, B.; Yang, S.; Jiang, L.; Wang, S.; Fan, X.; Yin, H.; Wong, K.; Miyazawa, T.; Chen, J.; et al. CSF-1 signaling mediates recovery from acute kidney injury. *J. Clin. Invest.* **2012**, *122*, 4519–4532. [CrossRef]

69. Baek, J.-H.; Zeng, R.; Weinmann-Menke, J.; Valerius, M.T.; Wada, Y.; Ajay, A.K.; Colonna, M.; Kelley, V.R. IL-34 mediates acute kidney injury and worsens subsequent chronic kidney disease. *J. Clin. Invest.* **2015**, *125*, 3198–3214. [CrossRef]

70. Lee, S.A.; Noel, S.; Sadasivam, M.; Hamad, A.R.A.; Rabb, H. Role of Immune Cells in Acute Kidney Injury and Repair. *Nephron* **2017**, *137*, 282–286. [CrossRef]

71. Kim, M.-G.; Koo, T.Y.; Yan, J.-J.; Lee, E.; Han, K.H.; Jeong, J.C.; Ro, H.; Kim, B.S.; Jo, S.-K.; Oh, K.H.; et al. IL-2/Anti-IL-2 Complex Attenuates Renal Ischemia-Reperfusion Injury through Expansion of Regulatory T Cells. *J. Am. Soc. Nephrol.* **2013**, *24*, 1529–1536. [CrossRef] [PubMed]

72. Gandolfo, M.T.; Jang, H.R.; Bagnasco, S.M.; Ko, G.-J.; Agreda, P.; Satpute, S.R.; Crow, M.T.; King, L.S.; Rabb, H. Foxp3[+] regulatory T cells participate in repair of ischemic acute kidney injury. *Kidney Int.* **2009**, *76*, 717–729. [CrossRef] [PubMed]

73. Baudoux, T.; Husson, C.; De Prez, E.; Jadot, I.; Antoine, M.-H.; Nortier, J.L.; Hougardy, J.-M. CD4+ and CD8+ T Cells Exert Regulatory Properties During Experimental Acute Aristolochic Acid Nephropathy. *Sci. Rep.* **2018**, *8*, 5334. [CrossRef] [PubMed]

74. Renner, B.; Strassheim, D.; Amura, C.R.; Kulik, L.; Ljubanovic, D.; Glogowska, M.J.; Takahashi, K.; Carroll, M.C.; Holers, V.M.; Thurman, J.M. B Cell Subsets Contribute to Renal Injury and Renal Protection after Ischemia/Reperfusion. *J. Immunol.* **2010**, *185*, 4393–4400. [CrossRef] [PubMed]

75. Klingberg, F.; Hinz, B.; White, E.S. The myofibroblast matrix: Implications for tissue repair and fibrosis: The myofibroblast matrix. *J. Pathol.* **2013**, *229*, 298–309. [CrossRef] [PubMed]

76. Mackensen-Haen, S.; Bader, R.; Grund, K.E.; Bohle, A. Correlations between renal cortical interstitial fibrosis, atrophy of the proximal tubules and impairment of the glomerular filtration rate. *Clin. Nephrol.* **1981**, *15*, 167–171. [PubMed]

77. Picken, M.; Long, J.; Williamson, G.A.; Polichnowski, A.J. Progression of Chronic Kidney Disease After Acute Kidney Injury: Role of Self-Perpetuating Versus Hemodynamic-Induced Fibrosis. *Hypertens. Dallas Tex 1979* **2016**, *68*, 921–928. [CrossRef] [PubMed]

78. Takaori, K.; Nakamura, J.; Yamamoto, S.; Nakata, H.; Sato, Y.; Takase, M.; Nameta, M.; Yamamoto, T.; Economides, A.N.; Kohno, K.; et al. Severity and Frequency of Proximal Tubule Injury Determines Renal Prognosis. *J. Am. Soc. Nephrol.* **2016**, *27*, 2393–2406. [CrossRef]

79. Sato, Y.; Mii, A.; Hamazaki, Y.; Fujita, H.; Nakata, H.; Masuda, K.; Nishiyama, S.; Shibuya, S.; Haga, H.; Ogawa, O.; et al. Heterogeneous fibroblasts underlie age-dependent tertiary lymphoid tissues in the kidney. *JCI Insight* **2016**, *1*, e87680. [CrossRef]

80. Allinovi, M.; de Chiara, L.; Angelotti, M.L.; Becherucci, F.; Romagnani, P. Anti-fibrotic treatments: A review of clinical evidence. *Matrix Biol.* **2018**, *68–69*, 333–354. [CrossRef]

81. De Chiara, L.; Romagnani, P. Tubule repair: With a little help from my "unexpected" friends. *Kidney Int.* **2019**, *95*, 487–489. [CrossRef] [PubMed]

82. Sharfuddin, A.A.; Molitoris, B.A. Pathophysiology of ischemic acute kidney injury. *Nat. Rev. Nephrol.* **2011**, *7*, 189–200. [CrossRef] [PubMed]

83. Funk, J.A.; Schnellmann, R.G. Persistent disruption of mitochondrial homeostasis after acute kidney injury. *Am. J. Physiol. Renal Physiol.* **2012**, *302*, 853–864. [CrossRef] [PubMed]

84. Wang, Y.; Chang, J.; Yao, B.; Niu, A.; Kelly, E.; Breeggemann, M.C.; Abboud Werner, S.L.; Harris, R.C.; Zhang, M.-Z. Proximal tubule-derived colony stimulating factor-1 mediates polarization of renal macrophages and dendritic cells, and recovery in acute kidney injury. *Kidney Int.* **2015**, *88*, 1274–1282. [CrossRef] [PubMed]

85. Huen, S.C.; Huynh, L.; Marlier, A.; Lee, Y.; Moeckel, G.W.; Cantley, L.G. GM-CSF Promotes Macrophage Alternative Activation after Renal Ischemia/Reperfusion Injury. *J. Am. Soc. Nephrol.* **2015**, *26*, 1334–1345. [CrossRef]

86. Kramann, R.; Kusaba, T.; Humphreys, B.D. Who regenerates the kidney tubule? *Nephrol. Dial. Transplant. Off. Publ. Eur. Dial. Transpl. Assoc. -Eur. Ren. Assoc.* **2015**, *30*, 903–910. [CrossRef] [PubMed]

87. Chang-Panesso, M.; Humphreys, B.D. Cellular plasticity in kidney injury and repair. *Nat. Rev. Nephrol.* **2017**, *13*, 39–46. [CrossRef]

88. Witzgall, R.; Brown, D.; Schwarz, C.; Bonventre, J.V. Localization of proliferating cell nuclear antigen, vimentin, c-Fos, and clusterin in the postischemic kidney. Evidence for a heterogenous genetic response among nephron segments, and a large pool of mitotically active and dedifferentiated cells. *J. Clin. Invest.* **1994**, *93*, 2175–2188. [CrossRef]

89. Grande, M.T.; Sánchez-Laorden, B.; López-Blau, C.; De Frutos, C.A.; Boutet, A.; Arévalo, M.; Rowe, R.G.; Weiss, S.J.; López-Novoa, J.M.; Nieto, M.A. Snail1-induced partial epithelial-to-mesenchymal transition drives renal fibrosis in mice and can be targeted to reverse established disease. *Nat. Med.* **2015**, *21*, 989–997. [CrossRef]

90. Lovisa, S.; LeBleu, V.S.; Tampe, B.; Sugimoto, H.; Vadnagara, K.; Carstens, J.L.; Wu, C.-C.; Hagos, Y.; Burckhardt, B.C.; Pentcheva-Hoang, T.; et al. Epithelial-to-mesenchymal transition induces cell cycle arrest and parenchymal damage in renal fibrosis. *Nat. Med.* **2015**, *21*, 998–1009. [CrossRef]

91. Vogetseder, A.; Karadeniz, A.; Kaissling, B.; Le Hir, M. Tubular cell proliferation in the healthy rat kidney. *Histochem. Cell Biol.* **2005**, *124*, 97–104. [CrossRef] [PubMed]

92. Vogetseder, A.; Picard, N.; Gaspert, A.; Walch, M.; Kaissling, B.; le Hir, M. Proliferation capacity of the renal proximal tubule involves the bulk of differentiated epithelial cells. *Am. J. Physiol.-Cell Physiol.* **2008**, *294*, 22–28. [CrossRef] [PubMed]

93. Yang, L.; Besschetnova, T.Y.; Brooks, C.R.; Shah, J.V.; Bonventre, J.V. Epithelial cell cycle arrest in G2/M mediates kidney fibrosis after injury. *Nat. Med.* **2010**, *16*, 535–543. [CrossRef] [PubMed]

94. Canaud, G.; Bonventre, J.V. Cell cycle arrest and the evolution of chronic kidney disease from acute kidney injury. *Nephrol. Dial. Transplant.* **2015**, *30*, 575–583. [CrossRef] [PubMed]

95. Lazzeri, E.; Angelotti, M.L.; Peired, A.; Conte, C.; Marschner, J.A.; Maggi, L.; Mazzinghi, B.; Lombardi, D.; Melica, M.E.; Nardi, S.; et al. Endocycle-related tubular cell hypertrophy and progenitor proliferation recover renal function after acute kidney injury. *Nat. Commun.* **2018**, *9*, 1344. [CrossRef] [PubMed]

96. Lazzeri, E.; Angelotti, M.L.; Conte, C.; Anders, H.-J.; Romagnani, P. Surviving Acute Organ Failure: Cell Polyploidization and Progenitor Proliferation. *Trends Mol. Med.* **2019**, *25*, 366–381. [CrossRef] [PubMed]

97. Lombardi, D.; Becherucci, F.; Romagnani, P. How much can the tubule regenerate and who does it? An open question. *Nephrol. Dial. Transplant.* **2016**, *31*, 1243–1250. [CrossRef] [PubMed]

98. Lindgren, D.; Boström, A.-K.; Nilsson, K.; Hansson, J.; Sjölund, J.; Möller, C.; Jirström, K.; Nilsson, E.; Landberg, G.; Axelson, H.; et al. Isolation and characterization of progenitor-like cells from human renal proximal tubules. *Am. J. Pathol.* **2011**, *178*, 828–837. [CrossRef] [PubMed]

99. Angelotti, M.L.; Ronconi, E.; Ballerini, L.; Peired, A.; Mazzinghi, B.; Sagrinati, C.; Parente, E.; Gacci, M.; Carini, M.; Rotondi, M.; et al. Characterization of renal progenitors committed toward tubular lineage and their regenerative potential in renal tubular injury. *Stem Cells Dayt. Ohio* **2012**, *30*, 1714–1725. [CrossRef]

100. Smeets, B.; Boor, P.; Dijkman, H.; Sharma, S.V.; Jirak, P.; Mooren, F.; Berger, K.; Bornemann, J.; Gelman, I.H.; Floege, J.; et al. Proximal tubular cells contain a phenotypically distinct, scattered cell population involved in tubular regeneration: Phenotypically distinct proximal tubular cells. *J. Pathol.* **2013**, *229*, 645–659. [CrossRef]

101. Kumar, S.; Liu, J.; Pang, P.; Krautzberger, A.M.; Reginensi, A.; Akiyama, H.; Schedl, A.; Humphreys, B.D.; McMahon, A.P. Sox9 Activation Highlights a Cellular Pathway of Renal Repair in the Acutely Injured Mammalian Kidney. *Cell Rep.* **2015**, *12*, 1325–1338. [CrossRef] [PubMed]

102. Kang, H.M.; Huang, S.; Reidy, K.; Han, S.H.; Chinga, F.; Susztak, K. Sox9-Positive Progenitor Cells Play a Key Role in Renal Tubule Epithelial Regeneration in Mice. *Cell Rep.* **2016**, *14*, 861–871. [CrossRef] [PubMed]

103. Berger, K.; Bangen, J.-M.; Hammerich, L.; Liedtke, C.; Floege, J.; Smeets, B.; Moeller, M.J. Origin of regenerating tubular cells after acute kidney injury. *Proc. Natl. Acad. Sci. USA* **2014**, *111*, 1533–1538. [CrossRef] [PubMed]

104. Romagnani, P.; Lasagni, L.; Remuzzi, G. Renal progenitors: An evolutionary conserved strategy for kidney regeneration. *Nat. Rev. Nephrol.* **2013**, *9*, 137–146. [CrossRef] [PubMed]

105. Rinkevich, Y.; Montoro, D.T.; Contreras-Trujillo, H.; Harari-Steinberg, O.; Newman, A.M.; Tsai, J.M.; Lim, X.; Van-Amerongen, R.; Bowman, A.; Januszyk, M.; et al. In Vivo Clonal Analysis Reveals Lineage-Restricted Progenitor Characteristics in Mammalian Kidney Development, Maintenance, and Regeneration. *Cell Rep.* **2014**, *7*, 1270–1283. [CrossRef] [PubMed]

106. Humphreys, B.D.; Valerius, M.T.; Kobayashi, A.; Mugford, J.W.; Soeung, S.; Duffield, J.S.; McMahon, A.P.; Bonventre, J.V. Intrinsic Epithelial Cells Repair the Kidney after Injury. *Cell Stem Cell* **2008**, *2*, 284–291. [CrossRef] [PubMed]

107. Shu, Z.; Row, S.; Deng, W.-M. Endoreplication: The Good, the Bad, and the Ugly. *Trends Cell Biol.* **2018**, *28*, 465–474. [CrossRef]

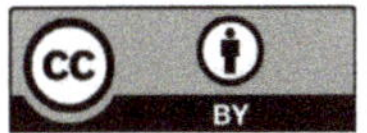

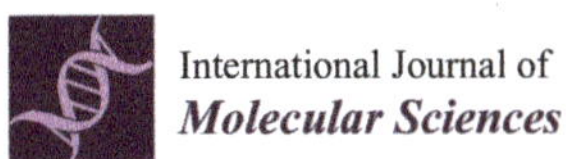

International Journal of
Molecular Sciences

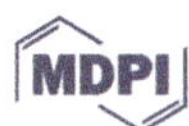

Review

Long Non-Coding RNAs in Kidney Disease

Michael Ignarski [1,2], Rashidul Islam [1,2] and Roman-Ulrich Müller [1,2,3,*]

1   Department II of Internal Medicine and Center for Molecular Medicine, University of Cologne,
    Faculty of Medicine and University Hospital Cologne, 50931 Cologne, Germany
2   Cologne Excellence Cluster on Cellular Stress Responses in Aging-Associated Diseases,
    University of Cologne, Faculty of Medicine and University Hospital Cologne, 50931 Cologne, Germany
3   Systems Biology of Ageing Cologne, University of Cologne, 50931 Cologne, Germany
*   Correspondence: roman-ulrich.mueller@uk-koeln.de; Tel.: +49-221-478-86288

Received: 31 May 2019; Accepted: 1 July 2019; Published: 3 July 2019

Abstract: Non-coding RNA species contribute more than 90% of all transcripts and have gained increasing attention in the last decade. One of the most recent members of this group are long non-coding RNAs (lncRNAs) which are characterized by a length of more than 200 nucleotides and a lack of coding potential. However, in contrast to this simple definition, lncRNAs are heterogenous regarding their molecular function—including the modulation of small RNA and protein function, guidance of epigenetic modifications and a role as enhancer RNAs. Furthermore, they show a highly tissue-specific expression pattern. These aspects already point towards an important role in cellular biology and imply lncRNAs as players in development, health and disease. This view has been confirmed by numerous publications from different fields in the last years and has raised the question as to whether lncRNAs may be future therapeutic targets in human disease. Here, we provide a concise overview of the current knowledge on lncRNAs in both glomerular and tubulointerstitial kidney disease.

Keywords: lncRNA; long non-coding RNA; miRNA; kidney; glomerulus; podocyte; acute kidney injury; AKI; diabetic nephropathy

1. Introduction

Most of the human genome is actively transcribed but less than 2% contains protein coding transcripts (mRNA). The other transcripts produced show no or low coding potential and have, therefore, been summarized in the large group of non-coding RNAs (ncRNA). This group contains the long known ribosomal RNAs (rRNAs) and transfer RNAs (tRNAs) involved in protein synthesis as well as two very diverse classes of ncRNAs mainly divided by their length: the class of small non-coding RNAs containing transcripts with lengths of less than 200 nucleotides consists of small interfering RNAs (siRNAs), small nuclear RNAs (snRNA), small nucleolar RNAs (snoRNAs), PIWI-interacting RNAs (piRNAs) and microRNAs (miRNAs). The role of miRNAs in kidney disease has been investigated extensively and reviewed multiple times over the last decades [1,2], therefore, we focus on the class of long non-coding RNAs (lncRNAs) with lengths of over 200 nucleotides. Like mRNAs most lncRNAs have their own promoters, are RNA polymerase II transcribed, 5'-capped, polyadenylated and subjected to splicing [3]. LncRNA genes are dispersed throughout the genome, they can be inter- or intragenic, in the latter case positioned in sense or antisense direction, inside exons, introns or overlapping both. Intergenic lncRNAs can be located at great distance from proteins coding genes, in close proximity or divergently transcribed from protein coding gene promoters. They can also be expressed from silencer, enhancer and insulator loci. For details on genomic location of lncRNAs refer to Laurent et al. [4]. So far, there is no formal classification with respect to lncRNA localization or function. Many lncRNAs were shown to act as nucleo- or cytoplasmic scaffolds providing platforms for interactions between other cellular components (e.g., DNA, proteins and other RNA species), which implies lncRNAs as central players in epigenetic processes and chromatin regulation. Another superordinate function of lncRNAs is the competition for binding sites, this can be the competitive binding to open chromatin leading to displacement of transcription factors or the sequestration of miRNAs leading to reduced inhibition of the target mRNA. Likewise, lncRNAs can act similarly to miRNAs to enhance or decrease the stability of mRNA. The great variety of lncRNA cellular functions was recently reviewed by Yao et al. [5].

Due to their generally low expression levels the vast majority of the 215,008 annotated human lncRNAs (RNAcentral, 5 May 2019) was only discovered within the last decade [6]. Whilst the existence of lncRNAs as a biotype is well conserved in mammals, identifying the actual homologues between species is more challenging than for protein-coding transcripts. LncRNAs are often not well-conserved on the sequence level but rather regarding structure and/or genomic position [7]. The expression pattern of lncRNA genes was shown to be far more tissue- and cell-type specific than is the case for protein coding genes [8,9]. Quantitative studies based mainly on RNA sequencing have led to a rapid growth of this field and have shown dysregulation of lncRNAs in many diseases [10]. Whilst before 2010 only few studies on this topic were published each year, this changed tremendously in the last decade and several thousand publications on lncRNAs are found for the year 2018. As to lncRNAs in the kidney, this rise in publication numbers occurred around five years later and resulted in about 100 studies in the year 2018. However, especially in the beginning much of this work was merely descriptive and did not focus on kidney disease but rather renal cell carcinoma due to the ease of analyses regarding RNA expression changes in tumors. Taking this into consideration, the aim of this review is filling the gap towards non-tumorous kidney diseases to lay a foundation for future studies building on existing data.

2. LncRNAs in Glomerular Disease

As to glomerular disease by far most publications have analyzed the role of lncRNAs in diabetic nephropathy (Figure 1). Consequently, this review contains a focused paragraph on diabetic nephropathy but also provides an insight into the publications on other glomerular disease entities such as focal segmental glomerulosclerosis and membranous nephropathy (Table 1).

2.1. Diabetic Nephropathy—The Link between MicroRNAs and LncRNAs

With the incidence of diabetes mellitus rising and diabetic nephropathy (DN) being a leading cause of end-stage renal disease in Western societies [11,12], it is clear that researchers chose this entity as a key topic to elucidate the role of lncRNAs in kidney disease. Most of the work that goes beyond a mere description of non-coding RNA expression in DN focused on miRNAs and a few annotated lncRNAs the function of which had been addressed in other diseases/organs before. Despite the fact that miRNAs are not the topic of this review, it is important to note the intricate connection between miRNAs and lncRNAs. Firstly, the latter can impact miRNA function, e.g., by serving as miRNA sponges that inhibit their binding to the actual mRNA targets [13]. This has been described in the context of DN for a number of miRNA—lncRNA interactions including work on the lncRNAs TUG1, NEAT1 and MALAT1 [14–16]. Furthermore, lncRNA genes can harbor miRNAs that are set free by posttranscriptional cleavage. Prominent examples are the lncRNA PVT1 serving as a host of miRNA 1207-5p and both non-coding RNAs having been implicated in DN [17]. Importantly, miRNAs are often organized as clusters with four more miRNAs having been localized to the *PVT1* locus [18] all of which are upregulated by high glucose levels and impact extracellular matrix (ECM) formation. MiRNA clusters contained in lncRNAs can get very large as demonstrated by a megacluster of more than 40 miRNAs harbored in lnc-MGC. This cluster is induced in the glomeruli of several mouse models of diabetic nephropathy through endoplasmic reticulum (ER) stress signaling and responds to both high glucose and TGFβ-activation [19]. Inhibition of lnc-MGC using a "Gapmers"—antisense oligonucleotides that induce the RNaseH-mediated degradation of their targets often used in the lncRNA field—ameliorates several histological signs of diabetic nephropathy in a mouse model pointing towards a therapeutic potential of these findings.

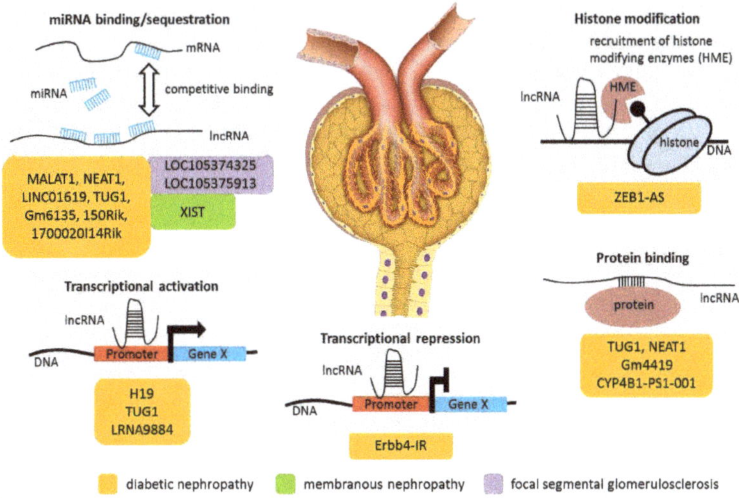

Figure 1. Long non-coding RNAs (lncRNAs) in glomerular disease and their reported molecular functions. Grey colored boxes depict the molecular mechanisms of lncRNA function (enhancer RNA, transcriptional repression, transcription activation, protein binding, miRNA binding/sequestration and histone modification) reported to play a role in glomerular disease. Orange, green and purple colored boxes indicate the disease: diabetic nephropathy, membranous nephropathy and focal segmental glomerulosclerosis, respectively. The lncRNAs associated with the particular mechanism and disease are specified by name. Glomerulus image obtained from: Aldona Griskieviciene/shutterstock.com.

2.2. Diabetic Nephropathy—Tthe Role of Specific Long Non-Coding RNAs (LncRNAs)

Regarding the involvement of specific lncRNAs we will focus on genes that have been implicated in DN by evidence from several publications.

The plasmacytoma variant translocation gene *PVT1* had been linked to diabetic nephropathy by the finding that variants in this gene are associated with the development of end-stage renal disease (ESRD) in both type 1 and 2 diabetes mellitus [20,21]. Soon after, it was noted that PVT1 was a non-coding RNA the expression of which was induced by high glucose in mesangial cells. Knockdown of PVT1 significantly decreased the upregulation of both ECM proteins and their transcriptional regulators PAI-1 and TGFβ1 [22], providing a functional link between the genomic data and the pathogenesis of DN. As described above, PVT1 hosts several miRNAs, one of which—miR-1207-5p—could be shown to regulate ECM formation in parallel to the lncRNA itself [17]. Zhang et al. provided further evidence on the role of PVT1 with a component from traditional Chinese medicine (Danggui Buxue Tang) alleviating glucose-indcued proliferation and ECM formation in mesangial cells through targeting PVT1 [23].

MALAT1 is another important example of an lncRNA involved in DN. MALAT1 is induced in the streptozocin-induced diabetic nephropathy mouse model [24]. Based on this finding and further work using cultured podocytes, Hu and colleagues hypothesized MALAT1 to play a role in high-glucose associated podocyte damage involving a feedback loop with beta-catenin employing the MALAT1-binding protein SRSF1 [24]. Furthermore, MALAT1 has been implicated in the damage of other renal cell types in DN. Regarding glomerular endothelial cells MALAT1 induction was accompanied by an epigenetically mediated decrease of Klotho expression [25]. The upregulation of this lncRNA upon glucose exposure led to increased IL1 and TNF-α levels suggesting this lncRNA to be involved in inflammatory processes of the endothelium [26]. In renal tubular epithelial cells MALAT1 induction by high glucose leads to increased pyroptosis by targeting miR-23c and consecutive upregulation of ELAVL1 and NLRP3 [16].

Mitochondrial dysfunction is one of the hallmarks in DN [27]. The modulation of mitochondrial metabolism was linked to the lncRNA TUG1 by an important study in 2016 [28]. TUG1 was differentially expressed in a murine DN model (db/db mice). Its podocyte-specific overexpression in this mouse model improved the glomerular phenotype both regarding albuminuria and histological changes. Mechanistically, TUG1 was linked to mitochondrial bioenergetics by showing that this lncRNA recruits PGC-1α to its own promoter [28]. Further studies corroborate the link of TUG1 to diabetic glomerulopathy. TUG1 both alleviated ECM deposition by acting as a sponge for miR-377 [14] and protected from podocyte apoptosis by modulating ER stress signaling, PGC-1α and TRAF5 [29,30] in different models of DN.

Besides, several lines of evidence point towards a functionally important involvement of the lncRNA NEAT1 in diabetic nephropathy. NEAT1 is induced in a streptozocin-mediated diabetic rat model and murine mesangial cells treated with high-glucose [15,31]. Increased expression of NEAT1 led to the activation of AKT/mTOR signalling accompanied by increased cellular proliferation and fibrosis [31]. Interestingly, this phenotype could be alleviated by knockdown of NEAT1, providing a therapeutic prospective. Additionally, NEAT1 served as a sponge for miR-27b-3p relieving ZEB1—a zinc finger transcription factor associated with epithelial-mesenchymal transition and ECM deposition—from miRNA-mediated repression [15].

CYP4B1-PS1-001 was first described in diabetic nephropathy in a microarray based-screen for dysregulated lncRNAs in the db/db mouse model [32]. Whilst this intergenic lncRNA was strongly downregulated in early phases of DN, its overexpression alleviated the increased proliferative tone in mesangial cells. This effect of CYP4B1-PS1-001 could later on be shown to be mediated by the proteasomal degradation of Nucleolin—a nucleolar ribosome biogenesis factor [33].

More than 20 additional lncRNAs have been implicated in diabetic nephropathy by single publications. Here, we summarize the most important findings. Several of these lncRNAs interact directly with miRNAs and inhibit their function. As examples, LINC01619 induces oxidative podocyte damage by serving as a sponge for miR-27a [34], Gm6135 protects from increased proliferation and apoptosis through impairing the miR-203-3p mediated downregulation of Toll-like receptor 4 [35], lincRNA1700020I14Rik reduces cellular proliferation via inhibition of miR-34-a-5p [36] and lncRNA 150Rik promotes proliferation by sponging miR-451 [37]. Apart from the inhibitory direct binding as described for these examples, lncRNA H19 induces the expression of miR-675 modulating vitamin D receptor expression [38] and lncRNA Erbb4-IR suppresses miR-29b on the transcriptional level [39]. The latter publication is a very good examples of a study taking lncRNAs in diabetic nephropathy beyond a mere description of expression changes by elucidating both the factor driving its expression (Smad3) as well as its downstream effects through mir-29b and by proving the therapeutic potential of Erbb4-IR inhibition in the db/db mouse model. Another lncRNA regulated by Smad3—LRNA9884—promotes DN through the stimulation of inflammation [40]. Similarly, lincRNA Gm4419 promotes inflammation in DN through the NLRP3 inflammasome [41]. Another layer of regulation through lncRNAs that has been found in other systems is epigenetic modifications. As to DN, lncRNA ZEB1-AS1 has been shown to enhance the expression of ZEB1 by promoting H3K4me3 histone modification on its promoter during high glucose treatment with increased ZEB1 exerting an anti-fibrotic role [42]. Importantly, since all of these data were primarily obtained in mouse models, a number of expression screens in DN have been able to show evolutionary conservation of lncRNA modulation in human datasets [43–45] indicating the future potential of data obtained in mouse models for the patient setting.

Table 1. LncRNAs involved in glomerular diseases.

Diabetic Nephropathy				
lncRNA	main disease model	suggested function	target	reference
TUG1	diabetic mice (db/db)	transcriptional activation	Ppargc1a promoter	[28]
	diabetic mice (db/db)	miRNA binding	miR-377	[14]
	streptozotocin treated rats	protein binding	TRAF5	[29]
MALAT1	streptozotocin treated rats	miRNA binding	miR-23	[16]
	streptozotocin treated mice	expression changed	IL-6 and TNF-α	[26]
	streptozotocin treated mice	expression changed	β-catenin, SRSF1	[24]
NEAT1	streptozotocin treated rats	miRNA binding	miR-27b-3p	[15]
	streptozotocin treated rats	expression changed	Akt/mTOR signaling	[31]
PVT1	high glucose treated CIHP-1	expression changed	ECM-related proteins	[22]
ZEB1-AS	streptozotocin treated mice	recruitment of histone modifications	ZEB1 promoter	[42]
LRNA9884	diabetic mice (db/db)	transcriptional activation	MCP-1	[40]
LINC01619	streptozotocin treated rats	miRNA binding	miR-27a	[34]
Gm6135	diabetic mice (db/db)	miRNA binding	miR-203-3p	[35]
CYP4B1-PS1-001	diabetic mice (db/db)	protein binding	NCL	[33]
1700020I14Rik	diabetic mice (db/db)	miRNA binding	miR-34	[36]
150Rik	diabetic mice (db/db)	miRNA binding	miR-451	[37]
H19	vitamin D3 treated CIHP-1	expression changed	miR-675	[38]
Erbb4-IR	diabetic mice (db/db)	transcriptional repression	miR-29b	[39]
Gm4419	high glucose treated mouse MCs	protein binding	p50	[41]
Focal-Segmental Glomerulosclerosis				
lncRNA	main disease model	suggested function	target	reference
LOC105374325	adriamycin treated podocytes	miRNA binding	miR-34c and miR-196a/b	[46]
LOC105375913	FSGS patient serum treated HK-2	miRNA binding	miR-27b	[47]
Membranous Nephropathy				
lncRNA	main disease model	suggested function	target	reference
XIST	angiotensin II treated AB8/13	miRNA binding	miR-217	[48]
Lupus Nephritis				
lncRNA	main disease model	suggested function	target	reference
RP11-2B6.2	IFN-I treated HeLa and HK-2	epigenetic inhibition	SOCS1	[49]

2.3. LncRNAs in Other Glomerular Diseases

In comparison to DN, little is known about the contribution of lncRNAs to other glomerular disease entitites. A Pubmed search for lncRNAs AND glomerulus revealed more than 80% of these publications to deal with DN. Fewer than 10 studies report results regarding different types of glomerulonephritis and focal-segmental glomerulosclerosis (FSGS). Due to the scarcity of data, all of these studies are discussed in the following paragraph independent from impact and approach. LncRNA LOC105375913 was found to be increased in tubular cells of 5 FSGS patients [47] and this upregulation was, based on cell culture results, induced by the C3a/p38/XBP-1s pathway. LOC105375913 exerted its profibrotic function through sequestration of miR-27b and consecutive overexpression of Snail. As to actual glomerular changes in FSGS lncRNA LOC105374325 has been described to be upregulated in podocytes of FSGS patients and to induce podocyte apoptosis. Again, the induction of this lncRNA (through p38 and C/EPBbeta) exerts its effects by serving as a sponge for two miRNAs (miR-34c, miR-196a/b) that normally regulate the expression of pro-apoptotic proteins [46]. Interestingly, the profibrotic function of LOC105375913 in the tubulointerstitium and the proapoptotic effect of LOC105374325 in podocytes could also be recapitulated in mouse models overexpressing the respective lncRNAs [46,47]. Regarding direct podocyte injury Fang et al. found the lncRNA GAS5 to be downregulated in a murine sepsis model (using lipopolysaccharide (LPS) injection) [50]. Loss of GAS5 led to a reduction of nephrin and an induction of both Snail/phosphorylated Snail and PI3K/AKT/GSK3β as potential harmful agents. In a descriptive approach Qin et al. reported 10 lncRNAs to be differentially expressed in glomeruli after treatment of mice with Adriamycin based on RNA-sequencing [51] and Gao at el. provided a similar analysis in whole kidney microarray analyses of two glomerulonephritis rat models (nephrotoxic serum nephritis and anti-glomerular basement membrane glomerulonephritis) [52]. As to human samples, two studies described the differential expression of numerous lncRNAs in either IgA-positive or -negative mesangio-proliferative glomerulonephritis [53,54]. The actual pathophysiological impact of this work remains to be determined. One of the longest-known lncRNAs—XIST, which is known for its role in the inactivation of the X-chromosome—has been linked to membranous nephropathy (MN) [48,55]. This lncRNA was found to be upregulated both in a mouse model of MN and in human samples [55]. Data in cell culture pointed towards XIST exerting its proapoptotic effect on podocytes through sequestration of miR-217 and consecutive upregulation of Toll-like receptor 4 [48]. Finally, in a recent report Liao et al. showed differential expression of lncRNAs in kidney biopsies of patients diagnosed with lupus nephritis (LN) [49]. LncRNA RP11-2B6.2 was found upregulated in kidney tissue of LN patients compared to healthy controls. Using HELA and HK-2 cell lines the authors showed that overexpression of RP11-2B6.2 led to inhibition of SOCS1, a known regulator of the IFN-1 signaling pathway and consequently increased the activity of the IFN-1 signaling pathway. They went on to evaluate chromatin accessibility of the SOCS1 locus in the presence and absence of RP11-2B6.2 and determined that downregulation of RP11-2B6.2 coincided with an open chromatin state in the promoter region of SOCS1. Based on this finding Liao et al. proposed that the inhibition of SOCS1 is conveyed by an undetermined epigenetic mechanism [49].

3. Tubulointerstitial Disease

To date, the majority of lncRNA studies on tubulointerstitial kidney disease were performed in the context of acute kidney injury (AKI) (Figure 2). Research on chronic kidney disease including genetic disorders such as autosomal dominant polycystic kidney disease (ADPKD) is still very scarce (Table 2).

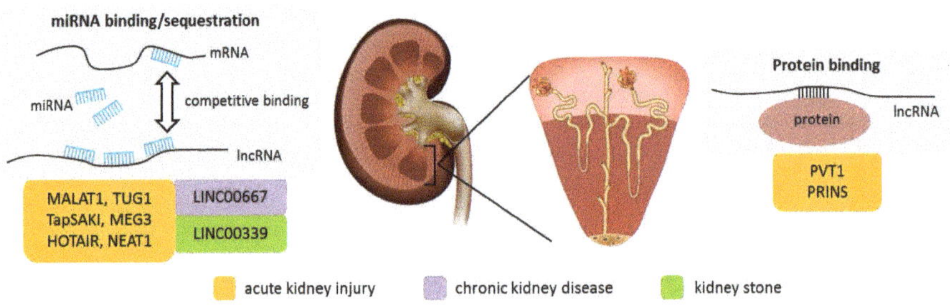

Figure 2. LncRNAs in tubulointerstitial disease and their reported molecular functions. Grey colored boxes depict the molecular mechanisms of lncRNA function (miRNA binding/sequestration and protein binding) reported to play a role in tubulointerstital disease. Orange, purple and green colored boxes indicate the disease: acute kidney injury, chronic kidney disease and kidney stone, respectively. The lncRNAs associated with the particular mechanism and disease are specified by name. Kidney image obtained from: Tefi/shutterstock.com.

3.1. LncRNAs and Acute Kidney Injury

AKI is a central problem in nephrology considering the high and increasing incidence associated with the demographic changes in Western societies and the lack of specific preventive and therapeutic strategies [56]. Consequently, it is crucial to gain an optimal understanding on the molecular mechanisms predisposing for and protecting from AKI and lncRNAs are an important novel layer of regulation in this context. Major triggers of AKI are sepsis, ischemia reperfusion injury and nephrotoxic agents. In recent years, based on transcriptomic data created from patient material as well as various animal models, a growing number of differentially expressed lncRNAs associated with AKI have been described. The majority of in vivo studies performed to examine AKI were carried out in mice or rats by the induction of ischemia reperfusion injury (IRI) [57–62], inflammation stimulated by lipopolysaccharide (LPS) [63,64], urine-derived sepsis [65,66] or exposure to hypoxia [67]. For in vitro models of AKI, the research community mainly relied on the HK-2 human tubular epithelial cell line either treated with LPS [64–66,68,69] or grown under hypoxic conditions [59–62,70]. However, when interpreting these data, it is important to note, that the comparability to the actual patient setting is limited especially for cell culture models. This highlights the importance of a confirmation of the findings in both rodents and especially using human biosamples.

Most evidence for an lncRNA to play a role in AKI has been presented for metastasis-associated lung adenocarcinoma transcript 1 (MALAT1). Initially identified as the most highly induced lncRNA gene in kidney and testis of hypoxic mice, MALAT1 was proposed to be hypoxia-inducible factor (HIF)-2 activated and postulated to function in renal proximal tubuli [67]. MALAT1 expression was suggested to inhibit the hypoxia-induced inflammatory response through the NF-κB pathway [57]. This idea was supported by the findings of Ding et al. who, in an LPS-induced model of AKI, found that MALAT1 interacts with mir-146a—a known regulator of the NF-κB signaling pathway [64]. In spite of these findings, no disease-specific phenotype was observed after challenging MALAT1 knockout mice with IRI-induced AKI [62]. Although the authors suggested that in vivo the impact of MALAT1 on signaling pathways might be minimal, it remains a potential biomarker of kidney IRI due to its high abundance in patient plasma and kidney biopsies [62].

Nuclear enriched abundant transcript 1 (NEAT1) was detected as significantly upregulated in the serum of patients with sepsis-induced as well as in patients with ischemia-induced AKI [71,72]. Using in vitro interaction assays both groups showed that NEAT1 interacts with several miRNAs. In the first case Chen et al. concluded that by binding to miR-204 NEAT1 reduces the cellular level of this miRNA, thereby alleviating the suppression of IL-6R and activating the NF-κB pathway with consecutive inflammation [71]. The second study conducted by Jiang et al. determined miR-27a-3p as a direct interactor of NEAT1 by RNA immunoprecipitation [72]. In knockdown and overexpression experiments the authors showed the negatively correlated influence of NEAT1 on miR-27a-3p levels leading to apoptosis.

Similar studies link the lncRNAs HOX transcript antisense RNA (HOTAIR) [66], taurine upregulated gene 1 (*TUG1*) [73], maternally expressed gene 3 (*MEG3*) [63] and transcript predicting survival in AKI (*TapSAKI*) [65] to a range of other miRNAs.

HOTAIR—known to play an important role in apoptosis—was upregulated in rats with sepsis caused by urinary tract infection [66]. The authors further observed a negative regulation of miR-22 and induction of apoptosis in HK-2 cells and related this regulation to the stabilization of high-mobility-group-protein B1 (HMGB1)—a key mediator of inflammation and a known target of miR-22. In a study using HOTAIR mimics in vivo in rats with sepsis induced AKI, Jiang et al. found that expression of HOTAIR declined serum serine—as well as blood urea nitrogen levels and reduced signs of apoptosis in kidney tissue [74]. These effects were attributed to the concomitant reduction of miR-34a and increase of B-cell leukemia/lymphoma 2 (Bcl-2) protein levels, with Bcl-2 being an anti-apoptotic factor and a target of miR-34a.

To unravel the role of the lncRNA TUG1, detected at lower levels in the serum of patients suffering from sepsis-associated AKI in comparison to healthy controls, a LPS based in vitro model was used [73]. Despite the fact that this study examined rat mesangial cells we report their results in this section due to the link to other LPS-induced AKI models. Liu et al. found that overexpression of TUG1 reversed the deteriorating effects of LPS on RMCs and showed that this was mediated by miR-142-3p. Furthermore, SIRT1 a known suppressor of the NF-κB signaling pathway, was identified as the direct target downregulated by miR-142-3p in the absence of TUG1. Consequently, these findings suggest that the lower levels of TUG1 observed in the serum of AKI patients may lead to activation of the NF-κB pathway driving inflammation. These findings are supported by a study of Xu et al. confirming the protective effect of overexpressed TUG1 on LPS-induced injury in HK-2 cells [68]. Although, the conveying factor between TUG1 and SIRT1 was found to be miR-223 in this study, the effects on the NF-κB pathway were similar. In addition, the authors suggested that the protective effects of TUG1 on renal tubular epithelial cells injury are associated with activation of the PI3K/AKT pathway.

In two individual studies MEG3 was found to be upregulated after LPS or hypoxia treatment, respectively and in both cases the authors report the sequestration of miRNAs by MEG3 [58,63]. Yang et al. showed that the higher levels of MEG3 lead to increased binding of miR-21 removing it from the pool available to inhibit the translation of programmed cell death protein 4 (PDCD4) [63]. The downregulation of MEG3 resulted in the inhibition of PDCD4 and attenuation of LPS-induced apoptosis. Likewise, data presented by Pang et al. suggested MEG3 to sequester mir-181b leading to upregulation of TNF-α in hypoxia-induced kidney injury in acute renal allografts [58].

TapSAKI, initially discovered as a circulating lncRNA upregulated in the plasma of AKI patients and their kidney tissue was proposed as a biomarker with predictive value for the survival of AKI patients [75]. Recently, Shen et al. using a urine-derived sepsis model of AKI in rats and LPS treated HK-2 cells, showed that TapSAKI interacts with miR-22 [65]. In a state of TapSAKI upregulation this interaction leads to increased levels of phosphatase and tensin homolog (PTEN) and activation of TLR4 and NF-κB pathway triggering inflammation.

In the section below we discuss lncRNAs which so far have only a single study connecting them to acute kidney injury—plasmacytoma variant translocation 1 (PVT1) [69], psoriasis-susceptibility-related RNA gene induced by stress (PRINS) [59], growth arrest-specific 5 (GAS5) [61], aspartyl-tRNA synthetase anti-sense 1 (DARS-AS1) [70], LINC00520 [60], UC.173 [76].

An involvement of PVT1 in kidney disease has been described previously for diabetic nephropathy [22] and is discussed above in the DN section. In their 2017 study on LPS-treated HK-2 cells, Huang et al. found PVT1 significantly upregulated compared to untreated control cells [69]. The authors reported PVT1 overexpression to decrease cell viability and to trigger inflammatory responses. Vice versa, downregulation of PVT1 resulted in suppression of inflammatory factors by regulation of the JNK/NF-κB signaling pathways. The authors suggested the binding of TNF-α by PVT1 to be the responsible mechanism leading to inhibition of JNK/NF-κB signaling pathways promoting inflammatory responses in sepsis-induced AKI.

The expression and secretion of RANTES/CCL5 (regulated on activation, normal T cell expressed and secreted) is known to recruit circulating leukocytes to sites of injury and to reinforce inflammatory reactions. In their report, Yu et al. showed that PRINS, a HIF-1α regulated lncRNA is potentially involved in RANTES production [59]. The study suggested a significant upregulation and direct interaction between PRINS and RANTES in hypoxic conditions leading to enhanced inflammation and AKI progression.

The hypoxia-responsive lncRNA GAS5 was reported to be upregulated in IRI treated mice by Geng et al. [61]. The increase of GAS5 was linked to induction of proapoptotic factors: p53, cIAP2 and TSP-1. Performing in vitro experiments in hypoxia treated HK-2 cells the authors confirmed this correlation for p53 and TSP-1 and in the reciprocal approach showed that knockdown of GAS5 led to downregulation of p53 and TSP-1, attenuating apoptosis.

The study conducted on HK-2 and primary renal proximal tubular epithelial cells (RPTEC) by Mimura et al. compared lncRNA expression patterns between hypoxic and normoxic cells [70]. DARS-AS1 containing hypoxia-responsive elements (HRE) in the promoter region was found upregulated as a consequence of HIF-1α binding in hypoxic conditions. The authors further showed that the expression of DARS-AS1 has inhibitory effects on cell death progression and therefore may be important for the survival of renal tubular cells during AKI.

Tian et al. observed an upregulation of LINC00520 in rat kidney tissue following IRI treatment [60]. Using HK-2 cells they determined a relation between LINC00520 and miR-27b and suggested that

LINC00520 may inhibit miR-27b by competitive binding. Reduction of miR-27b in the cellular pool resulted in the upregulation of Oncostatin M receptor (OSMR). Finally, the authors showed knockdown of LINC00520 to reduce levels of OSMR, reduction of PI3K/AKT and attenuation of renal injury in rats.

UC.173 belongs to a group of lncRNAs transcribed from an ultra-conserved region (T-UCR) shared between human, rat and mouse genomes and was initially reported as downregulated in lead-exposed human populations and animal models [77]. Qin et al. studied UC.173 in the context of lead-induced renal tubular epithelial cell apoptosis and showed that lead exposure reduced the levels of this lncRNA in HK-2 and HKC cells [76]. While the overexpression of UC.173 had no effect on cell viability, cell cycle or apoptotic factors in lead-unexposed HK-2 and HKC cells, its overexpression in lead treated cells increased cell survival and showed reduced signs of apoptosis.

Table 2. LncRNAs involved in tubulointerstitial disease.

Acute Kidney Injury				
lncRNA	main disease model	suggested function	target	reference
MEG3	IRI in renal allografts	miRNA binding	miR181b-5p	[58]
	LPS treated mice	miRNA binding	miR-21	[63]
NEAT1	LPS treated RMCs	miRNA binding	miR-204	[71]
	CoCl2 treated HK-2	miRNA binding	miR-27a-3p	[72]
MALAT1	LPS treated rats	miRNA binding	miR-146a	[64]
	hypoxia treated mice	expression changed	unknown	[67]
TapSAKI	Urine derived sepsis in rats	miRNA binding	miR-22	[65]
	AKI patients	circulating biomarker	unknown	[75]
HOTAIR	Urine derived sepsis in rats	miRNA binding	miR-22	[66]
	CLP induced sepsis in rats	expression changed	miR-34a and Bcl-2	[74]
TUG1	LPS treated RMCs	miRNA binding	miR-142-3p	[73]
	LPS treated HK-2	miRNA binding	miR-223	[68]
LINC00520	IRI in rats	miRNA binding	miR-27b-3p	[60]
PVT1	LPS treated HK-2	protein binding	TNF-α	[69]
PRINS	IRI in mice	protein binding	RANTES (CCL-5)	[59]
GAS5	IRI in mice	expression changed	mRNA of p53 and TCP1	[61]
DARS-AS1	hypoxia treated HK-2 and RPTECs	expression changed	unknown	[70]
UC.173	lead treated HK-2 and HKC	expression changed	unknown	[76]
Chronic kidney disease				
lncRNA	main disease model	suggested function	target	reference
LINC00667	CKD patients and rat model	miRNA binding	miR-19b-3p	[78]
LINC00963	CKD rat model	expression changed	mRNA of FoxO3a	[79]
Autosomal Dominant Polycystic Kidney Disease				
lncRNA	main disease model	suggested function	target	reference
Hoxb3os	Pkd1/2 knockout mice	expression changed	unknown	[80]
Kidney stone				
lncRNA	main disease model	suggested function	target	reference
LINC00339	COM treated HK-2	miRNA binding	miR-22-3p	[81]
CHCHD4P4	COM treated mice	expression changed	unknown	[82]
Uric Acid Nephropathy				
lncRNA	main disease model	suggested function	target	reference
ANRIL	uric acid treated HK-2	miRNA binding	miR-122-5p	[83]

3.2. LncRNAs Associated with Other Tubulointerstitial Diseases

In this section we give an overview of recent advances with regard to the function of lncRNAs in tubulointerstitial diseases other than acute kidney injury. We discuss the role of lncRNAs in 5/6 nephrectomy, autosomal dominant polycystic kidney disease (ADPKD) and kidney injury by crystal-formation (e.g., calcium oxalate).

To date, two lncRNAs have been associated with the transcriptional response in rat models of 5/6 nephrectomy [78,79]. LINC00963, studied by Chen et al. due to its upregulation in the context of renal interstitial fibrosis and oxidative stress, was determined to influence FoxO3a levels by an undetermined mechanism [79]. Lowered LINC00963 levels were associated with the activation of the FoxO signaling pathway, consequently leading to suppression of renal interstitial fibrosis and oxidative stress. The same group published a study investigating the role of LINC00667 [78]. LINC00667 was upregulated while miR-19b-3p was downregulated in kidney tissue of patients suffering from CKD (chronic kidney disease) of heterogenous etiology compared to normal renal tissue. The authors linked the downregulation of miR-19b-3b to a sequestration by LINC00667. In the 5/6 nephrectomy rat model used in this study, overexpression of miR-19b-3p decreased levels of TGF-β1, CTGF, α-SMA and TIMP-1 and improved the renal damage. A recent review provides a detailed view on the general role of non-coding RNAs in renal fibrosis [84].

To the best of our knowledge, so far only one lncRNA has been shown to have functional implications in ADPKD. Aboudehen et al. investigated the role of Hoxb3os, an lncRNA abundantly expressed in the kidney and evolutionary conserved with the human ortholog HOXB-AS1 [80]. The expression of HOXB-AS1 was decreased in the kidney tissue of ADPKD patients and likewise in *Pkd1* and *Pkd2* knockout mice, a genetic model of ADPKD, a downregulation of the mouse ortholog was observed. In a cell model using mIMCD3, the authors showed that knockout of Hoxb3os leads to mTORC1 activation and increase in mitochondrial respiration and that re-expression of Hoxb3os rescues this phenotype.

Recent findings have also shown that lncRNAs are associated with renal injury mediated by crystal formation. The studies - mainly based on HK-2 cell exposure to calcium oxalate monohydrate (COM), the major constituent of kidney stones [85], range from profiling changes in lncRNA expression upon COM stimulation to analysis of individual lncRNAs. Wang et al.—using the same cell model—profiled transcriptional changes by RNA sequencing and determined 25 differentially expressed lncRNAs [86]. Cao et al. used an ethylene glycol-induced rat model of kidney stone formation to profile expression changes and found 1440 lncRNAs differentially regulated in comparison to untreated controls [87]. In addition to an in vitro COM-HK-2 cell model, Zhang et al. used a mouse model of calcium oxalate-induced kidney damage and found 376 differentially regulated lncRNA in COM-treated animal in comparison to the control group. 15 of the regulated lncRNAs had homologous genes in the human genome. LncRNA AU015836 and the human homolog CHCHD4P4 were upregulated upon COM treatment in mouse kidney tissue and HK-2 cells, respectively. The authors further showed that CHCHD4P4 was involved in epithelial–mesenchymal transition (EMT) by regulation of EMT-related genes and the inhibited cell proliferation in COM-exposed HK-2 cells [82]. In their study on LINC00339 in COM-treated HK-2 cells, Song et al. linked the promotion of renal tubular epithelial pyroptosis to the activation of the NLRP3 inflammasome [81]. The inflammasome was activated due to increased levels of NLRP3 resulting from the sequestration of miR-22-3p—a regulator of NLRP3—by LINC00339. As a last example, antisense non-coding RNA in the INK4 locus ANRIL, a highly expressed lncRNA in the serum of patients suffering from uric acid nephropathy (UAN), was studied by Hu et al. in HK-2 cells and a rat model of UAN [83]. The authors report that downregulation of ANRIL in the animal model resulted in reduced signs of renal injury. According to the results from the in vitro studies in HK-2 cells this improvement was conveyed through the reduced sequestering of miR-122-5p by ANRIL, which in turn led to the downregulation of the BRCA1-BRCA2-containing complex subunit 3 (BRCC3) and as a consequence suppressed the activation of NLRP3 inflammasome.

4. Systemic Kidney Biomarkers

Regarding glomerular disease there are no reports on circulating lncRNAs as potential biomarkers. For membranous nephropathy lncRNA XIST has been hypothesized to be a potential urinary biomarker [55]. However, the increase of urinary XIST—which was originally described in kidneys of a mouse model of MN—was not specific to MN but rather reflected injury in different types of glomerulonephritis. Besides, the lncRNA TapSAKI was identified as a circulating factor with the potential to predict mortality among a cohort of 109 patients suffering from acute kidney injury [75]. A potential implementation of lncRNAs as biomarkers for standardized clinical use will require studies in larger cohorts including questions on specificity and predictive value regarding clinical outcome. Since for most renal disorders little is known regarding the impact of lncRNAs, screening studies describing differential expression of lncRNAs using state-of-the-art methodology (e.g., RNA and single cell RNA sequencing) are still an important asset but will require further complementation by targeted analyses elucidating the molecular function of specific lncRNAs (e.g., RNAscope for visualization, quantitative polymerase chain reaction (qPCR) for quantification and CHART-MS for the identification of binding partners.

5. Conclusion and Outlook

LncRNAs provide a fascinating new layer to pathophysiological studies and the search for novel therapeutic strategies in kidney disease. However, apart from few examples such as diabetic nephropathy and acute kidney injury, little is known about their impact in renal pathologies and most studies have remained primarily descriptive. Future work will need to close this gap in order to increase our understanding of this new class of non-coding RNAs in nephrology and to eventually elucidate how we can exploit the potential of lncRNA modulation for patients suffering from kidney disease. The inhibition of lncRNAs in vivo is technically no more challenging than the inhibition of messenger RNAs; therefore, with an increasing number of antisense oligonucleotide therapies coming into clinical use at the moment (e.g., RNAi for TTR-amyloidosis or modulation of splicing for spinal muscular atrophy) this concept could be of high interest for targeting lncRNAs in kidney disease [88–90]. Regarding the cell-type specific expression of RNAs in the kidney and specifically the glomerulus single cell or single nucleus RNA sequencing (scRNAseq) studies have started to add much to our knowledge in both conditions of health and disease including DN [91–94]. Importantly, since nearly all lncRNAs are polyadenylated, the commonly used 3′end sequencing approaches in scRNAseq do capture these sequences as well if samples are sequenced at a sufficient depth (due to comparably lower transcript counts of lncRNAs compared to other RNA species). These approaches will now need to be analyzed in detail regarding lncRNAs and transferred to human kidney biopsies using either scRNAseq itself (for an example regarding a first approach in Lupus nephritis see [95]) or targeted imaging of specific lncRNAs, e.g., by single-molecule FISH. When using model organisms, the difficulties in predicting evolutionary conservation are still a major challenge, which will make innovative bioinformatics solutions an essential asset. Furthermore, the function of lncRNAs can hardly be predicted and its elucidation requires continuous development of novel techniques. Taken together, it is time for nephrologists to team up with molecular and computational biologists and unravel the full impact of lncRNAs in kidney disease.

Author Contributions: M.I. and R.-U.M. drafted, wrote and revised the manuscript; R.I. performed the literature search.

Funding: R.-U.M was supported by the Nachwuchsgruppen.NRW program of the Ministry of Science North Rhine Westfalia (MIWF, to R.-U.M.) and the German Research Foundation (KFO329, MU3629/3-1).

Acknowledgments: We thank Petra Kleinwächter for excellent help with figure design.

Conflicts of Interest: The authors declare no conflict of interest.

Abbreviations

CIHP-1	human podocyte cell line
MC	mesangial cells
FSGS	focal-segmental glomerulosclerosis
HK-2	human proximal tubule epithelial cell line
AB8/13	human podocyte cell line
IRI	ischemia reperfusion injury
LPS	lipopolysaccharide
RMCs	rat mesangial cell line
HK-2	human proximal tubule epithelial cell line
CLP	cecal ligation puncture
RPTECs	human renal proximal tubular epithelial cell line
HKC	human kidney proximal tubular epithelial cell line
CKD	chronic kidney disease
COM	calcium oxalate monohydrate

References

1. Zhao, H.; Ma, S.X.; Shang, Y.Q.; Zhang, H.Q.; Su, W. MicroRNAs in chronic kidney disease. *Clin. Chim. Acta* **2019**, *491*, 59–65. [CrossRef] [PubMed]
2. Ledeganck, K.J.; Gielis, E.M.; Abramowicz, D.; Stenvinkel, P.; Shiels, P.G.; Van Craenenbroeck, A.H. MicroRNAs in AKI and Kidney Transplantation. *Clin. J. Am. Soc. Nephrol.* **2019**, *14*, 454–468. [CrossRef] [PubMed]
3. Quinn, J.J.; Chang, H.Y. Unique features of long non-coding RNA biogenesis and function. *Nat. Rev. Genet.* **2016**, *17*, 47–62. [CrossRef]
4. St Laurent, G.; Wahlestedt, C.; Kapranov, P. The Landscape of long noncoding RNA classification. *Trends Genet. Tig.* **2015**, *31*, 239–251. [CrossRef] [PubMed]
5. Yao, R.W.; Wang, Y.; Chen, L.L. Cellular functions of long noncoding RNAs. *Nat. Cell. Biol.* **2019**, *21*, 542–551. [CrossRef]
6. Cabili, M.N.; Trapnell, C.; Goff, L.; Koziol, M.; Tazon-Vega, B.; Regev, A.; Rinn, J.L. Integrative annotation of human large intergenic noncoding RNAs reveals global properties and specific subclasses. *Genes Dev.* **2011**, *25*, 1915–1927. [CrossRef]
7. Johnsson, P.; Lipovich, L.; Grander, D.; Morris, K.V. Evolutionary conservation of long non-coding RNAs; sequence, structure, function. *Biochim. Et. Biophys. Acta* **2014**, *1840*, 1063–1071. [CrossRef]
8. Derrien, T.; Johnson, R.; Bussotti, G.; Tanzer, A.; Djebali, S.; Tilgner, H.; Guernec, G.; Martin, D.; Merkel, A.; Knowles, D.G.; et al. The GENCODE v7 catalog of human long noncoding RNAs: Analysis of their gene structure, evolution, and expression. *Genome Res.* **2012**, *22*, 1775–1789. [CrossRef]
9. Gloss, B.S.; Dinger, M.E. The specificity of long noncoding RNA expression. *Biochim. Et. Biophys. Acta* **2016**, *1859*, 16–22. [CrossRef]
10. Maass, P.G.; Luft, F.C.; Bähring, S. Long non-coding RNA in health and disease. *J. Mol. Med.* **2014**, *92*, 337–346. [CrossRef]
11. Nathan, D.M. Diabetes: Advances in Diagnosis and Treatment. *JAMA* **2015**, *314*, 1052–1062. [CrossRef] [PubMed]
12. Fineberg, D.; Jandeleit-Dahm, K.A.; Cooper, M.E. Diabetic nephropathy: Diagnosis and treatment. *Nat. Rev. Endocrinol.* **2013**, *9*, 713–723. [CrossRef] [PubMed]
13. Paraskevopoulou, M.D.; Hatzigeorgiou, A.G. Analyzing MiRNA-LncRNA Interactions. *Methods Mol. Biol.* **2016**, *1402*, 271–286. [CrossRef] [PubMed]
14. Duan, L.J.; Ding, M.; Hou, L.J.; Cui, Y.T.; Li, C.J.; Yu, D.M. Long noncoding RNA TUG1 alleviates extracellular matrix accumulation via mediating microRNA-377 targeting of PPARgamma in diabetic nephropathy. *Biochem. Biophys. Res. Commun.* **2017**, *484*, 598–604. [CrossRef] [PubMed]
15. Wang, X.; Xu, Y.; Zhu, Y.C.; Wang, Y.K.; Li, J.; Li, X.Y.; Ji, T.; Bai, S.J. LncRNA NEAT1 promotes extracellular matrix accumulation and epithelial-to-mesenchymal transition by targeting miR-27b-3p and ZEB1 in diabetic nephropathy. *J. Cell Physiol.* **2019**, *234*, 12926–12933. [CrossRef]

16. Li, X.; Zeng, L.; Cao, C.; Lu, C.; Lian, W.; Han, J.; Zhang, X.; Zhang, J.; Tang, T.; Li, M. Long noncoding RNA MALAT1 regulates renal tubular epithelial pyroptosis by modulated miR-23c targeting of ELAVL1 in diabetic nephropathy. *Exp. Cell Res.* **2017**, *350*, 327–335. [CrossRef] [PubMed]

17. Alvarez, M.L.; Khosroheidari, M.; Eddy, E.; Kiefer, J. Role of microRNA 1207-5P and its host gene, the long non-coding RNA Pvt1, as mediators of extracellular matrix accumulation in the kidney: Implications for diabetic nephropathy. *PLoS ONE* **2013**, *8*, e77468. [CrossRef]

18. Huppi, K.; Volfovsky, N.; Runfola, T.; Jones, T.L.; Mackiewicz, M.; Martin, S.E.; Mushinski, J.F.; Stephens, R.; Caplen, N.J. The identification of microRNAs in a genomically unstable region of human chromosome 8q24. *Mol. Cancer Res.* **2008**, *6*, 212–221. [CrossRef]

19. Kato, M.; Wang, M.; Chen, Z.; Bhatt, K.; Oh, H.J.; Lanting, L.; Deshpande, S.; Jia, Y.; Lai, J.Y.; O'Connor, C.L.; et al. An endoplasmic reticulum stress-regulated lncRNA hosting a microRNA megacluster induces early features of diabetic nephropathy. *Nat. Commun.* **2016**, *7*, 12864. [CrossRef]

20. Millis, M.P.; Bowen, D.; Kingsley, C.; Watanabe, R.M.; Wolford, J.K. Variants in the plasmacytoma variant translocation gene (PVT1) are associated with end-stage renal disease attributed to type 1 diabetes. *Diabetes* **2007**, *56*, 3027–3032. [CrossRef]

21. Hanson, R.L.; Craig, D.W.; Millis, M.P.; Yeatts, K.A.; Kobes, S.; Pearson, J.V.; Lee, A.M.; Knowler, W.C.; Nelson, R.G.; Wolford, J.K. Identification of PVT1 as a candidate gene for end-stage renal disease in type 2 diabetes using a pooling-based genome-wide single nucleotide polymorphism association study. *Diabetes* **2007**, *56*, 975–983. [CrossRef] [PubMed]

22. Alvarez, M.L.; DiStefano, J.K. Functional characterization of the plasmacytoma variant translocation 1 gene (PVT1) in diabetic nephropathy. *PLoS ONE* **2011**, *6*, e18671. [CrossRef] [PubMed]

23. Zhang, R.; Li, J.; Huang, T.; Wang, X. Danggui buxue tang suppresses high glucose-induced proliferation and extracellular matrix accumulation of mesangial cells via inhibiting lncRNA PVT1. *Am. J. Transl. Res.* **2017**, *9*, 3732–3740. [PubMed]

24. Hu, M.; Wang, R.; Li, X.; Fan, M.; Lin, J.; Zhen, J.; Chen, L.; Lv, Z. LncRNA MALAT1 is dysregulated in diabetic nephropathy and involved in high glucose-induced podocyte injury via its interplay with beta-catenin. *J. Cell. Mol. Med.* **2017**, *21*, 2732–2747. [CrossRef] [PubMed]

25. Li, Y.; Ren, D.; Xu, G. Long noncoding RNA MALAT1 mediates high glucose-induced glomerular endothelial cell injury by epigenetically inhibiting klotho via methyltransferase G9a. *IUBMB Life* **2019**, *71*, 873–881. [CrossRef] [PubMed]

26. Puthanveetil, P.; Chen, S.; Feng, B.; Gautam, A.; Chakrabarti, S. Long non-coding RNA MALAT1 regulates hyperglycaemia induced inflammatory process in the endothelial cells. *J. Cell. Mol. Med.* **2015**, *19*, 1418–1425. [CrossRef]

27. Higgins, G.C.; Coughlan, M.T. Mitochondrial dysfunction and mitophagy: The beginning and end to diabetic nephropathy? *Br. J. Pharmacol.* **2014**, *171*, 1917–1942. [CrossRef]

28. Long, J.; Badal, S.S.; Ye, Z.; Wang, Y.; Ayanga, B.A.; Galvan, D.L.; Green, N.H.; Chang, B.H.; Overbeek, P.A.; Danesh, F.R. Long noncoding RNA Tug1 regulates mitochondrial bioenergetics in diabetic nephropathy. *J. Clin. Investig.* **2016**, *126*, 4205–4218. [CrossRef]

29. Lei, X.; Zhang, L.; Li, Z.; Ren, J. Astragaloside IV/lncRNA-TUG1/TRAF5 signaling pathway participates in podocyte apoptosis of diabetic nephropathy rats. *Drug Des. Devel.* **2018**, *12*, 2785–2793. [CrossRef]

30. Shen, H.; Ming, Y.; Xu, C.; Xu, Y.; Zhao, S.; Zhang, Q. Deregulation of long noncoding RNA (TUG1) contributes to excessive podocytes apoptosis by activating endoplasmic reticulum stress in the development of diabetic nephropathy. *J. Cell Physiol.* **2019**, *234*, 15123–15133. [CrossRef]

31. Huang, S.; Xu, Y.; Ge, X.; Xu, B.; Peng, W.; Jiang, X.; Shen, L.; Xia, L. Long noncoding RNA NEAT1 accelerates the proliferation and fibrosis in diabetic nephropathy through activating Akt/mTOR signaling pathway. *J. Cell Physiol.* **2019**, *234*, 11200–11207. [CrossRef] [PubMed]

32. Wang, M.; Wang, S.; Yao, D.; Yan, Q.; Lu, W. A novel long non-coding RNA CYP4B1-PS1-001 regulates proliferation and fibrosis in diabetic nephropathy. *Mol. Cell Endocrinol.* **2016**, *426*, 136–145. [CrossRef] [PubMed]

33. Wang, S.; Chen, X.; Wang, M.; Yao, D.; Chen, T.; Yan, Q.; Lu, W. Long Non-Coding RNA CYP4B1-PS1-001 Inhibits Proliferation and Fibrosis in Diabetic Nephropathy by Interacting with Nucleolin. *Cell Physiol. Biochem.* **2018**, *49*, 2174–2187. [CrossRef] [PubMed]

34. Bai, X.; Geng, J.; Li, X.; Wan, J.; Liu, J.; Zhou, Z.; Liu, X. Long Noncoding RNA LINC01619 Regulates MicroRNA-27a/Forkhead Box Protein O1 and Endoplasmic Reticulum Stress-Mediated Podocyte Injury in Diabetic Nephropathy. *Antioxid. Redox Signal* **2018**, *29*, 355–376. [CrossRef] [PubMed]

35. Ji, T.T.; Wang, Y.K.; Zhu, Y.C.; Gao, C.P.; Li, X.Y.; Li, J.; Bai, F.; Bai, S.J. Long noncoding RNA Gm6135 functions as a competitive endogenous RNA to regulate toll-like receptor 4 expression by sponging miR-203-3p in diabetic nephropathy. *J. Cell Physiol.* **2019**, *234*, 6633–6641. [CrossRef] [PubMed]

36. Li, A.; Peng, R.; Sun, Y.; Liu, H.; Peng, H.; Zhang, Z. LincRNA 1700020I14Rik alleviates cell proliferation and fibrosis in diabetic nephropathy via miR-34a-5p/Sirt1/HIF-1alpha signaling. *Cell Death Dis.* **2018**, *9*, 461. [CrossRef] [PubMed]

37. Zhang, Y.; Sun, Y.; Peng, R.; Liu, H.; He, W.; Zhang, L.; Peng, H.; Zhang, Z. The Long Noncoding RNA 150Rik Promotes Mesangial Cell Proliferation via miR-451/IGF1R/p38 MAPK Signaling in Diabetic Nephropathy. *Cell Physiol. Biochem.* **2018**, *51*, 1410–1428. [CrossRef]

38. Fan, W.; Peng, Y.; Liang, Z.; Yang, Y.; Zhang, J. A negative feedback loop of H19/miR-675/EGR1 is involved in diabetic nephropathy by downregulating the expression of the vitamin D receptor. *J. Cell Physiol.* **2019**, *234*, 17505–17513. [CrossRef]

39. Sun, S.F.; Tang, P.M.K.; Feng, M.; Xiao, J.; Huang, X.R.; Li, P.; Ma, R.C.W.; Lan, H.Y. Novel lncRNA Erbb4-IR Promotes Diabetic Kidney Injury in db/db Mice by Targeting miR-29b. *Diabetes* **2018**, *67*, 731–744. [CrossRef]

40. Zhang, Y.Y.; Tang, P.M.-K.; Tang, P.C.-T.; Xiao, J.; Huang, X.R.; Yu, C.; Ma, R.C.; Lan, H.Y. LRNA9884, a Novel Smad3-Dependent LncRNA, Promotes Diabetic Kidney Injury in db/db Mice Via Enhancing MCP-1-Dependent Renal Inflammation. *Diabetes* **2019**, *68*, 1485–1498. [CrossRef]

41. Yi, H.; Peng, R.; Zhang, L.Y.; Sun, Y.; Peng, H.M.; Liu, H.D.; Yu, L.J.; Li, A.L.; Zhang, Y.J.; Jiang, W.H.; et al. LincRNA-Gm4419 knockdown ameliorates NF-kappaB/NLRP3 inflammasome-mediated inflammation in diabetic nephropathy. *Cell Death Dis.* **2017**, *8*, e2583. [CrossRef] [PubMed]

42. Wang, J.; Pang, J.; Li, H.; Long, J.; Fang, F.; Chen, J.; Zhu, X.; Xiang, X.; Zhang, D. lncRNA ZEB1-AS1 Was Suppressed by p53 for Renal Fibrosis in Diabetic Nephropathy. *Mol. Ther. Nucleic Acids* **2018**, *12*, 741–750. [CrossRef] [PubMed]

43. Shang, J.; Wang, S.; Jiang, Y.; Duan, Y.; Cheng, G.; Liu, D.; Xiao, J.; Zhao, Z. Identification of key lncRNAs contributing to diabetic nephropathy by gene co-expression network analysis. *Sci. Rep.* **2019**, *9*, 3328. [CrossRef] [PubMed]

44. Wang, Y.Z.; Zhu, D.Y.; Xie, X.M.; Ding, M.; Wang, Y.L.; Sun, L.L.; Zhang, N.; Shen, E.; Wang, X.X. EA15, MIR22, LINC00472 as diagnostic markers for diabetic kidney disease. *J. Cell Physiol.* **2019**, *234*, 8797–8803. [CrossRef] [PubMed]

45. Tang, W.; Zhang, D.; Ma, X. RNA-sequencing reveals genome-wide long non-coding RNAs profiling associated with early development of diabetic nephropathy. *Oncotarget* **2017**, *8*, 105832–105847. [CrossRef] [PubMed]

46. Hu, S.; Han, R.; Shi, J.; Zhu, X.; Qin, W.; Zeng, C.; Bao, H.; Liu, Z. The long noncoding RNA LOC105374325 causes podocyte injury in individuals with focal segmental glomerulosclerosis. *J. Biol. Chem.* **2018**, *293*, 20227–20239. [CrossRef] [PubMed]

47. Han, R.; Hu, S.; Qin, W.; Shi, J.; Zeng, C.; Bao, H.; Liu, Z. Upregulated long noncoding RNA LOC105375913 induces tubulointerstitial fibrosis in focal segmental glomerulosclerosis. *Sci. Rep.* **2019**, *9*, 716. [CrossRef]

48. Jin, L.W.; Pan, M.; Ye, H.Y.; Zheng, Y.; Chen, Y.; Huang, W.W.; Xu, X.Y.; Zheng, S.B. Down-regulation of the long non-coding RNA XIST ameliorates podocyte apoptosis in membranous nephropathy via the miR-217-TLR4 pathway. *Exp. Physiol.* **2019**, *104*, 220–230. [CrossRef]

49. Liao, Z.; Ye, Z.; Xue, Z.; Wu, L.; Ouyang, Y.; Yao, C.; Cui, C.; Xu, N.; Ma, J.; Hou, G.; et al. Identification of Renal Long Non-coding RNA RP11-2B6.2 as a Positive Regulator of Type I Interferon Signaling Pathway in Lupus Nephritis. *Front Immunol.* **2019**, *10*, 975. [CrossRef]

50. Fang, Y.; Hu, J.F.; Wang, Z.H.; Zhang, S.G.; Zhang, R.F.; Sun, L.M.; Cui, H.W.; Yang, F. GAS5 promotes podocyte injury in sepsis by inhibiting PTEN expression. *Eur. Rev. Med. Pharm. Sci.* **2018**, *22*, 8423–8430. [CrossRef]

51. Qin, X.J.; Gao, J.R.; Xu, X.J.; Jiang, H.; Wei, L.B.; Jiang, N.N. LncRNAs expression in adriamycin-induced rats reveals the potential role of LncRNAs contributing to chronic glomerulonephritis pathogenesis. *Gene* **2019**, *687*, 90–98. [CrossRef] [PubMed]

52. Gao, J.R.; Qin, X.J.; Jiang, H.; Gao, Y.C.; Guo, M.F.; Jiang, N.N. Potential role of lncRNAs in contributing to pathogenesis of chronic glomerulonephritis based on microarray data. *Gene* **2018**, *643*, 46–54. [CrossRef] [PubMed]

53. Sui, W.; Li, H.; Ou, M.; Tang, D.; Dai, Y. Altered long non-coding RNA expression profile in patients with IgA-negative mesangial proliferative glomerulonephritis. *Int. J. Mol. Med.* **2012**, *30*, 173–178. [CrossRef] [PubMed]

54. Zuo, N.; Li, Y.; Liu, N.; Wang, L. Differentially expressed long noncoding RNAs and mRNAs in patients with IgA nephropathy. *Mol. Med. Rep.* **2017**, *16*, 7724–7730. [CrossRef] [PubMed]

55. Huang, Y.S.; Hsieh, H.Y.; Shih, H.M.; Sytwu, H.K.; Wu, C.C. Urinary Xist is a potential biomarker for membranous nephropathy. *Biochem. Biophys. Res. Commun.* **2014**, *452*, 415–421. [CrossRef] [PubMed]

56. Mehta, R.L.; Cerda, J.; Burdmann, E.A.; Tonelli, M.; Garcia-Garcia, G.; Jha, V.; Susantitaphong, P.; Rocco, M.; Vanholder, R.; Sever, M.S.; et al. International Society of Nephrology's 0by25 initiative for acute kidney injury (zero preventable deaths by 2025): A human rights case for nephrology. *Lancet* **2015**, *385*, 2616–2643. [CrossRef]

57. Tian, H.; Wu, M.; Zhou, P.; Huang, C.; Ye, C.; Wang, L. The long non-coding RNA MALAT1 is increased in renal ischemia-reperfusion injury and inhibits hypoxia-induced inflammation. *Ren. Fail.* **2018**, *40*, 527–533. [CrossRef] [PubMed]

58. Pang, X.; Feng, G.; Shang, W.; Liu, L.; Li, J.; Feng, Y.; Xie, H.; Wang, J. Inhibition of lncRNA MEG3 protects renal tubular from hypoxia-induced kidney injury in acute renal allografts by regulating miR-181b/TNF-α signaling pathway. *J. Cell Biochem.* **2019**, *120*, 12822–12831. [CrossRef] [PubMed]

59. Yu, T.M.; Palanisamy, K.; Sun, K.T.; Day, Y.J.; Shu, K.H.; Wang, I.K.; Shyu, W.C.; Chen, P.; Chen, Y.L.; Li, C.Y. RANTES mediates kidney ischemia reperfusion injury through a possible role of HIF-1α and LncRNA PRINS. *Sci. Rep.* **2016**, *6*, 18424. [CrossRef]

60. Tian, X.; Ji, Y.; Liang, Y.; Zhang, J.; Guan, L.; Wang, C. LINC00520 targeting miR-27b-3p regulates OSMR expression level to promote acute kidney injury development through the PI3K/AKT signaling pathway. *J. Cell Physiol.* **2019**, *234*, 14221–14233. [CrossRef]

61. Geng, X.; Xu, X.; Fang, Y.; Zhao, S.; Hu, J.; Xu, J.; Jia, P.; Ding, X.; Teng, J. Effect of long non-coding RNA growth arrest-specific 5 on apoptosis in renal ischaemia/reperfusion injury. *Nephrology* **2019**, *24*, 405–413. [CrossRef] [PubMed]

62. Kolling, M.; Genschel, C.; Kaucsar, T.; Hubner, A.; Rong, S.; Schmitt, R.; Sorensen-Zender, I.; Haddad, G.; Kistler, A.; Seeger, H.; et al. Hypoxia-induced long non-coding RNA Malat1 is dispensable for renal ischemia/reperfusion-injury. *Sci. Rep.* **2018**, *8*, 3438. [CrossRef] [PubMed]

63. Yang, R.; Liu, S.; Wen, J.; Xue, L.; Zhang, Y.; Yan, D.; Wang, G.; Liu, Z. Inhibition of maternally expressed gene 3 attenuated lipopolysaccharide-induced apoptosis through sponging miR-21 in renal tubular epithelial cells. *J. Cell Biochem.* **2018**, *119*, 7800–7806. [CrossRef] [PubMed]

64. Ding, Y.; Guo, F.; Zhu, T.; Li, J.; Gu, D.; Jiang, W.; Lu, Y.; Zhou, D. Mechanism of long non-coding RNA MALAT1 in lipopolysaccharide-induced acute kidney injury is mediated by the miR-146a/NF-kappaB signaling pathway. *Int. J. Mol. Med.* **2018**, *41*, 446–454. [CrossRef] [PubMed]

65. Shen, J.; Liu, L.; Zhang, F.; Gu, J.; Pan, G. LncRNA TapSAKI promotes inflammation injury in HK-2 cells and urine derived sepsis-induced kidney injury. *J. Pharm. Pharm.* **2019**, *71*, 839–848. [CrossRef] [PubMed]

66. Shen, J.; Zhang, J.; Jiang, X.; Wang, H.; Pan, G. LncRNA HOX transcript antisense RNA accelerated kidney injury induced by urine-derived sepsis through the miR-22/high mobility group box 1 pathway. *Life Sci.* **2018**, *210*, 185–191. [CrossRef] [PubMed]

67. Lelli, A.; Nolan, K.A.; Santambrogio, S.; Goncalves, A.F.; Schonenberger, M.J.; Guinot, A.; Frew, I.J.; Marti, H.H.; Hoogewijs, D.; Wenger, R.H. Induction of long noncoding RNA MALAT1 in hypoxic mice. *Hypoxia* **2015**, *3*, 45–52. [CrossRef]

68. Xu, Y.; Deng, W.; Zhang, W. Long non-coding RNA TUG1 protects renal tubular epithelial cells against injury induced by lipopolysaccharide via regulating microRNA-223. *Biomed. Pharmacother* **2018**, *104*, 509–519. [CrossRef]

69. Huang, W.; Lan, X.; Li, X.; Wang, D.; Sun, Y.; Wang, Q.; Gao, H.; Yu, K. Long non-coding RNA PVT1 promote LPS-induced septic acute kidney injury by regulating TNFalpha and JNK/NF-kappaB pathways in HK-2 cells. *Int. Immunopharmacol.* **2017**, *47*, 134–140. [CrossRef]

70. Mimura, I.; Hirakawa, Y.; Kanki, Y.; Kushida, N.; Nakaki, R.; Suzuki, Y.; Tanaka, T.; Aburatani, H.; Nangaku, M. Novel lnc RNA regulated by HIF-1 inhibits apoptotic cell death in the renal tubular epithelial cells under hypoxia. *Physiol. Rep.* **2017**, *5*. [CrossRef]

71. Chen, Y.; Qiu, J.; Chen, B.; Lin, Y.; Xie, G.; Tong, H.; Jiang, D. Long non-coding RNA NEAT1 plays an important role in sepsis-induced acute kidney injury by targeting miR-204 and modulating the NF-kappaB pathway. *Int. Immunopharmacol.* **2018**, *59*, 252–260. [CrossRef] [PubMed]

72. Jiang, X.; Li, D.; Shen, W.; Shen, X.; Liu, Y. LncRNA NEAT1 promotes hypoxia-induced renal tubular epithelial apoptosis through downregulating miR-27a-3p. *J. Cell Biochem.* **2019**. [CrossRef]

73. Liu, X.; Hong, C.; Wu, S.; Song, S.; Yang, Z.; Cao, L.; Song, T.; Yang, Y. Downregulation of lncRNA TUG1 contributes to the development of sepsis-associated acute kidney injury via regulating miR-142-3p/sirtuin 1 axis and modulating NF-kappaB pathway. *J. Cell Biochem.* **2019**. [CrossRef] [PubMed]

74. Jiang, Z.J.; Zhang, M.Y.; Fan, Z.W.; Sun, W.L.; Tang, Y. Influence of lncRNA HOTAIR on acute kidney injury in sepsis rats through regulating miR-34a/Bcl-2 pathway. *Eur Rev. Med. Pharm. Sci.* **2019**, *23*, 3512–3519. [CrossRef]

75. Lorenzen, J.M.; Schauerte, C.; Kielstein, J.T.; Hübner, A.; Martino, F.; Fiedler, J.; Gupta, S.K.; Faulhaber-Walter, R.; Kumarswamy, R.; Hafer, C.; et al. Circulating long noncoding RNATapSaki is a predictor of mortality in critically ill patients with acute kidney injury. *Inj. Clin. Chem.* **2015**, *61*, 191–201. [CrossRef] [PubMed]

76. Qin, J.; Ning, H.; Zhou, Y.; Hu, Y.; Huang, B.; Wu, Y.; Huang, R. LncRNA Uc.173 is a key molecule for the regulation of lead-induced renal tubular epithelial cell apoptosis. *Biomed. Pharm.* **2018**, *100*, 101–107. [CrossRef] [PubMed]

77. Nan, A.; Zhou, X.; Chen, L.; Liu, M.; Zhang, N.; Zhang, L.; Luo, Y.; Liu, Z.; Dai, L.; Jiang, Y. A transcribed ultraconserved noncoding RNA, Uc.173, is a key molecule for the inhibition of lead-induced neuronal apoptosis. *Oncotarget* **2016**, *7*, 112–124. [CrossRef]

78. Chen, W.; Zhou, Z.Q.; Ren, Y.Q.; Zhang, L.; Sun, L.N.; Man, Y.L.; Wang, Z.K. Effects of long non-coding RNA LINC00667 on renal tubular epithelial cell proliferation, apoptosis and renal fibrosis via the miR-19b-3p/LINC00667/CTGF signaling pathway in chronic renal failure. *Cell Signal.* **2019**, *54*, 102–114. [CrossRef]

79. Chen, W.; Zhang, L.; Zhou, Z.Q.; Ren, Y.Q.; Sun, L.N.; Man, Y.L.; Ma, Z.W.; Wang, Z.K. Effects of Long Non-Coding RNA LINC00963 on Renal Interstitial Fibrosis and Oxidative Stress of Rats with Chronic Renal Failure via the Foxo Signaling Pathway. *Cell Physiol. Biochem.* **2018**, *46*, 815–828. [CrossRef]

80. Aboudehen, K.; Farahani, S.; Kanchwala, M.; Chan, S.C.; Avdulov, S.; Mickelson, A.; Lee, D.; Gearhart, M.D.; Patel, V.; Xing, C.; et al. Long noncoding RNA Hoxb3os is dysregulated in autosomal dominant polycystic kidney disease and regulates mTOR signaling. *J. Biol. Chem.* **2018**, *293*, 9388–9398. [CrossRef]

81. Song, Z.; Zhang, Y.; Gong, B.; Xu, H.; Hao, Z.; Liang, C. Long noncoding RNA LINC00339 promotes renal tubular epithelial pyroptosis by regulating the miR-22-3p/NLRP3 axis in calcium oxalate-induced kidney stone. *J. Cell Biochem.* **2019**, *120*, 10452–10462. [CrossRef] [PubMed]

82. Zhang, C.; Yuan, J.; Hu, H.; Chen, W.; Liu, M.; Zhang, J.; Sun, S.; Guo, Z. Long non-coding RNA CHCHD4P4 promotes epithelial-mesenchymal transition and inhibits cell proliferation in calcium oxalate-induced kidney damage. *Braz. J. Med. Biol. Res.* **2017**, *51*, e6536. [CrossRef] [PubMed]

83. Hu, J.; Wu, H.; Wang, D.; Yang, Z.; Dong, J. LncRNA ANRIL promotes NLRP3 inflammasome activation in uric acid nephropathy through miR-122-5p/BRCC3 axis. *Biochimie* **2019**, *157*, 102–110. [CrossRef] [PubMed]

84. Van der Hauwaert, C.; Glowacki, F.; Pottier, N.; Cauffiez, C. Non-Coding RNAs as New Therapeutic Targets in the Context of Renal Fibrosis. *Int. J. Mol. Sci.* **2019**, *20*, 1977. [CrossRef] [PubMed]

85. Moe, O.W. Kidney stones: Pathophysiology and medical management. *Lancet* **2006**, *367*, 333–344. [CrossRef]

86. Wang, Z.; Zhang, J.W.; Zhang, Y.; Zhang, S.P.; Hu, Q.Y.; Liang, H. Analyses of long non-coding RNA and mRNA profiling using RNA sequencing in calcium oxalate monohydrate-stimulated renal tubular epithelial cells. *Urolithiasis* **2019**, *47*, 225–234. [CrossRef] [PubMed]

87. Cao, Y.; Gao, X.; Yang, Y.; Ye, Z.; Wang, E.; Dong, Z. Changing expression profiles of long non-coding RNAs, mRNAs and circular RNAs in ethylene glycol-induced kidney calculi rats. *BMC Genom.* **2018**, *19*, 660. [CrossRef]

88. Wan, L.; Dreyfuss, G. Splicing-Correcting Therapy for SMA. *Cell* **2017**, *170*, 5. [CrossRef]

89. Benson, M.D.; Waddington-Cruz, M.; Berk, J.L.; Polydefkis, M.; Dyck, P.J.; Wang, A.K.; Plante-Bordeneuve, V.; Barroso, F.A.; Merlini, G.; Obici, L.; et al. Inotersen Treatment for Patients with Hereditary Transthyretin Amyloidosis. *N. Engl. J. Med.* **2018**, *379*, 22–31. [CrossRef]

90. Adams, D.; Gonzalez-Duarte, A.; O'Riordan, W.D.; Yang, C.C.; Ueda, M.; Kristen, A.V.; Tournev, I.; Schmidt, H.H.; Coelho, T.; Berk, J.L.; et al. Patisiran, an RNAi Therapeutic, for Hereditary Transthyretin Amyloidosis. *N. Engl. J. Med.* **2018**, *379*, 11–21. [CrossRef]

91. Park, J.; Shrestha, R.; Qiu, C.; Kondo, A.; Huang, S.; Werth, M.; Li, M.; Barasch, J.; Susztak, K. Single-cell transcriptomics of the mouse kidney reveals potential cellular targets of kidney disease. *Science* **2018**, *360*, 758–763. [CrossRef] [PubMed]

92. Karaiskos, N.; Rahmatollahi, M.; Boltengagen, A.; Liu, H.; Hoehne, M.; Rinschen, M.; Schermer, B.; Benzing, T.; Rajewsky, N.; Kocks, C.; et al. A Single-Cell Transcriptome Atlas of the Mouse Glomerulus. *J. Am. Soc. Nephrol.* **2018**, *29*, 2060–2068. [CrossRef] [PubMed]

93. Fu, J.; Akat, K.M.; Sun, Z.; Zhang, W.; Schlondorff, D.; Liu, Z.; Tuschl, T.; Lee, K.; He, J.C. Single-Cell RNA Profiling of Glomerular Cells Shows Dynamic Changes in Experimental Diabetic Kidney Disease. *J. Am. Soc. Nephrol.* **2019**, *30*, 533–545. [CrossRef] [PubMed]

94. Wu, H.; Kirita, Y.; Donnelly, E.L.; Humphreys, B.D. Advantages of Single-Nucleus over Single-Cell RNA Sequencing of Adult Kidney: Rare Cell Types and Novel Cell States Revealed in Fibrosis. *J. Am. Soc. Nephrol.* **2019**, *30*, 23–32. [CrossRef] [PubMed]

95. Der, E.; Ranabothu, S.; Suryawanshi, H.; Akat, K.M.; Clancy, R.; Morozov, P.; Kustagi, M.; Czuppa, M.; Izmirly, P.; Belmont, H.M.; et al. Single cell RNA sequencing to dissect the molecular heterogeneity in lupus nephritis. *JCI Insight* **2017**, *2*. [CrossRef] [PubMed]

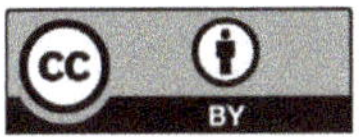

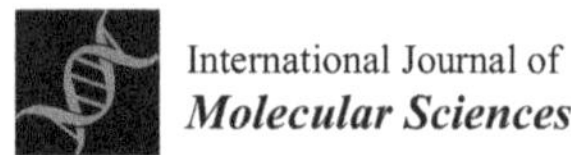

International Journal of
Molecular Sciences

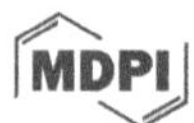

Review

Molecular Mechanisms of Kidney Injury and Repair in Arterial Hypertension

Laura Katharina Sievers [1,2,3,4,*] and Kai-Uwe Eckardt [1]

[1] Department of Nephrology and Medical Intensive Care, Charité-Universitätsmedizin Berlin, 13353 Berlin, Germany; kai-uwe.eckardt@charite.de
[2] Max-Delbrück Center for Molecular Medicine in the Helmholtz Association, 13125 Berlin, Germany
[3] Experimental and Clinical Research Center, a joint cooperation of Max-Delbrück Center for Molecular Medicine and Charité-Universitätsmedizin Berlin, 13125 Berlin, Germany
[4] Berlin Institute of Health (BIH), 10178 Berlin, Germany
[*] Correspondence: laura-katharina.sievers@charite.de

Received: 27 March 2019; Accepted: 28 April 2019; Published: 30 April 2019

Abstract: The global burden of chronic kidney disease is rising. The etiologies, heterogeneous, and arterial hypertension, are key factors contributing to the development and progression of chronic kidney disease. Arterial hypertension is induced and maintained by a complex network of systemic signaling pathways, such as the hormonal axis of the renin-angiotensin-aldosterone system, hemodynamic alterations affecting blood flow, oxygen supply, and the immune system. This review summarizes the clinical and histopathological features of hypertensive kidney injury and focusses on the interplay of distinct systemic signaling pathways, which drive hypertensive kidney injury in distinct cell types of the kidney. There are several parallels between hypertension-induced molecular signaling cascades in the renal epithelial, endothelial, interstitial, and immune cells. Angiotensin II signaling via the AT1R, hypoxia induced HIFα activation and mechanotransduction are closely interacting and further triggering the adaptions of metabolism, cytoskeletal rearrangement, and profibrotic TGF signaling. The interplay of these, and other cellular pathways, is crucial to balancing the injury and repair of the kidneys and determines the progression of hypertensive kidney disease.

Keywords: hypertension; kidney; molecular signaling

---

1. Introduction

Arterial hypertension has a large prevalence in the general population and is associated with a wide range of cardiovascular complications and chronic damage to the heart, brain, vasculature, eyes, kidney, and other organs. Hypertensive nephropathy is regarded as the second leading cause of end-stage renal disease (ESRD), outnumbered only by diabetic nephropathy. However, in many cases, it is hard to determine the primary underlying cause of chronic kidney disease (CKD). Arterial hypertension is a typical complication of CKD, irrespective of its etiology, and it is often difficult to differentiate whether increased blood pressure is the cause and/or consequence of impaired kidney function. In any case, coexisting arterial hypertension accelerates the progression of CKD and increases the cardiovascular risk in CKD patients [1]. The clinical course and histopathological characteristics of kidney injury in hypertensive kidney disease may vary, not only on comorbidities, but also in environmental factors and genetic predisposition. For example, patients of black ethnicity are at a much higher risk for rapidly progressing CKD. Given the importance of hypertension for the course of kidney disease, a thorough understanding of the molecular mechanisms of kidney injury and repair, in arterial hypertension, appears fundamental to the development of novel approaches against the progression of CKD worldwide. With the increasing availability of novel therapeutic strategies targeting molecular pathways, a classification of CKD, based on the predominant molecular pathology, rather than clinical correlations/etiologies might become a promising approach in the future.

Arterial hypertension is caused and sustained by a complex network of systemic signaling pathways. The renin-angiotensin-aldosterone-system (RAAS) is one important hormonal axis in hypertension. In addition, several other hormones, such as corticosteroids, catecholamines, thyroid hormones, sex hormones, and others contribute to the regulation of blood pressure. Furthermore, it has been shown that the immune system plays an important role in the development and maintenance of hypertension. For example, the balance between IL17 producing T lymphocytes (Th17) and regulatory T cells (Treg) is dysequilibrated in hypertensive patients, favoring Th17 cells. Other conditions favoring Th17 cells can drive hypertension. In this review we aim to provide a brief overview of clinical and histopathological characteristics of kidney injury in hypertensive kidney disease, and of the systemic signaling pathways and important aspects of the immune system, in arterial hypertension. Moreover, we will describe molecular mechanisms in hypertensive kidney injury and repair, including angiotensin II (Ang II) signaling in different cell types, hypoxia signaling, distinct pro-inflammatory pathways, and TGF-associated profibrotic signaling.

2. Clinical and Histopathological Characteristics of Kidney Injury in Arterial Hypertension

"Hypertensive nephropathy", also known as "hypertensive nephrosclerosis", is traditionally characterized by a combination of pathological changes of the pre- and intra-glomerular microvasculature and the tubulointerstitium. The histopathology can hardly distinguish whether arterial hypertension is the primary cause of kidney dysfunction or whether increased blood pressure occurs as a comorbidity, which drives CKD progression. Thus, the term hypertensive nephropathy summarizes both conditions. The severity of blood pressure elevation often correlates with the degree of renal damage. In many cases, hypertensive nephrosclerosis shows a slow progression, which is historically classified as "benign nephrosclerosis". In contrast, accelerated nephrosclerosis, histopathologically characterized by fibrinoid necrosis and/or myointimal cell proliferation, is classified as "malignant nephrosclerosis" and frequently leads to ESRD [2]. Hypertension-induced kidney damage involves different cell types and anatomical structures in the kidney, including the vasculature, glomeruli, tubulointerstitium, and immune cells. The muscular arteries and arterioles of the kidney parenchyma show progressive intimal thickening during aging, but besides age this process correlates with arterial hypertension [3]. The thickening is caused by collagen deposition and spreading of elastic fibers and myofibroblasts, and ultimately leads to more pulsatile blood flow in kidney arterioles [3]. Another histopathological characteristic of hypertensive nephrosclerosis is arteriosclerosis of the afferent arterioles, also referred to as "afferent arteriolar hyalinosis". These typical hyaline deposits are the consequence of a pathogenetic cascade of atrophy of vascular smooth muscle cells, increased endothelial leakiness and plasma protein extravasation, leading to sub-endothelial protein accumulation [3]. Although this process is associated with hypertension, to some extent, it occurs in all aging kidneys [3]. The glomerular involvement is heterogeneous; there is a side-by-side normal morphology, ischemic, obliterated glomeruli, with collapsed capillaries and focal-segmental-glomerular sclerosis-(FSGS)-like lesions, with partially sclerotic glomerular adhesions.

Another hallmark of hypertensive kidney injury is tubular atrophy, accompanied by interstitial fibrosis. Following a loss of functional nephrons, the surviving nephrons initially maintain total kidney function, but the concomitant hemodynamic adaptations results in an oxygen supply-demand mismatch and ultimately tubulointerstitial hypoxia [4]. Tubulointerstitial hypoxia presumably contributes to the progression of tubular damage and renal functional impairment [5,6]. This relative hypoxia is further aggravated by impaired oxygen delivery to the kidneys during hypertension, due to vasoconstriction hormones, including components of the RAAS, prostaglandins, and endothelin [5]. During the course of CKD, the loss of peritubular capillaries further aggravates tubulointerstitial hypoxia and damage. Hypoxic conditions trigger mitochondrial dysfunction [4] and can activate the transcription factor hypoxia-inducible factor (HIF) [7]. The signaling pathways which promote a maladaptive phenotype at the cellular level will be discussed below. Besides the characteristic vascular adaptations and glomerular pathology, kidney histology of hypertensive nephrosclerosis may also show trans-differentiation and apoptosis of tubular cells, increased peritubular fibrosis, fibroblasts proliferation, and increased interstitial inflammation.

3. Systemic Signaling Pathways and the Immune System in Arterial Hypertension

For decades, the pathophysiology of arterial hypertension has primarily been attributed to vasoconstriction hormones, including RAAS (Figure 1), prostaglandins, and endothelin 1 (ET1). Among these hormonal axes, the RAAS has received particular attention, and was shown to have a crucial influence on blood pressure and target organ damage. This important signaling axis includes several components that are activated stepwise: First, the 452 amino acid peptide pro-hormone angiotensinogen, which is synthesized and excreted by the liver, is cleaved to the ten amino acid peptide Angiotensin I by the protease renin (Figure 1). Angiotensin (Ang) I is then cleaved to the eight amino acid peptide hormone, Ang II, by angiotensin converting enzyme (ACE) (Figure 1). Although, the pro-hormone Ang I and other metabolites of angiontensinogen, such as Ang 1–7, which result from cleavage by other proteases, have effects on the vascular endothelia and other tissues. Here, we will focus on the canonical RAAS signaling and biological effects of Ang II. Ang II binds to the Ang II-receptor 1 (AT1R) in different cell types [8]: In the vasculature, Ang II leads to vasoconstriction and in the adrenal cortex, it increases the secretion of aldosterone (Figure 1). In the kidney, Ang II leads to tubular retention of NaCl and water (Figure 1). Further, Ang II increases the sympathetic activity, which also elevates blood pressure (Figure 1). The systemic vascular tone results from the interplay of many different vasoconstricting and vasodilating stimuli. Within this complex interplay, the pathophysiological relevance of the RAAS for blood pressure regulation is underlined by the clinical significance of RAAS inhibition. State-of-the-art clinical management of arterial hypertension includes, pharmacological targeting of the RAAS with ACE-inhibitors, AT1R blockers, direct renin inhibitors, and aldosterone antagonists [9]. The important pathophysiological contribution and clinical relevance of the RAAS, beyond blood pressure control, is underlined by the fact that treatment with ACE-inhibitors or AT1R blockers shows significant clinical benefits for cardiovascular morbidity and mortality.

ET1 expression may be regulated by inflammatory mediators, shear stress, and glucose. ET1 has an ambiguous role on the vascular tone. Binding of ET1 to the ET1 receptor A (ETA) of vascular smooth muscle cells causes vasoconstriction, while binding to the ET1 receptor B (ETB) has an indirect vasodilating effect via increased release of nitric oxide (NO). ETA antagonists are clinically used in pulmonary arterial hypertension. Further, ETA antagonists may slow the progression of diabetic nephropathy, but until recently, ET1 antagonists are not licensed in arterial hypertension. Sympathetic activity may be induced by central nervous regulation associated with stress, pain, or cold, It is affected by the RAAS and modifies peripheral resistance. In the last years, several non-pharmacological approaches addressing the autonomic nervous system in arterial hypertension have been developed. Renal sympathetic denervation, carotid baroreflex activation therapy, central iliac arteriovenous anastomosis, carotid body ablation, median nerve stimulation, vagal nerve stimulation, and deep brain stimulation continue to be evaluated with respect to their capacity to lower blood pressure and blood pressure associated target organ damage [10].

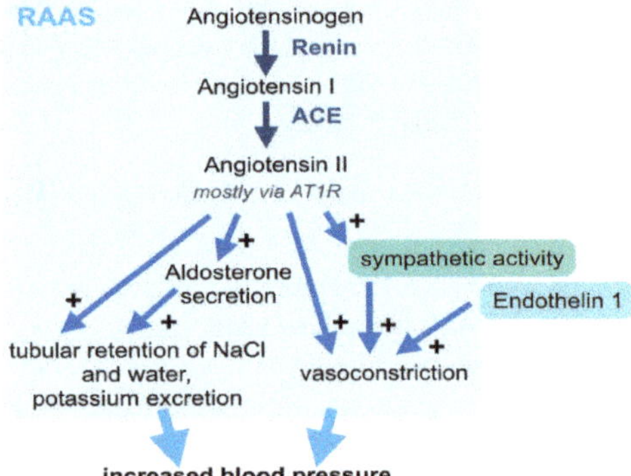

Figure 1. The renin-angiotensin-aldosterone system (RAAS) is a key hormonal axis in the pathogenesis of arterial hypertension. The RAAS combines a regulatory network, including angiotensin II (Ang II) and aldosterone, which increase systemic blood pressure through a concerted mechanism. Angiotensinogen is enzymatically cleaved by renin and angiotensin-converting enzyme (ACE) to generate Angiotensin II, which, mainly via the Ang II receptor 1 (AT1R), stimulates the secretion of aldosterone, acts as a vasoconstrictor and leads to renal tubular retention of NaCl and water. For simplification, the negative feedback loop, which physiologically limits an excess activation of these pathways, is not included in this graph. Besides Ang II, endothelin 1 and increased sympathetic activity, which may be induced by RAAS activation or independent stimuli, also contribute to systemic vasoconstriction and increased peripheral resistance.

Carotid baroreflex activation therapy resulted in a sustained reduction of arterial blood pressure in patients with resistant hypertension in the Rheos Pivotal Trial [11]. Since renal sympathetic over-activity is associated with the pathogenesis and progression of arterial hypertension and CKD, catheter-based renal denervation has been a promising approach in reducing blood pressure and attenuating renal functional decline in hypertensive CKD [12]. Further, meta-analyses have shown beneficial effects in patients with heart failure [12]. After promising animal studies and early trials in patients, subsequent clinical studies could not replicate the positive outcome [12–14]. There are ongoing trials, which aim to resolve the conflicting evidence and to provide data on the long-term safety and efficacy of renal denervation [15–18].

Besides the hormonal and autonomous axes, immune mechanisms play an important role in the pathogenesis of arterial hypertension by contributing to both, the development of hypertension and of hypertensive end-organ damage (Figure 2). CD4+ lymphocytes are key cell types involved in the balance between Treg and Th17 cells, which originate from naive CD4+ cells under specific skewing conditions. Several drivers of hypertension, including Ang II-induced signaling, dietary NaCl, the gut microbiome, at least partly exert their effect via immune mechanisms, and in particular, the regulation of the Treg/Th17 balance (Figure 2). Th17 cells are associated with hypertension and hypertensive end-organ damage, while a protective role is attributed to Treg. For example, it has been shown that Treg deficiency exaggerated Ang II-induced microvascular injury by enhancing immune responses [19]. Ang II was a driver of Treg infiltration in the aortic wall and renal cortex and, in a model of Treg deficient mice, the adoptive transfer of Treg cells prevented Ang II-induced hypertension and vascular injury [20]. Further, it has been demonstrated that Ang II increased the secretion of the pro- inflammatory cytokine IL17 by Th17 cells and that the activation Th17 cells in response to high salt was associated with accelerated fibrosis [21]. Notably, the cytokine IL17 has a differentiated function in diabetic kidney disease: Ablation of intrarenal Th17 cells ameliorated early diabetic nephropathy [22], while the administration of low-dose IL17A had beneficial effects [23]. The ambiguity of IL17 signaling in hypertensive kidney disease remains to be elucidated. Interestingly, the induction of Th17 cells seems to depend on gut microbiota, particularly salt-sensitive lactobacilli.

Increased dietary salt depleted these microbiota, increased Th17 cells, and increased the blood pressure in mice and humans [24]. Besides salt intake, intestinal metabolites, such as the short-chain fatty acid propionate have quantitative effects on the systemic composition of immune cell subsets and blood pressure [25] (Figure 2). Intracellular pathways, that balance the differentiation of Treg and Th17 include. TGFβ, IL6, RORγT, Hippo/TAZ, and HIF-1. All these pathways are directly influenced by Ang II/AT1R signaling. Besides the prominent role of the Treg/Th17 cells in hypertensive end-organ damage, innate immune cells contribute to hypertensive mechanisms. Neutrophils, monocytes/macrophages, dendritic cells, myeloid-derived suppressor cells and innate lymphoid cells may trigger both, blood pressure elevation on the one hand, and profibrotic inflammatory processes in end-organs on the other hand [26]. Innate and adaptive immune mechanisms closely interact in the pathogenesis of hypertension and hypertensive organ damage. For example, monocyte/macrophages and γδ T cells seem to play a crucial role in the initiation of hypertension by priming adaptive immune cells, thereby triggering vascular inflammation and blood pressure elevation or, if their signaling limits the inflammatory response, protecting against vascular injury [26].

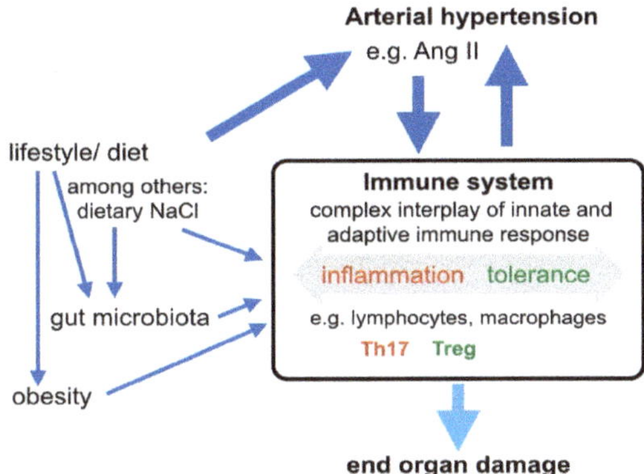

Figure 2. The immune system closely interacts with hormonal and environmental modifiers to control blood pressure. The immune system plays an important role in the pathogenesis of arterial hypertension and hypertensive end-organ damage. Lifestyle factors, such as the dietary nutrient composition and sodium intake directly, and via alterations in the gut microbiome, have influence on the cellular compositions of the immune system. Distinct immune cell subtypes, such as IL17 producing Th17 lymphocytes contribute to increased blood pressure. In parallel, existing arterial hypertension and Ang II favor Th17 polarization of T lymphocytes. Besides the effect of immune cells on blood pressure, the balance of various cells from the adaptive and innate immune system, including lymphocytes and macrophages is critical for end organ damage.

4. Molecular Mechanisms in Hypertensive Kidney Injury

Many different anatomical parts of the kidney, with distinct cell types, are affected by hypertensive kidney injury: Cells forming the nephron, including glomerular podocytes and tubular cells, the vasculature with endothelium and smooth muscle cells, interstital fibroblasts and resident, as well as circulating immune cells of adaptive and innate immune response, are involved (Figure 3). Although novel techniques, such as genome-wide association studies, single cell proteomics or deep sequencing are on the brink of their application in clinical studies, detailed reports scrutinizing cell-type specific molecular mechanisms of hypertensive kidney injury are still missing [27,28]. When subsequently discussing important molecular mechanisms in hypertensive kidney injury and repair, we will focus on the molecular signaling pathways of Ang II signaling, hypoxia, pro- inflammatory signaling, TGF, and profibrotic pathways. Although, the net effect of mechanisms promoting injury and repair is highly cell type- and context-dependent, there are several parallels with regard to the involved molecular signaling pathways across different cell types (Figure 3).

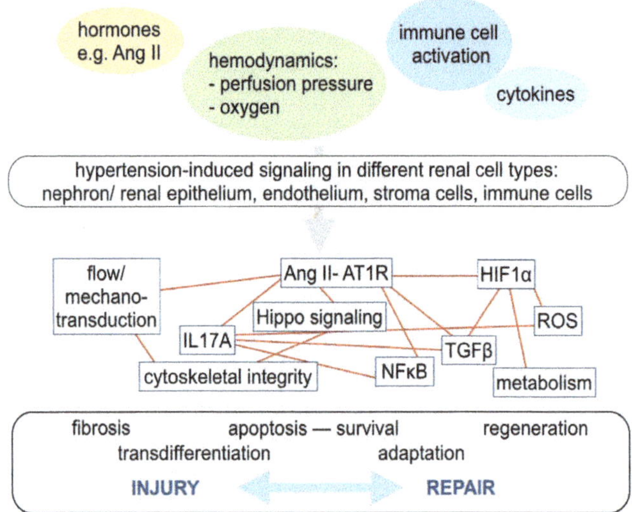

Figure 3. A complex network of various molecular pathways contributes to cellular adaptions, injury, and regenerative capacity in hypertensive kidney injury. In arterial hypertension, the cells in the kidney are exposed to various extracellular stimuli, including hormones, such as Ang II, altered hemodynamics with increased perfusion pressure, and potentially decreased oxygen supply and activated immune cells, which in turn secrete different cytokines. These stimuli affect all renal cell types: Nephron forming renal epithelial cells, endothelial cells, stroma, and immune cells. Although the net effect on injury and repair is highly cell type- and context-dependent, there are several parallels regarding the involved molecular signaling pathways. These pathways, or rather, signaling networks, are highly interrelated. For example, AT1R-mediated Ang II signaling, the Hippo pathway, pro- inflammatory signaling, including IL17 secretion and activation of TGFβ associated profibrotic signaling closely interact. Mechano-transduction and Hippo signaling, among others, influence the cytoskeletal integrity. Hypoxia-inducible factor (HIF) is stabilized by hypoxia, induces metabolic adaptions and may increase TGFβ- associated profibrotic pathways.

The peptide hormone Ang II is an important mediator in the pathophysiology of arterial hypertension, hypertensive end-organ damage, and also hypertensive kidney injury. The AT1R is expressed in various cell types, including podocytes, renal tubular cells, and immune cells. Further, Ang II exerts indirect effects via changes of the glomerular hemodynamics, leading to increased filtration pressure, increased filtration of NaCl and consecutive adaptations of the tubular salt and water handling. Furthermore, Ang II from the systemic circulation increases the tubular expression of angiotensinogen, ACE, renin and AT1R [29]. This feed-forward loop mechanism is at least partly driven by cytokines produced by activated T lymphocytes such as IL6 and IFNγ [30]. Consistent with the prominent glomerular histopathology and the clinical presentation of albuminuria in hypertensive kidney injury, elevated levels of Ang II lead to severe injury of glomerular podocytes with foot process effacement and ultimately podocyte loss. Podocyte depletion is an irreversible hallmark of glomerular injury in CKD, and the beneficial effect of Ang II blockade on the progression of hypertensive CKD correlates with attenuated podocyte loss [31]. Ang II causes podocyte injury via several pathways. Binding of Ang II to the G-protein-coupled AT1R activates an intracellular cascade of kinases, including the activation of phospholipase C, calcium-calmodulin binding, phosphorylation of the protein kinases extracellular-signal regulated kinases (ERK), ribosomal S6 kinase (RSK), protein kinase C (PKC), protein kinase A (PKA), and the activation of adenylate cyclase leading to the generation of cyclic AMP. Already decades ago, it has been demonstrated that a sustained intracellular rise in calcium, as induced by Ang II, has detrimental effects on podocyte viability [32,33]. The calcium influx may be aggravated by simultaneously increased expression of calcium channels, such as TRPC6 [34]. Further, Ang II signaling in podocytes is closely linked to the integrity of the actin cytoskeleton. It has been shown that short term treatment with Ang II regulates the phosphorylation of various actin-associated proteins in podocytes and that e.g., the increased phosphorylation of lymphocyte cytosolic protein 1 (LCP1) leads to alterations in actin bundling, increased filopodia and lamellipodia formation, and membrane ruffling [35]. Besides the regulation of intracellular cytoskeletal components, Ang II has a direct impact on nephrin, a fundamental extracellular adaptor protein crosslinking podocyte at the slit diaphragm. In models of Ang II induced hypertension and kidney injury, nephrin is dephosphorylated in a caveolin-1- [36] and c-Abl [37]-dependent way, ultimately leading to the disintegration of the slit diaphragm. Interestingly, it has been shown that Ang II also regulates the Hippo pathway, a conserved signaling pathway controlling cell proliferation and cell death via a kinase cascade, that regulates the nuclear shuttling of the transcription factors YAP and TAZ. Ang II inactivated the Hippo pathway by decreasing the activity of LATS kinase, consequently increasing the nuclear abundance of the transcription factor YAP in Human Embryonic Kidney cells [38] and TAZ is activated in the tubulointerstitium in mouse models of kidney injury [39]. At the same time, Ang II effects on YAP/TAZ were absent in podocytes, which are postmitotic cells with low baseline Hippo pathway activity [38]. Further, Ang II/AT1R signaling modifies the lipid metabolism and induced lipid droplet accumulation and expression of lipid droplet marker protein in podocytes [40]. The effects of Ang II on renal cells have been extensively studied, but the interrelation of different signaling networks is still not completely understood. Further, Ang II affects the infiltration of immune cells. AT1R signaling drives the differentiation of CD4 lymphocytes to Th17 cells: Silencing of AT1R with siRNA reduced the fraction of Th17 polarized cells and IL17 expression while Ang II treatment increased the secretion of the pro-inflammatory cytokine IL17 by Th17 [21] wheras, in the presence of ACE inhibition with lisinopril, Foxp3 positive Treg were enhanced [41]. Besides the significance of Th17/Treg cells for the development and progression of arterial hypertension and hypertensive end-organ damage, γδ T-cells contribute to Ang II-induced elevation of blood pressure, endothelial dysfunction, and the activation of innate and adaptive immune response [42]. Further, Ang II increased monocyte chemotactic protein-1 expression in the vasculature, accompanied by higher monocyte/macrophage infiltration and pro-inflammatory macrophage polarization in the renal cortex [19]. Ang II also acts as a pro-fibrogenic cytokine regulating renal cell proliferation, synthesis and degradation of the extracellular matrix by various pathways, e.g., TGFβ [43].

TGFβ is secreted by many different cell types, including monocytes/macrophages, and a key function is the regulation of inflammatory processes and profibrotic signaling. Increased systemic levels of TGFβ are associated with faster CKD progression and TGFβ polymorphisms have been identified as risk factors for ESRD [44,45]. However, the effect of TGFβ is highly context-dependent. Ang II induces the expression of the TGFβ downstream target connective tissue growth factor β (CTGF), which is associated with endothelial mesenchymal transition. The profibrotic action of Ang II may be aggravated by interaction with other pathways such as hypoxia, the activation of plasminogen activator inhibitor-1, or ET1 signaling. Interestingly, the Hippo pathway transcription factor, TAZ, was activated in the renal tubulointerstitium in different models of kidney injury. Nuclear accumulation of TAZ depended on TGFβ1-signaling and went along with fibrosis progression [39]. M2 macrophage polarization, which significantly correlates with kidney fibrosis, is driven by TGFβ1-induced activation of YAP/TAZ, too [46]. The action of bone morphogenetic protein (BMP), which also belongs to the TGF protein family, in the kidney is not completely understood. In healthy renal tubules, BMP is constitutively active and its reactivation, after an injury that suppressed BMP expression, correlates with functional recovery [47].

Ang II, ET1 and catecholamines both exert their function via G-protein coupled receptors (GPCRs), such as the AT1R, ETA, ETA and b-adrenergic receptors. Current pharmacological approaches mainly target these GPCRs. The sensitivity of hormone-induced GPCR activation is modified by G-protein coupled receptor kinases (GRKs), and the regulator of G-Protein Signaling proteins [48]. It has been demonstrated that the dysregulation of the GRK isoforms 2–6 correlates with increased blood pressure, poor response to antihypertensive treatment, and adverse cardiovascular outcomes [49]. Renal fibrosis could be alleviated by the inhibition of the G-protein βγ-subunit in mouse models of cardiorenal syndrome and ischemic acute kidney injury [50]. Further, inhibition of the downstream kinase PKA may reduce profibrotic signaling and profibrogenic epigenetic priming in diabetic kidney disease [51]. Pharmacological modification of GPCR downstream targets may be a promising approach in hypertensive CKD.

Another important mechanism, contributing to hypertensive nephrosclerosis, is hypoxia (Figure 3). Chronic ischemic tubulointerstitial damage, caused by altered hemodynamics, increased oxygen demand, and loss of peritubular capillaries is a hallmark of progressive CKD. Under hypoxic conditions, HIF, and its oxygen-regulated isoforms, HIF1α and HIF2α, are stabilized and promote cellular adaptation to the decreased oxygen supply and influence cell proliferation, survival and metabolism. The increased expression of HIF1α was reported to correlate with glomerular injury and promote hypertensive CKD [52]. HIF1α gene expression in renal endothelia was induced by Ang II in a Nuclear Factor-κB (NFκB)-dependent manner [52]. It has also been shown, that reciprocal positive transcriptional regulation leads to persistent activation of HIF1α and NFκB genes and drives disease progression [52]. The profibrotic action of HIF1α is partly mediated via induction of TGFβ and its proinflammatory downstream target CTGF [53]. Interestingly, HIF2α, which is primarily expressed in non-epithelial cells is associated with ambiguous effects on renal fibrosis: In early stages of CKD, activation of HIF2α worsened renal fibrosis but did not lead to renal functional impairment [54]. In another study, overexpression of HIF2α was sufficient to induce kidney fibrosis [55]. At later stages of CKD, HIF2α activation, in part, activated typical hypoxia-induced target genes of HIF1α such as VEGF, fibronectin, and type 1 collagen but restored the renal vasculature and thereby ameliorated renal dysfunction and fibrosis [54].

Besides the development of hypoxia, the hemodynamic changes associated with a defective renal autoregulation of blood pressure, during hypertensive nephropathy, and other types of chronic kidney disease, are associated with flow- and shear-stress dependent signaling in endothelial cells (Figure 3). In response to increased blood flow, endothelial cells release ATP, which in turn activates endothelial cells or adjacent immune cells, in a paracrine fashion via trinucleotide-receptors, from the ionotropic P2X and metabotropic P2Y receptor family. For example, hypertension correlates with overexpression and activation of the P2 × 7, P2Y12, and P2X1 receptors [56]. The blockade of these receptors inhibits renal vasoconstriction induced by Ang II, restores microvascular dysfunction, and improves the Ang II-associated regional hypoxia [56,57]. In addition to the microvascular implications, the release of inflammatory mediators, such as interleukins in the tubulointerstitium seems to be related to the activation of P2X/P2Y receptors [56]. Secondly, the increased filtration pressure may lead to higher urinary flow and flow-activated signaling pathways in tubular cells, which may lose epithelial characteristics, such as the in the expression of cell junctional proteins [58]. CKD goes along with secretion of pro-inflammatory cytokines by activated immune cells, interstitial cells, and tubular epithelial cells [59]. For example, hypertensive kidney injury correlates with phosphorylation of the cytoskeleton-associated protein cofilin 1, formation of actin stress fibers, nuclear translocation of NFκB and expression of downstream inflammatory factors in renal tubular epithelial cells. [59].

Further, infiltration of IL17 secreting T lymphocytes may lead to vascular dysfunction. IL17 acts on vascular smooth muscle cells and perivascular fibroblasts, in order to increase reactive oxygen species (ROS) production, collagen synthesis, and chemokine production. In parallel, IL 17 reduces the bioavailability of NO and, vasodilatation, enhances vascular stiffness and the recruitment of immune cells [30].

5. Approaches to Foster Regeneration and Repair in Hypertensive Nephropathy

Despite recent advances in the understanding of molecular mechanisms, contributing to hypertensive nephropathy, the interplay between the different signaling networks in each cell type and—even more complex—between distinct cell types, is still incompletely deciphered. However, "omics" approaches such as single-cell proteomics and metabolomics, in conjunction with advanced imaging techniques, comprise excellent opportunities to gain further insight into this complex signaling network. So far, clinical management of hypertensive CKD focusses on the deceleration of CKD progression. A major aim is to stop all comorbidities, which are known to drive the progression of hypertensive CKD: Blood pressure should ideally be normalized, blood glucose control should be excellent, dietary salt may be restricted, and nephrotoxic medications are to be avoided. Further, pharmacological Ang II blockade has beneficial effects on the progression of hypertensive end-organ damage. Therapeutic approaches to other signaling pathways, such as HIF stabilization, ET1 blockade, anti-inflammatory therapy or immunosuppression, have so far either not been tested or not proven safe and efficient. In pre-clinical research, stem cell based approaches are evaluated to improve kidney regeneration in CKD. However, in nephrology in general, and especially with regard to hypertensive nephropathy, regenerative medicine techniques are still in their children's shoes. Studies are carried out with embryonic stem cells, mesenchymal stem cells, adipose stem cells, amniotic fluid stem cells, and renal progenitors, but also pluripotent cells. So far, the results from these studies are conflicting. However, even if stem cells and multipotent cells might not directly differentiate and replace damaged cells, they might produce protective and regenerative factors, and thereby enable functional improvement [60,61].

The bench-to-bedside transition of insight into the molecular mechanisms of CKD in hypertensive patients, and also a profound understanding of the molecular pathogenesis of CKD with other/mixed etiology, may lead to the development novel treatment approaches. Classifying CKD, based on the individual predominant molecular pathology, rather than traditional clinical etiologies would be an important step in developing focused molecular treatments. There is still a long way ahead, but once achieved, personalized medicine holds promise in CKD.

Author Contributions: Conceptualization, L.K.S.; data curation of references, L.K.S. and K.-U.E.; writing—original draft preparation, L.K.S.; writing—review and editing, L.K.S. and K.-U.E.; visualization, L.K.S.; supervision, K.-U.E.

Funding: L.K.S was partly funded by the Berlin Institute of Health (BIH), 10178 Berlin, Germany.

Acknowledgments: We acknowledge support from the German Research Foundation (DFG) and the Open Access Publication Fund of Charité–Universitätsmedizin Berlin.

Conflicts of Interest: The authors declare no conflict of interest.

References

1. Scheppach, J.B.; Raff, U.; Toncar, S.; Ritter, C.; Klink, T.; Stork, S.; Wanner, C.; Schlieper, G.; Saritas, T.; Reinartz, S.D.; et al. Blood Pressure Pattern and Target Organ Damage in Patients with Chronic Kidney Disease. *Hypertension* **2018**, *72*, 929–936. [CrossRef] [PubMed]

2. Liang, S.; Le, W.; Liang, D.; Chen, H.; Xu, F.; Chen, H.; Liu, Z.; Zeng, C. Clinico-pathological characteristics and outcomes of patients with biopsy-proven hypertensive nephrosclerosis: A retrospective cohort study. *BMC Nephrol.* **2016**, *17*, 42. [CrossRef]

3. Hill, G.S. Hypertensive nephrosclerosis. *Curr. Opin. Nephrol. Hypertens.* **2008**, *17*, 266–270. [CrossRef]

4. Thomas, J.L.; Pham, H.; Li, Y.; Hall, E.; Perkins, G.A.; Ali, S.S.; Patel, H.H.; Singh, P. Hypoxia-inducible factor-1alpha activation improves renal oxygenation and mitochondrial function in early chronic kidney disease. *Am. J. Physiol. Renal. Physiol.* **2017**, *313*, F282–F290. [CrossRef] [PubMed]

5. Fu, Q.; Colgan, S.P.; Shelley, C.S. Hypoxia: The Force that Drives Chronic Kidney Disease. *Clin. Med. Res.* **2016**, *14*, 15–39. [CrossRef]

6. Venkatachalam, M.A.; Weinberg, J.M.; Kriz, W.; Bidani, A.K. Failed Tubule Recovery, AKI-CKD Transition, and Kidney Disease Progression. *J. Am. Soc. Nephrol.* **2015**, *26*, 1765–1776. [CrossRef]

7. Nangaku, M.; Rosenberger, C.; Heyman, S.N.; Eckardt, K.U. Regulation of hypoxia-inducible factor in kidney disease. *Clin. Exp. Pharmacol. Physiol.* **2013**, *40*, 148–157. [CrossRef]

8. Forrester, S.J.; Booz, G.W.; Sigmund, C.D.; Coffman, T.M.; Kawai, T.; Rizzo, V.; Scalia, R.; Eguchi, S. Angiotensin II Signal Transduction: An Update on Mechanisms of Physiology and Pathophysiology. *Physiol. Rev.* **2018**, *98*, 1627–1738. [CrossRef]

9. Reboussin, D.M.; Allen, N.B.; Griswold, M.E.; Guallar, E.; Hong, Y.; Lackland, D.T.; Miller, E.P.R., 3rd.; Polonsky, T.; Thompson-Paul, A.M.; Vupputuri, S. Systematic Review for the 2017 ACC/AHA/AAPA/ABC/ACPM/AGS/APhA/ASH/ASPC/NMA/PCNA Guideline for the Prevention, Detection, Evaluation, and Management of High Blood Pressure in Adults: A Report of the American College of Cardiology/American Heart Association Task Force on Clinical Practice Guidelines. *Circulation* **2018**, *138*, e595–e616.

10. Jordan, J. Device-Based Approaches for the Treatment of Arterial Hypertension. *Curr. Hypertens. Rep.* **2017**, *19*, 59. [CrossRef] [PubMed]

11. Bakris, G.L.; Nadim, M.K.; Haller, H.; Lovett, E.G.; Schafer, J.E.; Bisognano, J.D. Baroreflex activation therapy provides durable benefit in patients with resistant hypertension: Results of long-term follow-up in the Rheos Pivotal Trial. *J. Am. Soc. Hypertens.* **2012**, *6*, 152–158. [CrossRef]

12. Singh, R.R.; Denton, K.M. Renal Denervation. *Hypertension* **2018**, *72*, 528–536. [CrossRef] [PubMed]

13. Persu, A.; Kjeldsen, S.; Staessen, J.A.; Azizi, M. Renal Denervation for Treatment of Hypertension: A Second Start and New Challenges. *Curr. Hypertens. Rep.* **2016**, *18*, 6. [CrossRef]

14. Symplicity HTN-2 Investigators; Esler, M.D.; Krum, H.; Sobotka, P.A.; Schlaich, M.P.; Schmieder, R.E.; Bohm, M. Renal sympathetic denervation in patients with treatment-resistant hypertension (The Symplicity HTN-2 Trial): A randomised controlled trial. *Lancet* **2010**, *376*, 1903–1909.

15. Mahfoud, F.; Bohm, M.; Schmieder, R.; Narkiewicz, K.; Ewen, S.; Ruilope, L.; Schlaich, M.; Williams, B.; Fahy, M.; Mancia, G. Effects of renal denervation on kidney function and long-term outcomes: 3-year follow-up from the Global SYMPLICITY Registry. *Eur. Heart J.* **2019**. [CrossRef]

16. Townsend, R.R.; Mahfoud, F.; Kandzari, D.E.; Kario, K.; Pocock, S.; Weber, M.A.; Ewen, S.; Tsioufis, K.; Tousoulis, D.; Sharp, A.S.P.; et al. Catheter-based renal denervation in patients with uncontrolled hypertension in the absence of antihypertensive medications (SPYRAL HTN-OFF MED): A randomised, sham-controlled, proof-of-concept trial. *Lancet* **2017**, *390*, 2160–2170. [CrossRef]

17. Azizi, M.; Schmieder, R.E.; Mahfoud, F.; Weber, M.A.; Daemen, J.; Davies, J.; Basile, J.; Kirtane, A.J.; Wang, Y.; Lobo, M.D.; et al. Endovascular ultrasound renal denervation to treat hypertension (RADIANCE-HTN SOLO): A multicentre, international, single-blind, randomised, sham-controlled trial. *Lancet* **2018**, *391*, 2335–2345. [CrossRef]

18. Kandzari, D.E.; Bohm, M.; Mahfoud, F.; Townsend, R.R.; Weber, M.A.; Pocock, S.; Tsioufis, K.; Tousoulis, D.; Choi, J.W.; East, C.; et al. Effect of renal denervation on blood pressure in the presence of antihypertensive drugs: 6-month efficacy and safety results from the SPYRAL HTN-ON MED proof-of-concept randomised trial. *Lancet* **2018**, *391*, 2346–2355. [CrossRef]

19. Mian, M.O.; Barhoumi, T.; Briet, M.; Paradis, P.; Schiffrin, E.L. Deficiency of T-regulatory cells exaggerates angiotensin II-induced microvascular injury by enhancing immune responses. *J. Hypertens.* **2016**, *34*, 97–108. [CrossRef]

20. Barhoumi, T.; Kasal, D.A.; Li, M.W.; Shbat, L.; Laurant, P.; Neves, M.F.; Paradis, P.; Schiffrin, E.L. T regulatory lymphocytes prevent angiotensin II-induced hypertension and vascular injury. *Hypertension* **2011**, *57*, 469–476. [CrossRef]

21. Mehrotra, P.; Patel, J.B.; Ivancic, C.M.; Collett, J.A.; Basile, D.P. Th-17 cell activation in response to high salt following acute kidney injury is associated with progressive fibrosis and attenuated by AT-1R antagonism. *Kidney Int.* **2015**, *88*, 776–784. [CrossRef]

22. Kim, S.M.; Lee, S.H.; Lee, A.; Kim, D.J.; Kim, Y.G.; Kim, S.Y.; Jeong, K.H.; Lee, T.W.; Ihm, C.G.; Lim, S.J.; et al. Targeting T helper 17 by mycophenolate mofetil attenuates diabetic nephropathy progression. *Transl. Res.* **2015**, *166*, 375–383. [CrossRef]

23. Mohamed, R.; Jayakumar, C.; Chen, F.; Fulton, D.; Stepp, D.; Gansevoort, R.T.; Ramesh, G. Low-Dose IL-17 Therapy Prevents and Reverses Diabetic Nephropathy, Metabolic Syndrome, and Associated Organ Fibrosis. *J. Am. Soc. Nephrol.* **2016**, *27*, 745–765. [CrossRef]

24. Wilck, N.; Matus, M.G.; Kearney, S.M.; Olesen, S.W.; Forslund, K.; Bartolomaeus, H.; Haase, S.; Mahler, A.; Balogh, A.; Marko, L.; et al. Salt-responsive gut commensal modulates TH17 axis and disease. *Nature* **2017**, *551*, 585–589. [CrossRef] [PubMed]

25. Bartolomaeus, H.; Balogh, A.; Yakoub, M.; Homann, S.; Marko, L.; Hoges, S.; Tsvetkov, D.; Krannich, A.; Wundersitz, S.; Avery, E.G.; et al. The Short-Chain Fatty Acid Propionate Protects from Hypertensive Cardiovascular Damage. *Circulation* **2018**. [CrossRef] [PubMed]

26. Higaki, A.; Caillon, A.; Paradis, P.; Schiffrin, E.L. Innate and Innate-Like Immune System in Hypertension and Vascular Injury. *Curr. Hypertens. Rep.* **2019**, *21*, 4. [CrossRef]

27. Warren, H.R.; Evangelou, E.; Cabrera, C.P.; Gao, H.; Ren, M.; Mifsud, B.; Ntalla, I.; Surendran, P.; Liu, C.; Cook, J.P.; et al. Corrigendum: Genome-wide association analysis identifies novel blood pressure loci and offers biological insights into cardiovascular risk. *Nat. Genet.* **2017**, *49*, 1558. [CrossRef] [PubMed]

28. Delles, C.; Carrick, E.; Graham, D.; Nicklin, S.A. Utilizing proteomics to understand and define hypertension: Where are we and where do we go? *Expert Rev. Proteomics* **2018**, *15*, 581–592. [CrossRef]

29. Giani, J.F.; Janjulia, T.; Taylor, B.; Bernstein, E.A.; Shah, K.; Shen, X.Z.; McDonough, A.A.; Bernstein, K.E.; Gonzalez-Villalobos, R.A. Renal generation of angiotensin II and the pathogenesis of hypertension. *Curr. Hypertens. Rep.* **2014**, *16*, 477. [CrossRef] [PubMed]

30. McMaster, W.G.; Kirabo, A.; Madhur, M.S.; Harrison, D.G. Inflammation, immunity, and hypertensive end-organ damage. *Circ. Res.* **2015**, *116*, 1022–1033. [CrossRef]

31. Fukuda, A.; Wickman, L.T.; Venkatareddy, M.P.; Sato, Y.; Chowdhury, M.A.; Wang, S.Q.; Shedden, K.A.; Dysko, R.C.; Wiggins, J.E.; Wiggins, R.C. Angiotensin II-dependent persistent podocyte loss from destabilized glomeruli causes progression of end stage kidney disease. *Kidney Int.* **2012**, *81*, 40–55. [CrossRef]

32. Gloy, J.; Henger, A.; Fischer, K.G.; Nitschke, R.; Mundel, P.; Bleich, M.; Schollmeyer, P.; Greger, R.; Pavenstadt, H. Angiotensin II depolarizes podocytes in the intact glomerulus of the Rat. *J. Clin. Invest.* **1997**, *99*, 2772–2781. [CrossRef]

33. Henger, A.; Huber, T.; Fischer, K.G.; Nitschke, R.; Mundel, P.; Schollmeyer, P.; Greger, R.; Pavenstadt, H. Angiotensin II increases the cytosolic calcium activity in rat podocytes in culture. *Kidney Int.* **1997**, *52*, 687–693. [CrossRef] [PubMed]

34. Nijenhuis, T.; Sloan, A.J.; Hoenderop, J.G.; Flesche, J.; van Goor, H.; Kistler, A.D.; Bakker, M.; Bindels, R.J.; de Boer, R.A.; Moller, C.C.; et al. Angiotensin II contributes to podocyte injury by increasing TRPC6 expression via an NFAT-mediated positive feedback signaling pathway. *Am. J. Pathol.* **2011**, *179*, 1719–1732. [CrossRef]

35. Schenk, L.K.; Moller-Kerutt, A.; Klosowski, R.; Wolters, D.; Schaffner-Reckinger, E.; Weide, T.; Pavenstadt, H.; Vollenbroker, B. Angiotensin II regulates phosphorylation of actin-associated proteins in human podocytes. *FASEB J.* **2017**, *31*, 5019–5035. [CrossRef] [PubMed]

36. Ren, Z.; Liang, W.; Chen, C.; Yang, H.; Singhal, P.C.; Ding, G. Angiotensin II induces nephrin dephosphorylation and podocyte injury: Role of caveolin-1. *Cell Signal.* **2012**, *24*, 443–450. [CrossRef]

37. Yang, Q.; Ma, Y.; Liu, Y.; Liang, W.; Chen, X.; Ren, Z.; Wang, H.; Singhal, P.C.; Ding, G. Angiotensin II down-regulates nephrin-Akt signaling and induces podocyte injury: Roleof c-Abl. *Mol. Biol. Cell* **2016**, *27*, 197–208. [CrossRef] [PubMed]

38. Wennmann, D.O.; Vollenbroker, B.; Eckart, A.K.; Bonse, J.; Erdmann, F.; Wolters, D.A.; Schenk, L.K.; Schulze, U.; Kremerskothen, J.; Weide, T.; et al. The Hippo pathway is controlled by Angiotensin II signaling and its reactivation induces apoptosis in podocytes. *Cell Death Dis.* **2014**, *5*, e1519. [CrossRef]

39. Anorga, S.; Overstreet, J.M.; Falke, L.L.; Tang, J.; Goldschmeding, R.G.; Higgins, P.J.; Samarakoon, R. Deregulation of Hippo-TAZ pathway during renal injury confers a fibrotic maladaptive phenotype. *FASEB J.* **2018**, *32*, 2644–2657. [CrossRef]

40. Yang, Y.; Yang, Q.; Yang, J.; Ma, Y.; Ding, G. Angiotensin II induces cholesterol accumulation and injury in podocytes. *Sci. Rep.* **2017**, *7*, 10672. [CrossRef]

41. Platten, M.; Youssef, S.; Hur, E.M.; Ho, P.P.; Han, M.H.; Lanz, T.V.; Phillips, L.K.; Goldstein, M.J.; Bhat, R.; Raine, C.S.; et al. Blocking angiotensin-converting enzyme induces potent regulatory T cells and modulates TH1- and TH17-mediated autoimmunity. *Proc. Natl. Acad. Sci. USA* **2009**, *106*, 14948–14953. [CrossRef]

42. Caillon, A.; Mian, M.O.R.; Fraulob-Aquino, J.C.; Huo, K.G.; Barhoumi, T.; Ouerd, S.; Sinnaeve, P.R.; Paradis, P.; Schiffrin, E.L. gammadelta T Cells Mediate Angiotensin II-Induced Hypertension and Vascular Injury. *Circulation* **2017**, *135*, 2155–2162. [CrossRef]

43. Ruster, C.; Wolf, G. Angiotensin II as a morphogenic cytokine stimulating renal fibrogenesis. *J. Am. Soc. Nephrol.* **2011**, *22*, 1189–1199. [CrossRef]

44. Suthanthiran, M.; Li, B.; Song, J.O.; Ding, R.; Sharma, V.K.; Schwartz, J.E.; August, P. Transforming growth factor-beta 1 hyperexpression in African-American hypertensives: A novel mediator of hypertension and/or target organ damage. *Proc. Natl. Acad. Sci. USA* **2000**, *97*, 3479–3484. [CrossRef]

45. Suthanthiran, M.; Gerber, L.M.; Schwartz, J.E.; Sharma, V.K.; Medeiros, M.; Marion, R.; Pickering, T.G.; August, P. Circulating transforming growth factor-beta1 levels and the risk for kidney disease in African Americans. *Kidney Int.* **2009**, *76*, 72–80. [CrossRef]

46. Feng, Y.; Liang, Y.; Zhu, X.; Wang, M.; Gui, Y.; Lu, Q.; Gu, M.; Xue, X.; Sun, X.; He, W.; et al. The signaling protein Wnt5a promotes TGFbeta1-mediated macrophage polarization and kidney fibrosis by inducing the transcriptional regulators Yap/Taz. *J. Biol. Chem.* **2018**, *293*, 19290–19302. [CrossRef]

47. Vigolo, E.; Marko, L.; Hinze, C.; Muller, D.N.; Schmidt-Ullrich, R.; Schmidt-Ott, K.M. Canonical BMP signaling in tubular cells mediates recovery after acute kidney injury. *Kidney Int.* **2019**, *95*, 108–122. [CrossRef] [PubMed]

48. Brinks, H.L.; Eckhart, A.D. Regulation of GPCR signaling in hypertension. *Biochim. Biophys. Acta* **2010**, *1802*, 1268–1275. [CrossRef]

49. Yang, J.; Villar, V.A.; Armando, I.; Jose, P.A.; Zeng, C. G Protein-Coupled Receptor Kinases: Crucial Regulators of Blood Pressure. *J. Am. Heart Assoc.* **2016**, *5*, e003519. [CrossRef] [PubMed]

50. Kamal, F.A.; Travers, J.G.; Schafer, A.E.; Ma, Q.; Devarajan, P.; Blaxall, B.C. G Protein-Coupled Receptor-G-Protein betagamma-Subunit Signaling Mediates Renal Dysfunction and Fibrosis in Heart Failure. *J. Am. Soc. Nephrol.* **2017**, *28*, 197–208. [CrossRef]

51. Deb, D.K.; Bao, R.; Li, Y.C. Critical role of the cAMP-PKA pathway in hyperglycemia-induced epigenetic activation of fibrogenic program in the kidney. *FASEB J.* **2017**, *31*, 2065–2075. [CrossRef]

52. Luo, R.; Zhang, W.; Zhao, C.; Zhang, Y.; Wu, H.; Jin, J.; Zhang, W.; Grenz, A.; Eltzschig, H.K.; Tao, L.; et al. Elevated Endothelial Hypoxia-Inducible Factor-1alpha Contributes to Glomerular Injury and Promotes Hypertensive Chronic Kidney Disease. *Hypertension* **2015**, *66*, 75–84. [CrossRef]

53. Eckardt, K.U.; Bernhardt, W.M.; Weidemann, A.; Warnecke, C.; Rosenberger, C.; Wiesener, M.S.; Willam, C. Role of hypoxia in the pathogenesis of renal disease. *Kidney Int. Suppl.* **2005**, *99*, S46–S51. [CrossRef]

54. Kong, K.H.; Oh, H.J.; Lim, B.J.; Kim, M.; Han, K.H.; Choi, Y.H.; Kwon, K.; Nam, B.Y.; Park, K.S.; Park, J.T.; et al. Selective tubular activation of hypoxia-inducible factor-2alpha has dual effects on renal fibrosis. *Sci. Rep.* **2017**, *7*, 11351. [CrossRef]

55. Schietke, R.E.; Hackenbeck, T.; Tran, M.; Gunther, R.; Klanke, B.; Warnecke, C.L.; Knaup, K.X.; Shukla, D.; Rosenberger, C.; Koesters, R.; et al. Renal tubular HIF-2alpha expression requires VHL inactivation and causes fibrosis and cysts. *PLoS ONE* **2012**, *7*, e31034. [CrossRef]

56. Franco, M.; Bautista-Perez, R.; Perez-Mendez, O. Purinergic receptors in tubulointerstitial inflammatory cells: A pathophysiological mechanism of salt-sensitive hypertension. *Acta Physiol. (Oxf)* **2015**, *214*, 75–87. [CrossRef]

57. Menzies, R.I.; Howarth, A.R.; Unwin, R.J.; Tam, F.W.; Mullins, J.J.; Bailey, M.A. Inhibition of the purinergic P2X7 receptor improves renal perfusion in angiotensin-II-infused rats. *Kidney Int.* **2015**, *88*, 1079–1087. [CrossRef]

58. Maggiorani, D.; Dissard, R.; Belloy, M.; Saulnier-Blache, J.S.; Casemayou, A.; Ducasse, L.; Gres, S.; Belliere, J.; Caubet, C.; Bascands, J.L.; et al. Shear Stress-Induced Alteration of Epithelial Organization in Human Renal Tubular Cells. *PLoS ONE* **2015**, *10*, e0131416. [CrossRef] [PubMed]

59. Wang, Q.Z.; Gao, H.Q.; Liang, Y.; Zhang, J.; Wang, J.; Qiu, J. Cofilin1 is involved in hypertension-induced renal damage via the regulation of NF-kappaB in renal tubular epithelial cells. *J. Transl. Med.* **2015**, *13*, 323. [CrossRef]

60. Hickson, L.J.; Eirin, A.; Lerman, L.O. Challenges and opportunities for stem cell therapy in patients with chronic kidney disease. *Kidney Int.* **2016**, *89*, 767–778. [CrossRef] [PubMed]

61. Peired, A.J.; Sisti, A.; Romagnani, P. Mesenchymal Stem Cell-Based Therapy for Kidney Disease: A Review of Clinical Evidence. *Stem Cells Int.* **2016**, *2016*, 4798639. [CrossRef] [PubMed]

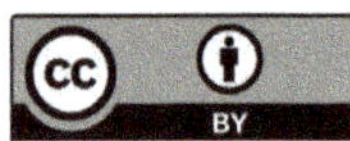

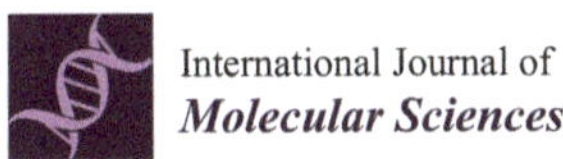
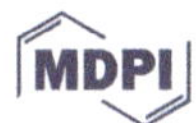

International Journal of
Molecular Sciences

Review

Salt Inducible Kinase Signaling Networks: Implications for Acute Kidney Injury and Therapeutic Potential

Mary Taub

Biochemistry Dept, Jacobs School of Medicine and Biomedical Sciences, University at Buffalo, 955 Main Street Suite 4102, Buffalo, NY 14203, USA; biochtau@buffalo.edu

Received: 28 May 2019; Accepted: 27 June 2019; Published: 30 June 2019

Abstract: A number of signal transduction pathways are activated during Acute Kidney Injury (AKI). Of particular interest is the Salt Inducible Kinase (SIK) signaling network, and its effects on the Renal Proximal Tubule (RPT), one of the primary targets of injury in AKI. The SIK1 network is activated in the RPT following an increase in intracellular Na^+ (Na^+_{in}), resulting in an increase in Na,K-ATPase activity, in addition to the phosphorylation of Class IIa Histone Deacetylases (HDACs). In addition, activated SIKs repress transcriptional regulation mediated by the interaction between cAMP Regulatory Element Binding Protein (CREB) and CREB Regulated Transcriptional Coactivators (CRTCs). Through their transcriptional effects, members of the SIK family regulate a number of metabolic processes, including such cellular processes regulated during AKI as fatty acid metabolism and mitochondrial biogenesis. SIKs are involved in regulating a number of other cellular events which occur during AKI, including apoptosis, the Epithelial to Mesenchymal Transition (EMT), and cell division. Recently, the different SIK kinase isoforms have emerged as promising drug targets, more than 20 new SIK2 inhibitors and activators having been identified by MALDI-TOF screening assays. Their implementation in the future should prove to be important in such renal disease states as AKI.

Keywords: kidney proximal tubule; acute kidney failure; signal transduction; transcription; CREB Regulated Transcriptional Coactivators (CRTC); cAMP Regulatory Element Binding Protein (CREB); Salt Inducible Kinase (SIK); Class IIa Histone Deacetylases (HDAC)

---

1. Introduction

Salt Inducible Kinase (SIK) was first discovered in the adrenal gland of rats on a high salt diet, where it plays a regulatory role in steroidogenesis [1]. Subsequently, a SIK network was identified that plays an important role in regulating Na^+ reabsorption in the Renal Proximal Tubule (RPT) [2]. SIK plays a number of additional roles, ranging from its roles in gene regulation, and the regulation of metabolism, to the roles played by SIK in cell survival, growth, the Epithelial to Mesenchymal Transition (EMT) as well as apoptosis. This report is concerned with the involvement of SIK in Acute Kidney Injury (AKI).

AKI is a heterogeneous group of conditions characterized by an abrupt decrease in the Glomerular Filtration Rate (GFR), followed by an increase in serum creatinine [3–5]. AKI arises as a consequence of ischemic and toxic insults, as well as radiation and ureteral obstruction [6,7]. Following the initiation and extension phases caused by the insults, the kidney goes through maintenance and recovery phases, during which repair occurs in cells that are sub-lethally damaged, in addition to the generation of new cells. There is a need to understand the underlying molecular changes that occur in the tubule epithelial cells during AKI, and the recovery period, so as to develop effective therapies. There is considerable evidence suggesting that signal transduction pathways that are activated during AKI involve different aspects of the SIK Networks, which opens up the possibility of new avenues for therapy.

2. Role of the Salt Inducible Kinase 1 (SIK1) Network in the Response of the Renal Proximal Tubule (RPT) to Injury

2.1. Initial Response of the Renal Proximal Tubule to Injury

Of particular interest in these regards, is the renal proximal tubule (RPT), one of the primary targets of injury in AKI [5]. The RPT primarily depends upon mitochondrial oxidative phosphorylation, rather than glycolysis [8]. Thus, ATP levels decline dramatically during hypoxia, resulting in a decrease in Na,K-ATPase activity, as well as an increase in intracellular Na^+ (Na^+_{in}). As a consequence, the capacity of the RPT to reabsorb Na^+ and other solutes is impaired. Impaired Na^+ reabsorption can present problems, because in order to survive, the body must retain Na^+ within an appropriate range (between 135 and 145 mEq/L). This level of Na^+ is necessary to maintain a normal blood pressure, support the function of muscles and nerves, and to preserve our body's fluid balance. One defense mechanism in the kidney, is Tubuloglomerular Feedback (TGF), which causes the Glomerular Filtration Rate (GFR) to decline when distal Na^+ levels increase, and in this manner acts so as to preserve Na^+ within a range compatible with renal tubular function (which may decline as a result of injury) [9]. In addition, tubule epithelial cells themselves possess defense mechanisms, including mechanisms that result in a response to changes in ionic balance. Although renal tubules are often viewed as being a central target in AKI, surprisingly little is known regarding these functional responses, which act to preserve renal tubule transport functions during AKI, including those in the RPT. Thus, it is important to gain an understanding of pertinent regulatory mechanisms involved in this nephron segment, and likely responses during AKI. Of particular interest in these regards is the SIK1 network, and its ability to regulate Na,K-ATPase, so as to maintain Na^+ homeostasis in the body.

2.2. Importance of Na,K-ATPase in Na^+ Reabsorption

As stated above, Na^+ plays a critical role in maintaining the homeostasis of bodily fluids, indirectly affecting the distribution of water in intravascular compartments, and ultimately, blood pressure [10]. Fluid as well as electrolyte disorders often develop during AKI, and fluid therapy (with its own inherent problems) is common [11]. Indeed, clinically employed saline solutions (154 mM) contain higher Na^+ levels than plasma (140 mM).

At the cellular level, the Na,K-ATPase is crucial in maintaining an appropriate Na^+/K^+ gradient across the plasma membrane (a requirement of all living cells). Presumably, the need for such a Na^+/K^+ gradient originated in primitive organisms, which were in an environment in which Na^+ was inhibitory, or even toxic, while K^+ was required for the activity of primitive enzymes (due to the preponderance of K^+ in the primitive environment) [12]. Thus, cells had to develop mechanisms to prevent the toxicity of intracellular Na^+. Indeed, if intracellular Na^+ levels are allowed to rise in mammalian cells, the intracellular environment risks intracellular "flooding" caused by a Donan equilibrium (i.e., intracellular swelling caused by an increase in the intracellular concentration of free cations over and above the extracellular level, due to the net negative charge of intracellular proteins). For this reason, mammalian cells have a Na,K-ATPase which ejects three intracellular Na^+ molecules in exchange for two extracellular K^+, at the expense of ATP [13]. Very importantly, the Na^+ gradient established by Na,K-ATPase provides the driving force for the cotransport of a number of solutes into the cell (amino acids, glucose, phosphate) with Na^+. In the case of the RPT, this is the first step in the transepithelial transport of these solutes.

Teleologically, it makes sense that cells are fortified to survive the continual changes in the ions in the extracellular milieu, including those that occur during exposure to a "toxic" environment. Protection from such external changes is provided by signaling systems that control the activity of membrane transporters, including Na,K-ATPase, and thereby permit renal cells to respond appropriately to changes not only in the external ionic environment, but also to metabolic challenges such as a decline in ATP levels, as well as oxidative stress and other toxic challenges. Of particular interest in these regards is the SIK Signaling Network and its role in the RPT during AKI.

2.3. SIK Structure and Function

SIKs are central components of a number of signaling pathways which are responsible for regulating a wide range of cellular processes in different organs. In subsequent studies, SIK1 was found to be homologous to AMP Kinase (AMPK), and for this reason, is included within the Sucrose Non-Fermenting 1 (SNF1)/AMPK family [14]. Three isoforms of SIK have been identified (SIK1, SIK2 and SIK3) which share common structural features, including a highly conserved, amino terminal kinase domain, a Sucrose Nonfermenting-1 Homology (SNH) domain, as well as a carboxy terminal phosphorylation domain (Figure 1). All three SIK isoforms are broadly expressed in a large number of tissues. Tissues which express amongst the highest levels of SIK1 include adipose tissue, as well as B and T cells. While heart and adipose tissue are amongst those with the highest level of SIK2 expression, other tissues, including the cerebral cortex and testes are amongst those with the highest levels of SIK3. However, the relative SIK expression level is not a necessary indicator of the importance of an individual SIK isoform in any particular tissue. When considering the kidney, SIK1 has been studied most extensively, although the kidney expresses moderate levels of all three SIK isoforms.

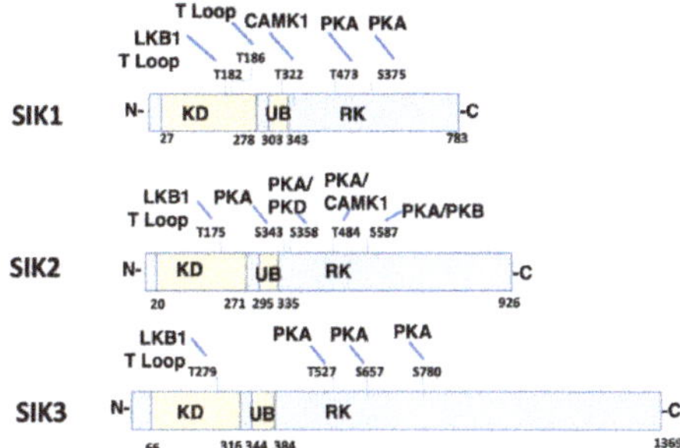

Figure 1. Domain Structure and Phosphorylation Sites of Salt Inducible Kinase (SIK) Isoforms. The domain structure of SIK1 (Uniprot P507059), SIK2 (Uniprot Q9Y2K2), and SIK3 (Uniprot Q9Y2K2) is shown including conserved Kinase Domain (KD), Ubiquitin Associated Domain (UB), and RK-rich region (RK). Identified phosphorylation sites are also illustrated, as well as the corresponding kinase (LKB1 (T182 SIK1, T175 SIK2, T221 SIK3), CaMK1 (T322 SIK1, T484 SIK2), PKA (T473 and S575 SIK1; S343, S358, T484 and S587 SIK2; T469, S551, S647 SIK3), and PKB (S587 SIK2)). T Loop indicates that the phosphorylation site is within the T activation loop. The amino and carboxy terminus of each SIK isoform are indicated by N- and C-, respectively. CaMK1, Calmodulin Activated Protein Kinase 1; PKA, Protein Kinase A; PKB, Protein Kinase B.

SIKs possess an activation loop within the kinase domain. Autophosphorylation occurs within the activation loop (Thr186 in SIK1), an event that is essential for kinase activity [15]. The catalytic activity of all SIK isoforms depends upon the phosphorylation of yet another residue within the activation loop (Thr182 in SIK1) by LKB1 [16]. LKB1 similarly phosphorylates all other members of the AMPK family. The activation loop of SIK1 and SIK2 is also phosphorylated by GSK-3β, although this phosphorylation event is not sufficient to activate SIK kinase activity [15]. Other domains of the SIKs also undergo phosphorylation by a number of protein kinases. For example, Calmodulin Activated Protein Kinase 1 (CaMK1) phosphorylates SIK1 within the UB domain, so as to increase SIK1 kinase activity. In contrast, CaMK1 phosphorylates SIK2 within the carboxy terminal domain, and in this manner similarly activates SIK kinase activity. Protein Kinase A (PKA) phosphorylates all three SIK isoforms in the carboxy terminal domain, depending upon the physiological condition [17].

A consequence of SIK phosphorylation by PKA is that SIKs become associated with cytoplasmic 14-3-3 proteins, which results in the sequestration of SIKs in the cytoplasm [17]. Thus, SIKs that have been phosphorylated by PKA can no longer phosphorylate nuclear proteins, including CRTCs, and class IIa HDACs.

2.4. SIK1 Signaling Network and Na,K-ATPase

2.4.1. Role of SIK1 in Na$^+$ Sensing: Acute Response

Of particular interest to this report, is the role of SIK1 in Na$^+$ sensing. In RPT cells, SIK1 is associated with a complex associated with the basolateral membrane, containing the Na, K-ATPase [12]. A number of proteins are associated with the SIK1/Na,K-ATPase complex, including Protein Phosphatase 2A (PP2A), and Protein Methylesterase-1 (PME-1), which constantly demethylates (and thus inactivates) PP2A. As illustrated in Figure 2, the increase in intracellular Na$^+$ (Na$^+_{in}$), which occurs following an increase in luminal Na$^+$, is followed by the activation of Na$^+$/Ca^{2+} exchange activity, and, as a consequence, an increase in intracellular Ca^{2+} (Ca$^{2+}_{in}$).

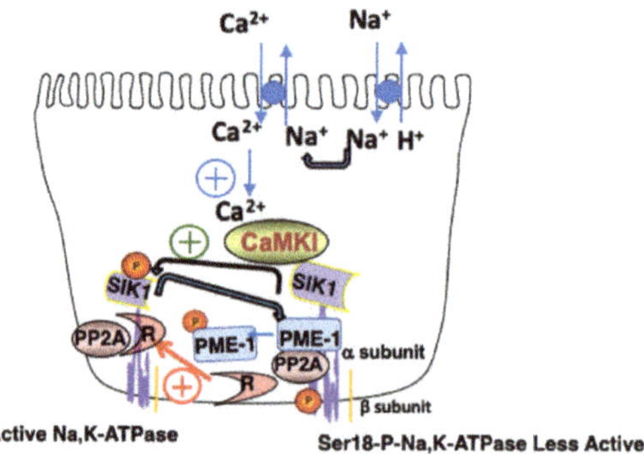

Figure 2. Model of the Basolateral SIK1 Network. An increase in luminal Na$^+$ results in an increase in Na$^+_{in}$, the activation of Na$^+$/Ca^{2+} exchange, and an increase in Ca$^{2+}_{in}$, which activates CaMK1. Activated CaMK1 phosphorylates SIK1 at Thr322 and activates basolateral SIK1, which as a consequence, phosphorylates PME-1, which dissociates from the Na,K-ATPase complex. PP2A remains demethylated, associates with its regulatory subunit (R), and in this activated state, dephosphorylates Ser18 of the catalytic subunit of Na,K-ATPase (i.e., the α subunit), activating the transporter. If the indicated reaction has a positive effect upon activity, it is indicated by a plus contained within a circle.

Ultimately, the increase in Ca$^{2+}_{in}$ results in CaMK1 activation, which in turn phosphorylates and activates SIK1. SIK1 then activates basolateral Na,K-ATPase, albeit indirectly [12]. Towards these ends, activated SIK1 phosphorylates PME1, which dissociates from the SIK1/Na,K-ATPase/PP2A complex. As a consequence, the PP2A catalytic subunit is no longer demethylated by PME1, and thus the activity of PP2A remains low. This is because PP2A only achieves its full catalytic activity following its demethylation, which allows the PP2A catalytic subunit to interact with the PP2A regulatory subunit, and dephosphorylate the catalytic subunit (i.e., the α subunit) of the Na,K-ATPase. The retention of the Na,K-ATPase in the basolateral membrane increases under these conditions, resulting in increased transport activity.

2.4.2. Relevance of the SIK1 Signaling Network and Na,K-ATPase to AKI

The SIK1 signaling network described above is responsible for eliciting the initial responses of the RPT to insults that result in AKI. An increase in luminal Na$^+$ (Na$^+_{in}$) occurs in response to a number of these insults, particularly when the GFR decreases (during the initiation phase of AKI), and luminal Na$^+$ increases. Intracellular ATP levels often decline during the initiation phase of AKI (often in response to hypoxia). A consequence of such a decline in intracellular ATP is reduced Na,K-ATPase activity, and, as a result, an increase in Na^+_{in} (which decreases the driving force for transepithelial transport). From our knowledge of the SIK1 network [12], such acute increases in Na^+_{in} rapidly activate the basolateral SIK1s, which are part of the Na,K-ATPase complex, and thereby initiate the events in the SIK1 network which counteract the tendency for Na^+ reabsorption to decline during AKI (by increasing the quantity of basolateral Na,K-ATPases).

In addition to these immediate effects of an increase in Na^+_{in} (which occurs during the initiation phase of AKI), during subsequent phases of AKI changes in gene expression occur which result in increased renal reabsorption, as well as other repair processes, due to changes occurring in other aspects of SIK networking.

2.5. Transcriptional Effects of SIK1 Involving Its HDAC Kinase Activity and Relevance to AKI

During the initiation phase of AKI, Na^+_{in} increases, resulting in SIK1 activation, which in turn results in a transcriptional response due to the Class IIa Histone Deacetylase (HDAC) kinase activity of SIK1 [18,19]. Class IIa HDACs associate with such transcription factors as Myocyte Enhancer Factor 2C (MEF2C) and Nuclear Factor of Activated T cells (NFAT) on chromosomal DNA, so as to repress transcription (Figure 3). However, when SIK1 is phosphorylated at Thr322 by CAMK1 (and activated), activated SIK1 phosphorylates Class IIa HDACs, which, as a consequence, a) dissociate from chromosomal MEF2 (as well as NFAT), and b) translocate to the cytoplasm, where they bind to cytoplasmic 14-3-3 proteins (Figure 3).

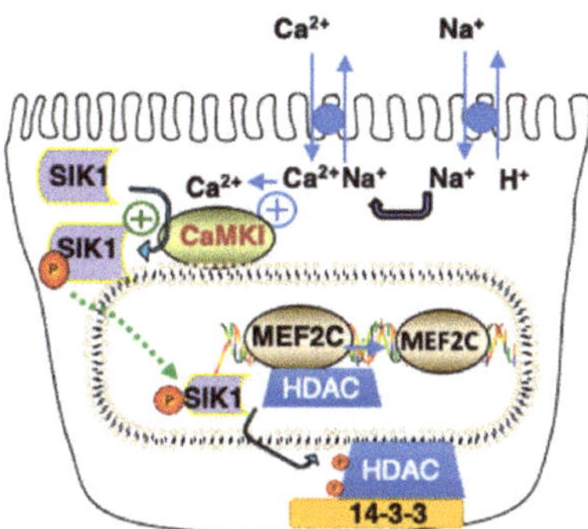

Figure 3. Model of Class IIa HDAC Kinase Phosphorylation by SIK1. An increase in Na^+_{in} results in an increase in Ca^{2+}_{in} due to activation of Na^+/Ca^{2+} exchange activity. SIK1 is phosphorylated at Thr322 by CAMK1 and activated, resulting in the phosphorylation of Class IIa HDACs associated with MEF2 transcriptions (as well as NFAT, not shown) on chromosomal DNA. As a consequence of their phosphorylation at two sites (Ser259 and Ser498 in the case of Human HDAC5), Class IIa HDACS translocate to the cytoplasm where they interact with 14-3-3 proteins. If the indicated reaction has a positive effect upon activity, it is indicated by a plus contained within a circle.

Following the dissociation of Class IIa HDACs from chromosomal DNA, transcription via MEF2 and NFAT is upregulated, increasing the expression of MEF2- (and NFAT-) regulated genes. Included amongst the genes upregulated following an increase in Na^+_{in} are those encoding for Atrial Natriuretic Peptide (ANP) as well as α and β Myosin Heavy Chains (MHCs) [18]. Of particular interest in these regards, is the increased expression of ANP A and B, as well as α and β MHCs which has been reported during AKI [20–22]. Such an increase in the expression of ANP, may very well promote recovery during AKI. Indeed, ANP has been used in the management of AKI [23–25].

2.6. Involvement of SIK1 in Transcriptional Events Mediated by cAMP and Ca^{2+}

SIKs are also involved in regulating transcriptional events mediated by the cAMP Regulatory Element Binding Protein (CREB) and CREB Regulated Transcriptional Coactivators (CRTCs) [26]. Prostaglandin E$_2$ (PGE$_2$) is an example of an effector that acts via such a mechanism [27,28]. In the kidney, PGs are synthesized from Arachidonic acid by Cyclooxygenases (COXs), including constitutive COX1 and inducible COX2. Of particular interest in these regards, COX-2 inhibitors are a major cause of drug-induced AKI, and exacerbate reductions in the GFR caused by other agents such as Lipopolysaccharides (LPS) [29]. In addition, chemokines and cytokines including PGE$_2$ are produced during AKI (as early as the initiation phase) [9,29]. While they may have beneficial effects on the GFR, chemokines and cytokines also contribute to the inflammatory response [29].

PGE$_2$ in particular is known to regulate renal Na$^+$ handling, in a manner which depends upon the nephron segment [9]. PGE$_2$ interacts with its specific G Protein Coupled Receptors (GPCRs) (i.e., Prostaglandin E (EP) receptors) which are differentially expressed in tubule epithelial cells. Included amongst the GPCRs for PGE$_2$ are EP2 and EP4 receptors (which are coupled to Gs, which activates adenylate cyclase (AC)), as well as EP1 receptors (which is coupled to Gq, which activates Phospholipase C (PLC)) [30]. Following the interaction of PGE$_2$ with Gs coupled EP2 and EP4 receptors, intracellular cAMP increases, resulting in the phosphorylation SIK1 at Thr475 (by PKA), and SIK1 inactivation [27,31,32], unlike increases in Na$^+_{in}$ which result in SIK1 phosphorylation at Thr322 (by CAMK1), and SIK activation.

The PGE$_2$-mediated increase in Na,K-ATPase activity in primary rabbit RPT cell cultures is an example of transcriptional regulation which involves inhibitory effects of cAMP on SIK1 [33]. The Na,K-ATPase is a heterodimer, consisting of an α subunit, responsible for the catalytic activity, as well as a β subunit, a chaperone which facilitates the insertion of the Na,K-ATPase into the basolateral membrane. Although both subunits are present in Na,K-ATPase, an increase in the level of the β subunit alone can cause an overall increase in the level the heterodimer [34]. This occurs when the level of the β subunit is limiting to heterodimer formation (excess α subunit being degraded). In this case, transcriptional regulation of the Na,K-ATPase β subunit gene *atp1b1* becomes a critical determinant of the overall Na,K-ATPase level, and activity. The observed increase in the overall level of the Na,K-ATPase in the RPT cells following a prolonged incubation with PGE$_2$, can be explained by this type of regulation by the *atp1b1* gene [35].

Transcriptional regulation of the *atp1b1* gene by PGE$_2$ involves CREB, which binds to Prostaglandin Regulatory Elements, PGREs, located in the *atp1b1* promoter [36,37]. CREB binds constitutively to PGREs, even in the absence of the binding of effectors such as PGE$_2$ to their receptors (i.e., EP receptors in the case of PGE$_2$) (Figure 4A). Under these conditions, CREB Regulated Transcriptional Coactivators (CRTCs) are localized in the cytoplasm. Transcriptional regulation by CREB on the *atp1b1* promoter involves increases in cAMP as well as Ca$^{2+}_{in}$. PGE$_2$ interacts with both EP2, as well as EP1 receptors in primary RPT cells. When PGE$_2$ interacts with EP2 receptors, AC is activated, and subsequently, PKA. Activated PKA phosphorylates CREB (localized on the PGRE1 and PGRE3 sites on the *atp1b1* promoter), resulting in the recruitment of CREB Binding Protein (CBP) to phospho-CREB (pCREB) [36]. In order to obtain a maximal transcriptional response, CREB Regulated Transcriptional Coactivators (CRTCs) also associate with CREB on the *atp1b1* promoter [27] (Figure 4B). However, a second signaling event (an increase in Ca^{2+}) must occur if CRTCs are to interact with CREB [27,38]. This second signaling event is initiated by the interaction of PGE$_2$ with EP1 receptors, the activation of Phospholipase C (PLC), and an increase in Ca$^{2+}_{in}$ [31].

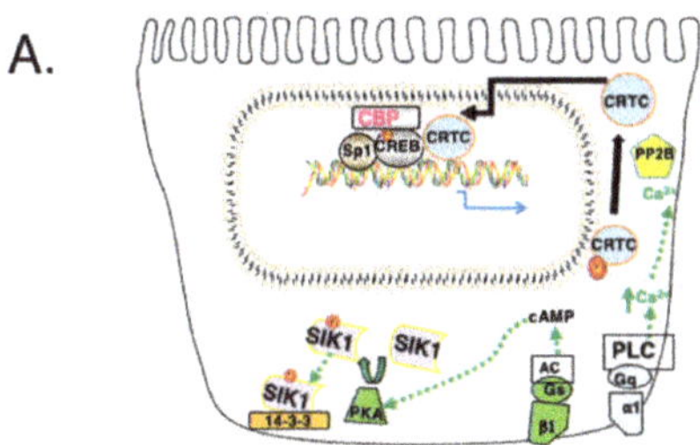

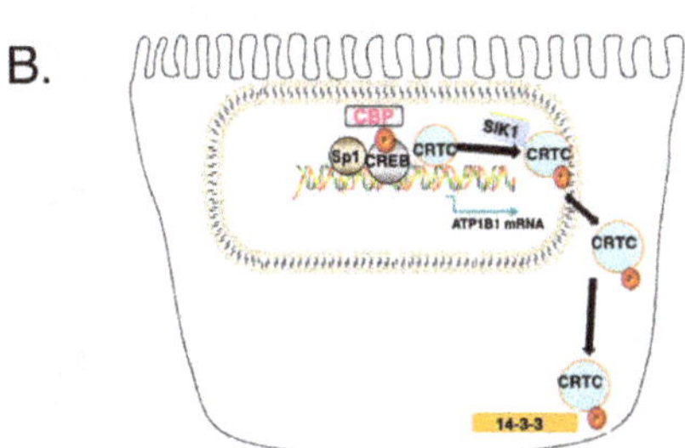

Figure 4. Establishment of a CREB/CRTC Interaction and its Disruption by SIK1. (**A**) Following a simultaneous increase in cAMP and Ca^{2+}_{in}, SIK1 is phosphorylated at Thr473 by PKA, which results in an interaction between PKA phosphorylated SIK1 and 14-3-3 proteins (which results in the sequestration of SIK1 in the cytoplasm, and which prevents the further phosphorylation of CRTCs by SIK1). CRTCs, which are phosphorylated (at Ser151 in the case of human CRTC1), are dephosphorylated by Calcineurin (i.e., Protein Phosphatase 2B (PP2B)). As a consequence, CRTCs translocate to the nucleus and interact with CREB, causing an increase in transcription, beyond that obtained with the Ser-133-pCREB/CBP interaction. (**B**) Following SIK1 activation (and its dephosphorylation at the PKA phosphorylation site), SIK1 no longer interacts with 14-3-3 proteins, which permits the nuclear translocation of SIK1. Once in the nucleus, SIK1 phosphorylates CRTCs, which translocate to the cytoplasm.

Notably, the binding of CRTCs to CREB on the *atp1b1* promoter is limited by SIK1 [27]. In order for CRTCs to interact with CREB, CRTCs must be in the nucleus (Figure 4A). However, activated SIK1 phosphorylates CRTCs, which causes CRTCs to translocate to the cytoplasm where they interact with 14-3-3 proteins (Figure 4B) [27].

Two simultaneous signaling events must occur in order for cytoplasmic CRTCs to reenter the nucleus (Figure 4A) [39]. First, intracellular cAMP must increase (due to the activation of AC, by Gs coupled EP2 in the case of PGE_2), and second, Ca^{2+}_{in} must increase (due to the activation of PLC, by Gq coupled EP1 in the case of PGE_2). Following an AC-mediated increase in cAMP, PKA (which is activated) phosphorylates SIK1 at Thr475, inactivating SIK1, which no longer phosphorylates CRTCs. CRTCs must in addition be dephosphorylated in order to enter the nucleus. The dephosphorylation of CRTCs depends upon the activation of Calcineurin, which occurs when Ca^{2+}_{in} increases. Calcineurin (i.e., Protein Phosphatase 2B (PP2B)), is a calcium- and calmodulin-dependent serine/threonine protein phosphatase.

2.7. Summary of the Three Major SIK1 Networks and Their Relevance to Acute Kidney Injury (AKI)

Thus, to summarize, the regulation of the transport and reabsorptive functions of the RPT depends upon three different signaling pathways involving SIK1. Two of these pathways are activated when Na^+_{in} increases (which occurs following increases in luminal Na^+), and involve on one hand, the direct phosphorylation of PME1 by activated SIK1 basolateral SIK1 (in the first pathway), and on the other hand the direct phosphorylation of class IIA HDACs by activated nuclear SIK1 (in the second pathway). As a consequence, 1) pre-existing Na,K-ATPases are retained in the basolateral membrane in the first pathway, and 2) transcriptional regulation by MEF2 and NFAT transcription factors increases in the second pathway. A third component of the SIK1 network, transcriptional regulation by CRTCs (and CREB), is inhibited when SIK1 is activated, due to the phosphorylation of CRTCs by SIK1. This latter event may occur in the absence of an increase in Na^+_{in} (i.e., when SIK1 is activated by LKB1 or CAMK).

The two SIK1 signal transduction pathways, which are activated following an increase in Na^+_{in}, both play a role during the initial phase of AKI. During this phase, a) luminal Na^+ increases due to TGF, and b) intracellular ATP levels may decline due to ischemia and/or a toxic insult. In this latter case, Na^+ extrusion by Na,K-ATPase declines, as this transporter depends upon cellular energy levels. As a consequence, Na^+_{in} increases further, resulting in a) a further activation of SIK1, and increase in Na,K-ATPase activity (via PP2A), as well as b) protective effects elicited as a consequence of the expression of NFAT-regulated genes (a result of the class IIa HDAC Kinase activity of SIK1). During these responses, activated SIK1 can also restrict chronic, transcriptional regulation of Na,K-ATPase by CREB (through the phosphorylation of CRTCs).

The restrictive effect of SIK1 on transcriptional regulation of Na,K-ATPase by CREB and CRTCs is alleviated, however, when SIK1 is phosphorylated, and inhibited by PKA. This occurs in response to cytokines (such as PGE_2) which are produced during the maintenance and recovery phases of AKI. During this time, the necessary increases in intracellular cAMP and Ca^{2+}_{in} required for the interaction of CRTCs with CREB on the *atp1b1* promoter must occur if RPT transport activity is to increase over the long term.

The SIK1 signaling networks described above are evolutionarily highly conserved, including the SIK1 signaling events responsible for maintaining cellular Na^+ homeostasis [40]. SIK1 orthologues have been reported in a diverse range of animal cells ranging from mouse, zebrafish, and drosophila, to Caenorhabditis elegans [12]. Even plants express the orthologous SOS2 and SOS3, which permit adaptions to drought, as well as increases in the salinity of the soil [41].

3. Other Roles of SIKs

3.1. Roles of SIK2 and SIK3 in Gluconeogenesis and Lipogenesis

SIKs are regulators of a diverse range of cellular functions which are much broader than those activated by ionic imbalances. Indeed, each of the three different SIK isoforms plays a variety of roles, in different tissues [26]. Examples discussed below include the role of SIK3 in hepatic gluconeogenesis [42], as well as the role of SIK2 in lipogenesis in adipocytes [43].

3.1.1. Role of SIK2 and SIK3 in Gluconeogenesis in the Liver

When blood glucose levels are high, insulin, which is produced, stimulates the phosphorylation and activation of Akt in the liver [38]. Akt in turn phosphorylates hepatic FOXO transcription factors, which become sequestered in the cytoplasm. Under these conditions, SIK3, which is activated by LKB1, phosphorylates CRTC2 and CRTC3 (as well as Class IIa HDACs), resulting in the sequestration of these proteins in the cytoplasm. As a consequence, gluconeogenic gene expression is repressed.

In contrast, during fasting, glucagon is produced, with a resultant increase in hepatocyte cAMP, the activation of AC, which as a consequence, phosphorylates (and inactivates) SIK3 [38]. Subsequently, CRTC2 and CRTC3 are dephosphorylated by calcineurin, and translocate to the nucleus, where they interact with pCREB (and CBP) on the promoters of gluconeogenic genes, including genes encoding for Phosphoenol Pyruvate Carboxykinase (PEPCK) and Glucose 6 Phosphatase (G6Pase).

At the same time (i.e., during fasting), hepatic class IIa HDACs and FOXO1 become dephosphorylated (due to the inhibition of SIK3), and translocate to the nucleus [44]. HDAC4 and HDAC5 (Class IIa HDACs) interact with FOXO1 on IRE sites in the PEPCK and G6Pase promoters, where they recruit HDAC3 (a Class I HDAC), which deacetylates FOXO1, thereby stimulating transcription. Thus, both CRTCs and Class IIa HDACs act so as to stimulate the expression of these hepatic gluconeogenic genes.

3.1.2. Role of SIK2 and Activating Transcription Factor 3 (ATF3) in Lipid Metabolism in Adipocytes

SIKs, HDACs and CRTCs similarly play a role in transcriptional regulation in other insulin-sensitive tissues, including adipocytes [38]. In white adipocytes, catecholamines (which are produced by the hypothalamus during fasting) stimulate lipolysis by activating β adrenergic receptors (and thus PKA) resulting in the phosphorylation of hormone-sensitive lipase [45]. Activated PKA also phosphorylates, and inactivates SIK2, which results in an increase in the transcription of ATF3 (ATF3 being a CREB, and CRTC dependent gene). ATF3 acts as a transcriptional repressor of the insulin responsive GLUT4 gene, as well as the adiponectin gene. In contrast, in the fed state SIK2 becomes dephosphorylated and activated, which results in the phosphorylation of CRTC2 (as well as HDAC4), and reduced expression of ATF3. The ultimate result is increased expression of GLUT4 and glucose uptake, promoting lipogenesis.

3.1.3. Relevance to the Kidney

Although the kidney is not generally noted as being an insulin-sensitive tissue, the RPT nevertheless does have gluconeogenic capacity, that is reportedly inhibited by insulin as well as glucose, by a mechanism which involves the inactivation of FOXO1 [46]. Very likely this mechanism involves SIK3, which very likely phosphorylates class IIa HDACs in the kidney (as in the liver), thereby preventing the interaction of class IIa HDACs (and HDAC3, a Class I HDAC) with FOXO1 on IREs in the PEPCK and G6Pase promoters (an interaction which is very likely just as necessary for the activation of FOXO1 in the kidney, in addition to the liver). Little is known about the effects of catecholamines on ATF3 expression in the kidney. However, ATF3 is rapidly induced during ischemia/reperfusion injury, and suppresses the expression of inflammatory cytokines (including IL-6 and IL-12b) during AKI (as indicated by studies with AFT3 deficient mice) [47]. Catecholamines (or other renal effectors that activate PKA) may be responsible for the induction of ATF3 in the kidney during AKI by stimulating the phosphorylation and inactivation of SIK2 by PKA (as observed in white adipocytes), thereby resulting in increased transcription of AFT3 (due to a CREB/CRTC1 interaction in the kidney as occurs in white adipocytes).

3.2. Role of SIK2 in Mitochondrial Biogenesis and Its Relevance to AKI

During AKI, the ability of the RPT to carry out is reabsorptive functions is impaired in part due to a reduced capacity to generate sufficient levels of ATP. In addition, Reactive Oxygen Species (ROS) are generated due to injuries affecting the mitochondria. These problems can be alleviated by means of mitochondrial biogenesis, which depends upon the expression of the Peroxisome Proliferator-Activated Receptor γ Co-activator-1α (PGC-1α) gene, which in turn depends upon SIKs.

3.2.1. Role of SIK2 in Regulating PGC-1α Adipocytes

In adipocytes, the PKA mediated activation of CREB, and its interaction with CRTC2 (which occurs following the inhibition of SIK2), results in increased expression of PGC-1α [48]. PGC-1α functions to induce Uncoupling protein 1 (UCP-1), as well as other mitochondrial genes and transcription factors. The ultimate result is mitochondrial biogenesis, and an increased oxidative capacity. In white adipocytes, inducers of PGC-1α include β adrenergic agonists, thyroid hormone, and in brown adipocytes, insulin. Insulin acts as an inducer in brown adipocytes by activating Phosphoinositol 3-Kinase (PI3K) as well as Akt, and ultimately phosphorylating SIK2 (at Ser587). In contrast, SIK1 has been implicated in regulating the expression of PGC-1α in skeletal muscle [49]. In skeletal muscle, important promoter elements for the PGC-1α gene include a regulatory element for CREB (i.e., a CRE), as well as MEF2. Thus, SIK1 regulates PGC-1α gene expression via its ability to phosphorylate CRTCs [50], as well as class IIA HDACs [19].

3.2.2. Regulation of Mitochondrial Biogenesis during AKI

In the RPT, mitochondrial biogenesis is particularly important in maintaining the energy demands of the RPT after injury, including injuries that result in AKI [51]. This is because the RPT primarily depends upon mitochondrial oxidative metabolism to produce the ATP necessary to carry out its reabsorptive functions, having a very limited capacity for glycolysis [29]. Thus, following injuries to the RPT, the remaining viable, transporting RPT cells may very well require additional mitochondria in order to meet their energy requirements.

Several small molecules such as resveratrol and isoflavone-derived compounds, induce mitochondrial biogenesis in the RPT, and have been used to alleviate deleterious effects of injuries to the RPT [52]. While resveratrol has been observed to increase mitochondrial biogenesis through the activation of AMPK in fibroblasts, a similar AMPK activation has not been observed in RPT cells [52]. Thus, the SIK network may be involved. Indeed, a recent report indicates that the mitochondrial biogenesis that occurs after the formoterol-induced recovery from ischemia-reperfusion injury is mediated by β adrenergic receptors [53]. Similarly, mitochondrial biogenesis occurs in brown adipocytes in response to catecholamines and occurs via a mechanism which involves the phosphorylation and inhibition of SIK2 [48].

The induction of mitochondrial biogenesis following injury to the RPT is also an important means of overcoming damage caused by Reactive Oxygen Species (ROS). ROS production occurs more often when the mitochondrial electron transport chain becomes more reduced as a consequence of cellular injuries [4,54,55]. This problem is alleviated when mitochondrial biogenesis occurs, which causes oxidative substrates to be distributed to more mitochondria. As a consequence, the degree to which the electron transport chain becomes reduced in individual mitochondria (and hence the degree that ROS production occurs) decreases.

As stated above, mitochondrial biogenesis is mediated by PGC-1α, whose expression depends upon the interaction of CRTCs with CREB, which in turn depends upon SIK. Following its induction, PGC-1α interacts with FOXO3 so as to increase the expression of the antioxidant genes CAT, SOD2, and GPX1 (which encode for catalase, superoxide dismutase and glutathione peroxidase, respectively) [55,56]. Indeed, these same antioxidant enzymes are induced in the kidney response to AKI [57,58]. Therefore, an understanding of the role of the SIK network in this process is important.

3.3. Yet Other Roles Known to Be Played by SIKs in Events Which Occur during AKI

A number of other metabolic events and cellular processes that occur during AKI are also known to involve SIKs. Included amongst the metabolic events is the decline in Fatty Acid (FA) oxidation in the RPT, which results in the Epithelial to Mesenchymal Transition (EMT). In addition, lethal damage during AKI results in apoptosis, and sublethal damage in repair processes, and ultimately cell division. The decline in FA oxidation, and apoptosis, as well as the progression of cells through the cell cycle, and ultimately, cell division involve SIKs.

3.3.1. Fatty Acid Oxidation

ATP Production in the RPT Is Generated by FA Oxidation, Which Declines in AKI

As stated above, RPT cells are included amongst the most energy demanding cells in the body, expending extensive quantities of ATP in order to meet their reabsorptive requirements. However, following a hypoxic or toxic insult, there is a major decline in cellular ATP and metabolism. ATP production by the RPT is primarily generated by the oxidation of FAs in mitochondria as well as peroxisomes. This process is largely shut down during AKI and for a lengthy period thereafter [54]. The FAs utilized by RPT cells are generated by their uptake by FA transporters such as CD36, the deacylation of phospholipids, and other metabolic events. Free FAs are first metabolized by Carnitine Palmitoyl-Transferase 1 (CPT-1), so as to form acyl carnitine derivatives, which enter mitochondria and peroxisomes [54]. After entering mitochondria and peroxisomes, the metabolism of FAs then depends upon enzymes including mitochondrial medium chain acyl COA dehydrogenase (MCAD) and peroxisomal acyl-CoA oxidase (ACOX1). However, both CPT-1 and ACOX1 enzymatic activity declines following ischemia/reperfusion injury, and MCAD activity declines as a consequence of cisplatin-induced AKI [54]. RPT cells have only a limited capacity to metabolize glucose in lieu of FAs. Thus, the decline in ATP levels that occurs in the RPT during AKI can be prolonged, with severe consequences.

SIK2 Regulates FA Oxidation in Other Tissues

Of particular interest in these regards, are the studies indicating that SIK2 regulates FA oxidation, in the liver, skeletal muscle, as well as in adipocytes [45]. Indeed, the levels of ACOX1, CPT1 and MCAD all decline in SIK2 KO mice. Thus, inactivation of SIK2 is an explanation for the decline in FA oxidation in RPT cells during AKI. Presumably then, interventions which specifically result in SIK2 activation would be expected to counteract the decline in FA oxidation (and resulting reductions in ATP levels).

Decreased FA Oxidation Results in EMT in the RPT

A number of studies indicate that the decrease in FA Oxidation that occurs during AKI results in EMT [54]. For example, studies with HK2 cells indicate that such a decrease in FA oxidation, and lipid accumulation precedes a glucose-induced morphological change typical of the EMT. Similarly, RPT cell cultures treated with the CPT-1 inhibitor Etoxmoxir undergo EMT. However, an alternative explanation for the EMT observed in the RPT during AKI (as well as during a decline in FA oxidation) is that it is a result of a TGFβ-mediated downregulation of cell–cell junctional constituents including E-cadherin.

Involvement of SIK1 in EMT

The studies of Vanlandewijck et al. [59] indicate that TGFβ downregulates E-cadherin through the activation of SIK1, which phosphorylates the polarity complex protein Par3 (a regulator of tight junction assembly), resulting in the degradation of Par3 by the proteasomes and lysosomes, an event which ultimately results in EMT. In addition, other kinases such as LKB1 maintain epithelial cell polarity, by activating SIKs, causing transcriptional repressors such as Snail1 to be downregulated (thereby preventing repression of E-Cadherin) [60].

TGFβ is a key profibrotic factor that is activated during AKI, and promotes EMT in the RPT [61]. Following repeated injury, RPT cells which have undergone EMT may fail to either re-differentiate, or to regain normal mitochondrial and metabolic function. Instead, these damaged RPT cells produce large quantities of TGFβ, which perpetuates the EMT, and prevents the proliferation necessary for repair. As a consequence, events can be initiated which result in Chronic Kidney Disease (CKD) [61]. Presumably, TGFβ production is responsible for perpetuating these problems. Conceivably, this cycle of events may be prevented by the use of SIK1 inhibitors to prevent signal transduction events which have been initiated via TGFβ receptors.

3.3.2. Role of SIKs in Apoptosis

Transient ischemia which occurs as a result of hypovolemia, hypotension and/or heart failure is a common cause of AKI. As stated above, the RPT is particularly susceptible to ischemic damage, which results in their detachment from their substratum, and death (either by apoptosis or necrosis) [62]. The apoptosis which occurs in the RPT during ischemia is a means of removing damaged, dysfunctional cells from the kidney. A number of studies indicate that p53 plays an important role in the apoptosis, cell cycle arrest and autophagy that occurs in the RPT when AKI is induced by ischemia, cisplatin and even folic acid [62]. Of particular interest in these regards are recent studies indicating that p53-dependent anoikis (a subtype of apoptosis resulting from a lack of cell adhesion) is mediated by SIK1 [63].

3.3.3. Pro-Survival Roles of SIKs and Epigenetics

Prosurvival Role of SIK1 in Myocytes Involves SIK1's HDAC Kinase Activity

A number of studies indicate that in addition, SIK1 has a pro-survival role (pertinent to cells which have been damaged, but are not destined to undergo apoptosis). Studies with transgenic mice with the targeted expression of a dominant negative CREB (ACREB), indicated that the survival of the differentiated cells in the targeted tissues decreased in the absence of functional CREB protein [19,64–66]. Initially, investigators thought that CREB was directly responsible for increasing cell survival and differentiation in the targeted tissues. However, subsequent studies indicated that CREB promoted cell survival (and differentiation) indirectly, by inducing the expression of the Snf1lk gene (encoding SIK1), resulting in an elevated level of activated SIK1 [19]. The activated SIK1 was observed to phosphorylate Class IIa HDACs, an event which was lost in vitro when the SIK1 phosphorylation site was removed by mutation [67]. The ultimate result of SIK1 phosphorylation in vivo was increased cell survival.

The initial studies indicating that SIK1 promoted cell survival were conducted with mice in which ACREB was targeted to skeletal muscle [67]. In skeletal muscle, previous studies indicated that the myogenic program depends upon MEF2 transcriptional activity. The binding of Class IIa HDACs to MEF2 transcription factors on chromosomal DNA inhibits MEF2-mediated transcription, and thus myogenesis. However, CREB activation was observed to induce SIK1 expression (which no longer occurred in ACREB skeletal muscle). Normally, the phosphorylation of Class IIa HDACs by SIK1 (and their translocation to the cytoplasm), results in increased MEF2 transcriptional activity and myogenesis (events which are impaired in ACREB mice). The discovery of that SIK1 is a pro-survival factor that promotes myogenesis, resulting in a reassessment of many previous studies.

Involvement of Epigenetics and Class IIa HDACs in Regeneration of Damaged Kidneys

A number of recent studies indicate that a number of epigenetic events, including histone acetylation, are important in the regeneration of damaged kidneys [68]. Indeed, a decrease in histone acetylation has been reported in RPTs subjected to energy depletion, while during the subsequent recovery period HDAC5 (a class IIa HDAC) was downregulated, and histone acetylation increased [69]. SIK1 may very well play a role in this process.

3.3.4. Role of SIKs in Cell Growth and Hypertrophy

Cell Division and Hypertrophy during AKI

In the normal kidney, RPT cells divide very slowly [70]. Cell division only occurs as a means to replace tubule epithelial cells, which are lost very slowly into the urine. However, following an ischemic or toxic insult, many RPT cells, which were previously quiescent, enter the cell cycle (even when there is massive necrosis and apoptosis). Many of the tubule epithelial cells which enter the cell cycle immediately after an ischemic or toxic insult spend a lengthy period in G2/M, secreting factors such as TGFβ, which result in fibrosis [71]. A large proportion of the epithelial cells which enter the cell cycle immediately after an ischemic or toxic insult have extensive DNA damage, leading to a mitotic catastrophe [70].

Subsequently, during the recovery period of AKI, additional RPT cells, including those which are sub-lethally injured, enter the cell cycle, and may divide [29]. The newly generated RPT cells migrate to regions which have been denuded as a consequence of injury, where they assume the polarized morphology required for transepithelial transport.

In recent studies, Lazzeri et al. [72] tracked the fate of individual tubular cells in conditional Pax8/Confetti mice during AKI. The results indicate that regeneration of new tubule epithelial cells during AKI is not as extensive as previously thought, even though kidney function recovers. Renal functional recovery could be attributed to some of the original tubule epithelial cells, in addition to limited progenitor driven regeneration. A number of the original tubule epithelial cells (or remnant cells) which were in the cell cycle, actually, went through endocycles (i.e., alternative cell cycles without cell division). Tubule epithelial cells which had undergone endoreplication cycles were often polyploid, and had undergone hypertrophy. Notably, endocycling cells and hypertrophy was also observed in the kidneys of patients after AKI.

Role of SIKs in Hypertrophy and Cell Division

As discussed above, the hypertrophy of atrial myocytes has been attributed to the activation of SIK1, in particular following an increase in intracellular Na^+ [18]. Recent studies by Popov et al. [73] indicate that SIK2 activation also causes hypertrophy in cardiac myocytes. In rats expressing a hypertensive variant of the α-adducin gene, the expression of SIK2 is elevated, as well as genes associated with left ventricle hypertrophy (LVH). Similarly, in mice on a high salt diet, LVH can be prevented by the ablation of sik2. Although not reported in the case of cardiac tissue, the SIK3 isoform is essential for chondrocyte hypertrophy during skeletal development [74]. However, the SIK Isoform(s) involved in renal hypertrophy have not been identified.

A number of recent studies indicate that SIKs regulate cell proliferation, particularly under conditions of stress. SIK2 promotes G1/S progression presumably due to its ability to phosphorylate the p85 α subunit of Phosphoinositide 3 Kinase (PI3K) [75], which mediates signaling in response to a number of growth factors. In addition, SIK2 is localized in centrosomes, where it acts as a "centrosome kinase" required for mitotic spindle formation [76]. The SIK3 isoform similarly is a mitotic regulator [77,78]. Indeed, mitosis is extended following a SIK3 knockdown. The increased duration of mitosis following a SIK3 knockdown has been attributed to a SIK3 requirement for mitotic exit. Although the metaphase plate forms normally when SIK3 is depleted, the onset of anaphase is delayed.

4. Summary and Therapeutic Potential

All three SIK isoforms are expressed in the RPT, and most likely play distinct roles in the preservation and reacquisition of renal function during AKI. Presently, the role played by each of the SIK isoforms during AKI can be surmised from investigations conducted with the renal SIK1 network, as well as with the SIK2 and SIK3 isoforms in other tissues, as summarized below.

During the initiation and extension phases of AKI, renal reabsorptive function declines and cytokines are produced. Activation of the SIK1 network during this time period results in an acute increase in the number of basolateral Na,K-ATPases (due to a SIK1 mediated decrease in basolateral PME activity, and an increase in dephosphorylated Na,K-ATPase (by activated PP2A)). The SIK1 activation caused by an increase in Ca^{2+}_{in}, also results in an increase in the phosphorylation of Class IIa HDACs by SIK1, transcriptional activation of NFAT2, which positively regulates the expression of the ANP and MHC genes. Thus, the development of SIK1 activators is needed so as to promote the expression of the SIK1 network during the early stages of AKI. The use of physiologic activators such as norepinephrine may have similar effects.

Needless to say, SIK1 activation may not always be beneficial. TGFβ (whose production starts during the early stages AKI) activates SIK1, and in this manner induces EMT. TGFβ production has the potential to continue for prolonged periods during AKI [61]. Thus, SIK1 inhibitors can presumably be employed to alleviate the long-term deleterious effects of TGFβ, including EMT and fibrosis.

PGE_2 is also produced during AKI. PGE_2 is a known mediator of inflammatory responses. Nevertheless, AKI was aggravated when microsomal Prostaglandin Synthase 2 (i.e., mPGES-2, which is responsible for renal PGE_2 production) was down-regulated, and this was associated with increased apoptosis [79]. These latter results suggest that PGE_2 promotes recovery from AKI. This can presumably be explained by a) the PKA-mediated inhibition of SIK1 which occurs as a consequence of the interaction of PGE_2 with either EP2 or EP4 receptors, as well as b) the Ca^{2+}-mediated activation of calcineurin, which results in the dephosphorylation of CRTC1, and its interaction with pCREB in RPT cells. As a consequence, not only does the expression of the *atp1b1* gene increase, as well the level of the Na,K-ATPase in RPT cells, but in addition, ATF3 expression increases. Such an increase in the expression of ATF3 (observed in vivo when ATF3 is overexpressed in mice by adenoviral mediated gene transfer) has been observed to result in a reduction of ischemia-reperfusion injury [80]. Thus, SIK1 inhibition at least during the latter stages of AKI presumably promotes recovery.

An increase in mitochondrial biogenesis during the initial phases of AKI is expected to cause an increase in reabsorption, as well as a decrease in the level of ROS. As summarized above, the SIK2 isoform has been observed to restrict mitochondrial biogenesis, due to its ability to phosphorylate CRTCs, thereby preventing the interaction of CRTCs with CREB, and reducing transcription of the PGC1-α gene. This limitation can be overcome, presumably by the inhibition of the SIK2 isoform per se during the initiation phase of AKI.

However, the cell cycle progression which occurs during subsequent phases of AKI depends upon SIK2. Not only is the p85 α subunit of PI3 Kinase is a substrate of SIK2 (PI3K promoting cell cycle entry) [81], but, in addition, SIK2 is required for cell division itself, being a centrosome kinase [76]. Similarly, the SIK3 isoform is required for mitotic exit. These processes would be promoted by targeting either SIK2 or SIK3 via an activating drug.

Studies conducted both in vitro with cultured renal cells as well as in vivo with transgenic animals are needed in order to evaluate whether the different SIK isoforms participate as anticipated in the events occurring during the different phases of AKI. In addition to employing siRNA and CRISPR technology, a number of expression vectors can be employed, including kinase dead SIK K56M [16], as well as SIK phosphomutants which cannot be phosphorylated by either LKB1, CaMK1 or PKA, the mutants being T182A, T322A, or T577A, respectively in the case of SIK1 [12,16,67]. Similar SIK mutants have been employed in studies with the other SIK isoforms [82,83]. In addition to employing the in vitro approach, studies conducted in vivo with mice possessing targeted knockouts should also prove to be invaluable when studying the role of SIKs in AKI. For example, the use of a mouse strain which expresses CRE recombinase under the control of the SGLT2 promoter will permit targeting of specific SIK knockouts to the RPT [84].

5. Development of Clinical Kinase Drugs

Protein kinases have emerged as major drug targets, because their functions within signaling networks are deregulated in a number of disease states [85]. Currently, more than 37 kinase inhibitors have been approved for human use, and the number is expected to increase dramatically, because more than 250 kinase inhibitors are undergoing clinical trials [85]. A number of these drugs target the ATP binding site, which has led to concerns of selectivity. This has led to chemoproteomic target screens of a multitude of kinase inhibitors [85]. Although a number of clinical kinase inhibitors have been found to be nonselective, at the same time other inhibitors were found to be extremely selective, including drugs targeting Mitogen Activated Protein Kinase (MAPK) and the Epidermal Growth Factor Receptor (EGFR). In addition, chemoproteomics have found some unexpected, yet promising drug targets, including SIK2.

SIK2 became of interest as a drug target when a small-molecule screening found that a number of kinase inhibitors that enhanced IL-10 production (and inhibited TNFα production) by murine bone-marrow-derived dendritic cells (including the FDA approved drugs dasatinib and bosutinib) actually targeted SIK2 [86]. The SIK inhibitor HG-9-91-01 was observed to have similar effects. In order to identify additional SIK2 inhibitors, MALDI-TOF screening assays have been conducted. In such studies, Heap et al. [87] were able to screen for SIK2 inhibitors, while assaying the phosphorylation of CHKtide, a peptide derived from CHK1 protein kinase involved in DNA repair (CHKtide had been previously identified in a kinase screen as being a good SIK substrate). Not only did Heap et al. [87] successfully identify SIK2 inhibitors, but in addition obtained evidence of activators [87]. Using a similar chemoproteomic screening approach, 21 additional SIK2 inhibitors were identified by Klaeger et al. [85]. Further progress is needed in validating the newly identified SIK2 inhibitors and activators, in addition to identifying drugs specifically targeting the other SIK isoforms.

Funding: This work was funded by NHLBI 1RO1 HL6976-01 to Mary Taub.

Acknowledgments: The author thanks Sudha Garimella, Dongwook Kim, Trivikram Rajkhowa, and Facundo Cutuli for their experimental work that inspired this review.

Conflicts of Interest: The author declares no conflict of interest.

References

1. Okamoto, M.; Takemori, H.; Katoh, Y. Salt-inducible kinase in steroidogenesis and adipogenesis. *Trends Endocrinol. Metab.* **2004**, *15*, 21–26. [CrossRef] [PubMed]
2. Jaitovich, A.; Bertorello, A.M. Intracellular sodium sensing: SIK1 network, hormone action and high blood pressure. *Biochim. Et Biophys. Acta* **2010**, *1802*, 1140–1149. [CrossRef] [PubMed]
3. Makris, K.; Spanou, L. Acute Kidney Injury: Definition, Pathophysiology and Clinical Phenotypes. *Clin. Biochem. Rev.* **2016**, *37*, 85–98. [PubMed]
4. Pavlakou, P.; Liakopoulos, V.; Eleftheriadis, T.; Mitsis, M.; Dounousi, E. Oxidative Stress and Acute Kidney Injury in Critical Illness: Pathophysiologic Mechanisms-Biomarkers-Interventions, and Future Perspectives. *Oxid Med. Cell Longev.* **2017**, *2017*, 6193694. [CrossRef] [PubMed]
5. Zuk, A.; Bonventre, J.V. Acute Kidney Injury. *Annu. Rev. Med.* **2016**, *67*, 293–307. [CrossRef]
6. Moore, P.K.; Hsu, R.K.; Liu, K.D. Management of Acute Kidney Injury: Core Curriculum 2018. *Am. J. Kidney Dis.* **2018**, *72*, 136–148. [CrossRef] [PubMed]
7. Levey, A.S.; James, M.T. Acute Kidney Injury. *Ann. Intern. Med.* **2017**, *167*, ITC66–ITC80. [CrossRef]
8. Lan, R.; Geng, H.; Singha, P.K.; Saikumar, P.; Bottinger, E.P.; Weinberg, J.M.; Venkatachalam, M.A. Mitochondrial Pathology and Glycolytic Shift during Proximal Tubule Atrophy after Ischemic AKI. *J. Am. Soc. Nephrol.* **2016**, *27*, 3356–3367. [CrossRef]
9. Morrell, E.D.; Kellum, J.A.; Hallows, K.R.; Pastor-Soler, N.M. Epithelial transport during septic acute kidney injury. *Nephrol. Dial. Transpl.* **2014**, *29*, 1312–1319. [CrossRef]
10. Strazzullo, P.; Leclercq, C. Sodium. *Adv. Nutr.* **2014**, *5*, 188–190. [CrossRef]
11. Ding, X.; Cheng, Z.; Qian, Q. Intravenous Fluids and Acute Kidney Injury. *Blood Purif.* **2017**, *43*, 163–172. [CrossRef] [PubMed]
12. Sjostrom, M.; Stenstrom, K.; Eneling, K.; Zwiller, J.; Katz, A.I.; Takemori, H.; Bertorello, A.M. SIK1 is part of a cell sodium-sensing network that regulates active sodium transport through a calcium-dependent process. *Proc. Natl. Acad. Sci. USA.* **2007**, *104*, 16922–16927. [CrossRef] [PubMed]
13. Skou, J.C.; Esmann, M. The Na,K-ATPase. *J. Bioenerg. Biomembr.* **1992**, *24*, 249–261. [PubMed]
14. Sakamoto, K.; Bultot, L.; Goransson, O. The Salt-Inducible Kinases: Emerging Metabolic Regulators. *Trends Endocrinol Metab.* **2018**, *29*, 827–840. [CrossRef] [PubMed]
15. Hashimoto, Y.K.; Satoh, T.; Okamoto, M.; Takemori, H. Importance of autophosphorylation at Ser186 in the A-loop of salt inducible kinase 1 for its sustained kinase activity. *J. Cell Biochem.* **2008**, *104*, 1724–1739. [CrossRef] [PubMed]
16. Katoh, Y.; Takemori, H.; Lin, X.Z.; Tamura, M.; Muraoka, M.; Satoh, T.; Tsuchiya, Y.; Min, L.; Doi, J.; Miyauchi, A.; et al. Silencing the constitutive active transcription factor CREB by the LKB1-SIK signaling cascade. *Febs. J.* **2006**, *273*, 2730–2748. [CrossRef] [PubMed]
17. Sonntag, T.; Vaughan, J.M.; Montminy, M. 14-3-3 proteins mediate inhibitory effects of cAMP on salt-inducible kinases (SIKs). *Febs. J.* **2018**, *285*, 467–480. [CrossRef] [PubMed]
18. Popov, S.; Venetsanou, K.; Chedrese, P.J.; Pinto, V.; Takemori, H.; Franco-Cereceda, A.; Eriksson, P.; Mochizuki, N.; Soares-da-Silva, P.; Bertorello, A.M. Increases in intracellular sodium activate transcription and gene expression via the salt-inducible kinase 1 network in an atrial myocyte cell line, American journal of physiology. *Heart Circ. Physiol.* **2012**, *303*, H57–H65. [CrossRef]
19. Berdeaux, R.; Goebel, N.; Banaszynski, L.; Takemori, H.; Wandless, T.; Shelton, G.D.; Montminy, M. SIK1 is a class II HDAC kinase that promotes survival of skeletal myocytes. *Nat. Med.* **2007**, *13*, 597–603. [CrossRef]
20. Vesely, D.L. Natriuretic peptides and acute renal failure. *Am. J. Physiol. Ren. Physiol.* **2003**, *285*, F167–F177. [CrossRef]
21. Kim, S.W.; Lee, J.; Park, J.W.; Hong, J.H.; Kook, H.; Choi, C.; Choi, K.C. Increased expression of atrial natriuretic peptide in the kidney of rats with bilateral ureteral obstruction. *Kidney Int.* **2001**, *59*, 1274–1282. [CrossRef] [PubMed]

22. Takei, Y.; Sims, T.N.; Urmson, J.; Halloran, P.F. Central role for interferon-gamma receptor in the regulation of renal MHC expression. *J. Am. Soc. Nephrol.* **2000**, *11*, 250–261. [PubMed]

23. Arulkumaran, N.; Prowle, J.R. Natriuretic Peptides: A Role in Early Septic Acute Kidney Injury? *Anesthesiology* **2018**, *129*, 235–237. [CrossRef] [PubMed]

24. Ueda, K.; Hirahashi, J.; Seki, G.; Tanaka, M.; Kushida, N.; Takeshima, Y.; Nishikawa, Y.; Fujita, T.; Nangaku, M. Successful treatment of acute kidney injury in patients with idiopathic nephrotic syndrome using human atrial natriuretic Peptide. *Intern. Med.* **2014**, *53*, 865–869. [CrossRef] [PubMed]

25. Nigwekar, S.U.; Navaneethan, S.D.; Parikh, C.R.; Hix, J.K. Atrial natriuretic peptide for management of acute kidney injury: A systematic review and meta-analysis. *Clin. J. Am. Soc. Nephrol.* **2009**, *4*, 261–272. [CrossRef]

26. Wein, M.N.; Foretz, M.; Fisher, D.E.; Xavier, R.J.; Kronenberg, H.M. Salt-Inducible Kinases: Physiology, Regulation by cAMP, and Therapeutic Potential. *Trends Endocrinol Metab.* **2018**, *29*, 723–735. [CrossRef] [PubMed]

27. Taub, M.; Garamella, S.; Kim, D.; Rajkhowa, T.; Cutuli, F. Renal Proximal Tubule Na,K-ATPase is Controlled by CREB Regulated Transcriptional CoActivators as well as Salt Inducible Kinase 1. *Cell. Signal.* **2015**, *27*, 2568–2578. [CrossRef]

28. MacKenzie, K.F.; Clark, K.; Naqvi, S.; McGuire, V.A.; Noehren, G.; Kristariyanto, Y.; van den Bosch, M.; Mudaliar, M.; McCarthy, P.C.; Pattison, M.J.; et al. PGE(2) induces macrophage IL-10 production and a regulatory-like phenotype via a protein kinase A-SIK-CRTC3 pathway. *J. Immunol.* **2013**, *190*, 565–577. [CrossRef]

29. Basile, D.P.; Anderson, M.D.; Sutton, T.A. Pathophysiology of acute kidney injury. *Compr. Physiol.* **2012**, *2*, 1303–1353.

30. Breyer, M.D.; Breyer, R.M. Prostaglandin E receptors and the kidney. *Am. J. Physiol. Ren. Physiol.* **2000**, *279*, F12–F23. [CrossRef]

31. Matlhagela, K.; Taub, M. Involvement of EP1 and EP2 receptors in the regulation of the Na,K-ATPase by prostaglandins in MDCK cells. *Prostaglandins Other Lipid Mediat.* **2006**, *79*, 101–113. [CrossRef] [PubMed]

32. Herman, M.B.; Rajkhowa, T.; Cutuli, F.; Springate, J.E.; Taub, M. Regulation of renal proximal tubule Na-K-ATPase by prostaglandins. *Am. J. Physiol. Ren. Physiol.* **2010**, *298*, F1222–F1234. [CrossRef] [PubMed]

33. Taub, M.; Borsick, M.; Geisel, J.; Rajkhowa, T.; Allen, C. Regulation of the Na,K-ATPase in MDCK cells by prostaglandin E1: A role for calcium as well as cAMP. *Exp. Cell Res.* **2004**, *299*, 1–14. [CrossRef] [PubMed]

34. Geering, K. The functional role of the beta-subunit in the maturation and intracellular transport of sodium-potassium ATPase. *FEBS Lett.* **1991**, *285*, 189–193. [CrossRef]

35. Taub, M. Gene Level Regulation of Na,K-ATPase in the Renal Proximal Tubule Is Controlled by Two Independent but Interacting Regulatory Mechanisms Involving Salt Inducible Kinase 1 and CREB-Regulated Transcriptional Coactivators. *Int. J. Mol. Sci.* **2018**, *19*, 2086–2095. [CrossRef] [PubMed]

36. Matlhagela, K.; Borsick, M.; Rajkhowa, T.; Taub, M. Identification of a Prostaglandin-responsive Element in the Na,K-ATPase {beta}1 Promoter That Is Regulated by cAMP and Ca2+: Evidence for an interactive role of cAMP regulatory element-bindin protein and Sp1. *J. Biol. Chem.* **2005**, *280*, 334–346. [CrossRef]

37. Matlhagela, K.; Taub, M. Regulation of the Na-K-ATPase beta(1)-subunit promoter by multiple prostaglandin-responsive elements. *Am. J. Physiol. - Ren. Physiol.* **2006**, *291*, F635–F646. [CrossRef]

38. Altarejos, J.Y.; Montminy, M. CREB and the CRTC co-activators: Sensors for hormonal and metabolic signals, Nature reviews. *Mol. Cell Biol.* **2011**, *12*, 141–151.

39. Nakajima, T.; Uchida, C.; Anderson, S.F.; Parvin, J.D.; Montminy, M. Analysis of a cAMP-responsive activator reveals a two-component mechanism for transcriptional induction via signal-dependent factors. *Genes Dev.* **1997**, *11*, 738–747. [CrossRef]

40. Bertorello, A.M.; Zhu, J.K. SIK1/SOS2 networks: Decoding sodium signals via calcium-responsive protein kinase pathways. *Pflug. Arch. - Eur. J. Physiol.* **2009**, *458*, 613–619. [CrossRef]

41. Ji, H.; Pardo, J.M.; Batelli, G.; Van Oosten, M.J.; Bressan, R.A.; Li, X. The Salt Overly Sensitive (SOS) pathway: Established and emerging roles. *Mol. Plant.* **2013**, *6*, 275–286. [CrossRef] [PubMed]

42. Itoh, Y.; Sanosaka, M.; Fuchino, H.; Yahara, Y.; Kumagai, A.; Takemoto, D.; Kagawa, M.; Doi, J.; Ohta, M.; Tsumaki, N.; et al. Salt-inducible Kinase 3 Signaling Is Important for the Gluconeogenic Programs in Mouse Hepatocytes. *J. Biol. Chem.* **2015**, *290*, 17879–17893. [CrossRef] [PubMed]

43. Du, J.; Chen, Q.; Takemori, H.; Xu, H. SIK2 can be activated by deprivation of nutrition and it inhibits expression of lipogenic genes in adipocytes. *Obes. (Silver Spring)* **2008**, *16*, 531–538. [CrossRef] [PubMed]

44. Liu, Y.; Dentin, R.; Chen, D.; Hedrick, S.; Ravnskjaer, K.; Schenk, S.; Milne, J.; Meyers, D.J.; Cole, P.; Yates III, J.; et al. A fasting inducible switch modulates gluconeogenesis via activator/coactivator exchange. *Nature* **2008**, *456*, 269–273. [CrossRef] [PubMed]

45. Park, J.; Yoon, Y.S.; Han, H.S.; Kim, Y.H.; Ogawa, Y.; Park, K.G.; Lee, C.H.; Kim, S.T.; Koo, S.H. SIK2 is critical in the regulation of lipid homeostasis and adipogenesis *in vivo*. *Diabetes* **2014**, *63*, 3659–3673. [CrossRef] [PubMed]

46. Sasaki, M.; Sasako, T.; Kubota, N.; Sakurai, Y.; Takamoto, I.; Kubota, T.; Inagi, R.; Seki, G.; Goto, M.; Ueki, K.; et al. Dual Regulation of Gluconeogenesis by Insulin and Glucose in the Proximal Tubules of the Kidney. *Diabetes* **2017**, *66*, 2339–2350. [CrossRef] [PubMed]

47. Li, H.F.; Cheng, C.F.; Liao, W.J.; Lin, H.; Yang, R.B. ATF3-mediated epigenetic regulation protects against acute kidney injury. *J. Am. Soc. Nephrol.* **2010**, *21*, 1003–1013. [CrossRef] [PubMed]

48. Muraoka, M.; Fukushima, A.; Viengchareun, S.; Lombes, M.; Kishi, F.; Miyauchi, A.; Kanematsu, M.; Doi, J.; Kajimura, J.; Nakai, R.; et al. Involvement of SIK2/TORC2 signaling cascade in the regulation of insulin-induced PGC-1alpha and UCP-1 gene expression in brown adipocytes. *Am. J. Physiol. Endocrinol. Metab.* **2009**, *296*, E1430–E1439. [CrossRef] [PubMed]

49. Nixon, M.; Stewart-Fitzgibbon, R.; Fu, J.; Akhmedov, D.; Rajendran, K.; Mendoza-Rodriguez, M.G.; Rivera-Molina, Y.A.; Gibson, M.; Berglund, E.D.; Justice, N.J.; et al. Skeletal muscle salt inducible kinase 1 promotes insulin resistance in obesity. *Mol. Metab.* **2016**, *5*, 34–46. [CrossRef]

50. Wu, Z.; Huang, X.; Feng, Y.; Handschin, C.; Feng, Y.; Gullicksen, P.S.; Bare, O.; Labow, M.; Spiegelman, B.; Stevenson, S.C. Transducer of regulated CREB-binding proteins (TORCs) induce PGC-1alpha transcription and mitochondrial biogenesis in muscle cells. *Proc. Natl. Acad. Sci. USA.* **2006**, *103*, 14379–14384. [CrossRef]

51. Rasbach, K.A.; Schnellmann, R.G. PGC-1alpha over-expression promotes recovery from mitochondrial dysfunction and cell injury. *Biochem. Biophys. Res. Commun.* **2007**, *355*, 734–739. [CrossRef] [PubMed]

52. Funk, J.A.; Odejinmi, S.; Schnellmann, R.G. SRT1720 induces mitochondrial biogenesis and rescues mitochondrial function after oxidant injury in renal proximal tubule cells. *J. Pharm. Exp.* **2010**, *333*, 593–601. [CrossRef] [PubMed]

53. Cameron, R.B.; Gibbs, W.S.; Miller, S.R.; Dupre, T.V.; Megyesi, J.; Beeson, C.C.; Schnellmann, R.G. Proximal Tubule beta 2-Adrenergic Receptor Mediates Formoterol-Induced Recovery of Mitochondrial and Renal Function after Ischemia-Reperfusion Injury. *J. Pharm. Exp.* **2019**, *369*, 173–180. [CrossRef] [PubMed]

54. Simon, N.; Hertig, A. Alteration of Fatty Acid Oxidation in Tubular Epithelial Cells: From Acute Kidney Injury to Renal Fibrogenesis. *Front. Med. (Lausanne)* **2015**, *2*, 52. [CrossRef] [PubMed]

55. Weinberg, J.M. Mitochondrial biogenesis in kidney disease. *J. Am. Soc. Nephrol.* **2011**, *22*, 431–436. [CrossRef]

56. Olmos, Y.; Valle, I.; Borniquel, S.; Tierrez, A.; Soria, E.; Lamas, S.; Monsalve, M. Mutual dependence of Foxo3a and PGC-1alpha in the induction of oxidative stress genes. *J. Biol. Chem.* **2009**, *284*, 14476–14484. [CrossRef] [PubMed]

57. Singh, I.; Gulati, S.; Orak, J.K.; Singh, A.K. Expression of antioxidant enzymes in rat kidney during ischemia-reperfusion injury. *Mol. Cell Biochem.* **1993**, *125*, 97–104. [CrossRef]

58. Tran, M.; Parikh, S.M. Mitochondrial biogenesis in the acutely injured kidney. *Nephron Clin. Pr.* **2014**, *127*, 42–45. [CrossRef]

59. Vanlandewijck, M.; Dadras, M.S.; Lomnytska, M.; Mahzabin, T.; Lee Miller, M.; Busch, C.; Brunak, S.; Heldin, C.H.; Moustakas, A. The protein kinase SIK downregulates the polarity protein Par3. *Oncotarget* **2018**, *9*, 5716–5735. [CrossRef]

60. Goodwin, J.M.; Svensson, R.U.; Lou, H.J.; Winslow, M.M.; Turk, B.E.; Shaw, R.J. An AMPK-independent signaling pathway downstream of the LKB1 tumor suppressor controls Snail1 and metastatic potential. *Mol Cell* **2014**, *55*, 436–450. [CrossRef]

61. Gewin, L.S. Transforming Growth Factor-beta in the Acute Kidney Injury to Chronic Kidney Disease Transition. *Nephron* **2019**, 1–4. [CrossRef] [PubMed]

62. Havasi, A.; Borkan, S.C. Apoptosis and acute kidney injury. *Kidney Int.* **2011**, *80*, 29–40. [CrossRef] [PubMed]

63. Cheng, H.; Liu, P.; Wang, Z.C.; Zou, L.; Santiago, S.; Garbitt, V.; Gjoerup, O.V.; Iglehart, J.D.; Miron, A.; Richardson, A.L.; et al. SIK1 couples LKB1 to p53-dependent anoikis and suppresses metastasis. *Sci. Signal.* **2009**, *2*, ra35. [CrossRef] [PubMed]

64. Watson, P.A.; Birdsey, N.; Huggins, G.S.; Svensson, E.; Heppe, D.; Knaub, L. Cardiac-specific overexpression of dominant-negative CREB leads to increased mortality and mitochondrial dysfunction in female mice. *Am. J. Physiol. Heart Circ. Physiol.* **2010**, *299*, H2056–H2068. [CrossRef]

65. Jhala, U.S.; Canettieri, G.; Screaton, R.A.; Kulkarni, R.N.; Krajewski, S.; Reed, J.; Walker, J.; Lin, X.; White, M.; Montminy, M. cAMP promotes pancreatic beta-cell survival via CREB-mediated induction of IRS2. *Genes Dev.* **2003**, *17*, 1575–1580. [CrossRef]

66. Sakamoto, K.; Karelina, K.; Obrietan, K. CREB: A multifaceted regulator of neuronal plasticity and protection. *J. Neurochem.* **2011**, *116*, 1–9. [CrossRef] [PubMed]

67. Stewart, R.; Akhmedov, D.; Robb, C.; Leiter, C.; Berdeaux, R. Regulation of SIK1 abundance and stability is critical for myogenesis. *Proc. Natl. Acad. Sci. USA.* **2013**, *110*, 117–122. [CrossRef]

68. Dressler, G.R.; Patel, S.R. Epigenetics in kidney development and renal disease. *Transl. Res.* **2015**, *165*, 166–176. [CrossRef]

69. Marumo, T.; Hishikawa, K.; Yoshikawa, M.; Fujita, T. Epigenetic regulation of BMP7 in the regenerative response to ischemia. *J. Am. Soc. Nephrol.* **2008**, *19*, 1311–1320. [CrossRef]

70. Thomasova, D.; Anders, H.J. Cell cycle control in the kidney. *Nephrol. Dial. Transpl.* **2015**, *30*, 1622–1630. [CrossRef]

71. Wu, C.F.; Chiang, W.C.; Lai, C.F.; Chang, F.C.; Chen, Y.T.; Chou, Y.H.; Wu, T.H.; Linn, G.R.; Ling, H.; Wu, K.D.; et al. Transforming growth factor beta-1 stimulates profibrotic epithelial signaling to activate pericyte-myofibroblast transition in obstructive kidney fibrosis. *Am. J. Pathol.* **2013**, *182*, 118–131. [CrossRef] [PubMed]

72. Lazzeri, E.; Angelotti, M.L.; Peired, A.; Conte, C.; Marschner, J.A.; Maggi, L.; Mazzinghi, B.; Lombardi, D.; Melica, M.E.; Nardi, S.; et al. Endocycle-related tubular cell hypertrophy and progenitor proliferation recover renal function after acute kidney injury. *Nat. Commun.* **2018**, *9*, 1344. [CrossRef] [PubMed]

73. Popov, S.; Takemori, H.; Tokudome, T.; Mao, Y.; Otani, K.; Mochizuki, N.; Pires, N.; Pinho, M.J.; Franco-Cereceda, A.; Torielli, L.; et al. Lack of salt-inducible kinase 2 (SIK2) prevents the development of cardiac hypertrophy in response to chronic high-salt intake. *PLoS ONE* **2014**, *9*, e95771. [CrossRef] [PubMed]

74. Sasagawa, S.; Takemori, H.; Uebi, T.; Ikegami, D.; Hiramatsu, K.; Ikegawa, S.; Yoshikawa, H.; Tsumaki, N. SIK3 is essential for chondrocyte hypertrophy during skeletal development in mice. *Development* **2012**, *139*, 1153–1163. [CrossRef] [PubMed]

75. Miranda, F.; Mannion, D.; Liu, S.; Zheng, Y.; Mangala, L.S.; Redondo, C.; Herrero-Gonzalez, S.; Xu, R.; Taylor, C.; Chedom, D.F.; et al. Salt-Inducible Kinase 2 Couples Ovarian Cancer Cell Metabolism with Survival at the Adipocyte-Rich Metastatic Niche. *Cancer Cell* **2016**, *30*, 273–289. [CrossRef] [PubMed]

76. Ahmed, A.A.; Lu, Z.; Jennings, N.B.; Etemadmoghadam, D.; Capalbo, L.; Jacamo, R.O.; Barbosa-Morais, N.; Le, X.F.; Australian Ovarian Cancer Study Group; Vivas-Mejia, P.; et al. SIK2 is a centrosome kinase required for bipolar mitotic spindle formation that provides a potential target for therapy in ovarian cancer. *Cancer Cell* **2010**, *18*, 109–121. [CrossRef] [PubMed]

77. Wehr, M.C.; Holder, M.V.; Gailite, I.; Saunders, R.E.; Maile, T.M.; Ciirdaeva, E.; Instrell, R.; Jiang, M.; Howell, M.; Rossner, M.J.; et al. Salt-inducible kinases regulate growth through the Hippo signalling pathway in Drosophila. *Nat. Cell Biol.* **2013**, *15*, 61–71. [CrossRef]

78. Chen, H.; Huang, S.; Han, X.; Zhang, J.; Shan, C.; Tsang, Y.H.; Ma, H.T.; Poon, R.Y. Salt-inducible kinase 3 is a novel mitotic regulator and a target for enhancing antimitotic therapeutic-mediated cell death. *Cell Death Dis.* **2014**, *5*, e1177. [CrossRef]

79. Li, Y.; Xia, W.; Zhao, F.; Wen, Z.; Zhang, A.; Huang, S.; Jia, Z.; Zhang, Y. Prostaglandins in the pathogenesis of kidney diseases. *Oncotarget* **2018**, *9*, 26586–26602. [CrossRef]

80. Yoshida, T.; Sugiura, H.; Mitobe, M.; Tsuchiya, K.; Shirota, S.; Nishimura, S.; Shiohira, S.; Ito, H.; Nobori, K.; Gullans, S.R.; et al. ATF3 protects against renal ischemia-reperfusion injury. *J. Am. Soc. Nephrol.* **2008**, *19*, 217–224. [CrossRef]

81. Chen, F.; Chen, L.; Qin, Q.; Sun, X. Salt-Inducible Kinase 2: An Oncogenic Signal Transmitter and Potential Target for Cancer Therapy. *Front. Oncol.* **2019**, *9*, 18. [CrossRef] [PubMed]

82. Patel, K.; Foretz, M.; Marion, A.; Campbell, D.G.; Gourlay, R.; Boudaba, N.; Tournier, E.; Titchenell, P.; Peggie, M.; Deak, M.; et al. The LKB1-salt-inducible kinase pathway functions as a key gluconeogenic suppressor in the liver. *Nat. Commun.* **2014**, *5*, 4535. [CrossRef] [PubMed]

83. Honda, T.; Fujiyama, T.; Miyoshi, C.; Ikkyu, A.; Hotta-Hirashima, N.; Kanno, S.; Mizuno, S.; Sugiyama, F.; Takahashi, S.; Funato, H.; et al. A single phosphorylation site of SIK3 regulates daily sleep amounts and sleep need in mice. *Proc. Natl. Acad. Sci. USA.* **2018**, *115*, 10458–10463. [CrossRef] [PubMed]
84. Igarashi, P. Kidney-specific gene targeting. *J. Am. Soc. Nephrol.* **2004**, *15*, 2237–2239. [CrossRef] [PubMed]
85. Klaeger, S.; Heinzlmeir, S.; Wilhelm, M.; Polzer, H.; Vick, B.; Koenig, P.A.; Reinecke, M.; Ruprecht, B.; Petzoldt, S.; Meng, C.; et al. The target landscape of clinical kinase drugs. *Science* **2017**, *358*. [CrossRef] [PubMed]
86. Sundberg, T.B.; Choi, H.G.; Song, J.H.; Russell, C.N.; Hussain, M.M.; Graham, D.B.; Khor, B.; Gagnon, J.; O'Connell, D.J.; Narayan, K.; et al. Small-molecule screening identifies inhibition of salt-inducible kinases as a therapeutic strategy to enhance immunoregulatory functions of dendritic cells. *Proc. Natl. Acad. Sci. USA.* **2014**, *111*, 12468–12473. [CrossRef]
87. Heap, R.E.; Hope, A.G.; Pearson, L.A.; Reyskens, K.; McElroy, S.P.; Hastie, C.J.; Porter, D.W.; Arthur, J.S.C.; Gray, D.W.; Trost, M. Identifying Inhibitors of Inflammation: A Novel High-Throughput MALDI-TOF Screening Assay for Salt-Inducible Kinases (SIKs). *Slas. Discov.* **2017**, *22*, 1193–1202. [CrossRef] [PubMed]

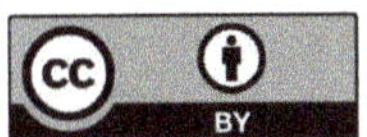

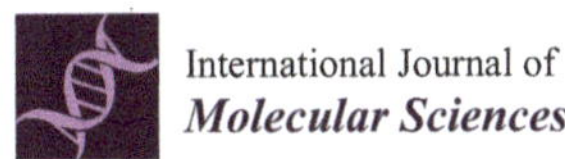

International Journal of
Molecular Sciences

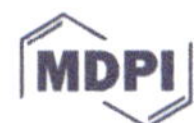

Review

The Anti-Inflammatory, Anti-Oxidative, and Anti-Apoptotic Benefits of Stem Cells in Acute Ischemic Kidney Injury

Kuo-Hua Lee [1,2,3], Wei-Cheng Tseng [1,2,3], Chih-Yu Yang [1,2,3] and Der-Cherng Tarng [1,2,3,4,*]

[1] Division of Nephrology, Department of Medicine, Taipei Veterans General Hospital, Taipei 11217, Taiwan
[2] Institute of Clinical Medicine, National Yang-Ming University, Taipei 11217, Taiwan
[3] Center for Intelligent Drug Systems and Smart Bio-devices (IDS2B), Hsinchu 30010, Taiwan
[4] Department and Institute of Physiology, National Yang-Ming University, Taipei 11217, Taiwan
* Correspondence: dctarng@vghtpe.gov.tw; Tel.: +886-2-2875-7517; Fax: +886-2-2875-7841

Received: 2 July 2019; Accepted: 18 July 2019; Published: 19 July 2019

Abstract: Ischemia-reperfusion injury (IRI) plays a significant role in the pathogenesis of acute kidney injury (AKI). The complicated interaction between injured tubular cells, activated endothelial cells, and the immune system leads to oxidative stress and systemic inflammation, thereby exacerbating the apoptosis of renal tubular cells and impeding the process of tissue repair. Stem cell therapy is an innovative approach to ameliorate IRI due to its antioxidative, immunomodulatory, and anti-apoptotic properties. Therefore, it is crucial to understand the biological effects and mechanisms of action of stem cell therapy in the context of acute ischemic AKI to improve its therapeutic benefits. The recent finding that treatment with conditioned medium (CM) derived from stem cells is likely an effective alternative to conventional stem cell transplantation increases the potential for future therapeutic uses of stem cell therapy. In this review, we discuss the recent findings regarding stem cell-mediated cytoprotection, with a focus on the anti-inflammatory effects via suppression of oxidative stress and uncompromised immune responses following AKI. Stem cell-derived CM represents a favorable approach to stem cell-based therapy and may serve as a potential therapeutic strategy against acute ischemic AKI.

Keywords: ischemia-reperfusion; acute kidney injury; stem cell; conditioned medium; inflammation

---

1. Introduction

Acute kidney injury (AKI) involves a complex interaction between the kidney parenchyma and immune system that leads to inflammation at the site of the injured tissue and impaired renal function [1]. Renal ischemia is a significant cause of AKI and is characterized by reduced tissue perfusion, which leads to acute tubular injury. Re-establishing the blood supply after prolonged ischemia activates vascular endothelial cells and enhances the generation of reactive oxygen species (ROS). This triggers a myriad of inflammatory consequences and induces apoptosis of tubular epithelial cells (TECs) [2]. This phenomenon is referred to as ischemia-reperfusion induced AKI (IR-AKI) and is characterized by elevated oxidative stress and activation of the immune system in response to ischemic tissue injury [3,4].

In the early stages of renal ischemia, the circulating neutrophils and monocytes rapidly infiltrate the ischemic kidney and release lysosomal enzymes, leading to tubular epithelial cell injury [2]. Subsequent crosstalk between the injured TECs, activated endothelial cells, and tissue macrophages induces oxidative stress and complement activation, aggravating cell damaging processes, such as mitochondrial dysfunction and lipid peroxidation [5].

Furthermore, the extensive release of pro-inflammatory cytokines, such as tumor necrosis factor (TNF)-α, interleukin (IL)-6, and monocyte chemoattractant protein 1 (MCP-1), attract an immune response involving monocytes, dendritic cells (DC), natural killer (NK) cells, and lymphocytes [6]. Subsequent ROS-mediated mitogen-activated protein kinase (MAPK) and nuclear factor (NF)-κB cascades amplify the inflammatory response. The signaling transduction pathways induce extensive TEC apoptosis and upregulate several important inflammatory mediators, such as IL-6, TNF-α, IL-1β, interferon (IFN)-γ, and IL-17 [2,4,7]. These immune reactions establish a continuous positive feedback loop, or a vicious circle, resulting in constant stimulation. As a consequence, IR-AKI is not merely a localized kidney insult, but also a trigger for a cascade of systemic inflammation (Figure 1).

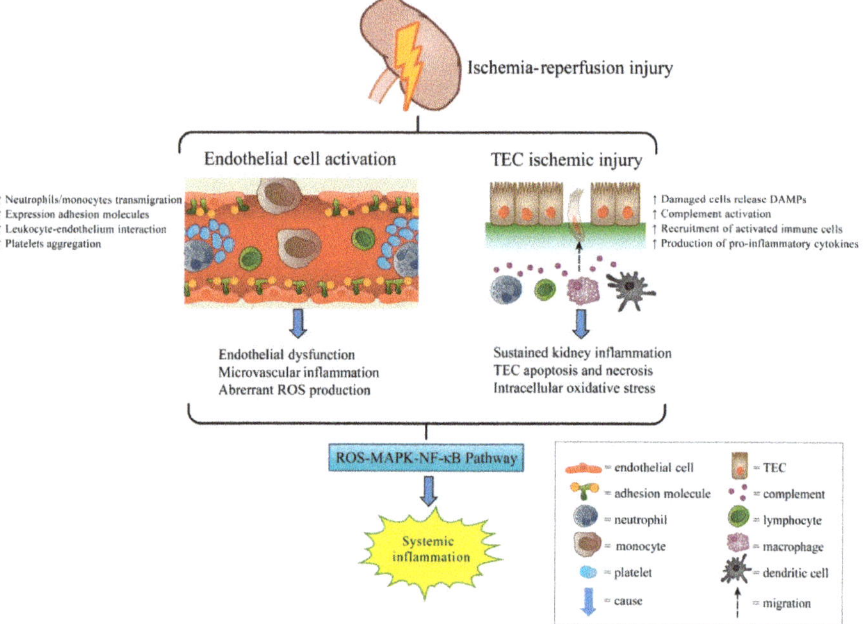

Figure 1. Pathogenesis of ischemia-reperfusion induced acute kidney injury. Ischemia-reperfusion-induced acute kidney injury involves endothelial cell activation (1). The increased leukocyte adhesion molecules on the activated endothelial cells induce leukocyte transmigration and platelet aggregation, which both cause microvascular inflammation. In tubular epithelial cell injury (2), the injured tubular cells release danger signals, which activate immune cells involved in local and systemic inflammation. The substantial amount of reactive oxygen species generated by this process activates the MAPK-NF-κB pathway and induces systemic inflammation. Abbreviations: DAMPs, damage-associated molecular patterns; TECs, tubular epithelial cells; ROS, reactive oxygen species; MAPK, mitogen-activated protein kinase; NF-κB, nuclear factor-κB.

In contrast to previous therapeutic approaches for AKI, which were mainly supportive, innovative treatments targeting AKI-induced inflammation, including stem cell therapy, have elicited a great deal of interest. In experimental models, administration of stem cells has proven effective in the treatment of AKI. One of the critical mechanisms of stem cell therapy is the anti-inflammatory effect caused by interaction with immune cells in the inflamed microenvironment [8–10]. Furthermore, stem cells may minimize the magnitude of tissue damage by secreting soluble cytoprotective factors in a paracrine manner [11,12].

Given that oxidative stress and inflammation have been implicated in the pathogenesis of IR-AKI, it is imperative to discuss these anti-inflammatory and immunoregulatory properties of stem cells. In this review, we focus on the therapeutic potential of stem cells in IR-AKI and illustrate the underlying antioxidant and anti-inflammatory mechanisms of this therapy. Because stem cells release soluble factors and microvesicles in a paracrine manner [13], we also discuss the effectiveness of stem cell-derived conditioned medium (CM) as an alternative to stem cell transplantation in the treatment of IR-AKI.

2. Immune Responses and Inflammation in IR-AKI

In IR-AKI, damaged cells are thought to be the critical trigger of inflammation. During the reperfusion phase, TECs are vulnerable to oxidative stress, and apoptotic and necrotic TECs release damage-associated molecular patterns (DAMPs) into the extracellular space. Endogenous DAMP molecules include DNA, RNA, and several intracellular proteins such as S100, heat-shock proteins, and high-mobility group box 1 (HMGB1) [14]. The so-called "danger signals" stimulate pattern recognition receptors (PRRs) expressed on renal parenchyma and immune cells, like epithelial and endothelial cells, DCs, lymphocytes, and macrophages. This recognition process initiates the host's defense mechanisms and further produces various cytokines that attract neutrophils and macrophages [15]. Signaling pathways activated by DAMP ligation of PRRs also result in activation of NF-κB, which further promotes the expression of pro-inflammatory cytokines and perpetuates the inflammatory response in IR-AKI.

The balance between pro-inflammatory (e.g., TNF-α, IFN-γ, IL-6, IL-1β, IL-17, C3, C5a, and C5b) and anti-inflammatory (e.g., IL-4, TGF-β, IL-10, and heme oxygenase-1 (HO-1)) mediators secreted by the participating cell populations determines the status of injury and repair [16]. HO-1 is an endogenous stress-inducible enzyme, which modulates leukocyte adhesion and migration, immune cell maturation, and production of inflammatory cytokines following ischemia. Up-regulation of HO-1 represents an anti-inflammatory and anti-oxidative defense capacity against IRI [17]. Under ideal conditions, a regulated balance between inflammatory and anti-inflammatory mediators ensures healthy tissue regeneration and reversal of homeostatic conditions. However, AKI often results in impeded tissue repair attributed to sustained inflammation and secretion of profibrotic cytokines (e.g., IL-13 and TGF-β1), which triggers myofibroblast activation and progressive kidney fibrosis [18].

Immunomodulatory Effects of Stem Cells

Considered an innovative anti-inflammatory treatment, the immunomodulatory effects of mesenchymal stem cells (MSCs) have been extensively investigated among other types of stem cells [19–21]. Firstly, MSCs are hypoimmunogenic as a result of reduced major histocompatibility complex (MHC) class I expression and a complete lack of expression of MHC class II and costimulatory molecules CD80 and CD86 [22]. This indicates that they can likely evade innate immunity processes, such as NK cell-mediated cytotoxicity, and lack the antigen presentation pathway essential for activation of the adaptive immune system [23]. To elicit an immunological balance, MSCs act as an immunomodulator by reducing the functional capacities and proliferation of all types of immune cells. MSCs have been proven to suppress lymphocyte activation and regulate their survival in a quiescent state [24]. Inhibition of T cell proliferation occurs through expression of inducible nitric oxide synthase (iNOS) and indoleamine 2,3-dioxygenase (IDO) in rodent and human MSCs, respectively [25]. More specifically, MSCs suppress CD4$^+$ T helper (Th) cells from differentiating into their Th1 and Th17 subsets, which are the causal agents in the pathogenesis of autoimmunity [26]. On the other hand, MSCs enhance the proliferation of regulatory T cells (Tregs) and strengthen their immune modulating capacities [27,28]. MSCs also inhibit the differentiation, maturation, and activation of DCs by downregulating the surface expression of CD80, CD86, and MHC class II molecules, retaining the DCs in a tolerogenic phenotype. In this state, they express various factors, such as IDO and prostaglandin E2 (PGE2), which lower DC immunogenicity, reduce T cell proliferation, and induce Treg differentiation [29,30]. Simultaneously,

MSCs induce macrophages to secrete immunosuppressive cytokines, like IL-4, IL-10 and transforming growth factor-β (TGF-β). It has also been shown that MSCs suppress NK cell proliferation and protect against perforin/granzyme-mediated cytotoxicity [31]. Furthermore, MSCs have inhibitory effects on B-cell proliferation, differentiation, and antibody production [32]. Given that HO-1 has significant anti-inflammatory therapeutic potential, recent research has pointed out HO-1-modified MSCs have an enhanced ability to attenuate inflammatory responses in ischemic heart disease [33], acute ischemic liver failure [34], lipopolysaccharide (LPS)-induced microvascular injury [35], and cisplatin-induced AKI [36]. Taken together, the administration of MSCs prevents immune cell activation and modulates kidney inflammation progression by managing cytokine secretion to promote anti-inflammatory processes.

It is noteworthy that the environment surrounding the MSCs is of critical importance to regulate the immunomodulatory effects. Liu et al. reported that MSCs derived from inflamed periodontal ligaments exhibit an impaired immunosuppressive capacity, with less inhibition of T cell proliferation, less induction of regulatory T cell, and less IL-10 production. The inflamed microenvironment also diminishes the immunomodulatory benefits of MSCs by reducing Th17 differentiation and IL-17 production [37]. Furthermore, Waterman et al. disclosed that MSCs could undergo functional polarization by differential Toll-like receptor (TLR) downstream signaling. Activation through TLR4 induced the pro-inflammatory MSC1, mostly producing pro-inflammatory mediators (IL-6, IL-8, and IFN-γ), can induce T cell activation. On the other hand, the TLR3-primed MSC2 mainly express anti-inflammatory factors such as IDO, PGE2, and HO-1, leading to T cell inhibition [38,39]. Moreover, to explain the diverse response of MSCs to TLR activation, Levin et al. suggested the level of co-cultured LPS-binding protein as a predictive factor in determining the secretomes of MSCs in response to TLR activation [40].

Similar to MSCs, Schnabel et al. found that induced pluripotent stem cells (iPSCs) possess immunomodulatory capacities evidenced by reducing responder T-cell proliferation in modified mixed leukocyte reactions in vitro [41]. Their findings echo our previous study [42], in which iPSCs without c-Myc were introduced into IR-AKI rat kidneys. This approach was not only safe, but also resulted in a substantial decrease in the levels of ROS and inflammatory cytokines. Furthermore, iPSCs have been shown to have strong immunomodulation effects through suppression of lymphocyte proliferation, NK cell-directed cytotoxicity, and DC differentiation and function [43–45]. This information is critical in considering the use of iPSCs in place of MSCs for both regenerative medicine and transplant medicine.

3. Oxidative Stress in IR-AKI

After the occurrence of acute ischemia, restoration of renal perfusion rapidly activates vascular endothelial cells, which trigger the production of pro-inflammatory cytokines and ROS, including superoxide ($\bullet O2^-$), hydrogen peroxide (HOOH), and hydroxyl radical ($\bullet OH$) [46]. Following IR-AKI, defective antioxidant processes cause depletion of endogenous antioxidants and reduced activity of redox-regulated enzymes, exacerbating the accumulation of intracellular ROS. This increased ROS production associated with reduced antioxidant capacity leads to a state of oxidative stress, which ultimately results in mitochondrial damage, depletion of ATP, increased lipid peroxidation, and activation of cell death pathways. Another harmful effect of ROS is oxidative modification of cell membrane proteins; this impairs ion and nutrient transport, energy metabolism, and organelle function essential for cellular homeostasis [47]. Furthermore, ROS-mediated activation of NF-κB continues to exacerbate systemic inflammation, triggering TEC apoptosis and kidney fibrosis, which have a detrimental impact on renal function [48].

Antioxidant Effects of Stem Cells

As a promising regenerative approach, stem cell therapy has been demonstrated to ameliorate various inflammatory diseases via its antioxidative activity [49–52]. MSCs can be isolated from bone marrow, umbilical cord blood, adipose tissue, placenta, periosteum, trabecular bone, synovium, skeletal muscle, and deciduous teeth [53], and their administration has been widely reported to upregulate the expression of the antioxidative enzyme HO-1 [35,54–57]. Increased HO-1 enzymatic activity is not only essential for MSC maturation, but is also cytoprotective against oxidative stress [58,59]. The antioxidant effects of HO-1 arise from its ability to increase reduced glutathione levels and degrade heme, as well as its ability to increase biliverdin and bilirubin, which have potent antioxidant properties [60,61]. In IR-AKI models, the increased production of HO-1 after MSC administration correlated with decreased levels of 8-hydroxy-2-deoxyguanosine (8-OHdG) and ROS [62]. The pro-angiogenic effects of MSCs lacking HO-1 expression are impaired; this triggers post-ischemic neovascularization and tissue repair, demonstrated by decreased secretion of several crucial pro-angiogenic growth factors, such as stromal cell-derived factor-1, vascular endothelial growth factor-A (VEGF-A), and hepatocyte growth factor (HGF) [36]. Similarly, CM derived from HO-1 knockout MSCs lacked therapeutic effects and failed to restore the functional and morphological changes in AKI [63]. A recent study also showed that modification with HO-1 significantly attenuated cell-cycle arrest, activated the PI3K/Akt and MEK/ERK pathways, and enhanced the survival of MSCs, all of which improved the therapeutic effects of MSCs against IR- AKI [64].

In addition to its impact on HO-1, IR-AKI also reduces the activity of antioxidant enzymes that scavenge ROS, including superoxide dismutase (SOD), catalase (CAT), glutathione-S-transferase (GST), and glutathione peroxidase (GPX), in post-ischemic kidney tissue [65]. MSC therapy increases the antioxidant capacity of post-ischemic kidney tissue by enhancing the activity of these ROS-scavenging enzymes, thereby reducing the levels of tissue malondialdehyde (MDA) [66–68]. Zhang et al. applied MSC-derived extracellular vesicles (MSC-EV) into an IR-AKI model and found that MSC-EV treatment reduced oxidative stress, and subsequently attenuated IR-AKI. This antioxidant effect is likely a result of activation of the NF-E2-related factor 2 (Nrf2)/antioxidant responsive element (ARE) pathway [69], but may also be due to decreased expression of NADPH oxidase 2 (NOX2) and ROS in injured kidney tissues [57,70].

In addition to MSCs, induced pluripotent stem cells (iPSC) are also equipped with antioxidative properties. In rats with IR- AKI, our previous study showed that the administration of iPSCs into kidneys via an intrarenal arterial route not only ameliorated the severity of tubular damage and kidney failure by reducing the expression of oxidative markers, pro-inflammatory cytokines, and apoptotic factors, but also improved the survival of IR-AKI rats [42]. We further showed that treatment of iPSC-CM in rats with IR-AKI significantly diminished oxidative stress and protected tubular cells against apoptosis [71], supporting the innovation occurring in this field of research.

4. Apoptosis of TEC in IR-AKI

Apoptosis is known to be a relevant mechanism of tubular cell death in IR-AKI. Kidney biopsies from IR-AKI animal models and humans have consistently shown apoptotic changes in TECs. There are several mechanisms of the pathogenesis of apoptosis of TECs. During ischemia, the pro-apoptotic protein Bax is upregulated in TECs, which results in a reduction of the anti-apoptotic protein Bcl-2, thus, promoting the initiation of apoptosis [72]. Another important stress kinase activated in the setting of ischemia is glycogen synthase kinase 3-β (GSK3β), which has been linked to mitochondrial dysfunction after exposure to oxidative stress [73]. During ischemia and ATP depletion, GSK3β upregulates Bax to activate caspase cascades, thus, promoting TEC apoptosis. Active GSK3β also positively regulates NF-κB leading to the inhibition of TNF-mediated apoptosis [74].

Other mechanisms of the activation of apoptotic pathways during IR-AKI have been proposed. The extrinsic apoptotic pathway is triggered by the binding of TNF-α and Fas ligands to death receptors, including Fas, tumor necrosis factor receptor 1 (TNFR1), and TNF-related apoptosis-inducing ligand receptors (TRAIL-Rs), expressed on TECs. Binding to these ligands results in receptor aggregation and recruitment of adaptor proteins, which, in turn, initiates a proteolytic cascade by activating initiator caspase-8 and caspase-10 [75]. The intrinsic apoptotic pathway is characterized by permeabilization of the mitochondrial outer membrane, resulting in the release of cytochrome c into the cytoplasm [76]. Cytochrome c then forms a multiprotein complex known as the "apoptosome" and initiates activation of the caspase cascade through caspase-9 [77]. Due to the significant consequences of TEC apoptosis and the complexity of its pathogenesis, reduction of tubular apoptosis is an essential requirement for the successful treatment of IR-AKI by stem cell therapy.

Anti-Apoptotic Effects of Stem Cells

To date, the anti-apoptotic property of stem cells seems to be the most widely recognized beneficial effect of MSCs [49,78–80]. In experimental models of AKI, administration of MSCs displayed a renoprotective effect by preventing tissue apoptosis, which accelerated the repair of injured tissue. MSC-treated AKI mice showed increased expression of the anti-apoptotic gene BCL2 and downregulation of the pro-apoptotic gene BAX [81]. Regarding the mechanisms of these treatment processes, MSCs modulate tubular apoptosis and regeneration through production of soluble paracrine factors and trophic growth factors, including VEGF, HGF, insulin-like growth factor 1 (IGF-1), stanniocalcin-1, TGF-β, and fibroblast growth factor 2 [82,83]. Cumulating evidence indicates that MSCs release extracellular vesicles (EVs) that deliver genes, microRNAs, exosomes, and proteins to recipient cells, thus, acting as mediators of MSC paracrine action and conferring resistance to apoptosis [84,85]. These EVs are also thought to communicate intercellularly and influence the function of progenitor cells to stimulate angiogenesis and other reparative processes and, consequently, accelerate tissue repair [11,86].

iPSCs present a promising new therapeutic approach for AKI [87], and several studies have illustrated their anti-apoptotic effects against IR-AKI. Subcapsular transplantation of human-iPSCs in rodent kidneys attenuated TEC apoptosis and ameliorated histological alterations resulting in renal function improvements following IR-AKI [88]. Li et al. also demonstrated the therapeutic effect of iPSC-derived renal progenitor cells (RPC) in IR-AKI; they observed the reduction of tubular apoptosis and renal function recovery in a rat model of IR-AKI. Simultaneously, increased expression of anti-inflammatory mediators and growth factors involved in kidney repair were observed after transplantation of iPSC-derived RPCs and MSCs in injured kidneys [88–90]. Shen et al. also showed that iPSC-derived endothelial progenitor cells ameliorated apoptosis of TECs and cardiomyocytes while treating IR-AKI in mice [91]. Regarding the mechanisms of the anti-apoptotic properties of stem cells, our previous study suggested that iPSC-derived CM provided a protective effect against IR-AKI by reducing ROS generation, suppressing p38-MAPK activation, and inhibiting TNF-induced cell death and its downstream effect of NF-κB-induced systemic inflammation [71]. Therefore, we have demonstrated that iPSCs exerted renoprotective effects via the secretion of paracrine factors and suggest that iPSC-CM is a potential resource for stem cell-based therapy against IR-AKI.

The therapeutic potential of spermatogonial stem cells (SSC) in AKI has been explored in the preclinical setting. Unlike the production of soluble cytokines and growth factors by MSCs and iPSCs, the mechanism governing SSCs to accelerate tissue regeneration is through direct differentiation into renal parenchymal cells. To prove this phenomenon, Wu et al. injected mouse SSCs into adult female mice kidneys. Three months after SSC administration, the histological analysis revealed the transplanted SSCs migrated to the basement membrane and trans-differentiated into mature renal TECs. The most convincing evidence for self-renewal and multipotency of SSCs came from the presence of the Y chromosome in the nucleolus of TECs and glomerular podocytes isolated from the SSC-transplanted kidneys in female mice [92].

Under specific conditions, SSCs can spontaneously transform into germline cell-derived pluripotent stem cells (GPSCs), which can be readily frozen and thawed without loss of cell viability. Using a novel renal epithelial differentiation protocol, Chiara et al. generated GPSC-derived tubular-like cells (GTCs) resembling renal TEC phenotypes and biological functions. After administration of GTCs intravenously in IR-AKI mice, these cells were able to home in on sites of inflammation and showed long-term engraftment in the injured kidney. Histological analysis disclosed less extent of cortical damage, inflammatory infiltrate, and interstitial fibrosis in the GTC-treated kidney. The GTCs also elicit cytoprotective functions in reducing renal oxidative stress, tubular apoptosis, and upregulation tubular expression of HO-1. Accordingly, GPSCs could be considered as a potential stem cell therapy against IR-AKI and subsequent chronic kidney damage [93].

5. Stem Cells in the Context of Clinical Use

Clinical applications of stem cell therapy are widely under investigation, as they possess anti-inflammatory, anti-fibrotic, and anti-apoptotic properties. However, clinical trials evaluating the therapeutic potentials of stem cells in AKI are still in the evolving stage, and their promise in preclinical models is yet to be translated. Dating back to 2008, the first phase 1 clinical trial (NTC00733876) evaluated the safety and efficacy of MSCs in AKI initiated with open-heart surgery. This study enrolled 16 open-heart surgical patients, and bone marrow-derived MSCs were administered into the suprarenal aorta through a femoral catheter after completion of surgery. The inclusion criteria were patients at high risk for postoperative AKI, such as old age, underlying diabetes mellitus, congestive heart failure, chronic obstructive lung disease, and pre-existing CKD stage 1-4. The exclusion criteria were active infection, evolving myocardial infarction, cardiogenic shock, history of malignancy, or advanced CKD stage 5/5D. The primary outcome was the absence of MSC-specific adverse events. During the six-month follow-up period, there were no specific or serious adverse effects observed, and this study concluded that infusions of MSCs might provide a novel and safe approach for inducing renal protection [94]. Based on this positive result, a subsequent multicenter randomized controlled trial in 2017 (NCT01602328) was conducted to determine the efficacy of allogeneic human MSCs in accelerating kidney recovery from established AKI. This phase 2 study enrolled patients who developed AKI within 48 h after cardiac surgery, and they randomized a total 156 participants to receive allogeneic MSCs (AC607, in a single dose of 2×10^6 cells/kg) or placebo administration through an intra-aortic route. The primary outcome was the time to recovery of kidney function. At the end of follow-up, although treatment with MSCs was found to be safe and tolerated well, this study concluded that administration of MSCs did not decrease the time to renal function recovery or provision for dialysis. Besides, the 30-day all-cause mortality was comparable between MSCs group and placebo group, and the rates of other major adverse kidney events were similar [95]. From these two early-phase clinical trials, the role of administering allogeneic MSCs for postcardiac surgery AKI is initially recognized. Although MSCs may be of no value as a therapy to recover renal function in established AKI, the preliminary analysis showed that MSC administration is safe at all tested doses. Unfortunately, there are no other ongoing registered clinical trials for the treatment of postcardiac surgery AKI, thus leaving unexplored the possibility of a potential beneficial effect of MSC therapy at doses higher than those reported so far.

Other clinical trials regarding AKI situation include administration of MSC to kidney transplant recipients. In a single-site, prospective, open-label, randomized study in China (NCT00658073), a total of 159 adult subjects underwent kidney transplants with allografts from living donors were divided into three groups: The standard dose ($n = 53$) and lower dose (80% of standard, $n = 52$) calcineurin inhibitors (CNI), in combination with a double intravenous infusion of autologous bone marrow-derived MSCs ($1–2 \times 10^6$/kg) at kidney reperfusion and 2 weeks later. Patients ($n = 51$) in the control group were given the anti-IL-2 receptor antibody basiliximab induction therapy, plus standard dose CNI. The main outcome included the one-year incidence of acute rejection, adverse events, patient and graft survival. Compared to the basiliximab group, this study demonstrated that the use of autologous MSC resulted in a lower incidence of acute rejection, lower risk of opportunistic infection, and better graft function at one year [96]. Another trial also suggested MSCs enable 50% reduction of CNI maintenance immunosuppression in living donor kidney transplant recipients [97]. Therefore, MSC-based therapy has proven to reduce induction and maintenance of immunosuppressive drugs without compromising patient safety and graft outcome. This may be due to the immunomodulatory activity of MSCs, but these studies, unfortunately, did not address the underlying mechanism.

A clinical trial using stem cells in treating AKI receiving continuous renal replacement therapy (CRRT) is ongoing (NCT03015623) [98]. AKI participants were treated with extracorporeal therapy with hemofiltration device containing millions of allogeneic MSCs (SBI-101) up to 24 h, designed to regulate inflammation and promote repair of injured tissue. Instead of intravenous infusion of allogeneic MSCs that are diluted rapidly throughout the body, SBI-101 allows delivery of a stable dose of cells by exposing the blood ultrafiltrate to MSCs that are immobilized on the extraluminal side of membranes within the hollow fiber dialyzer. This provides AKI patients with both standard-of-care hemofiltration as well as MSC-mediated blood conditioning in a single session. The conditioned ultrafiltrate is then delivered back to the subject, which allows for continuous exposure of the MSCs to patient blood during the CRRT treatment. In this trial, the recruitment is currently active, and subjects will be randomized into three different doses: Low dose SBI-101 containing 250 million MSCs, high dose SBI-101 containing 750 million MSCs, or sham control to characterize the pharmacokinetics and pharmacodynamics of SBI-101. In this first-in-human clinical trial, the primary outcome is its safety and tolerability. Measures of SBI-101 efficacy could be reduced patient time on dialysis or reduced patient time in the ICU.

There are still some barriers in the utilization of stem cells in clinical settings for AKI. Although MSC therapy has multiple benefits with no detrimental side effects, so far it still lacks both long-term follow-up data and the consensus in therapeutic protocols. Furthermore, the collection of MSCs from bone marrow is relatively invasive and the source is not available in a large volume. Similarly, SSC-based therapies in AKI have some limitations. Although SSCs are recognized to differentiate into renal lineages, their promise in preclinical AKI models is not yet translated in humans. Furthermore, even though SSCs can be administered in both genders, they can only be harvested from the testis and require a somewhat invasive procedure on male donors. In regard to iPSCs, c-Myc, one of the reprogramming factors to induce pluripotency, is a well-known oncogene leading to tumorigenesis. Therefore, the adverse effect of teratoma or tumor formation derived from iPSC treatment warrants significant concern. Our previous study demonstrated that rats treated with iPSCs without c-Myc effectively blocked the teratoma formation [42]. Alternatively, therapy utilizing iPSC-CM showed the promising anti-inflammatory benefits for IR-AKI and eliminated the concern of tumorigenesis as well [71]. Until now, there are few clinical trials of iPSC or stem cell-derived CM containing soluble factors and EVs in the treatment of AKI, and the future outcomes are highly expected [99].

6. Conclusions

In summary, animal experiments have provided compelling evidence to support a renoprotective role for stem cells in rescuing IR-AKI. Multiple mechanisms have been proposed to explain the beneficial effects of stem cells and their derived CM, including antioxidant, immunomodulatory, and anti-apoptotic effects (Figure 2). Another essential component of the beneficial effects of stem cells is their production of soluble paracrine factors and trophic growth factors. Moreover, recent investigations have found that stem cell-derived EVs may carry pro-regenerative micro-RNA molecules that stabilize vascular and tubular function, which has therapeutic potential for rescuing IR-AKI. Although the majority of studies in the field of IR-AKI show remarkable benefits of stem cell therapy, they are mostly confined to experimental animal models. More translational studies are needed to provide a more comprehensive understanding of stem cell-based therapies and to ensure their safety for future clinical applications.

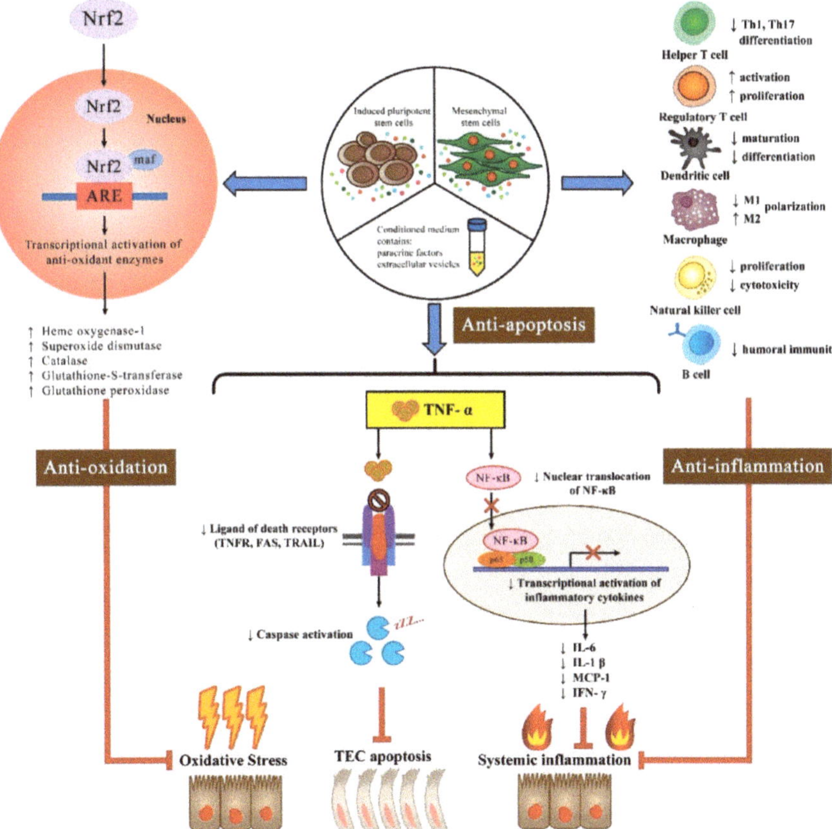

Figure 2. Illustration of proposed mechanisms of stem cell therapy in rescuing ischemia-reperfusion induced acute kidney injury. The therapeutic effects of mesenchymal stem cells, induced pluripotent stem cells, and their conditioned medium containing soluble factors and extracellular vesicles include: (1) Anti-oxidation, which may act through activation of the Nrf2/ARE pathway and, subsequently, upregulation of antioxidative enzymes against oxidative stress; (2) anti-inflammation, via immunosuppressive effects on immune cells and inhibition of NF-κB transcriptional activity; and (3) anti-apoptosis, possibly through decreased tumor necrosis factor-induced intrinsic apoptosis signaling. Abbreviations: Nrf2, NF-E2-related factor 2; ARE, antioxidant responsive element; TNF-α, tumor necrosis factor-α; TNFR, tumor necrosis factor receptor; TRAIL, TNF-related apoptosis-inducing ligand; TEC, tubular epithelial cell; NF-κB, nuclear factor-κB; MCP-1, monocyte chemoattractant protein 1; IFN-γ, Interferon-γ.

Author Contributions: K.-H.L. and D.-C.T. were involved in the planning and data collection for this review. K.-H.L., W.-C.T., C.-Y.Y., and D.-C.T. all participated in the drafting/editing of the manuscript. All of the abovementioned authors have approved the final draft of the manuscript.

Funding: This work was supported by grants from the Ministry of Science and Technology, R.O.C. (MOST 105-2628-B-010-017-MY3, MOST 106-2314-B-010-039-MY3, and MOST 107-2314-B-075-064-MY3), and projects from Taipei Veterans General Hospital (V107C-127, V108C-103, and V108D42-004-MY3-1). This work was also financially supported by the "Center for Intelligent Drug Systems and Smart Bio-devices (IDS2B)" from The Featured Areas Research Center Program within the framework of the Higher Education Sprout Project by the Ministry of Education (MOE) in Taiwan.

Conflicts of Interest: The authors declare no conflict of interest. The founders of the study had no role in the study design, data collection, data analysis, data interpretation, or writing of the report.

References

1. Rabb, H.; Griffin, M.D.; McKay, D.B.; Swaminathan, S.; Pickkers, P.; Rosner, M.H.; Kellum, J.A.; Ronco, C.; Acute Dialysis Quality Initiative Consensus, X.W.G. Inflammation in AKI: Current Understanding, Key Questions, and Knowledge Gaps. *J. Am. Soc. Nephrol.* **2016**, *27*, 371–379. [CrossRef] [PubMed]

2. Malek, M.; Nematbakhsh, M. Renal ischemia/reperfusion injury; from pathophysiology to treatment. *J. Ren. Inj. Prev.* **2015**, *4*, 20–27. [CrossRef] [PubMed]

3. Bonventre, J.V.; Yang, L. Cellular pathophysiology of ischemic acute kidney injury. *J. Clin. Investig.* **2011**, *121*, 4210–4221. [CrossRef] [PubMed]

4. Mulay, S.R.; Holderied, A.; Kumar, S.V.; Anders, H.J. Targeting Inflammation in So-Called Acute Kidney Injury. *Semin. Nephrol.* **2016**, *36*, 17–30. [CrossRef] [PubMed]

5. Huen, S.C.; Cantley, L.G. Macrophages in Renal Injury and Repair. *Annu. Rev. Physiol.* **2017**, *79*, 449–469. [CrossRef] [PubMed]

6. Bonavia, A.; Singbartl, K. A review of the role of immune cells in acute kidney injury. *Pediatr. Nephrol.* **2018**, *33*, 1629–1639. [CrossRef]

7. Chen, L.; Deng, H.; Cui, H.; Fang, J.; Zuo, Z.; Deng, J.; Li, Y.; Wang, X.; Zhao, L. Inflammatory responses and inflammation-associated diseases in organs. *Oncotarget* **2018**, *9*, 7204–7218. [CrossRef]

8. Pino, C.J.; Humes, H.D. Stem cell technology for the treatment of acute and chronic renal failure. *Transl. Res.* **2010**, *156*, 161–168. [CrossRef]

9. Pavyde, E.; Usas, A.; Maciulaitis, R. Regenerative pharmacology for the treatment of acute kidney injury: Skeletal muscle stem/progenitor cells for renal regeneration? *Pharmacol. Res.* **2016**, *113*, 802–807. [CrossRef]

10. Zhao, H.; Alam, A.; Soo, A.P.; George, A.J.T.; Ma, D. Ischemia-Reperfusion Injury Reduces Long Term Renal Graft Survival: Mechanism and Beyond. *EBioMedicine* **2018**, *28*, 31–42. [CrossRef]

11. Aghajani Nargesi, A.; Lerman, L.O.; Eirin, A. Mesenchymal stem cell-derived extracellular vesicles for kidney repair: Current status and looming challenges. *Stem Cell Res. Ther.* **2017**, *8*, 273. [CrossRef] [PubMed]

12. Hu, H.; Zou, C. Mesenchymal Stem Cells in Renal Ischemia-Reperfusion Injury: Biological and Therapeutic Perspectives. *Curr. Stem Cell Res. Ther.* **2017**, *12*, 183–187. [CrossRef] [PubMed]

13. Yang, Y.; Song, M.; Liu, Y.; Liu, H.; Sun, L.; Peng, Y.; Liu, F.; Venkatachalam, M.A.; Dong, Z. Renoprotective approaches and strategies in acute kidney injury. *Pharmacol. Ther.* **2016**, *163*, 58–73. [CrossRef] [PubMed]

14. Agarwal, A.; Dong, Z.; Harris, R.; Murray, P.; Parikh, S.M.; Rosner, M.H.; Kellum, J.A.; Ronco, C.; Acute Dialysis Quality Initiative XIII Working Group. Cellular and Molecular Mechanisms of AKI. *J. Am. Soc. Nephrol.* **2016**, *27*, 1288–1299. [CrossRef] [PubMed]

15. Lu, L.; Zhou, H.; Ni, M.; Wang, X.; Busuttil, R.; Kupiec-Weglinski, J.; Zhai, Y. Innate Immune Regulations and Liver Ischemia-Reperfusion Injury. *Transplantation* **2016**, *100*, 2601–2610. [CrossRef] [PubMed]

16. Mulay, S.R.; Kumar, S.V.; Lech, M.; Desai, J.; Anders, H.J. How Kidney Cell Death Induces Renal Necroinflammation. *Semin. Nephrol.* **2016**, *36*, 162–173. [CrossRef] [PubMed]

17. Bolisetty, S.; Zarjou, A.; Agarwal, A. Heme Oxygenase 1 as a Therapeutic Target in Acute Kidney Injury. *Am. J. Kidney Dis.* **2017**, *69*, 531–545. [CrossRef]

18. Chung, S.; Overstreet, J.M.; Li, Y.; Wang, Y.; Niu, A.; Wang, S.; Fan, X.; Sasaki, K.; Jin, G.N.; Khodo, S.N.; et al. TGF-beta promotes fibrosis after severe acute kidney injury by enhancing renal macrophage infiltration. *JCI Insight* **2018**, *3*. [CrossRef]

19. Yi, T.; Song, S.U. Immunomodulatory properties of mesenchymal stem cells and their therapeutic applications. *Arch. Pharm. Res.* **2012**, *35*, 213–221. [CrossRef]

20. Casiraghi, F.; Perico, N.; Cortinovis, M.; Remuzzi, G. Mesenchymal stromal cells in renal transplantation: Opportunities and challenges. *Nat. Rev. Nephrol.* **2016**, *12*, 241–253. [CrossRef]

21. Gao, F.; Chiu, S.M.; Motan, D.A.; Zhang, Z.; Chen, L.; Ji, H.L.; Tse, H.F.; Fu, Q.L.; Lian, Q. Mesenchymal stem cells and immunomodulation: Current status and future prospects. *Cell Death Dis.* **2016**, *7*, e2062. [CrossRef] [PubMed]

22. Ankrum, J.A.; Ong, J.F.; Karp, J.M. Mesenchymal stem cells: Immune evasive, not immune privileged. *Nat. Biotechnol.* **2014**, *32*, 252–260. [CrossRef] [PubMed]

23. McTaggart, S.J.; Atkinson, K. Mesenchymal stem cells: Immunobiology and therapeutic potential in kidney disease. *Nephrology* **2007**, *12*, 44–52. [CrossRef] [PubMed]

24. Benvenuto, F.; Ferrari, S.; Gerdoni, E.; Gualandi, F.; Frassoni, F.; Pistoia, V.; Mancardi, G.; Uccelli, A. Human mesenchymal stem cells promote survival of T cells in a quiescent state. *Stem Cells* **2007**, *25*, 1753–1760. [CrossRef] [PubMed]

25. Su, J.; Chen, X.; Huang, Y.; Li, W.; Li, J.; Cao, K.; Cao, G.; Zhang, L.; Li, F.; Roberts, A.I.; et al. Phylogenetic distinction of iNOS and IDO function in mesenchymal stem cell-mediated immunosuppression in mammalian species. *Cell Death Differ.* **2014**, *21*, 388–396. [CrossRef] [PubMed]

26. Castro-Manrreza, M.E.; Montesinos, J.J. Immunoregulation by mesenchymal stem cells: Biological aspects and clinical applications. *J. Immunol. Res.* **2015**, *2015*, 394917. [CrossRef] [PubMed]

27. Duffy, M.M.; Ritter, T.; Ceredig, R.; Griffin, M.D. Mesenchymal stem cell effects on T-cell effector pathways. *Stem Cell Res. Ther.* **2011**, *2*, 34. [CrossRef] [PubMed]

28. Fitzsimmons, R.E.B.; Mazurek, M.S.; Soos, A.; Simmons, C.A. Mesenchymal Stromal/Stem Cells in Regenerative Medicine and Tissue Engineering. *Stem Cells Int.* **2018**, *2018*, 8031718. [CrossRef] [PubMed]

29. Cahill, E.F.; Tobin, L.M.; Carty, F.; Mahon, B.P.; English, K. Jagged-1 is required for the expansion of CD4$^+$ CD25$^+$ FoxP3$^+$ regulatory T cells and tolerogenic dendritic cells by murine mesenchymal stromal cells. *Stem Cell Res. Ther.* **2015**, *6*, 19. [CrossRef]

30. Ethokic, J.M.; Tomic, S.Z.; Colic, M.J. Cross-Talk Between Mesenchymal Stem/Stromal Cells and Dendritic Cells. *Curr. Stem Cell Res. Ther.* **2016**, *11*, 51–65.

31. Reinders, M.E.; Hoogduijn, M.J. NK Cells and MSCs: Possible Implications for MSC Therapy in Renal Transplantation. *J. Stem Cell Res. Ther.* **2014**, *4*, 1000166. [CrossRef] [PubMed]

32. Rosado, M.M.; Bernardo, M.E.; Scarsella, M.; Conforti, A.; Giorda, E.; Biagini, S.; Cascioli, S.; Rossi, F.; Guzzo, I.; Vivarelli, M.; et al. Inhibition of B-cell proliferation and antibody production by mesenchymal stromal cells is mediated by T cells. *Stem Cells Dev.* **2015**, *24*, 93–103. [CrossRef] [PubMed]

33. Jiang, Y.B.; Zhang, X.L.; Tang, Y.L.; Ma, G.S.; Shen, C.X.; Wei, Q.; Zhu, Q.; Yao, Y.Y.; Liu, N.F. Effects of heme oxygenase-1 gene modulated mesenchymal stem cells on vasculogenesis in ischemic swine hearts. *Chin. Med. J.* **2011**, *124*, 401–407. [PubMed]

34. Wang, X.; Wang, S.; Zhou, Y.; Obulkasim, H.; Zhang, Z.H.; Dai, B.; Zhu, W.; Shi, X.L. BMMSCs protect against liver ischemia/reperfusion injury via HO1 mediated autophagy. *Mol. Med. Rep.* **2018**, *18*, 2253–2262. [CrossRef] [PubMed]

35. Chen, X.; Zhang, Y.; Wang, W.; Liu, Z.; Meng, J.; Han, Z. Mesenchymal Stem Cells Modified with Heme Oxygenase-1 Have Enhanced Paracrine Function and Attenuate Lipopolysaccharide-Induced Inflammatory and Oxidative Damage in Pulmonary Microvascular Endothelial Cells. *Cell. Physiol. Biochem.* **2018**, *49*, 101–122. [CrossRef]

36. Zarjou, A.; Kim, J.; Traylor, A.M.; Sanders, P.W.; Balla, J.; Agarwal, A.; Curtis, L.M. Paracrine effects of mesenchymal stem cells in cisplatin-induced renal injury require heme oxygenase-1. *Am. J. Physiol. Ren. Physiol.* **2011**, *300*, F254–F262. [CrossRef]

37. Liu, D.; Xu, J.; Liu, O.; Fan, Z.; Liu, Y.; Wang, F.; Ding, G.; Wei, F.; Zhang, C.; Wang, S. Mesenchymal stem cells derived from inflamed periodontal ligaments exhibit impaired immunomodulation. *J. Clin. Periodontol.* **2012**, *39*, 1174–1182. [CrossRef]

38. Najar, M.; Krayem, M.; Meuleman, N.; Bron, D.; Lagneaux, L. Mesenchymal Stromal Cells and Toll-Like Receptor Priming: A Critical Review. *Immune Netw.* **2017**, *17*, 89–102. [CrossRef]

39. Waterman, R.S.; Tomchuck, S.L.; Henkle, S.L.; Betancourt, A.M. A new mesenchymal stem cell (MSC) paradigm: Polarization into a pro-inflammatory MSC1 or an Immunosuppressive MSC2 phenotype. *PLoS ONE* **2010**, *5*, e10088. [CrossRef]

40. Levin, S.; Pevsner-Fischer, M.; Kagan, S.; Lifshitz, H.; Weinstock, A.; Gataulin, D.; Friedlander, G.; Zipori, D. Divergent levels of LBP and TGFbeta1 in murine MSCs lead to heterogenic response to TLR and proinflammatory cytokine activation. *Stem Cell Rev.* **2014**, *10*, 376–388. [CrossRef]

41. Schnabel, L.V.; Abratte, C.M.; Schimenti, J.C.; Felippe, M.J.; Cassano, J.M.; Southard, T.L.; Cross, J.A.; Fortier, L.A. Induced pluripotent stem cells have similar immunogenic and more potent immunomodulatory properties compared with bone marrow-derived stromal cells in vitro. *Regen. Med.* **2014**, *9*, 621–635. [CrossRef]

42. Lee, P.Y.; Chien, Y.; Chiou, G.Y.; Lin, C.H.; Chiou, C.H.; Tarng, D.C. Induced pluripotent stem cells without c-Myc attenuate acute kidney injury via downregulating the signaling of oxidative stress and inflammation in ischemia-reperfusion rats. *Cell Transplant.* **2012**, *21*, 2569–2585. [CrossRef]

43. Yen, B.L.; Chang, C.J.; Liu, K.J.; Chen, Y.C.; Hu, H.I.; Bai, C.H.; Yen, M.L. Brief report—Human embryonic stem cell-derived mesenchymal progenitors possess strong immunosuppressive effects toward natural killer cells as well as T lymphocytes. *Stem Cells* **2009**, *27*, 451–456. [CrossRef]

44. Gao, W.X.; Sun, Y.Q.; Shi, J.; Li, C.L.; Fang, S.B.; Wang, D.; Deng, X.Q.; Wen, W.; Fu, Q.L. Effects of mesenchymal stem cells from human induced pluripotent stem cells on differentiation, maturation, and function of dendritic cells. *Stem Cell Res. Ther.* **2017**, *8*, 48. [CrossRef]

45. Tan, Z.; Su, Z.Y.; Wu, R.R.; Gu, B.; Liu, Y.K.; Zhao, X.L.; Zhang, M. Immunomodulative effects of mesenchymal stem cells derived from human embryonic stem cells in vivo and in vitro. *J. Zhejiang Univ. Sci. B* **2011**, *12*, 18–27. [CrossRef]

46. Korthuis, R.J. Mechanisms of I/R-Induced Endothelium-Dependent Vasodilator Dysfunction. *Adv. Pharmacol.* **2018**, *81*, 331–364. [CrossRef]

47. Gonzalez-Vicente, A.; Garvin, J.L. Effects of Reactive Oxygen Species on Tubular Transport along the Nephron. *Antioxidants* **2017**, *6*, 23. [CrossRef]

48. Marko, L.; Vigolo, E.; Hinze, C.; Park, J.K.; Roel, G.; Balogh, A.; Choi, M.; Wubken, A.; Cording, J.; Blasig, I.E.; et al. Tubular Epithelial NF-kappaB Activity Regulates Ischemic AKI. *J. Am. Soc. Nephrol.* **2016**, *27*, 2658–2669. [CrossRef]

49. Shih, Y.C.; Lee, P.Y.; Cheng, H.; Tsai, C.H.; Ma, H.; Tarng, D.C. Adipose-derived stem cells exhibit antioxidative and antiapoptotic properties to rescue ischemic acute kidney injury in rats. *Plast. Reconstr. Surg.* **2013**, *132*, 940e–951e. [CrossRef]

50. Zhang, J.B.; Wang, X.Q.; Lu, G.L.; Huang, H.S.; Xu, S.Y. Adipose-derived mesenchymal stem cells therapy for acute kidney injury induced by ischemia-reperfusion in a rat model. *Clin. Exp. Pharmacol. Physiol.* **2017**, *44*, 1232–1240. [CrossRef]

51. Havakhah, S.; Sankian, M.; Kazemzadeh, G.H.; Sadri, K.; Bidkhori, H.R.; Naderi-Meshkin, H.; Ebrahimzadeh Bideskan, A.; Niazmand, S.; Bahrami, A.R.; Khajavi Rad, A. In vivo effects of allogeneic mesenchymal stem cells in a rat model of acute ischemic kidney injury. *Iran. J. Basic Med. Sci.* **2018**, *21*, 824–831. [CrossRef]

52. Lee, K.W.; Kim, T.M.; Kim, K.S.; Lee, S.; Cho, J.; Park, J.B.; Kwon, G.Y.; Kim, S.J. Renal Ischemia-Reperfusion Injury in a Diabetic Monkey Model and Therapeutic Testing of Human Bone Marrow-Derived Mesenchymal Stem Cells. *J. Diabetes Res.* **2018**, *2018*, 5182606. [CrossRef]

53. Orbay, H.; Tobita, M.; Mizuno, H. Mesenchymal stem cells isolated from adipose and other tissues: Basic biological properties and clinical applications. *Stem Cells Int.* **2012**, *2012*, 461718. [CrossRef]

54. Zhang, Z.H.; Zhu, W.; Ren, H.Z.; Zhao, X.; Wang, S.; Ma, H.C.; Shi, X.L. Mesenchymal stem cells increase expression of heme oxygenase-1 leading to anti-inflammatory activity in treatment of acute liver failure. *Stem Cell Res. Ther.* **2017**, *8*, 70. [CrossRef]

55. Sung, P.H.; Chang, C.L.; Tsai, T.H.; Chang, L.T.; Leu, S.; Chen, Y.L.; Yang, C.C.; Chua, S.; Yeh, K.H.; Chai, H.T.; et al. Apoptotic adipose-derived mesenchymal stem cell therapy protects against lung and kidney injury in sepsis syndrome caused by cecal ligation puncture in rats. *Stem Cell Res. Ther.* **2013**, *4*, 155. [CrossRef]

56. Du, T.; Cheng, J.; Zhong, L.; Zhao, X.F.; Zhu, J.; Zhu, Y.J.; Liu, G.H. The alleviation of acute and chronic kidney injury by human Wharton's jelly-derived mesenchymal stromal cells triggered by ischemia-reperfusion injury via an endocrine mechanism. *Cytotherapy* **2012**, *14*, 1215–1227. [CrossRef]

57. Zhang, D.; Fu, L.; Wang, L.; Lin, L.; Yu, L.; Zhang, L.; Shang, T. Therapeutic benefit of mesenchymal stem cells in pregnant rats with angiotensin receptor agonistic autoantibody-induced hypertension: Implications for immunomodulation and cytoprotection. *Hypertens. Pregnancy* **2017**, *36*, 247–258. [CrossRef]

58. Camara, N.O.; Soares, M.P. Heme oxygenase-1 (HO-1), a protective gene that prevents chronic graft dysfunction. *Free Radic. Biol. Med.* **2005**, *38*, 426–435. [CrossRef]

59. Liu, N.; Wang, H.; Han, G.; Tian, J.; Hu, W.; Zhang, J. Alleviation of apoptosis of bone marrow-derived mesenchymal stem cells in the acute injured kidney by heme oxygenase-1 gene modification. *Int. J. Biochem. Cell Biol.* **2015**, *69*, 85–94. [CrossRef]

60. Turkseven, S.; Kruger, A.; Mingone, C.J.; Kaminski, P.; Inaba, M.; Rodella, L.F.; Ikehara, S.; Wolin, M.S.; Abraham, N.G. Antioxidant mechanism of heme oxygenase-1 involves an increase in superoxide dismutase and catalase in experimental diabetes. *Am. J. Physiol. Heart Circ. Physiol.* **2005**, *289*, H701–H707. [CrossRef]

61. Tsai, M.T.; Tarng, D.C. Beyond a Measure of Liver Function-Bilirubin Acts as a Potential Cardiovascular Protector in Chronic Kidney Disease Patients. *Int. J. Mol. Sci.* **2018**, *20*, 117. [CrossRef]

62. Liu, H.; McTaggart, S.J.; Johnson, D.W.; Gobe, G.C. Anti-oxidant pathways are stimulated by mesenchymal stromal cells in renal repair after ischemic injury. *Cytotherapy* **2012**, *14*, 162–172. [CrossRef]

63. Agarwal, A.; Bolisetty, S. Adaptive responses to tissue injury: Role of heme oxygenase-1. *Trans. Am. Clin. Climatol. Assoc.* **2013**, *124*, 111–122.

64. Liu, N.; Wang, H.; Han, G.; Cheng, J.; Hu, W.; Zhang, J. Enhanced proliferation and differentiation of HO-1 gene-modified bone marrow-derived mesenchymal stem cells in the acute injured kidney. *Int. J. Mol. Med.* **2018**, *42*, 946–956. [CrossRef]

65. Mates, J.M. Effects of antioxidant enzymes in the molecular control of reactive oxygen species toxicology. *Toxicology* **2000**, *153*, 83–104. [CrossRef]

66. Zhuo, W.; Liao, L.; Xu, T.; Wu, W.; Yang, S.; Tan, J. Mesenchymal stem cells ameliorate ischemia-reperfusion-induced renal dysfunction by improving the antioxidant/oxidant balance in the ischemic kidney. *Urol. Int.* **2011**, *86*, 191–196. [CrossRef]

67. Fahmy, S.R.; Soliman, A.M.; El Ansary, M.; Elhamid, S.A.; Mohsen, H. Therapeutic efficacy of human umbilical cord mesenchymal stem cells transplantation against renal ischemia/reperfusion injury in rats. *Tissue Cell* **2017**, *49*, 369–375. [CrossRef]

68. Inan, M.; Bakar, E.; Cerkezkayabekir, A.; Sanal, F.; Ulucam, E.; Subasi, C.; Karaoz, E. Mesenchymal stem cells increase antioxidant capacity in intestinal ischemia/reperfusion damage. *J. Pediatr. Surg.* **2017**, *52*, 1196–1206. [CrossRef]

69. Zhang, G.; Zou, X.; Huang, Y.; Wang, F.; Miao, S.; Liu, G.; Chen, M.; Zhu, Y. Mesenchymal Stromal Cell-Derived Extracellular Vesicles Protect Against Acute Kidney Injury Through Anti-Oxidation by Enhancing Nrf2/ARE Activation in Rats. *Kidney Blood Press. Res.* **2016**, *41*, 119–128. [CrossRef]

70. Zhang, G.; Zou, X.; Miao, S.; Chen, J.; Du, T.; Zhong, L.; Ju, G.; Liu, G.; Zhu, Y. The anti-oxidative role of micro-vesicles derived from human Wharton-Jelly mesenchymal stromal cells through NOX2/gp91(phox) suppression in alleviating renal ischemia-reperfusion injury in rats. *PLoS ONE* **2014**, *9*, e92129. [CrossRef]

71. Tarng, D.C.; Tseng, W.C.; Lee, P.Y.; Chiou, S.H.; Hsieh, S.L. Induced Pluripotent Stem Cell-Derived Conditioned Medium Attenuates Acute Kidney Injury by Downregulating the Oxidative Stress-Related Pathway in Ischemia-Reperfusion Rats. *Cell Transplant.* **2016**, *25*, 517–530. [CrossRef]

72. Borkan, S.C. The Role of BCL-2 Family Members in Acute Kidney Injury. *Semin. Nephrol.* **2016**, *36*, 237–250. [CrossRef]

73. Plotnikov, E.Y.; Kazachenko, A.V.; Vyssokikh, M.Y.; Vasileva, A.K.; Tcvirkun, D.V.; Isaev, N.K.; Kirpatovsky, V.I.; Zorov, D.B. The role of mitochondria in oxidative and nitrosative stress during ischemia/reperfusion in the rat kidney. *Kidney Int.* **2007**, *72*, 1493–1502. [CrossRef]

74. Jacobs, K.M.; Bhave, S.R.; Ferraro, D.J.; Jaboin, J.J.; Hallahan, D.E.; Thotala, D. GSK-3beta: A Bifunctional Role in Cell Death Pathways. *Int. J. Cell Biol.* **2012**, *2012*, 930710. [CrossRef]

75. Devarapu, S.K.; Grill, J.F.; Xie, J.; Weidenbusch, M.; Honarpisheh, M.; Vielhauer, V.; Anders, H.J.; Mulay, S.R. Tumor necrosis factor superfamily ligand mRNA expression profiles differ between humans and mice during homeostasis and between various murine kidney injuries. *J. Biomed. Sci.* **2017**, *24*, 77. [CrossRef]

76. Wu, C.C.; Bratton, S.B. Regulation of the intrinsic apoptosis pathway by reactive oxygen species. *Antioxid. Redox Signal.* **2013**, *19*, 546–558. [CrossRef]

77. Dorstyn, L.; Akey, C.W.; Kumar, S. New insights into apoptosome structure and function. *Cell Death Differ.* **2018**, *25*, 1194–1208. [CrossRef]

78. Humphreys, B.D.; Cantaluppi, V.; Portilla, D.; Singbartl, K.; Yang, L.; Rosner, M.H.; Kellum, J.A.; Ronco, C.; Acute Dialysis Quality Initiative XIII Working Group. Targeting Endogenous Repair Pathways after AKI. *J. Am. Soc. Nephrol.* **2016**, *27*, 990–998. [CrossRef]

79. Rowart, P.; Erpicum, P.; Detry, O.; Weekers, L.; Gregoire, C.; Lechanteur, C.; Briquet, A.; Beguin, Y.; Krzesinski, J.M.; Jouret, F. Mesenchymal Stromal Cell Therapy in Ischemia/Reperfusion Injury. *J. Immunol. Res.* **2015**, *2015*, 602597. [CrossRef]

80. Fleig, S.V.; Humphreys, B.D. Rationale of mesenchymal stem cell therapy in kidney injury. *Nephron Clin. Pract.* **2014**, *127*, 75–80. [CrossRef]

81. Bianchi, F.; Sala, E.; Donadei, C.; Capelli, I.; La Manna, G. Potential advantages of acute kidney injury management by mesenchymal stem cells. *World J. Stem Cells* **2014**, *6*, 644–650. [CrossRef]

82. Naji, A.; Favier, B.; Deschaseaux, F.; Rouas-Freiss, N.; Eitoku, M.; Suganuma, N. Mesenchymal stem/stromal cell function in modulating cell death. *Stem Cell Res. Ther.* **2019**, *10*, 56. [CrossRef]

83. Gnecchi, M.; Danieli, P.; Malpasso, G.; Ciuffreda, M.C. Paracrine Mechanisms of Mesenchymal Stem Cells in Tissue Repair. *Methods Mol. Biol.* **2016**, *1416*, 123–146. [CrossRef]

84. Borger, V.; Bremer, M.; Ferrer-Tur, R.; Gockeln, L.; Stambouli, O.; Becic, A.; Giebel, B. Mesenchymal Stem/Stromal Cell-Derived Extracellular Vesicles and Their Potential as Novel Immunomodulatory Therapeutic Agents. *Int. J. Mol. Sci.* **2017**, *18*, 1450. [CrossRef]

85. Li, N.; Long, B.; Han, W.; Yuan, S.; Wang, K. microRNAs: Important regulators of stem cells. *Stem Cell Res. Ther.* **2017**, *8*, 110. [CrossRef]

86. Nargesi, A.A.; Lerman, L.O.; Eirin, A. Mesenchymal Stem Cell-derived Extracellular Vesicles for Renal Repair. *Curr. Gene Ther.* **2017**, *17*, 29–42. [CrossRef]

87. Osafune, K. Cell therapy for kidney injury: Different options and mechanisms–kidney progenitor cells. *Nephron Exp. Nephrol.* **2014**, *126*, 64. [CrossRef]

88. Toyohara, T.; Mae, S.; Sueta, S.; Inoue, T.; Yamagishi, Y.; Kawamoto, T.; Kasahara, T.; Hoshina, A.; Toyoda, T.; Tanaka, H.; et al. Cell Therapy Using Human Induced Pluripotent Stem Cell-Derived Renal Progenitors Ameliorates Acute Kidney Injury in Mice. *Stem Cells Transl. Med.* **2015**, *4*, 980–992. [CrossRef]

89. Li, Q.; Tian, S.F.; Guo, Y.; Niu, X.; Hu, B.; Guo, S.C.; Wang, N.S.; Wang, Y. Transplantation of induced pluripotent stem cell-derived renal stem cells improved acute kidney injury. *Cell Biosci.* **2015**, *5*, 45. [CrossRef]

90. Ko, S.F.; Chen, Y.T.; Wallace, C.G.; Chen, K.H.; Sung, P.H.; Cheng, B.C.; Huang, T.H.; Chen, Y.L.; Li, Y.C.; Chang, H.W.; et al. Inducible pluripotent stem cell-derived mesenchymal stem cell therapy effectively protected kidney from acute ischemia-reperfusion injury. *Am. J. Transl. Res.* **2018**, *10*, 3053–3067.

91. Shen, W.C.; Chou, Y.H.; Huang, H.P.; Sheen, J.F.; Hung, S.C.; Chen, H.F. Induced pluripotent stem cell-derived endothelial progenitor cells attenuate ischemic acute kidney injury and cardiac dysfunction. *Stem Cell Res. Ther.* **2018**, *9*, 344. [CrossRef]

92. Wu, D.P.; He, D.L.; Li, X.; Liu, Z.H. Differentiations of transplanted mouse spermatogonial stem cells in the adult mouse renal parenchyma in vivo. *Acta Pharmacol. Sin.* **2008**, *29*, 1029–1034. [CrossRef]

93. De Chiara, L.; Fagoonee, S.; Ranghino, A.; Bruno, S.; Camussi, G.; Tolosano, E.; Silengo, L.; Altruda, F. Renal cells from spermatogonial germline stem cells protect against kidney injury. *J. Am. Soc. Nephrol.* **2014**, *25*, 316–328. [CrossRef]

94. Togel, F.E.; Westenfelder, C. Kidney protection and regeneration following acute injury: Progress through stem cell therapy. *Am. J. Kidney Dis.* **2012**, *60*, 1012–1022. [CrossRef]

95. Swaminathan, M.; Stafford-Smith, M.; Chertow, G.M.; Warnock, D.G.; Paragamian, V.; Brenner, R.M.; Lellouche, F.; Fox-Robichaud, A.; Atta, M.G.; Melby, S.; et al. Allogeneic Mesenchymal Stem Cells for Treatment of AKI after Cardiac Surgery. *J. Am. Soc. Nephrol.* **2018**, *29*, 260–267. [CrossRef]

96. Tan, J.; Wu, W.; Xu, X.; Liao, L.; Zheng, F.; Messinger, S.; Sun, X.; Chen, J.; Yang, S.; Cai, J.; et al. Induction therapy with autologous mesenchymal stem cells in living-related kidney transplants: A randomized controlled trial. *JAMA* **2012**, *307*, 1169–1177. [CrossRef]

97. Pan, G.H.; Chen, Z.; Xu, L.; Zhu, J.H.; Xiang, P.; Ma, J.J.; Peng, Y.W.; Li, G.H.; Chen, X.Y.; Fang, J.L.; et al. Low-dose tacrolimus combined with donor-derived mesenchymal stem cells after renal transplantation: A prospective, non-randomized study. *Oncotarget* **2016**, *7*, 12089–12101. [CrossRef]

98. Miller, B.L.K.; Garg, P.; Bronstein, B.; LaPointe, E.; Lin, H.; Charytan, D.M.; Tilles, A.W.; Parekkadan, B. Extracorporeal Stromal Cell Therapy for Subjects With Dialysis-Dependent Acute Kidney Injury. *Kidney Int. Rep.* **2018**, *3*, 1119–1127. [CrossRef]

99. Rota, C.; Morigi, M.; Imberti, B. Stem Cell Therapies in Kidney Diseases: Progress and Challenges. *Int. J. Mol. Sci.* **2019**, *20*, 2790. [CrossRef]

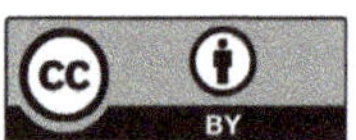

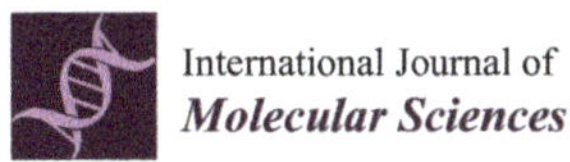

International Journal of
Molecular Sciences

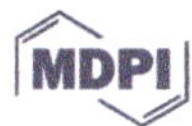

Review

Mesenchymal Stem Cells—Potential Applications in Kidney Diseases

Benjamin Bochon [1,†], Magdalena Kozubska [2,†], Grzegorz Surygała [3,†], Agnieszka Witkowska [4], Roman Kuźniewicz [5], Władysław Grzeszczak [5] and Grzegorz Wystrychowski [5,*]

1   Psychiatric Services of Thurgovia, Academic Teaching Hospital of the Medical University of Salzburg, 8596 Münsterlingen, Switzerland; benjaminbochon@yahoo.com
2   General Practice, 43-426 Dębowiec, Poland; magdalena.kozubska@interia.eu
3   Regional Blood Donation and Blood Treatment Centre, 40-074 Katowice, Poland; gregorian08@wp.pl
4   DaVita Dialysis, 42-700 Lubliniec, Poland; witkowskaaga@op.pl
5   Department of Internal Medicine, Diabetology and Nephrology, School of Medicine with the Division of Dentistry in Zabrze, Medical University of Silesia in Katowice, 41-800 Zabrze, Poland; rkuzniewicz@sum.edu.pl (R.K.); wgrzeszczak@sum.edu.pl (W.G.)
*   Correspondence: gwystrychowski@sum.edu.pl; Tel.: +48-32-3704462
†   These authors contributed equally to this paper.

Received: 29 March 2019; Accepted: 16 May 2019; Published: 18 May 2019

Abstract: Mesenchymal stem cells constitute a pool of cells present throughout the lifetime in numerous niches, characteristic of unlimited replication potential and the ability to differentiate into mature cells of mesodermal tissues in vitro. The therapeutic potential of these cells is, however, primarily associated with their capabilities of inhibiting inflammation and initiating tissue regeneration. Owing to these properties, mesenchymal stem cells (derived from the bone marrow, subcutaneous adipose tissue, and increasingly urine) are the subject of research in the settings of kidney diseases in which inflammation plays the key role. The most advanced studies, with the first clinical trials, apply to ischemic acute kidney injury, renal transplantation, lupus and diabetic nephropathies, in which beneficial clinical effects of cells themselves, as well as their culture medium, were observed. The study findings imply that mesenchymal stem cells act predominantly through secreted factors, including, above all, microRNAs contained within extracellular vesicles. Research over the coming years will focus on this secretome as a possible therapeutic agent void of the potential carcinogenicity of the cells.

Keywords: mesenchymal stem cell; mesodermal stem cell; renal ischemia-reperfusion; inflammation; kidney transplantation; microRNA; extracellular vesicles; exosomes

---

1. Introduction

Chronic kidney disease (CKD) affects ~10% of the general population, leading to the deterioration of the quality of life and premature death due to cardiovascular complications. On one hand, chronic renal insufficiency arises as a consequence of continuous insidious kidney damage and scarring in such common diseases as high blood pressure, diabetes, or nephrolithiasis, and, fortunately not as frequent, various forms of chronic glomerulonephritis. On the other, CKD gets instigated or aggravated with incidents of acute kidney injury (AKI), due to such insults as ischemia, infection, autoimmune reaction or toxins like radiological contrast or drugs. The possibilities of pharmacological prevention or attenuation of chronic renal failure are limited to controlling cardiovascular risk factors (usually not optimal), avoidance of potential renal toxins (often unfeasible), or causal treatment of AKI whenever possible (with variable efficiency and frequent complications). In the light of medical advances in other areas, this shortage of therapeutic options raises understandable frustration among patients and their physicians. Stem cell-based therapies may lead to the expected breakthrough in the treatment of kidney diseases.

2. Mesenchymal Stem Cells

2.1. Types of Stem Cells

Stem cells, owing to their unique ability to replicate and differentiate into specialized organ cells, provide the tissues with the ability to regenerate and survive most injuries [1]. Four types of these cells are defined according to their differentiation potential. In the embryonic period, the early stages of ontogenesis occur owing to the unlimited abilities of totipotent zygotic cells, replaced over time by pluripotent embryonic cells that differentiate into cells of all three germ layers, but no longer have the ability to differentiate into placental cells [2]. Beyond this phase, pluripotent cells that resemble the embryonic stem cells can be obtained by dedifferentiation of fibroblasts or epithelial cells in vitro (induced pluripotent stem cells) [3]. Throughout the lifetime, somatic stem cells are preserved within numerous niches—multipotent ones, which transform into all cells of a given tissue (e.g., bone marrow progenitor cells) or unipotent ones that can only differentiate into one type of mature cell (e.g., cells of the basal layer of the epidermis) [4].

At present, the cells under the most extensive investigations in experimental biology and medicine are mesenchymal (mesodermal) stem cells (MSC) that occur in the human body in mesodermal tissues, including placenta, amniotic fluid, umbilical cord tissues, bone marrow, adipose tissue, testis or lungs [5].

2.2. Regenerative Properties of MSC

MSC exhibit multipotent properties in vitro—when treated with appropriate chemical compounds they have the ability to differentiate into all mesodermal lineage cells, such as fibroblasts, osteocytes, chondrocytes, adipocytes or myocytes [6]. Few studies indicate that they can also transform into cells of endodermal or ectodermal origin [7]. Whereas this vast differentiation potential is of interest and conceivable use in the ex vivo generation of injured tissue replacements, there is only scarce evidence that MSC takes advantage of it in vivo [8]. Most data show that they rather promote tissue repair processes by the means of cell-to-cell interactions or secreted biomaterial, including antioxidant, antiapoptotic and growth factors (GF), such as Epithelial GF, Vascular Endothelial GF (VEGF), Transforming GF (TGF) α and β, Fibroblast GF, Insulin-like GF type 1, and others [9] that stimulate divisions of local progenitor cells. Studies show that these compounds are released from MSC in the free state or contained within spherical vesicles of a 30–100 nm diameter—exosomes of an endosomal origin or microvesicles budding from the cellular membrane. These extracellular vesicles allow signal transmission between the cells not only through the transported proteins, but also mRNAs and microRNAs [10]. Multiple microRNA particles have been identified within MSC extracellular vesicles and their patterns differ considerably between experimental models of different ischemic/inflammatory diseases [11]. Of great importance is homing of MSC to the ischemic, necrotic or inflamed sites, as a result of their membrane expression of chemokine receptors and integrins [5], responsiveness to damage associated molecular patterns [12] or mitochondria released from dead cells with their engulfment [13]. This tropism reduces the distance of secreted products to their target locations and allows an additional way of restoring local homeostasis by MSC—intercellular transfer of mitochondria [14]. Substituting defective native mitochondria with MSC-derived fully operational ones provides ATP for most needed anabolic reactions [15] and has been shown to revive damaged alveolar or corneal epithelia [16,17]. According to most reports mitochondria are moved to the damaged cells by means of nanotube tunneling [18], microvesicles [19] or cellular fusion, as recently comprehensively reviewed [20].

MSC are increasingly used in reconstructive surgery. In countries with less stringent legal restrictions (such as Japan and South Korea), they are used as a replicative matrix for renewal of joint surfaces and regeneration of facial defects (which requires collagen scaffolding) or as a source of cytokines and GFs stimulating natural healing in periodontal disease and skin wounds [21]. Their usefulness is examined in experimental models of corneal damage, lung, spinal cord and brain injuries [22].

2.3. Immunomodulatory Properties of MSC

Beside their regenerative potential, MSC are characterized by the ability to modulate immune responses. Of note, they are characterized by low expression of MHC class I antigens and no expression of MHC class II antigens or B7-1, B7-2 and CD40 costimulatory molecules. This implies that the infusion of allogeneic stem cells does not induce a clinically significant immune response [23]. Most importantly, exposure to MSC in vitro or their systemic administration in large amounts ($\sim 10^6$–10^8 cells) inhibits Th17 lymphocytes, augments the pool and activity of regulatory T-cells, and increases expression of anti-inflammatory cytokines like IL-10, subsequently blunting inflammatory reaction [24]. Their use in the treatment of autoimmune diseases, such as inflammatory diseases of the joints [25] or intestines [26] has been tested with good results. Contrary to initial assumptions, studies with infusions of exogenous MSC showed that their anti-inflammatory effect is not primarily the result of the direct interaction with immune cells in the target inflamed tissue, but they can act from distance by the means of their secretome, at least partially contained within exosomes or microvesicles [27]. Meticulously isolated extracellular vesicles of umbilical cord MSC (by means of size-exclusion chromatography) have been shown to exert a potent immunosuppressant effect in vitro, in contrast to other fractions of the MSC conditioned medium [28].

A British group has recently found that immunosuppressive activity of human bone marrow MSC in the experimental model of an established severe inflammatory reaction (MSC intravenous infusion on the third day of graft-versus-host disease in mice) relies on their apoptosis. The reductions of the lung and spleen pools of graft-versus-host disease effector T-cells were detectable either when MSC were lysed and engulfed by recipient's NK or CD8+ T cells in an antigen-independent way or when apoptosis was induced in MSC prior to their infusion. Based on the results with the additional use of an inhibitor of indoleamine 2,3-dioxygenase, the authors concluded that increased expression and release of this anti-inflammatory cytokine by recipient's phagocytes upon MSC apoptosis is the mediator of the immunosuppressive effect [29]. However, it can be reasoned that this very mechanism does not exclude the role of extracellular vesicles and microRNAs which can be extensively released from the apoptotic cells. Somewhat in line with the latter study, the key role of apoptosis of MSC with the self-activation of IL-1/IL-1R/NFκB pathway induced by caspases, has been implicated in the increased secretion of Prostaglandin E2 by MSC and consequential proinflammatory M1→ anti-inflammatory M2 macrophage transition [30].

2.4. Source of MSC for Research Purposes

Mesenchymal stem cells can be obtained from fetal tissues, umbilical cord blood or Wharton's Jelly, which for obvious reasons limits this route of acquisition to the perinatal period. In males, they may be acquired throughout a lifetime from testis [31], but due to greater accessibility, MSC for research purposes are derived mostly from bone marrow or subcutaneous adipose tissue. Fat may become preferential as a source of MSC not only owing to less invasive procurement, but also due to higher MSC concentration than in bone marrow, lesser expression of MHC class I antigens, and greater replicative and secretory potential of MSC [32,33] (Table 1). MSC can also be obtained from induced pluripotent stem cells by their differentiation in vitro [34], which constitutes another life-long, yet technically much more challenging way of acquisition.

Table 1. Differences in the properties of bone marrow and fat mesenchymal stem cells.

Differentiating Characteristic	Bone Marrow MSC	Adipose MSC
Stability in culture	Lower	Higher
Aging	More advanced	Less advanced
Replicative potential	Lower	Higher
Immunomodulatory properties	Lower	Higher

2.5. Kidney as a Source of MSC

A promising method of a non-invasive collection of MSC is their isolation from urine. In 2008, for the first time, Zhang et al. from North Carolina identified cells present in the urine in the amount of 2–7/100 mL that adhere to plastic and form colonies of differentiated daughter cells expressing membrane markers characteristic of urothelial, endothelial, and interstitial cells, or myocytes [35]. In further studies, the differentiation of these cells in appropriate culture media to the endo, ecto- and mesodermal lineage was achieved [36]. In contrast to MSC, urine-derived cells (up to 75% of them) show telomerase activity, which is associated with their higher replicative potential, apparently not associated with an increased risk of tumorigenesis [37]. The origin of these cells is most likely glomerular—MSC-like cells with a vast differentiation potential were isolated from the renal cortical decapsulated glomeruli [38] and shown nephroprotective in the renal ischemia-reperfusion injury (IRI) [39]. These cells seem distinct from the renal perivascular MSC-like cells that possess lesser differentiating capabilities (no adipogenesis), but also compelling kidney reparative properties confirmed in the tubular epithelial cell line injury in vitro or non-ischemic AKI in mice [40].

3. Research on the Use of Mesenchymal Stem Cells in Kidney Diseases

Potential applications of MSC in kidney diseases primarily take advantage of their secretory capabilities and aim to enhance the natural regenerative processes in the settings of AKI, and in the bolder perspective, even induce such processes in CKD. On the other hand, MSC can be used to grow renal cells in vitro to replace damaged native cells. In this context, cultures of kidney fragments (organoids) with subsequent implantations are to be considered, despite all technical complexity. Thirdly, the use of immunomodulatory properties of MSC can play an important role in the treatment of inflammatory kidney disease, such as primary and secondary glomerulonephritis, or in the prevention of rejection of the transplanted kidney. Finally, urinary isolation of cells that are functionally similar to MSC can significantly increase the availability of the material for all these therapeutic options.

3.1. Attempts to Replace Damaged Kidney Tissue

Kidney organogenesis includes mutually stimulating processes of the growth and differentiation of the intermediate mesoderm cells—to the ureteric bud (mesonephric duct protrusion) and to the metanephric blastema. They further transform respectively into the urinary tract system (up to connecting tubules), or nephrons, renal interstitium and endothelium [41]. Development of a new kidney by recapitulating organogenesis in whole or in part in vitro is an intensively studied area of tissue engineering. As research from the 1990s showed, appropriate sets of GFs can induce early stages of the development of an isolated ureteric bud, as well as metanephric blastema [42,43]. However, it remains problematic to derive cells with fetal characteristics from an adult, as well as to provide vascularization of the developing tissue. The first issue is currently being investigated with the use of induced pluripotent cells obtained from fibroblasts. In several cases, these cells (as well as embryonic MSC) were successfully cultured over <4 weeks into three-dimensional organoids with structural and functional characteristics of nephron complexes. The applied protocols included the use of such stimulants as Fibroblast GF-9, WNT-signaling pathway agonist, and activin [44,45]. Recent works by van den Berg et al. showed that renal organoids generated from human embryonic or induced pluripotent stem cells, became efficiently vascularized upon kidney subcapsular implantation in mice. Compared to organoids cultured continuously in vitro, those that were placed in vivo on the 18th day of the three-dimensional growth featured a more advanced structural maturation regarding glomerular endothelium, filtration barrier (slit diaphragm formation), tubular epithelium polarization and differentiation, as well as peritubular vascularization, when assessed on the 28th day since implantation [46].

A different way of generating a kidney replacement is through colonization of an acellular connective tissue scaffold with cells of a high replicative and differentiating potential or mature renal cells. The use of mature renal cells would eliminate the possible risk of cancer associated with stem cell divisions, but is much more technically difficult. A more feasible approach is through intra-arterial and intra-ureteral infusions of multipotent cells, which in response to the scaffold environment and native or exogenous GFs would differentiate into glomerular endothelial and epithelial or tubular cells, respectively. In order to obtain an intact acellular, sterile connective tissue scaffold of the kidney, an organ retrieved from another organism is infused with detergents like sodium lauryl sulfate or nonionic surfactants [47]. A successful repopulation of digested rat kidneys with rat fetal cells has been reported by the authors from Boston in 2013. The umbilical vein endothelial cells infused into renal artery produced endothelial layer in the entire renal circulation, whereas neonatal kidney cell suspension administered into the ureter resulted in the settlement of cells in their physiological niches of the urinary tract, beginning from podocytes down to connecting tubules. Such regenerated kidneys perfused in vitro with a solution containing crystalloids, glucose, albumin, amino acids, creatinine and urea showed partial functionality in the production of "urine", creatinine filtration (10–25% of the physiological level) and albumin retention (47% of the physiological level). In contrast, after orthotopic implantation, despite adequate blood flow and absence of bleeding or clotting and urine production of ~1/3 of physiological volume, they featured only a negligible excretion of urea and creatinine [48]. Similar results were obtained by another team of researchers from China [49]. On the other hand, Italian researchers did not manage to obtain sealed layers of cells in the distal parts of the renal circulation and proximal sections of the nephrons despite various protocols of embryonic MSC administration [50]. This area of research is awaiting verification of the usefulness of bone marrow or adipose MSC.

In the context of kidney regeneration, it is of note, that Iranian authors intend to assess effects of intravenous infusion of autologous bone marrow MSC on the course of autosomal dominant polycystic kidney disease [51].

3.2. Induction of Repair Processes after Acute Kidney Injury

One of the major study areas of MSC has been their influence on the course of renal IRI, being the most frequent cause of AKI and occurring in the clinical settings of shock, cardiac arrest, extracorporeal circulation and peritransplantation period. In addition to apoptosis caused by an energy deficiency and acidosis during ischemia, reperfusion results in further tissue damage, due to oxidative stress and inflammatory reaction. Studies conducted so far have shown that MSC infusion alleviates IRI of the kidney. Regardless of the mode of MSC administration (to the renal artery or intravenously, at various times in relation to IRI), the animal models showed a milder course of acute kidney failure [52], with reductions of oxidative damage and local expression of inflammatory cytokines [53], increased renal pool of regulatory T lymphocytes [54], faster regeneration of renal tubular epithelium [55], and reduction of subsequent fibrosis of the renal interstitium [56].

Intravenous infusion of MSC (derived from induced pluripotent stem cells) was equally nephroprotective in the model of toxin-induced AKI. In mice 2×10^5 MSC, injected 2 h after administration of Adriamycin, mitigated proteinuria and renal failure present on day 7 in controls. This could be attributed to the observed inhibition of oxidative stress and apoptosis in the tubular cells [57].

As already mentioned, these beneficial effects of MSC result from their secretory properties, not replicative-differentiating potential. In an experiment conducted by a German-American team, rats subjected to 40-min ischemia of both kidneys were administered labelled allogenic bone marrow-derived

MSC (10^6 cells) to the aorta immediately after or 24 h after renal reperfusion. In both cases, two hours after the end of the infusion, MSC were found in the renal tissue (within the glomerular and peritubular capillaries), but were not detected, neither did differentiate to other cells, during the subsequent 22 and 70 h of observation. Nevertheless, faster normalization of renal excretory function, reduced renal expression of proinflammatory cytokines (Interleukin-1β, Tumor Necrosis Factor α, Interferon γ) and higher renal expression of anti-inflammatory and antiapoptotic factors, such as Interleukin-10, basic Fibroblast GF, TGF α and Bcl-2 were observed at the conclusion of observation [58].

The fraction of MSC secretome responsible for this nephroprotective effect may be largely RNA, as shown by Italian researchers. Microvesicles isolated from human bone marrow MSC medium (30 µg), administered intravenously to rats after a 45-min ischemia of the sole kidney, attenuated acute renal failure and atrophy of tubular cells, whereas subjecting these microvesicles to RNase abolished their beneficial effects in this experimental model [59]. Further studies in rodents and cell lines by this largely Torino-based group revealed that the nephroprotective effect of microvesicles derived from bone marrow MSC in AKI may be owing to high contents of a few microRNA families (miR-483–5p, -191, -28–3p, -423–5p, -744, -129–3p, -24, and miR-148a) that get transferred to tubular epithelial cells. This results in altered expression of at least 165 genes involved in cellular adhesion and extracellular matrix remodeling, including downregulation of the transcription of fibrinogen-α subunit [60]. Furthermore, extracellular vesicles secreted by the bone marrow MSC were shown by this group to be heterogeneous in size and contents, with the exosomal fraction to diminish apoptosis and enhance proliferation of tubular cells undergoing hypoxia/reperfusion in vitro. This fraction was rich in the microRNA families involved in kidney regeneration (miR-100, -21, -24, -214, -34a, -127, -30c, -29a, -125b, -10b, -let-7c, -99a, -17 and miR-20a) [61]. Another study showed that also the above mentioned glomerular MSC-like cells (obtained from human renal cortex) and their extracellular vesicles alleviate AKI in mice by promoting tubular cell proliferation when infused intravenously at reperfusion following a 35-min sole kidney ischemia (10^5 cells or 400×10^6 vesicles, respectively). Interestingly, the injected vesicles were homing to the injured tubular cells (and not glomeruli) where they were visible for up to 6 h after infusion, contrary to the administered vesicles obtained from dermal fibroblasts, which did not accumulate in the kidney and consequently showed no effects whatsoever. In line with earlier studies, the nephroprotective properties of the vesicles derived from the glomerular MSC-like cells were eliminated in case they had been pretreated with high-concentration RNase and 62 microRNAs were found to be specifically abundant in these extracellular vesicles [39].

Similar to MSC, the MSC-derived extracellular vesicles were found to protect kidneys also from a toxic injury. The above quoted Italian group of Camussi showed that human bone marrow MSC (75×10^3) or their microvesicles (15 µg) alleviated AKI to the same extent when administered intravenously on the third day after glycerol injection in mice. Moreover MSC microvesicles were homing and getting incorporated into tubular cells in vivo only in glycerol-exposed animals, and not in controls, and their antiapoptotic effects were RNA-dependent [62]. Correspondingly positive renal outcomes were obtained by these authors in the mouse model of cisplatin-induced lethal AKI, in which MSC-secreted microvesicles (100 µg) were infused 8 h after cisplatin injection. Importantly, nearly half of the animals were alive after three weeks, and when injections of the microvesicles were repeated every four days, 80% of mice survived [63].

The very same model of toxic AKI was used by German investigators to show that the renoprotective properties of MSC secretome can be enhanced by hypoxic preconditioning of the MSC culture. Such treatment of mouse adipose MSC (0.5% oxygen for 48 h) increased their expression of VEGF and by >2-fold its secretion, as well as that of other 63 proteins. This corresponded with a moderately alleviated course of AKI following infusion of the hypoxia-preconditioned MSC medium (at 24 h after cisplatin injection), as compared to the non-manipulated MSC medium [64]. Significantly positive renal outcomes were obtained by another group in the rat model of renal IRI with the administration of hypoxia-preconditioned (1% oxygen for 24 h) human adipose MSC at reperfusion.

Like in the former study, these cells showed higher expression of VEGF than naïve MSC. Furthermore, in vivo they featured greater antioxidant and antiapoptotic properties [65].

More light on the possible cellular mechanisms of the regenerative properties of the MSC extracellular vesicles was shed by Chinese groups. In studies conducted in the rat models of renal IRI, urologists from Shanghai have shown that 100 μg microvesicles derived from the human umbilical cord mesenchyme alleviated kidney macrophage infiltration, tubular apoptosis and AKI when intravenously infused at reperfusion. This may be due to the revealed attenuation of the renal expression of fractalkine (itself a potent chemoattractant), likely mediated by a transfer of certain microRNAs to renal cells [66]. RNA transfer from MSC extracellular vesicles to tubular cells was also shown by these authors to underlie the increase of tubular VEGF synthesis and attenuation of AKI, as well as renal fibrosis, in rats that were administered the vesicles at reperfusion of the solitary kidney [67]. Other experiments showed that additional effectors of the MSC vesicles in the tubular cell nuclei of the kidneys subjected to IRI may be Nrf2/antioxidant response element with subsequent overexpression of antioxidant enzymes [68] or the Sox9 transcription factor enhancing tubular cell proliferation and diminishing kidney fibrosis [69] (one of the few studies with the use of human adipose-derived MSC and their vesicles).

On the other hand, another group from the same university have convincingly shown that a transfer of protein may also take part in the nephroprotective effects of MSC and their vesicles. It was found by these researchers that extracellular vesicles derived from human induced pluripotent stem cell-derived MSC exert a potent nephroprotective effect in the renal IRI by a transfer of protein that inhibits programmed inflammatory cell death (necroptosis) [70]. 10^{12} extracellular vesicles delivered intravenously 1 h before bilateral 30-min kidney ischemia decreased the kidney histological damage and the degree of renal failure in rats at 48 h after ischemia. Analyses in vitro showed that this phenomenon relied on a transfer of the transcription factor Specificity protein-1 to the renal proximal tubule cells with subsequent activation of nuclear expression of sphingosine kinase-1. This enzyme phosphorylates dihydrosphingosine into sphinganine-1-phosphate, a compound shown to alleviate the extent of IRI [71].

The use of MSC in the clinical setting of renal ischemia (not related to kidney transplantation) was the subject of a study conducted by researchers from Minnesota. Fourteen patients with unilateral renal artery stenosis were administered autologous adipose-derived MSC (10^5 or 2.5×10^5 cells/kg body weight) to the stenotic renal artery. After the subsequent three months blood flows increased in both the stenotic and the contralateral kidney, and glomerular filtration was higher by 21% compared to the control group [72]. Somewhat contrary to these results, MSC were ineffective in the setting of postoperative AKI that occurred within 24 h from cardiac surgery. Intraaortic infusion of allogenic bone marrow-derived MSC (2×10^6 cells / kg body weight within 48 h from the operation) in 67 patients did not improve kidney function nor 30-day mortality. In fact, patients who received the MSC suspension showed a tendency to a worse prognosis in the postoperative period [73]. As noted by the authors, such results indicate that MSC may not be as effective in the environment of an established inflammatory reaction as in its prevention, like with the pretreatment of anticipated ischemic AKI. Nevertheless, a clinical trial is planned by a team from Massachusetts in patients with AKI treated with continuous renal replacement therapy, in which patient's blood will be exposed to MSC across a semipermeable membrane of a hollow fiber extracorporeal device inserted into the hemodiafiltration circuit [74]. This would prevent any MSC-induced immunization, eliminate the risk of uncontrolled MSC replication, but expectantly provide a constant influx of the cells' beneficial products into the patient.

3.3. Immunomodulation of Kidney Transplantation

IRI is an inherent element of kidney transplantation and is manifested in the peritransplant period as the delayed graft function. The therapeutic potential of MSC in this setting is additionally related to a possible immunosuppressive effect, which may increase the effectiveness of pharmacological prophylaxis of the transplant rejection. The animal studies and scarce observations in humans, despite varying protocols of application, encourage the use of MSC-based therapies in kidney transplant patients, with no clear preference of any of the cell sources (autologous, donor-derived, third-party).

In rats in which allogeneic or syngeneic kidney transplantation was performed, infusion of allogeneic bone marrow MSC into the graft artery during reperfusion reduced the organ infiltration with CD8+ lymphocytes and monocytes, and alleviated failure of the rejected graft [75]. MSC were likewise effective with intravenous administrations. Syngeneic MSC infused in this way during kidney transplantation reduced the expression of inflammatory cytokines in the graft in rats [76]. In mice MSC administered intravenously 24 h before kidney transplantation increased the pool of regulatory T-cells in the spleen and prolonged survival of the transplanted kidney (which was not observed with the infusion performed at 24 h post-transplantation) [77]. In addition, Spanish researchers reported that MSCs can also be effective in the treatment of chronic graft nephropathy—intravenous infusion at 11 weeks after renal transplantation in rats resulted in reduced proteinuria, diminished inflammatory infiltration of the interstitium, and lesser interstitial fibrosis/tubular atrophy at 24 weeks after organ transplantation [78].

In one of the pioneer studies of human MSC use in renal transplantation, adipose MSC derived from the perirenal fat of the living kidney donor or the third-party MSC, inhibited similarly both pre- and post-transplant anti-donor and anti-third party alloreactivity of recipient's T lymphocytes [79]. This finding was followed by the first clinical studies of the MSC use in the living-donor kidney transplant recipients conducted in Italy. In total, two patients underwent intravenous administration of autologous bone marrow MSC at one week after transplantation (1.7×10^6 and 2.0×10^6 cells per kg body weight, respectively), while the other two were given autologous MSC 24 h prior to kidney graft implantation (2.0×10^6 cells per kg body weight intravenously). Over the five- to seven-year follow-up the mean renal function yearly decline rate was lower by ~70% than in non-MSC treated transplanted patients [80]. However, the MSC recipients showed considerable variability in the clinical course with one patient developing calcineurin inhibitor-free graft tolerance, whilst the other one experiencing acute graft rejection at two weeks after transplantation—both patients being ones that were given MSC before kidney implantation. Nevertheless, there was no elevation in the frequency of infections or neoplasms in the MSC-treated subjects. With the exception of one patient, a ~50% reduction in the blood percentage of memory CD8+ T cells was observed at 12 months post-transplantation compared with the pre-transplant levels, a phenomenon not seen in any of the controls [80].

In another pilot study, authors from China infused donor-derived bone marrow MSC into the graft renal artery during reperfusion and intravenously at one month after kidney transplantation in six recipients. This allowed the reduction of tacrolimus dosing by ~50% (with C0 ~4 vs. ~7 μg/L in controls) without episodes of rejection within 12 months of observation [81]. The immunosuppressive efficacy of MSC in the late post-transplant period was studied by Dutch researchers, who applied autologous bone marrow MSC in six kidney transplant recipients with subclinical rejection or histological progression of graft nephropathy at six months after transplantation. Two intravenous infusions of 10^6 cells/kg body weight each, in a week interval, eliminated peri-tubular cellular infiltrates at 12 months after transplantation, and patients' blood monocytes were characterized by diminished replication in vitro. It is notable, however, that CMV or BKV infection occurred in three of these patients [82].

In the largest clinical trial conducted so far 105 Chinese renal transplant recipients were administered autologous MSC at graft reperfusion and again after two weeks in place of anti-IL-2 receptor antibodies. Such induction of immunosuppression was associated with faster organ regeneration in the first month after transplantation, as well as a lower rate of cellular rejection (7.6% vs. 21.6% in the control group) and its milder course in the six-month follow-up [83].

On the other hand, studies appeared that denied effects of intravenous infusions of MSC on the kidney transplant outcome—improvement of renal allograft function and rat survival was found only when allogeneic fat MSC were injected into the graft artery, and not when they were administered intravenously at implantation [84]. Even more discouraging are the recent findings of another Chinese team of researchers, who injected allogeneic umbilical cord blood MSC to 21 recipients intravenously immediately prior to transplantation (2×10^6/kg body weight) and, additionally, to graft artery at reperfusion (5×10^6), on top of the standard immunosuppression. In the period of one-year follow-up, no statistically significant differences were found against the controls in terms of postoperative and infectious complications, renal function, frequency of rejection nor survival time of the kidney transplant [85]. Of note, one experimental study from Germany also found unfavorable effects of MSC infusion in the peritransplant period—rats given syngeneic or donor-derived bone marrow MSC intravenously four days before kidney transplantation showed symptoms of more severe cellular and humoral rejection and worse graft function on the 10th day after graft implantation [86].

3.4. Immunomodulation of Primary Glomerulonephritis

Inflammatory glomerulopathies constitute another area of potential clinical applications of the MSC. The few conducted experimental studies have shown their beneficial effect on the course of these diseases. For example, in an animal model of membranoproliferative glomerulonephritis, intravenous infusion of allogeneic fetal MSC reduced glomerular expression of proinflammatory cytokines, decreased monocyte infiltrates, mesangial hyperplasia, synthesis of connective tissue matrix and proteinuria. Interestingly, in this study the MSC culture medium inhibited mesangial expression of TNFα and monocyte chemoattractant protein 1 (MCP-1) in vitro [87]. Likewise, in the rat model of focal segmental glomerulosclerosis (doxorubicin-induced nephropathy), several intravenous infusions of bone marrow MSC increased glomerular VEGF synthesis, which was accompanied by attenuations of: Glomerular monocyte infiltration, apoptosis of the podocytes, and the extent of podocyte-parietal epithelial bridging [88].

A key role of MSC secretome in their actions was revealed in a rat model of experimental anti-glomerular basement membrane disease, in which intraperitoneal administration of human MSC medium over the 10 days since induction of disease reduced renal proinflammatory cytokine expression, increased plasma MCP-1 concentration and shifted the glomerular macrophage infiltration into the dominance of the anti-inflammatory M2 cells. This was associated with the lesser formation of crescents, reduction of proteinuria and improvement of glomerular filtration [89]. Similar favorable results were obtained in rats that received human MSC intravenously on the fourth day of the same type of rapidly progressive glomerulonephritis. Beside a smaller degree of histological and functional renal disorders, increased expression of anti-inflammatory cytokines, as well as reduced TGF β, collagen I and III mRNA concentrations in the kidney cortex were found in these rats on day 13 of the disease [90].

The use of MSC in primary glomerulonephritis in human patients has been described in two case reports from Italy. In the first one, a 13-year-old boy experienced a relapse of focal segmental glomerulosclerosis in the kidney graft on the second day after the transplantation. Intensification of immunosuppressive therapy with rituximab did not bring remission and the patient underwent weekly plasmapheresis, which only temporarily reduced the amount of proteinuria. Therefore, at month 7 after the transplantation, the patient was given two intravenous infusions of allogeneic bone marrow MSC (1×10^6 cells/kg body weight each), which was repeated after further three and seven months. In the 22-month follow-up from the first infusion, proteinuria remained stable without the need to perform plasmapheresis, the plasma concentration of Epidermal GF and TGF α decreased, and serum creatinine oscillated around 0.9 mg/dL [91]. In the second case, autologous bone marrow MSC (1.5×10^6 cells/kg body weight) were given intravenously to a 73-year-old patient with pANCA-positive rapidly progressive glomerulonephritis, whose treatment with steroid and cyclophosphamide was ineffective, and rituximab was discontinued due to severe oral candidiasis. Seven days after administration of MSC, serum creatinine decreased from 7.8 to 2.2 mg/dL, which was accompanied by normalization of urinary sediment, a significant reduction in the pANCA titer, and decrease in serum cytokine concentrations, as well as an increase in the regulatory T-cell pool in the blood. The MSC infusion was repeated after eight months, due to the recurrence of the disease with similar efficiency (serum creatinine 1.9 mg/dL), and over the next 11 months of observation, the patient's condition was good and did not require any treatment [92].

3.5. Immunomodulation of Lupus Nephritis

Systemic lupus erythematosus is a multisystem condition that involves kidneys in approximately 60% of cases. Since the standard immunosuppressive treatment is mostly insufficient in patients with severe proliferative lupus nephritis [93], the cell-based therapies are a promising alternative owing to their immunomodulatory properties. To date, many pre-clinical studies regarding the use of MSC transplantation in the context of lupus nephritis therapy have been performed giving mostly positive outcomes in terms of proteinuria and renal histopathology, as reviewed lately [94]. In one of the most recent experimental studies, Tani et al. applied systemic treatment with low-dose allogenic bone marrow MSC (10^6 cells/kg body weight intravenously) in a mouse model of spontaneously developing lupus with co-occurring glomerulonephritis. The therapeutic strategy was the early MSC administration (18–22 weeks of age) in order to investigate its potential interference with the developing disease, as well as to compare the outcomes of a single and multiple cell infusions. MSC treatment resulted in a significant delay of proteinuria appearance with the most beneficial results in mice that received multiple cell administrations. Nevertheless, histopathological nephritis scores did not differ from the controls and some harmful effects of MSC were observed, such as significantly higher B-cell deposition in kidneys of mice that received multiple MSC doses and decreased levels of regulatory T-cells after both single and multiple MSC injections [95].

The MSC-based therapies are used increasingly in Chinese patients with lupus nephritis, and often with good outcomes in terms of clinical remission [96] or blood Treg/Th17 balance [97]. However, there is still a shortage of randomized, double-blind, placebo-controlled trials. In 2017 Deng et al. presented a randomized clinical study comparing the efficacy of a standard immunosuppressive treatment (methylprednisolone and cyclophosphamide applied intravenously, followed by maintenance oral prednisolone and mycophenolate mofetil) with ($n = 12$) or without ($n = 6$) a co-administration of human umbilical cord MSC (two intravenous injections of 2×10^8 cells in total) [98]. The primary endpoint was remission of nephritis (combined partial and complete remission) defined with specified values of serum creatinine, urinary red blood cells and proteinuria in the 12-month follow-up. Remission was noted in 75% of patients in the MSC-treated group and in 83% of patients in the placebo group. The reduction of proteinuria was comparable and no significant difference in serum creatinine levels between the two groups was noted. When it comes to secondary endpoints (clinical symptom scores, complement concentration, anti-dsDNA antibody and ANA titers, death and commencement of permanent dialysis or renal transplantation), no significant differences were observed, either, and the trial was terminated ahead of schedule. The newest report regarding the application of MSC in the lupus nephritis came from Spain and suggests the efficacy of the cells in the most severe cases. Three patients who demonstrated class IV active proliferative lupus nephritis, were treated with allogenic bone marrow MCS (9×10^7 of cells infused intravenously) at the exacerbation of the disease [99]. One week after MSC infusion a considerable decrease of proteinuria was observed in all patients and maintained throughout the course of a nine-month follow-up. The complete clinical symptom remission in two patients and partial remission to the mild activity of the disease in the third patient were noted and call for a randomized and controlled trial in such patients.

Of note, so far no animal or clinical studies have been reported with the application of MSC extracellular vesicles in the lupus nephropathy, although the rationale for such investigations have been formulated [100,101].

3.6. Therapeutic Potential in Diabetic Kidney Disease

Glomerular microinflammation takes part in the pathogenesis of diabetic nephropathy, albeit is not the target of standard immunosuppressive treatment, due to its small intensity and possible metabolic complications of such therapies. Not surprisingly, the interest of researchers has recently focused on MSC and the studies of their use in diabetic nephropathy are consequently, and somewhat paradoxically, more advanced than in gross inflammatory glomerulopathies.

On one hand, MSC can indirectly prevent kidney damage or inhibit its progression by improving glycemic control of diabetes, as shown in experimental and clinical studies. In the mouse model of established streptozotocin-induced type 1 diabetes, intravenous administrations of human bone marrow MSC or their medium induced regeneration of pancreatic islets and subsequently reduced blood glucose levels by 30–35% [102,103]. MSC may also hinder type 2 diabetes: Myoblasts pre-exposed to the MSC medium featured lower expression of proinflammatory cytokines, increased synthesis and expression of the GLUT4 glucose transporter, and consequently less compromised insulin sensitivity upon 24-h exposure to a palmitate solution. MSC medium was as effective in this regard as a metformin solution [104]. The influence of MSC on the course of type 2 diabetes in humans has been evaluated so far in several studies conducted in small groups of patients, and with considerable methodological differences—in terms of the origin of administered cells, dose and route of administration (intravenous, pancreatic artery), or the use of controls. In the majority of these works, increases in the blood C-peptide concentrations and reductions of hemoglobin A1c levels were observed for several months after the MSC infusions, with no effects on the peripheral insulin resistance [105,106].

The nephroprotective properties of MSC in diabetic nephropathy have been revealed in experimental models of type 1 diabetes. Intravenous infusion of allogeneic bone marrow MSC in the late phase of streptozotocin-induced diabetes resulted in the reduction of albuminuria and the degree of glomerular filtration impairment in rodents. In the renal tissue of these animals, reduced oxidative stress, as well as diminished expressions of proinflammatory cytokines, apoptotic proteins and TGF β were observed, whereas expressions of nephrin, podocin, bone morphogenetic protein 7 and VEGF were augmented [107,108].

The immunomodulatory effects of MSC-secreted factors, rather than the cells themselves, have been implicated by a study in mice with streptozotocin-induced or high-fat diet-induced diabetes. In both models, intravenous infusions of both rat bone marrow MSC or their medium reduced alike renal proinflammatory cytokine expression and macrophage infiltration. This was accompanied by attenuated albuminuria and diminished interstitial fibrosis [109]. The key role of the MSC-secreted extracellular vesicles could be deduced from only scarce renal localization of the administered MSC and the fact of obtaining comparable beneficial histological effects in the kidney after subcapsular administration of exosomes previously isolated from MSC [109]. The nephroprotective effects of factors secreted by the MSC were also indicated by the results of a study in rats with streptozotocin-induced diabetes that were injected intravenously with exosomes derived from the aforementioned pluripotent MSC-like cells isolated from human urine. In these animals, no mesangial expansion, reduced renal expression of apoptotic proteins, as well as diminished albuminuria were found in comparison to the control group [110]. Recently, Ebrahim et al. succeeded in clarifying the mechanisms of the beneficial effects of bone marrow MSC exosomes in type 1 diabetic nephropathy in rats, showing their capability of improving tubular cell autophagy, as seen with the electron microscopy and reflected in the reduced renal expression of the mechanistic target of rapamycin. This was accompanied by significantly reduced expression of fibronectin and TGF β with diminished fibrosis and improved function of the kidneys [111].

In the years 2015–2016, the first reports emerged on the use of allogeneic multipotent mesenchymal precursor cells in patients with type 2 diabetes. The cellular suspension was obtained from the bone marrow by a selection of cells with membrane expression of alkaline phosphatase STRO-3 (rexlemestrocel-L, currently in the second phases of clinical verification in groups of patients with various medical conditions). In the first of these works, these cells were given in the amount of 0.3–2×10^6/kg body weight to 45 patients with inadequately controlled type 2 diabetes. In the second one the same preparation was given to patients with diabetic renal insufficiency (eGFR 20–50 mL/min/1.73 m^2) at a dose of 150×10^6 or 300×10^6 cells (both groups numbering 10 patients). During the 12 weeks following infusions, no significant side effects or immunization of patients with donor antigens were noted. In this relatively short period of observation, there was however no significant effect of the tested preparation on the clinical parameters related to diabetes and renal failure [112,113].

4. Conclusions

The presented review of published works on the use of mesenchymal stem cells in kidney diseases shows the greatest advancement of experimental research in the fields of AKI, kidney transplantation, and diabetic or lupus nephropathies (Table 2). The majority of results indicate the reparative, immunosuppressive and antifibrotic effects of factors released from MSC in the environment of low-grade inflammation (as in the case of diabetic glomerulopathy) or in prevention/alleviation of a developing inflammatory injury (as with pretreatment of the anticipated ischemic AKI, early treatment of ischemic or toxic tubular injury or administration preceding/concurrent with kidney graft implantation). The efficacy of MSC secretome in the milieu of an established renal inflammation or injury (as with post-IRI administration) seems less uniform.

Table 2. Intensity and outcomes of the studies of MSC or MSC secretome in the major renal settings.

Kidney Disease Setting		Animal Studies		Human Studies	
		MSC	MSC Medium or EVs	MSC	MSC Medium or EVs
Acute kidney injury	ischemic	↑↑↑	↑↑↑	↑↓	○
	non-ischemic	↑↑	↑↑	○	○
Kidney transplantation	pre-/intra-implantation	↑↑	○	↑↑	○
	post-implantation	↓	○	↑	○
Chronic allograft nephropathy		↑	○	↑	○
Glomerulo-nephritis	primary	↑↑	↑	↑	○
	lupus	↑↑↑	○	↑↓	○
Diabetic kidney disease		↑↑	↑↑	○	○

MSC—mesenchymal stem cells; EVs—extracellular vesicles; ○ no conducted studies; ↑ single conducted study or a few case reports, positive outcomes; ↑↑ several conducted studies, mostly positive outcomes; ↑↑↑ numerous conducted studies, mostly positive outcomes; ↑↓ several conducted studies, conflicting outcomes; ↓ single conducted study, negative outcomes.

The most promising MSC product in the context of renal regeneration/immunosuppression appears to be microRNAs contained within extracellular vesicles (Figure 1). Membranous protection enables their homing to the injured tissue and subsequent epigenetic modulation of the local expression of reparative cytokines and transcription/growth factors. Studies show that also MSC-secreted proteins or mitochondria take part in tissue regeneration. However, the role of freely released transcription/growth factors or cell-to-cell mitochondrial transfer may be limited to MSC infused to the aorta or renal artery, for the assured proximity to the injured cells. On the other hand, the intravenously administered MSC, which largely get trapped and apoptotic in the lungs, may dispatch both proteins and mitochondria within extracellular vesicles that shall be able to reach the injured or inflamed kidneys. Of importance for the future clinical applications, the secretory reparative potential of MSC can be enhanced in culture, as with hypoxic preconditioning.

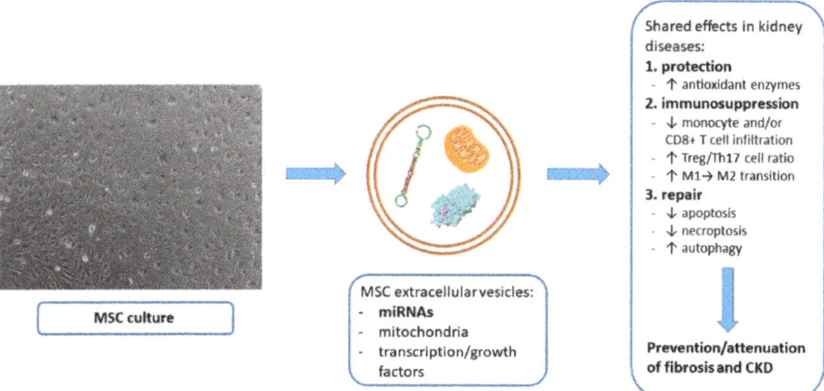

Figure 1. Shared major mechanisms of nephroprotection with exogenous MSC/MSC-derived products in renal diseases.

It is striking that the number of clinical trials with the use of MSC in kidney diseases so far has remained disproportionately low considering their therapeutic potential emerging from experimental studies (placebo-controlled trials are particularly in demand). For example, in the last three years there has been only one reported use of MSC in renal transplant recipients [85]. This may be related to the fact that the outcomes of the pioneer uses of MSC in patients have not been uniformly favorable. Also, and likely more importantly, shortage of trials can be attributed to reservations that both scientists and bioethical boards may have towards applications of allogenic cells with high mitotic potential, as such associated with the risk of immunization or cancer.

Thus far, there have been findings of MSC enhancing divisions in cancer cell lines [114] and augmenting the metastatic potential of co-administered cancerous cells in animals [115]. Nevertheless, there has been no report of de novo carcinogenesis in vivo following MSC infusion, neither in animals nor in humans. One reported case of angiomyeloproliferative renal lesions was related to percutaneous renal injections of not MSC, but peripheral blood-derived autologous hematopoietic cells [116]. Moreover, it has been shown that MSC can actually inhibit the progression of cancerous tumors. In hamsters with induced premalignant stages of squamous cell carcinoma of the mouth cavity, they decreased the progression of lesions (except for the largest doses) [117]. Less optimistic are the latest discoveries in the field of MSC immunogenicity. Contrary to the assumptions of its negligibility due to lack of expression of HLA class II antigens, equine bone marrow stromal cells treated with a proinflammatory cytokine (Interferon γ) expressed MHC class II antigens on their cellular membrane and stimulated the proliferation of T lymphocytes in vitro [118]. It is not certain whether this process also takes place in vivo—current applications in humans do not indicate significant immunogenicity of allogeneic MSC, although it is necessary to bear in mind the relatively short periods of observation in the conducted studies [119].

All these objections direct the researchers' interest into microvesicles or exosomes secreted by MSC. In particular, microRNAs contained within are considered equally efficient, but potentially not tumorigenic and less immunogenic therapeutic objects. Although increasingly used in animal models, their applicability in clinical trials is dulled by the lack of sufficient knowledge of the consequences of administering exogenous molecules with such high stability as microRNAs [120]. On the other hand, it has to be noted that this very characteristic may constitute the observed effectiveness of systemically administered MSC-derived vesicles in kidney disease models.

Regardless of all question marks, the secretory products of mesenchymal stem cells deserve further research in experimental and subsequently clinical studies, providing a chance for the most awaited breakthrough in the treatment of the inflammatory and, especially, ever more frequent autoimmune diseases with renal involvement. Finally, commenting on the concerns of possible side effects of MSC-based therapies, it can be questioned whether the widely used classical immunosuppressive drugs—source of common infectious, metabolic and cancerous complications—would ever be approved for the clinical use at the present-day level of safety expectations.

Author Contributions: Concept, writing—review and editing, G.W.; literature search, writing—original draft preparation, B.B., M.K., G.S., A.W., R.K., and G.W.; supervision, W.G. and G.W.

Funding: The APC was funded by the Medical University of Silesia in Katowice, Poland (KNW-1-008/K/8/K).

Acknowledgments: We acknowledge Wojciech Wystrychowski for providing an image of human adipose MSC culture in a subconfluent state, as well as Krzysztof Gajdzik for his assistance in editing the paper.

Conflicts of Interest: The authors declare no conflict of interest.

Abbreviations

ANA	Anti-Nuclear Antibody
AKI	Acute Kidney Injury
CKD	Chronic Kidney Disease
dsDNA	double stranded Deoxyribonucleic Acid
eGFR	estimated Glomerular Filtration Rate
HLA	Human Leukocyte Antigen
IRI	Ischemia-Reperfusion Injury
MCP	Monocyte Chemoattractant Protein
MHC	Major Histocompatibility Complex
MSC	Mesenchymal (mesodermal) stem cells
pANCA	perinuclear Anti-Neutrophil Cytoplasmic Antibody
RNA	Ribonucleic Acid
TGF	Transforming Growth Factor
VEGF	Vascular Endothelial Growth Factor

References

1. Bonaventura, G.; Chamayou, S.; Liprino, A.; Guglielmino, A.; Fichera, M.; Caruso, M.; Barcellona, M.L. Different Tissue-Derived Stem Cells: A Comparison of Neural Differentiation Capability. *PLoS ONE* **2015**, *10*, e0140790. [CrossRef] [PubMed]

2. Mitalipov, S.; Wolf, D. Totipotency, pluripotency and nuclear reprogramming. *Adv. Biochem. Eng. Biotechnol.* **2009**, *114*, 185–199.

3. Yu, J.; Vodyanik, M.A.; Smuga-Otto, K.; Antosiewicz-Bourget, J.; Frane, J.L.; Tian, S.; Nie, J.; Jonsdottir, G.A.; Ruotti, V.; Stewart, R.; et al. Induced pluripotent stem cell lines derived from human somatic cells. *Science* **2007**, *318*, 1917–1920. [CrossRef]

4. Biehl, J.K.; Russell, B. Introduction to stem cell therapy. *J. Cardiovasc Nurs* **2009**, *24*, 98–103; quiz 104–105. [CrossRef] [PubMed]

5. Kim, N.; Cho, S.-G. Clinical applications of mesenchymal stem cells. *Korean J. Intern. Med.* **2013**, *28*, 387–402. [CrossRef]

6. Kariminekoo, S.; Movassaghpour, A.; Rahimzadeh, A.; Talebi, M.; Shamsasenjan, K.; Akbarzadeh, A. Implications of mesenchymal stem cells in regenerative medicine. *Artif. Cells Nanomed. Biotechnol.* **2016**, *44*, 749–757. [CrossRef]

7. Jeon, B.-G.; Jang, S.-J.; Park, J.-S.; Subbarao, R.B.; Jeong, G.-J.; Park, B.-W.; Rho, G.-J. Differentiation potential of mesenchymal stem cells isolated from human dental tissues into non-mesodermal lineage. *Animal Cells and Systems* **2015**, *19*, 321–331. [CrossRef]

8. Seo, M.J.; Suh, S.Y.; Bae, Y.C.; Jung, J.S. Differentiation of human adipose stromal cells into hepatic lineage in vitro and in vivo. *Biochem. Biophys. Res. Commun.* **2005**, *328*, 258–264. [CrossRef]

9. Murphy, M.B.; Moncivais, K.; Caplan, A.I. Mesenchymal stem cells: environmentally responsive therapeutics for regenerative medicine. *Exp. Mol. Med.* **2013**, *45*, e54. [CrossRef]

10. Belting, M.; Wittrup, A. Nanotubes, exosomes, and nucleic acid-binding peptides provide novel mechanisms of intercellular communication in eukaryotic cells: implications in health and disease. *J. Cell Biol.* **2008**, *183*, 1187–1191. [CrossRef]

11. Qiu, G.; Zheng, G.; Ge, M.; Wang, J.; Huang, R.; Shu, Q.; Xu, J. Mesenchymal stem cell-derived extracellular vesicles affect disease outcomes via transfer of microRNAs. *Stem Cell Res. Ther.* **2018**, *9*, 320. [CrossRef] [PubMed]

12. Lotfi, R.; Eisenbacher, J.; Solgi, G.; Fuchs, K.; Yildiz, T.; Nienhaus, C.; Rojewski, M.T.; Schrezenmeier, H. Human mesenchymal stem cells respond to native but not oxidized damage associated molecular pattern molecules from necrotic (tumor) material. *Eur. J. Immunol.* **2011**, *41*, 2021–2028. [CrossRef]

13. Mahrouf-Yorgov, M.; Augeul, L.; Da Silva, C.C.; Jourdan, M.; Rigolet, M.; Manin, S.; Ferrera, R.; Ovize, M.; Henry, A.; Guguin, A.; et al. Mesenchymal stem cells sense mitochondria released from damaged cells as danger signals to activate their rescue properties. *Cell Death Differ.* **2017**, *24*, 1224–1238. [CrossRef]

14. Spees, J.L.; Olson, S.D.; Whitney, M.J.; Prockop, D.J. Mitochondrial transfer between cells can rescue aerobic respiration. *Proc. Natl. Acad. Sci. USA* **2006**, *103*, 1283–1288. [CrossRef] [PubMed]

15. Wang, X.; Gerdes, H.-H. Transfer of mitochondria via tunneling nanotubes rescues apoptotic PC12 cells. *Cell Death Differ.* **2015**, *22*, 1181–1191. [CrossRef] [PubMed]

16. Jiang, D.; Gao, F.; Zhang, Y.; Wong, D.S.H.; Li, Q.; Tse, H.-F.; Xu, G.; Yu, Z.; Lian, Q. Mitochondrial transfer of mesenchymal stem cells effectively protects corneal epithelial cells from mitochondrial damage. *Cell Death Dis.* **2016**, *7*, e2467. [CrossRef] [PubMed]

17. Islam, M.N.; Das, S.R.; Emin, M.T.; Wei, M.; Sun, L.; Westphalen, K.; Rowlands, D.J.; Quadri, S.K.; Bhattacharya, S.; Bhattacharya, J. Mitochondrial transfer from bone-marrow-derived stromal cells to pulmonary alveoli protects against acute lung injury. *Nat. Med.* **2012**, *18*, 759–765. [CrossRef] [PubMed]

18. Liu, K.; Ji, K.; Guo, L.; Wu, W.; Lu, H.; Shan, P.; Yan, C. Mesenchymal stem cells rescue injured endothelial cells in an in vitro ischemia-reperfusion model via tunneling nanotube like structure-mediated mitochondrial transfer. *Microvasc. Res.* **2014**, *92*, 10–18. [CrossRef] [PubMed]

19. Phinney, D.G.; Di Giuseppe, M.; Njah, J.; Sala, E.; Shiva, S.; St Croix, C.M.; Stolz, D.B.; Watkins, S.C.; Di, Y.P.; Leikauf, G.D.; et al. Mesenchymal stem cells use extracellular vesicles to outsource mitophagy and shuttle microRNAs. *Nat. Commun.* **2015**, *6*, 8472. [CrossRef]

20. Torralba, D.; Baixauli, F.; Sánchez-Madrid, F. Mitochondria Know No Boundaries: Mechanisms and Functions of Intercellular Mitochondrial Transfer. *Front. Cell Dev. Biol.* **2016**, *4*, 107. [CrossRef]

21. Kim, Y.-J.; Jeong, J.-H. Clinical application of adipose stem cells in plastic surgery. *J. Korean Med. Sci.* **2014**, *29*, 462–467. [CrossRef]

22. Wei, X.; Yang, X.; Han, Z.; Qu, F.; Shao, L.; Shi, Y. Mesenchymal stem cells: A new trend for cell therapy. *Acta Pharmacol. Sin.* **2013**, *34*, 747–754. [CrossRef]

23. Le Blanc, K. Immunomodulatory effects of fetal and adult mesenchymal stem cells. *Cytotherapy* **2003**, *5*, 485–489. [CrossRef] [PubMed]

24. Luz-Crawford, P.; Kurte, M.; Bravo-Alegría, J.; Contreras, R.; Nova-Lamperti, E.; Tejedor, G.; Noël, D.; Jorgensen, C.; Figueroa, F.; Djouad, F.; et al. Mesenchymal stem cells generate a CD4+CD25+Foxp3+ regulatory T cell population during the differentiation process of Th1 and Th17 cells. *Stem Cell Res. Ther.* **2013**, *4*, 65. [CrossRef]

25. Maumus, M.; Guérit, D.; Toupet, K.; Jorgensen, C.; Noël, D. Mesenchymal stem cell-based therapies in regenerative medicine: applications in rheumatology. *Stem Cell Res. Ther.* **2011**, *2*, 14. [CrossRef]

26. Duran, N.E.; Hommes, D.W. Stem cell-based therapies in inflammatory bowel disease: Promises and pitfalls. *Therap Adv. Gastroenterol.* **2016**, *9*, 533–547. [CrossRef]

27. Zhang, B.; Yin, Y.; Lai, R.C.; Tan, S.S.; Choo, A.B.H.; Lim, S.K. Mesenchymal stem cells secrete immunologically active exosomes. *Stem Cells Dev.* **2014**, *23*, 1233–1244. [CrossRef] [PubMed]

28. Monguió-Tortajada, M.; Roura, S.; Gálvez-Montón, C.; Pujal, J.M.; Aran, G.; Sanjurjo, L.; la Franquesa, M.; Sarrias, M.-R.; Bayes-Genis, A.; Borràs, F.E. Nanosized UCMSC-derived extracellular vesicles but not conditioned medium exclusively inhibit the inflammatory response of stimulated T cells: implications for nanomedicine. *Theranostics* **2017**, *7*, 270–284. [CrossRef] [PubMed]

29. Galleu, A.; Riffo-Vasquez, Y.; Trento, C.; Lomas, C.; Dolcetti, L.; Cheung, T.S.; von Bonin, M.; Barbieri, L.; Halai, K.; Ward, S.; et al. Apoptosis in mesenchymal stromal cells induces in vivo recipient-mediated immunomodulation. *Sci. Transl. Med.* **2017**, *9*. [CrossRef]

30. Bartosh, T.J.; Ylöstalo, J.H.; Bazhanov, N.; Kuhlman, J.; Prockop, D.J. Dynamic compaction of human mesenchymal stem/precursor cells into spheres self-activates caspase-dependent IL1 signaling to enhance secretion of modulators of inflammation and immunity (PGE2, TSG6, and STC1). *Stem Cells* **2013**, *31*, 2443–2456. [CrossRef] [PubMed]

31. De Chiara, L.; Famulari, E.S.; Fagoonee, S.; van Daalen, S.K.M.; Buttiglieri, S.; Revelli, A.; Tolosano, E.; Silengo, L.; van Pelt, A.M.M.; Altruda, F. Characterization of Human Mesenchymal Stem Cells Isolated from the Testis. *Stem Cells Int.* **2018**, *2018*, 4910304. [CrossRef] [PubMed]

32. Strioga, M.; Viswanathan, S.; Darinskas, A.; Slaby, O.; Michalek, J. Same or not the same? Comparison of adipose tissue-derived versus bone marrow-derived mesenchymal stem and stromal cells. *Stem Cells Dev.* **2012**, *21*, 2724–2752. [CrossRef]

33. Melief, S.M.; Zwaginga, J.J.; Fibbe, W.E.; Roelofs, H. Adipose tissue-derived multipotent stromal cells have a higher immunomodulatory capacity than their bone marrow-derived counterparts. *Stem Cells Transl. Med.* **2013**, *2*, 455–463. [CrossRef]

34. Lian, Q.; Zhang, Y.; Zhang, J.; Zhang, H.K.; Wu, X.; Zhang, Y.; Lam, F.F.-Y.; Kang, S.; Xia, J.C.; Lai, W.-H.; et al. Functional mesenchymal stem cells derived from human induced pluripotent stem cells attenuate limb ischemia in mice. *Circulation* **2010**, *121*, 1113–1123. [CrossRef]

35. Zhang, Y.; McNeill, E.; Tian, H.; Soker, S.; Andersson, K.-E.; Yoo, J.J.; Atala, A. Urine derived cells are a potential source for urological tissue reconstruction. *J. Urol.* **2008**, *180*, 2226–2233. [CrossRef]

36. Bharadwaj, S.; Liu, G.; Shi, Y.; Wu, R.; Yang, B.; He, T.; Fan, Y.; Lu, X.; Zhou, X.; Liu, H.; et al. Multipotential differentiation of human urine-derived stem cells: potential for therapeutic applications in urology. *Stem Cells* **2013**, *31*, 1840–1856. [CrossRef]

37. Zhang, D.; Wei, G.; Li, P.; Zhou, X.; Zhang, Y. Urine-derived stem cells: A novel and versatile progenitor source for cell-based therapy and regenerative medicine. *Genes Dis.* **2014**, *1*, 8–17. [CrossRef] [PubMed]

38. Bruno, S.; Bussolati, B.; Grange, C.; Collino, F.; di Cantogno, L.V.; Herrera, M.B.; Biancone, L.; Tetta, C.; Segoloni, G.; Camussi, G. Isolation and characterization of resident mesenchymal stem cells in human glomeruli. *Stem Cells Dev.* **2009**, *18*, 867–880. [CrossRef]

39. Ranghino, A.; Bruno, S.; Bussolati, B.; Moggio, A.; Dimuccio, V.; Tapparo, M.; Biancone, L.; Gontero, P.; Frea, B.; Camussi, G. The effects of glomerular and tubular renal progenitors and derived extracellular vesicles on recovery from acute kidney injury. *Stem Cell Res. Ther.* **2017**, *8*, 24. [CrossRef]

40. Leuning, D.G.; Reinders, M.E.J.; Li, J.; Peired, A.J.; Lievers, E.; de Boer, H.C.; Fibbe, W.E.; Romagnani, P.; van Kooten, C.; Little, M.H.; et al. Clinical-Grade Isolated Human Kidney Perivascular Stromal Cells as an Organotypic Cell Source for Kidney Regenerative Medicine. *Stem Cells Transl. Med.* **2017**, *6*, 405–418. [CrossRef] [PubMed]

41. Grobstein, C. Inductive epitheliomesenchymal interaction in cultured organ rudiments of the mouse. *Science* **1953**, *118*, 52–55. [CrossRef]

42. Barasch, J.; Yang, J.; Ware, C.B.; Taga, T.; Yoshida, K.; Erdjument-Bromage, H.; Tempst, P.; Parravicini, E.; Malach, S.; Aranoff, T.; et al. Mesenchymal to epithelial conversion in rat metanephros is induced by LIF. *Cell* **1999**, *99*, 377–386. [CrossRef]

43. Sakurai, H.; Bush, K.T.; Nigam, S.K. Identification of pleiotrophin as a mesenchymal factor involved in ureteric bud branching morphogenesis. *Development* **2001**, *128*, 3283–3293.

44. Takasato, M.; Er, P.X.; Chiu, H.S.; Little, M.H. Generation of kidney organoids from human pluripotent stem cells. *Nat. Protoc.* **2016**, *11*, 1681–1692. [CrossRef]

45. Morizane, R.; Lam, A.Q.; Freedman, B.S.; Kishi, S.; Valerius, M.T.; Bonventre, J.V. Nephron organoids derived from human pluripotent stem cells model kidney development and injury. *Nat. Biotechnol.* **2015**, *33*, 1193–1200. [CrossRef] [PubMed]

46. van den Berg, C.W.; Ritsma, L.; Avramut, M.C.; Wiersma, L.E.; van den Berg, B.M.; Leuning, D.G.; Lievers, E.; Koning, M.; Vanslambrouck, J.M.; Koster, A.J.; et al. Renal Subcapsular Transplantation of PSC-Derived Kidney Organoids Induces Neo-vasculogenesis and Significant Glomerular and Tubular Maturation In Vivo. *Stem Cell Reports* **2018**, *10*, 751–765. [CrossRef]

47. Caralt, M.; Uzarski, J.S.; Iacob, S.; Obergfell, K.P.; Berg, N.; Bijonowski, B.M.; Kiefer, K.M.; Ward, H.H.; Wandinger-Ness, A.; Miller, W.M.; et al. Optimization and critical evaluation of decellularization strategies to develop renal extracellular matrix scaffolds as biological templates for organ engineering and transplantation. *Am. J. Transplant.* **2015**, *15*, 64–75. [CrossRef]

48. Song, J.J.; Guyette, J.P.; Gilpin, S.E.; Gonzalez, G.; Vacanti, J.P.; Ott, H.C. Regeneration and experimental orthotopic transplantation of a bioengineered kidney. *Nat. Med.* **2013**, *19*, 646–651. [CrossRef] [PubMed]

49. Guan, Y.; Liu, S.; Sun, C.; Cheng, G.; Kong, F.; Luan, Y.; Xie, X.; Zhao, S.; Zhang, D.; Wang, J.; et al. The effective bioengineering method of implantation decellularized renal extracellular matrix scaffolds. *Oncotarget* **2015**, *6*, 36126–36138. [CrossRef]

50. Remuzzi, A.; Figliuzzi, M.; Bonandrini, B.; Silvani, S.; Azzollini, N.; Nossa, R.; Benigni, A.; Remuzzi, G. Experimental Evaluation of Kidney Regeneration by Organ Scaffold Recellularization. *Sci Rep.* **2017**, *7*, 43502. [CrossRef] [PubMed]

51. Makhlough, A.; Shekarchian, S.; Moghadasali, R.; Einollahi, B.; Hosseini, S.E.; Jaroughi, N.; Bolurieh, T.; Baharvand, H.; Aghdami, N. Safety and tolerability of autologous bone marrow mesenchymal stromal cells in ADPKD patients. *Stem Cell Res. Ther.* **2017**, *8*, 116. [CrossRef]

52. Sheashaa, H.; Lotfy, A.; Elhusseini, F.; Aziz, A.A.; Baiomy, A.; Awad, S.; Alsayed, A.; El-Gilany, A.-H.; Saad, M.-A.A.A.; Mahmoud, K.; et al. Protective effect of adipose-derived mesenchymal stem cells against acute kidney injury induced by ischemia-reperfusion in Sprague-Dawley rats. *Exp. Ther. Med.* **2016**, *11*, 1573–1580. [CrossRef]

53. Chen, Y.-T.; Sun, C.-K.; Lin, Y.-C.; Chang, L.-T.; Chen, Y.-L.; Tsai, T.-H.; Chung, S.-Y.; Chua, S.; Kao, Y.-H.; Yen, C.-H.; et al. Adipose-derived mesenchymal stem cell protects kidneys against ischemia-reperfusion injury through suppressing oxidative stress and inflammatory reaction. *J. Transl. Med.* **2011**, *9*, 51. [CrossRef] [PubMed]

54. Hu, J.; Zhang, L.; Wang, N.; Ding, R.; Cui, S.; Zhu, F.; Xie, Y.; Sun, X.; Wu, D.; Hong, Q.; et al. Mesenchymal stem cells attenuate ischemic acute kidney injury by inducing regulatory T cells through splenocyte interactions. *Kidney Int.* **2013**, *84*, 521–531. [CrossRef] [PubMed]

55. Cao, H.; Qian, H.; Xu, W.; Zhu, W.; Zhang, X.; Chen, Y.; Wang, M.; Yan, Y.; Xie, Y. Mesenchymal stem cells derived from human umbilical cord ameliorate ischemia/reperfusion-induced acute renal failure in rats. *Biotechnol. Lett.* **2010**, *32*, 725–732. [CrossRef]

56. Donizetti-Oliveira, C.; Semedo, P.; Burgos-Silva, M.; Cenedeze, M.A.; Malheiros, D.M.A.C.; Reis, M.A.; Pacheco-Silva, A.; Câmara, N.O.S. Adipose tissue-derived stem cell treatment prevents renal disease progression. *Cell Transplant.* **2012**, *21*, 1727–1741. [CrossRef]

57. Wu, H.J.; Yiu, W.H.; Wong, D.W.L.; Li, R.X.; Chan, L.Y.Y.; Leung, J.C.K.; Zhang, Y.; Lian, Q.; Lai, K.N.; Tse, H.F.; et al. Human induced pluripotent stem cell-derived mesenchymal stem cells prevent adriamycin nephropathy in mice. *Oncotarget* **2017**, *8*, 103640–103656. [CrossRef]

58. Tögel, F.; Hu, Z.; Weiss, K.; Isaac, J.; Lange, C.; Westenfelder, C. Administered mesenchymal stem cells protect against ischemic acute renal failure through differentiation-independent mechanisms. *Am. J. Physiol. Renal Physiol.* **2005**, *289*, F31–F42. [CrossRef] [PubMed]

59. Gatti, S.; Bruno, S.; Deregibus, M.C.; Sordi, A.; Cantaluppi, V.; Tetta, C.; Camussi, G. Microvesicles derived from human adult mesenchymal stem cells protect against ischaemia-reperfusion-induced acute and chronic kidney injury. *Nephrol. Dial. Transplant.* **2011**, *26*, 1474–1483. [CrossRef]

60. Collino, F.; Bruno, S.; Incarnato, D.; Dettori, D.; Neri, F.; Provero, P.; Pomatto, M.; Oliviero, S.; Tetta, C.; Quesenberry, P.J.; et al. AKI Recovery Induced by Mesenchymal Stromal Cell-Derived Extracellular Vesicles Carrying MicroRNAs. *J. Am. Soc. Nephrol.* **2015**, *26*, 2349–2360. [CrossRef]

61. Collino, F.; Pomatto, M.; Bruno, S.; Lindoso, R.S.; Tapparo, M.; Sicheng, W.; Quesenberry, P.; Camussi, G. Exosome and Microvesicle-Enriched Fractions Isolated from Mesenchymal Stem Cells by Gradient Separation Showed Different Molecular Signatures and Functions on Renal Tubular Epithelial Cells. *Stem Cell Rev.* **2017**, *13*, 226–243. [CrossRef]

62. Bruno, S.; Grange, C.; Deregibus, M.C.; Calogero, R.A.; Saviozzi, S.; Collino, F.; Morando, L.; Busca, A.; Falda, M.; Bussolati, B.; et al. Mesenchymal stem cell-derived microvesicles protect against acute tubular injury. *J. Am. Soc. Nephrol.* **2009**, *20*, 1053–1067. [CrossRef] [PubMed]

63. Bruno, S.; Grange, C.; Collino, F.; Deregibus, M.C.; Cantaluppi, V.; Biancone, L.; Tetta, C.; Camussi, G. Microvesicles derived from mesenchymal stem cells enhance survival in a lethal model of acute kidney injury. *PLoS ONE* **2012**, *7*, e33115. [CrossRef]

64. Overath, J.M.; Gauer, S.; Obermüller, N.; Schubert, R.; Schäfer, R.; Geiger, H.; Baer, P.C. Short-term preconditioning enhances the therapeutic potential of adipose-derived stromal/stem cell-conditioned medium in cisplatin-induced acute kidney injury. *Exp. Cell Res.* **2016**, *342*, 175–183. [CrossRef]

65. Zhang, W.; Liu, L.; Huo, Y.; Yang, Y.; Wang, Y. Hypoxia-pretreated human MSCs attenuate acute kidney injury through enhanced angiogenic and antioxidative capacities. *BioMed Res. Int.* **2014**, *2014*, 462472. [CrossRef]

66. Zou, X.; Zhang, G.; Cheng, Z.; Yin, D.; Du, T.; Ju, G.; Miao, S.; Liu, G.; Lu, M.; Zhu, Y. Microvesicles derived from human Wharton's Jelly mesenchymal stromal cells ameliorate renal ischemia-reperfusion injury in rats by suppressing CX3CL1. *Stem Cell Res. Ther.* **2014**, *5*, 40. [CrossRef] [PubMed]

67. Zou, X.; Gu, D.; Xing, X.; Cheng, Z.; Gong, D.; Zhang, G.; Zhu, Y. Human mesenchymal stromal cell-derived extracellular vesicles alleviate renal ischemic reperfusion injury and enhance angiogenesis in rats. *Am. J. Transl. Res.* **2016**, *8*, 4289–4299.

68. Zhang, G.; Zou, X.; Huang, Y.; Wang, F.; Miao, S.; Liu, G.; Chen, M.; Zhu, Y. Mesenchymal Stromal Cell-Derived Extracellular Vesicles Protect Against Acute Kidney Injury Through Anti-Oxidation by Enhancing Nrf2/ARE Activation in Rats. *Kidney Blood Press. Res.* **2016**, *41*, 119–128. [CrossRef] [PubMed]

69. Zhu, F.; Chong Lee Shin, O.L.S.; Pei, G.; Hu, Z.; Yang, J.; Zhu, H.; Wang, M.; Mou, J.; Sun, J.; Wang, Y.; et al. Adipose-derived mesenchymal stem cells employed exosomes to attenuate AKI-CKD transition through tubular epithelial cell dependent Sox9 activation. *Oncotarget* **2017**, *8*, 70707–70726. [CrossRef]

70. Yuan, X.; Li, D.; Chen, X.; Han, C.; Xu, L.; Huang, T.; Dong, Z.; Zhang, M. Extracellular vesicles from human-induced pluripotent stem cell-derived mesenchymal stromal cells (hiPSC-MSCs) protect against renal ischemia/reperfusion injury via delivering specificity protein (SP1) and transcriptional activating of sphingosine kinase 1 and inhibiting necroptosis. *Cell Death Dis.* **2017**, *8*, 3200.

71. Awad, A.S.; Ye, H.; Huang, L.; Li, L.; Foss, F.W.; Macdonald, T.L.; Lynch, K.R.; Okusa, M.D. Selective sphingosine 1-phosphate 1 receptor activation reduces ischemia-reperfusion injury in mouse kidney. *Am. J. Physiol. Renal Physiol.* **2006**, *290*, F1516–F1524. [CrossRef]

72. Saad, A.; Dietz, A.B.; Herrmann, S.M.S.; Hickson, L.J.; Glockner, J.F.; McKusick, M.A.; Misra, S.; Bjarnason, H.; Armstrong, A.S.; Gastineau, D.A.; et al. Autologous Mesenchymal Stem Cells Increase Cortical Perfusion in Renovascular Disease. *J. Am. Soc. Nephrol.* **2017**, *28*, 2777–2785. [CrossRef] [PubMed]

73. Swaminathan, M.; Stafford-Smith, M.; Chertow, G.M.; Warnock, D.G.; Paragamian, V.; Brenner, R.M.; Lellouche, F.; Fox-Robichaud, A.; Atta, M.G.; Melby, S.; et al. Allogeneic Mesenchymal Stem Cells for Treatment of AKI after Cardiac Surgery. *J. Am. Soc. Nephrol.* **2018**, *29*, 260–267. [CrossRef]

74. Miller, B.L.K.; Garg, P.; Bronstein, B.; LaPointe, E.; Lin, H.; Charytan, D.M.; Tilles, A.W.; Parekkadan, B. Extracorporeal Stromal Cell Therapy for Subjects With Dialysis-Dependent Acute Kidney Injury. *Kidney Int Rep.* **2018**, *3*, 1119–1127. [CrossRef]

75. De Martino, M.; Zonta, S.; Rampino, T.; Gregorini, M.; Frassoni, F.; Piotti, G.; Bedino, G.; Cobianchi, L.; Dal Canton, A.; Dionigi, P.; et al. Mesenchymal stem cells infusion prevents acute cellular rejection in rat kidney transplantation. *Transplant. Proc.* **2010**, *42*, 1331–1335. [CrossRef]

76. Hara, Y.; Stolk, M.; Ringe, J.; Dehne, T.; Ladhoff, J.; Kotsch, K.; Reutzel-Selke, A.; Reinke, P.; Volk, H.-D.; Seifert, M. In vivo effect of bone marrow-derived mesenchymal stem cells in a rat kidney transplantation model with prolonged cold ischemia. *Transpl. Int.* **2011**, *24*, 1112–1123. [CrossRef]

77. Casiraghi, F.; Azzollini, N.; Todeschini, M.; Cavinato, R.A.; Cassis, P.; Solini, S.; Rota, C.; Morigi, M.; Introna, M.; Maranta, R.; et al. Localization of mesenchymal stromal cells dictates their immune or proinflammatory effects in kidney transplantation. *Am. J. Transplant.* **2012**, *12*, 2373–2383. [CrossRef] [PubMed]

78. Franquesa, M.; Herrero, E.; Torras, J.; Ripoll, E.; Flaquer, M.; Gomà, M.; Lloberas, N.; Anegon, I.; Cruzado, J.M.; Grinyó, J.M.; et al. Mesenchymal stem cell therapy prevents interstitial fibrosis and tubular atrophy in a rat kidney allograft model. *Stem Cells Dev.* **2012**, *21*, 3125–3135. [CrossRef] [PubMed]

79. Crop, M.J.; Baan, C.C.; Korevaar, S.S.; Ijzermans, J.N.M.; Alwayn, I.P.J.; Weimar, W.; Hoogduijn, M.J. Donor-derived mesenchymal stem cells suppress alloreactivity of kidney transplant patients. *Transplantation* **2009**, *87*, 896–906. [CrossRef]

80. Perico, N.; Casiraghi, F.; Todeschini, M.; Cortinovis, M.; Gotti, E.; Portalupi, V.; Mister, M.; Gaspari, F.; Villa, A.; Fiori, S.; et al. Long-Term Clinical and Immunological Profile of Kidney Transplant Patients Given Mesenchymal Stromal Cell Immunotherapy. *Front. Immunol.* **2018**, *9*, 1359. [CrossRef] [PubMed]

81. Peng, Y.; Ke, M.; Xu, L.; Liu, L.; Chen, X.; Xia, W.; Li, X.; Chen, Z.; Ma, J.; Liao, D.; et al. Donor-derived mesenchymal stem cells combined with low-dose tacrolimus prevent acute rejection after renal transplantation: A clinical pilot study. *Transplantation* **2013**, *95*, 161–168. [CrossRef] [PubMed]

82. Reinders, M.E.J.; de Fijter, J.W.; Roelofs, H.; Bajema, I.M.; de Vries, D.K.; Schaapherder, A.F.; Claas, F.H.J.; van Miert, P.P.M.C.; Roelen, D.L.; van Kooten, C.; et al. Autologous bone marrow-derived mesenchymal stromal cells for the treatment of allograft rejection after renal transplantation: Results of a phase I study. *Stem Cells Transl. Med.* **2013**, *2*, 107–111. [CrossRef] [PubMed]

83. Tan, J.; Wu, W.; Xu, X.; Liao, L.; Zheng, F.; Messinger, S.; Sun, X.; Chen, J.; Yang, S.; Cai, J.; et al. Induction therapy with autologous mesenchymal stem cells in living-related kidney transplants: A randomized controlled trial. *JAMA* **2012**, *307*, 1169–1177. [CrossRef] [PubMed]

84. Iwai, S.; Sakonju, I.; Okano, S.; Teratani, T.; Kasahara, N.; Yokote, S.; Yokoo, T.; Kobayash, E. Impact of ex vivo administration of mesenchymal stem cells on the function of kidney grafts from cardiac death donors in rat. *Transplant. Proc.* **2014**, *46*, 1578–1584. [CrossRef]

85. Sun, Q.; Huang, Z.; Han, F.; Zhao, M.; Cao, R.; Zhao, D.; Hong, L.; Na, N.; Li, H.; Miao, B.; et al. Allogeneic mesenchymal stem cells as induction therapy are safe and feasible in renal allografts: Pilot results of a multicenter randomized controlled trial. *J. Transl Med.* **2018**, *16*, 52. [CrossRef]

86. Seifert, M.; Stolk, M.; Polenz, D.; Volk, H.-D. Detrimental effects of rat mesenchymal stromal cell pre-treatment in a model of acute kidney rejection. *Front. Immunol* **2012**, *3*, 202. [CrossRef]

87. Tsuda, H.; Yamahara, K.; Ishikane, S.; Otani, K.; Nakamura, A.; Sawai, K.; Ichimaru, N.; Sada, M.; Taguchi, A.; Hosoda, H.; et al. Allogenic fetal membrane-derived mesenchymal stem cells contribute to renal repair in experimental glomerulonephritis. *Am. J. Physiol. Renal Physiol.* **2010**, *299*, F1004–F1013. [CrossRef]

88. Zoja, C.; Garcia, P.B.; Rota, C.; Conti, S.; Gagliardini, E.; Corna, D.; Zanchi, C.; Bigini, P.; Benigni, A.; Remuzzi, G.; et al. Mesenchymal stem cell therapy promotes renal repair by limiting glomerular podocyte and progenitor cell dysfunction in adriamycin-induced nephropathy. *Am. J. Physiol. Renal Physiol.* **2012**, *303*, F1370–F1381. [CrossRef] [PubMed]

89. Iseri, K.; Iyoda, M.; Ohtaki, H.; Matsumoto, K.; Wada, Y.; Suzuki, T.; Yamamoto, Y.; Saito, T.; Hihara, K.; Tachibana, S.; et al. Therapeutic effects and mechanism of conditioned media from human mesenchymal stem cells on anti-GBM glomerulonephritis in WKY rats. *Am. J. Physiol. Renal Physiol.* **2016**, *310*, F1182–F1191. [CrossRef] [PubMed]

90. Suzuki, T.; Iyoda, M.; Shibata, T.; Ohtaki, H.; Matsumoto, K.; Shindo-Hirai, Y.; Kuno, Y.; Wada, Y.; Yamamoto, Y.; Kawaguchi, M.; et al. Therapeutic effects of human mesenchymal stem cells in Wistar-Kyoto rats with anti-glomerular basement membrane glomerulonephritis. *PLoS ONE* **2013**, *8*, e67475. [CrossRef]

91. Belingheri, M.; Lazzari, L.; Parazzi, V.; Groppali, E.; Biagi, E.; Gaipa, G.; Giordano, R.; Rastaldi, M.P.; Croci, D.; Biondi, A.; et al. Allogeneic mesenchymal stem cell infusion for the stabilization of focal segmental glomerulosclerosis. *Biologicals* **2013**, *41*, 439–445. [CrossRef]

92. Gregorini, M.; Maccario, R.; Avanzini, M.A.; Corradetti, V.; Moretta, A.; Libetta, C.; Esposito, P.; Bosio, F.; Dal Canton, A.; Rampino, T. Antineutrophil cytoplasmic antibody-associated renal vasculitis treated with autologous mesenchymal stromal cells: Evaluation of the contribution of immune-mediated mechanisms. *Mayo Clin. Proc.* **2013**, *88*, 1174–1179. [CrossRef]

93. Jiménez, S.; Cervera, R.; Font, J.; Ingelmo, M. The epidemiology of systemic lupus erythematosus. *Clin. Rev. Allergy Immunol.* **2003**, *25*, 3–12. [CrossRef]

94. Sattwika, P.D.; Mustafa, R.; Paramaiswari, A.; Herningtyas, E.H. Stem cells for lupus nephritis: A concise review of current knowledge. *Lupus* **2018**, *27*, 1881–1897. [CrossRef]

95. Tani, C.; Vagnani, S.; Carli, L.; Querci, F.; Kühl, A.A.; Spieckermann, S.; Cieluch, C.P.; Pacini, S.; Fazzi, R.; Mosca, M. Treatment with Allogenic Mesenchymal Stromal Cells in a Murine Model of Systemic Lupus Erythematosus. *Int J. Stem Cells* **2017**, *10*, 160–168. [CrossRef] [PubMed]

96. Gu, F.; Wang, D.; Zhang, H.; Feng, X.; Gilkeson, G.S.; Shi, S.; Sun, L. Allogeneic mesenchymal stem cell transplantation for lupus nephritis patients refractory to conventional therapy. *Clin. Rheumatol.* **2014**, *33*, 1611–1619. [CrossRef] [PubMed]

97. Wang, D.; Huang, S.; Yuan, X.; Liang, J.; Xu, R.; Yao, G.; Feng, X.; Sun, L. The regulation of the Treg/Th17 balance by mesenchymal stem cells in human systemic lupus erythematosus. *Cell. Mol. Immunol.* **2017**, *14*, 423–431. [CrossRef]

98. Deng, D.; Zhang, P.; Guo, Y.; Lim, T.O. A randomised double-blind, placebo-controlled trial of allogeneic umbilical cord-derived mesenchymal stem cell for lupus nephritis. *Ann. Rheum. Dis.* **2017**, *76*, 1436–1439. [CrossRef]

99. Barbado, J.; Tabera, S.; Sánchez, A.; García-Sancho, J. Therapeutic potential of allogeneic mesenchymal stromal cells transplantation for lupus nephritis. *Lupus* **2018**, *27*, 2161–2165. [CrossRef]

100. Sharma, J.; Hampton, J.M.; Valiente, G.R.; Wada, T.; Steigelman, H.; Young, M.C.; Spurbeck, R.R.; Blazek, A.D.; Bösh, S.; Jarjour, W.N.; et al. Therapeutic Development of Mesenchymal Stem Cells or Their Extracellular Vesicles to Inhibit Autoimmune-Mediated Inflammatory Processes in Systemic Lupus Erythematosus. *Front. Immunol.* **2017**, *8*, 526. [CrossRef]

101. Perez-Hernandez, J.; Redon, J.; Cortes, R. Extracellular Vesicles as Therapeutic Agents in Systemic Lupus Erythematosus. *Int. J. Mol. Sci* **2017**, *18*, 717. [CrossRef]

102. Gao, X.; Song, L.; Shen, K.; Wang, H.; Qian, M.; Niu, W.; Qin, X. Bone marrow mesenchymal stem cells promote the repair of islets from diabetic mice through paracrine actions. *Mol. Cell. Endocrinol.* **2014**, *388*, 41–50. [CrossRef]

103. Lee, R.H.; Seo, M.J.; Reger, R.L.; Spees, J.L.; Pulin, A.A.; Olson, S.D.; Prockop, D.J. Multipotent stromal cells from human marrow home to and promote repair of pancreatic islets and renal glomeruli in diabetic NOD/scid mice. *Proc. Natl. Acad. Sci. USA* **2006**, *103*, 17438–17443. [CrossRef]

104. Shree, N.; Bhonde, R.R. Conditioned Media From Adipose Tissue Derived Mesenchymal Stem Cells Reverse Insulin Resistance in Cellular Models. *J. Cell. Biochem.* **2017**, *118*, 2037–2043. [CrossRef]

105. Liu, X.; Zheng, P.; Wang, X.; Dai, G.; Cheng, H.; Zhang, Z.; Hua, R.; Niu, X.; Shi, J.; An, Y. A preliminary evaluation of efficacy and safety of Wharton's jelly mesenchymal stem cell transplantation in patients with type 2 diabetes mellitus. *Stem Cell Res. Ther.* **2014**, *5*, 57. [CrossRef]

106. Hu, J.; Li, C.; Wang, L.; Zhang, X.; Zhang, M.; Gao, H.; Yu, X.; Wang, F.; Zhao, W.; Yan, S.; et al. Long term effects of the implantation of autologous bone marrow mononuclear cells for type 2 diabetes mellitus. *Endocr. J.* **2012**, *59*, 1031–1039. [CrossRef]

107. Ezquer, F.; Giraud-Billoud, M.; Carpio, D.; Cabezas, F.; Conget, P.; Ezquer, M. Proregenerative Microenvironment Triggered by Donor Mesenchymal Stem Cells Preserves Renal Function and Structure in Mice with Severe Diabetes Mellitus. *BioMed Res. Int.* **2015**, *2015*, 164703. [CrossRef]

108. Abdel Aziz, M.T.; Wassef, M.A.A.; Ahmed, H.H.; Rashed, L.; Mahfouz, S.; Aly, M.I.; Hussein, R.E.; Abdelaziz, M. The role of bone marrow derived-mesenchymal stem cells in attenuation of kidney function in rats with diabetic nephropathy. *Diabetol. Metab. Syndr.* **2014**, *6*, 34. [CrossRef] [PubMed]

109. Nagaishi, K.; Mizue, Y.; Chikenji, T.; Otani, M.; Nakano, M.; Konari, N.; Fujimiya, M. Mesenchymal stem cell therapy ameliorates diabetic nephropathy via the paracrine effect of renal trophic factors including exosomes. *Sci. Rep.* **2016**, *6*, 34842. [CrossRef]

110. Jiang, Z.; Liu, Y.; Niu, X.; Yin, J.; Hu, B.; Guo, S.; Fan, Y.; Wang, Y.; Wang, N. Exosomes secreted by human urine-derived stem cells could prevent kidney complications from type I diabetes in rats. *Stem Cell Res. Ther.* **2016**, *7*, 24. [CrossRef] [PubMed]

111. Ebrahim, N.; Ahmed, I.A.; Hussien, N.I.; Dessouky, A.A.; Farid, A.S.; Elshazly, A.M.; Mostafa, O.; Gazzar, W.B.E.; Sorour, S.M.; Seleem, Y.; et al. Mesenchymal Stem Cell-Derived Exosomes Ameliorated Diabetic Nephropathy by Autophagy Induction through the mTOR Signaling Pathway. *Cells* **2018**, *7*, 226. [CrossRef]

112. Packham, D.K.; Fraser, I.R.; Kerr, P.G.; Segal, K.R. Allogeneic Mesenchymal Precursor Cells (MPC) in Diabetic Nephropathy: A Randomized, Placebo-controlled, Dose Escalation Study. *EBioMedicine* **2016**, *12*, 263–269. [CrossRef]

113. Skyler, J.S.; Fonseca, V.A.; Segal, K.R.; Rosenstock, J. MSB-DM003 Investigators Allogeneic Mesenchymal Precursor Cells in Type 2 Diabetes: A Randomized, Placebo-Controlled, Dose-Escalation Safety and Tolerability Pilot Study. *Diabetes Care* **2015**, *38*, 1742–1749. [CrossRef]

114. Sasser, A.K.; Mundy, B.L.; Smith, K.M.; Studebaker, A.W.; Axel, A.E.; Haidet, A.M.; Fernandez, S.A.; Hall, B.M. Human bone marrow stromal cells enhance breast cancer cell growth rates in a cell line-dependent manner when evaluated in 3D tumor environments. *Cancer Lett.* **2007**, *254*, 255–264. [CrossRef]

115. Zhu, W.; Xu, W.; Jiang, R.; Qian, H.; Chen, M.; Hu, J.; Cao, W.; Han, C.; Chen, Y. Mesenchymal stem cells derived from bone marrow favor tumor cell growth in vivo. *Exp. Mol. Pathol.* **2006**, *80*, 267–274. [CrossRef]

116. Thirabanjasak, D.; Tantiwongse, K.; Thorner, P.S. Angiomyeloproliferative lesions following autologous stem cell therapy. *J. Am. Soc. Nephrol.* **2010**, *21*, 1218–1222. [CrossRef]

117. Bruna, F.; Plaza, A.; Arango, M.; Espinoza, I.; Conget, P. Systemically administered allogeneic mesenchymal stem cells do not aggravate the progression of precancerous lesions: A new biosafety insight. *Stem Cell Res. Ther.* **2018**, *9*, 137. [CrossRef]
118. Schnabel, L.V.; Pezzanite, L.M.; Antczak, D.F.; Felippe, M.J.B.; Fortier, L.A. Equine bone marrow-derived mesenchymal stromal cells are heterogeneous in MHC class II expression and capable of inciting an immune response in vitro. *Stem Cell Res. Ther.* **2014**, *5*, 13. [CrossRef]
119. Lohan, P.; Treacy, O.; Griffin, M.D.; Ritter, T.; Ryan, A.E. Anti-Donor Immune Responses Elicited by Allogeneic Mesenchymal Stem Cells and Their Extracellular Vesicles: Are We Still Learning? *Front. Immunol.* **2017**, *8*, 1626. [CrossRef]
120. Sohel, M.H. Extracellular/Circulating MicroRNAs: Release Mechanisms, Functions and Challenges. *Achiev. Life Sci.* **2016**, *10*, 175–186. [CrossRef]

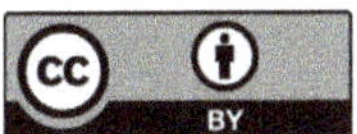

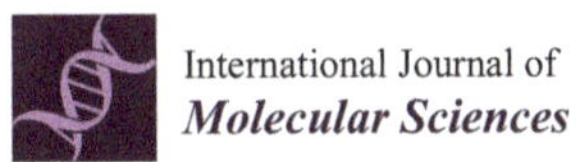
International Journal of
Molecular Sciences

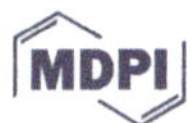

Review

Potential and Therapeutic Efficacy of Cell-based Therapy Using Mesenchymal Stem Cells for Acute/chronic Kidney Disease

Chul Won Yun [1] and Sang Hun Lee [1,2,*]

[1] Medical Science Research Institute, Soonchunhyang University Seoul Hospital, Seoul 04401, Korea; skydbs113@naver.com

[2] Department of Biochemistry, Soonchunhyang University College of Medicine, Cheonan 34538, Korea

* Correspondence: ykckss1114@nate.com; Tel.: +82-02-709-2029

Received: 2 March 2019; Accepted: 28 March 2019; Published: 1 April 2019

Abstract: Kidney disease can be either acute kidney injury (AKI) or chronic kidney disease (CKD) and it can lead to the development of functional organ failure. Mesenchymal stem cells (MSCs) are derived from a diverse range of human tissues. They are multipotent and have immunomodulatory effects to assist in the recovery from tissue injury and the inhibition of inflammation. Numerous studies have investigated the feasibility, safety, and efficacy of MSC-based therapies for kidney disease. Although the exact mechanism of MSC-based therapy remains uncertain, their therapeutic value in the treatment of a diverse range of kidney diseases has been studied in clinical trials. The use of MSCs is a promising therapeutic strategy for both acute and chronic kidney disease. The mechanism underlying the effects of MSCs on survival rate after transplantation and functional repair of damaged tissue is still ambiguous. The paracrine effects of MSCs on renal recovery, optimization of the microenvironment for cell survival, and control of inflammatory responses are thought to be related to their interaction with the damaged kidney environment. This review discusses recent experimental and clinical findings related to kidney disease, with a focus on the role of MSCs in kidney disease recovery, differentiation, and microenvironment. The therapeutic efficacy and current applications of MSC-based kidney disease therapies are also discussed.

Keywords: mesenchymal stem cells; acute and chronic kidney disease; exosome; natural products

---

1. Introduction

Kidney disease, including acute kidney injury (AKI) and chronic kidney disease (CKD), is a significant global public health problem, with incidence and mortality rates increasing in recent decades [1,2]. AKI is experienced by one fifth of all adults and one third of all children worldwide. It is characterized by sudden kidney failure or a rapid loss of kidney function [3]. AKI has many potential causes, including renal ischemia from low blood pressure, crush injury, inflammation, and urinary tract obstruction or infection [4,5]. It is diagnosed based on elevated blood urea nitrogen (BUN) and creatinine concentrations, or decreased urine output [5]. Chronic kidney disease (CKD) is characterized by a progressive loss of kidney function, leading to end-stage renal disease (ESRD) and the accumulation of collagen, caused by inflammation, resulting in fibrosis [6,7]. At the end stage of CKD, an irreversible loss of renal function is treated with dialysis or kidney transplantation. AKI can also result in ESRD, leading to an increased risk of CKD or worsening of CKD symptoms [8]. Additionally, CKD is a progressive disease, causing significant morbidity and mortality. Although pharmaceutical or surgical therapies may improve overall kidney function, they cannot enhance the regeneration and functional recovery of the surrounding tissues affected by kidney damage. Therefore, there is a need to develop more effective strategies for treating kidney injury.

Human mesenchymal stem cells (MSCs) are isolated from diverse tissues, including bone marrow and adipose tissue. They have the characteristics of multipotent cells, with multi-lineage differentiation, self-renewal, and proliferative potential [9–11]. There is some evidence indicating that MSCs originate from renal pericytes, which form a network around the microvasculature [12]. In addition, MSCs can secrete many different cytokines and growth factors, which regulate immune activity and enhance the potential of expansion and differentiation of host cells, thus promoting the recovery of damaged tissues [13]. They also play critical roles in the modulation of renal blood flow, capillary permeability, endothelial cell survival, and immunological responses [14]. Therefore, MSCs with potential angiogenic and immunomodulatory properties, are also a promising source of cells for the recovery of damaged sites and the treatment of various pathological conditions, such as renal injury and renal failure, making them an ideal therapeutic strategy for regenerative kidney therapy [15,16]. For effective MSC-based treatment of kidney disease, it is important to study the therapeutic mechanisms of MSCs and explore ways of enhancing the efficiency of MSC-based therapy.

In this review, we first summarize the various types of kidney disease and then explore the application of MSC-based therapies. The potential therapeutic effects of MSCs, their mechanisms of action, and techniques for enhancing MSC functionality are then discussed.

2. The Mechanisms of MSC-based Therapy for Kidney Disease

MSCs may have several origins, such as bone-morrow [17], adipose [18], and umbilical cord [19], and can be used to treat various renal diseases. The therapeutic effects of MSC-based therapy are associated with characteristics including multipotency, self-renewal, secretion of factors related to proliferation and survival, immunomodulation, and homing [20–22]. MSCs differentiate into various organ lineages, such as bone, cartilage, and adipose [23]. The differentiation potential of MSCs has increasing interest due to the potential to treat diverse diseases and improve novel clinical perspectives on MSC function. Recent evidence indicates that MSCs differentiate into epithelial-like cells. One study has demonstrated that MSCs generate keratinocytes and multiple skin cell types, which can then be processed for use in wound repair procedures [24]. In a mouse model of ischemia/kidney reperfusion injury, administered MSCs differentiated into renal tubular epithelium, which induced tissue structural integrity and tissue recovery [25]. In addition, recent studies have indicated that the benefits of MSC injection are related to the ability of MSCs to secrete several cytokines, chemokines, and growth factors. Several observations have revealed that the major role of MSCs include secretion of multiple biologically active factors that exert effects on local cellular environments. Other studies have demonstrated that these factors protected against apoptosis of adjacent cells and induced cell proliferation, as well as promoting the regeneration of damaged renal tissue [26]. There is also much evidence that has demonstrated that MSCs injected into damaged tissue sites for repair interacted closely with local microenvironments, including inflammatory responses and hypoxic tissues, and stimulated cells to secrete several growth factors related to tissue regeneration factors [5,27].

In addition, modulation of the immune system is another characteristic of MSCs and these cells were effective in treating several immune disorders in humans and animal models [28,29]. Although the mechanism of immunomodulatory function is not fully clear, cell-to-cell contact, and/or the secretion of soluble immunosuppressive factors is thought to contribute. Several studies have revealed that MSCs interact with multiple immune cells and display an ability to suppress excessive inflammatory responses [30,31]. Furthermore, inflammation induced tissue damage is a critical process triggered in response to injury and disease, MSCs could be used for the treatment of tissue or organ injury associated with intense inflammatory activity, such as kidney failure, heart injury. Finally, the homing mechanism of MSCs is related to their ability to reach damaged sites via interaction with signal molecules secreted by injured tissue and MSC receptors [32]. Some studies have revealed that MSCs migrate to areas of inflammation [33,34], and then further promote homing into damaged tissues by enhancing paracrine effects. Furthermore some studies have suggested that overexpression by MSCs of CXCR4, or serine protease kallikrein, which are homing receptors, improved renal function and enhanced anti-inflammatory effects in renal injury [35,36]. Another study confirmed that IGF1-pretreated MSCs displayed increased expression of IGF1 and CXCR4 in bmMSCs, and enhanced cell migration and renal protective effects [37]. Therefore, several mechanisms and complex signaling contribute to the therapeutic effects of MSC-based therapy, and further studies are necessary to enhance the efficacy of MSC-based therapy to treat kidney disease.

3. MSC-based Therapy for Kidney Disease

The promising properties of MSCs, such as regeneration and differentiation, has generated considerable interest and spurred numerous studies in various diseases. Preclinical results have demonstrated the therapeutic efficacy of MSCs in reducing acute and chronic kidney injuries in animal models. Therefore, early-phase clinical trials have been performed to investigate the safety and efficacy of allogenic MSC infusion [38] (Figure 1).

A symptom of AKI is acute renal failure, which is the sudden loss of kidney function. Mesenchymal stem cells (MSCs) are one option for the treatment of AKI [39], due to their physiological activities related to inflammation, apoptosis, angiogenesis, and immunomodulation [40]. The administration of MSCs has been shown to improve renal function and protect against tubular injury in a mouse model of AKI [41]. This was accompanied by an increase in M2 macrophage infiltration and the conversion of activated macrophages to an anti-inflammatory phenotype. These findings suggest that MSCs can protect against AKI through the anti-inflammatory activation of macrophages, which assists in the recovery from tubular injury. MSCs have also been shown to contribute to improved renal function in an in vivo canine acute kidney injury model, by decreasing BUN and creatinine levels and recovering renal lesions [42]. Another study has suggested that MSCs treatment improves glomerular filtration, renal function, and alleviates oxidative stress-induced cell senescence and inflammation and increases the proliferation of kidney cells in an ischemia/reperfusion injury (IRI)-induced acute kidney injury model [43].

In addition, numerous studies in a range of different mouse models have suggested that novel therapeutic strategies using MSCs can be developed to treat AKI. One such study showed AKI-protective effects when using MSC-based therapy, but failed to confirm that the injected MSCs were incorporated into tubules, vessels, or other specific compartments of the kidney [44]. Further studies demonstrated that the subcellular mechanisms of MSC-mediated protection did not act directly at the sites of damage. One study indicated that the protective effects of MSCs are due to the secretion of factors that have paracrine effects [22]. Another study suggested that MSCs produce and secrete extracellular vesicles, which then lead to renal-protective effects [45]. The mortality rate in AKI patients is approximately 50%. Most surviving patients recover full renal function, but some develop CKD, requiring further treatment, such as dialysis and renal transplantation [46]. Clinical trials using MSC-based therapies are currently underway to investigate the safety and efficacy of allogenic MSC administration. One such trial (NCT00733876), performed in 2013, was a phase I exploratory study of 16 patients [5,26] aimed at estimating the safety and efficacy of bone marrow-derived MSC injection in patients at high risk of developing AKI after on-pump cardiac surgery [47]. No specific or serious adverse effects were observed during a six-month follow-up period during this trial. These observations indicate that the administration of MSCs is safe at the doses used and has protective effects on renal function. Another clinical trial (NCT01275612) performed in oncology patients with cisplatin-mediated AKI, has completed phase II. This study aims to test the feasibility and safety of ex vivo proliferative MSCs as a treatment to recover kidney function.

CKD is diagnosed based on increased serum creatinine levels, low estimated glomerular filtration rate (eGFR), or urinary abnormalities for at least three months [48]. CKD is associated with a significant increase in the risk of atherosclerosis and type 2 diabetes [49]. Moreover, CKD is closely related to cardiovascular disease, which is the cause of mortality in almost 50% of CKD patients [50]. Some patients with CKD develop ESRD and show increased risk factors for cardiovascular disease.

Considering the high cost of renal replacement therapy, effective treatment of progressive CKD is required, [49]. Therefore, there is a need to develop novel therapeutic strategies to treat CKD.

CKD is a global public health problem, due to the high cost of treatment and its major impact on the health of affected patients [51]. CKD is associated with a high risk of diabetics, hypertension, and cardiovascular disease and results in the loss of kidney function [52]. The kidneys play an important role in eliminating toxic metabolites, such as uremic toxins. When the function of kidney is weakened, these toxic substances accumulate in the blood and result in biochemically toxic effects in numerous tissues and organs, which results in additional complications, including cardiovascular disease, anemia, and neurological disorders [53,54]. The administration of MSCs induces anti-inflammatory and anti-fibrotic effects in CKD models [17,55] and is a promising cell-based therapy for chronic kidney disease. Uremic toxins, such as p-cresol (PC) and indoxyl sulfate (IS), reduce the functionality of MSCs in CKD patients [18]. A recent study has suggested that the toxic product, p-cresol, leads to mitochondrial dysfunction in adipose-derived (ad) MSCs from CKD patients and inhibits the therapeutic effects of cell-based therapy. Pioglitazone, which is used to treat CKD, protects against PC-induced apoptosis and improves mitochondrial function via upregulation of PINK1 [19]. In addition, the transplantation of MSCs enhances renal function and increases the expression and activity of ATPase in a rat model of CKD with renovascular hypertension. Moreover, MSCs improve renal morphology and reduce fibrosis in the kidney [20]. MSC treatment alleviates renal fibrosis and chronic inflammation by reducing collagen deposition and modulating chemokine and cytokine expression in a CKD model [56]. These results demonstrate that MSC treatment has protective effects by regulating inflammation and proliferation and, thus, reducing renal damage and improving kidney function.

A major symptom of CKD is the reduced regenerative capacity of the kidney. Several studies have indicated that MSCs induce regenerative effects in animal CKD models [21]. Some studies have suggested that the administration of MSCs provides significant renal protection by decreasing inflammatory infiltrates, fibrosis, and glomerulosclerosis [22]. In addition, four clinical trials are currently assessing the safety and efficacy of MSC-based therapies to treat CKD. One clinical trial using autologous bone-marrow (bm) was performed in 2014 and phase I exploratory study of six patients (NCT02166489). This study is aimed to evaluate the safety and tolerability of bmMSC administration in CKD patients. No cell-related adverse effects was observed during 12 months after bmMSC administration. This study is limited the therapeutic effects of MSCs due to small sample size, the lack of a control group, and a short follow-up; further study is necessary to confirm the efficacy of bmMSC to treat CKD [57]. Another clinical trial using adMSC was performed in 2013 and phase I exploratory study of six patients (NCT01840540). This study is aimed to test the safety and toxicity of adMSC administration in CKD paitents. adMSC is confirmed the potential of clinical usage and characteristics of MSC marker [58]. Other clinical trials are using autologous bmMSCs (NCT02195323) and using AD-MSCs (NCT02266394 and NCT01840540). These clinical studies are either ongoing or are completed, but the results are not yet published.

Diabetes mellitus usually progresses to CKD, despite recent developments in its clinical management [59]. In addition, diabetic kidney disease (DKD), also known as diabetic nephropathy (DN), can cause kidney damage [60]. DKD is caused by a complex mechanism involving the kidney and other organs and tissues. The five-year mortality rate for DKD patients is approximately 39%, which is similar to the mortality rates of many cancers. However, there have been no successful, specific therapies developed to treat DKD. The current treatment involves early detection, glycemic control, and regulation of blood pressure. Several studies have indicated that MSC administration improves DKD symptoms, including elevated serum creatinine and BUN levels and glomerular hypertrophy [24,25,61]. These results indicate that the systemic administration of MSCs induces beneficial effects via their anti-inflammatory properties in animal models of DKD. MSCs have been shown to reduce the levels of inflammatory factors, such as TNFa, IL-6, and IL-1b and the infiltration of macrophages [25,61]. A clinical trial, aimed at developing novel treatments for DKD using MSC-based therapies, is ongoing

(NCT02585622). This clinical study is investigating the safety, feasibility, tolerability, and efficacy of bmMSC therapy in a diabetic mouse model [62] (Table 1).

Table 1. The effects of mesenchymal stem cells (MSCs) in the treatment of kidney disease.

Pathological Condition	Type of Source	Findings	Reference
Acute Kidney Injury (AKI)	BM-derived MSC	Protection against kidney tubular injury, M2 macrophage infiltration and reduction of inflammatory responses, improvement of renal function	[41]
AKI	UC-derived MSC	Decrease in BUN and creatinine levels, recovery of renal lesions and cell senescence, improvement of glomerular filtration, induction of proliferation	[42,43]
Clinical trial (AKI)	BM-derived MSC	Phase I, exploratory study of 16 patients, estimating safety and efficacy of MSC administration	NCT00733876 [5,26,47]
Clinical trial (AKI)	BM-derived MSC	Phase II, oncology patients with cisplatin-mediated AKI, testing of the feasibility and safety of MSC therapy, treatment to recover kidney function	NCT01275612
Chronic kidney disease (CKD)	AD-derived MSC	Recovery of MSC functionality, such as mitochondrial dysfunction via treatment of pioglitazone, reduction of p-cresol mediated apoptosis	[19]
CKD with renovascular hypertension	BM-derived MSC	Enhancement of renal function, increase of ATPase activity, improvement of renal morphology, decrease of renal fibrosis	[20]
CKD	BM-derived MSC	Alleviation of renal fibrosis and chronic inflammation, reduction of collagen deposition, modulation of chemokine and cytokine expression	[56]
Clinical trial (CKD)	BM-derived MSC	Phase I, evaluation of safety and tolerability of MSC administration, improvement of renal function	NCT02166489 [57]
Clinical trial (CKD)	BM-derived MSC	Phase I, test of safety of MSC administration	NCT02195323
Clinical trial (CKD)	AD-derived MSC	Phase I, investigation of safety and toxicity of MSC administration, confirmation of the characteristics of MSC markers, classical and non-classical markers.	NCT01840540 [58]
Clinical trial (CKD)	AD-derived MSC	Phase I, ongoing clinical trial, measurement of blood and urinary markers for kidney function	NCT02266394
Diabetic kidney disease (DKD)	BM-derived MSC	Reduction of creatinine and BUN levels, improvement of glomerular hypertrophy, anti-inflammatory effects	[61]
Clinical trial (DKD)	BM-derived MSC	Phase I, Phase II, ongoing clinical trial, investigation of the safety, feasibility, tolerability, and efficacy of MSC therapy	NCT02585622 [62]

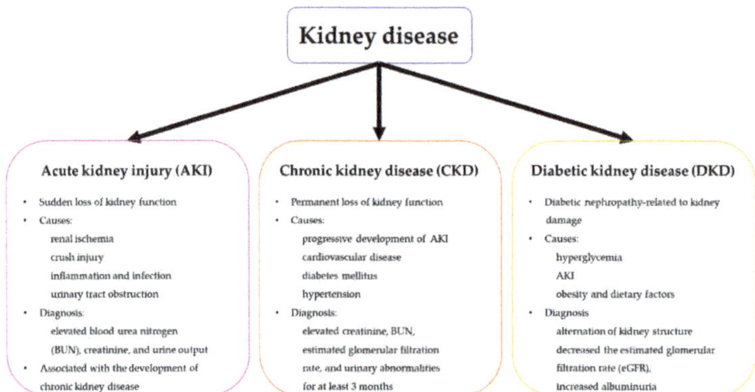

Figure 1. A schema illustrating an overview of kidney disease, with its diverse symptoms.

4. The Therapeutic Strategy of Exosomes Derived MSCs in the Treatment of Kidney Disease

Extracellular vesicles (EVs) are small vesicles secreted by MSCs and endocytic compartments. Exosomes are a type of EV, 30–100 nm in diameter, that are derived from the plasma membrane and micro-vesicles (100–1000 nm), and are released into the extracellular environment. Some studies have suggested that exosomes contain cytokines, proteins, mRNAs, miRNAs, and rRNAs [27–30]. In addition, a recent study demonstrated that miRNAs, mRNAs, and proteins from EVs are able to regulate cellular signaling pathways in recipient cells [31]. Indeed, there is a considerable amount of data indicating that the administration of MSC-derived EVs is safe and can enhance kidney function in numerous animal models of AKI and CKD. Therefore, MSC-derived EVs may be a potential therapeutic agent for renal disease (Figure 2).

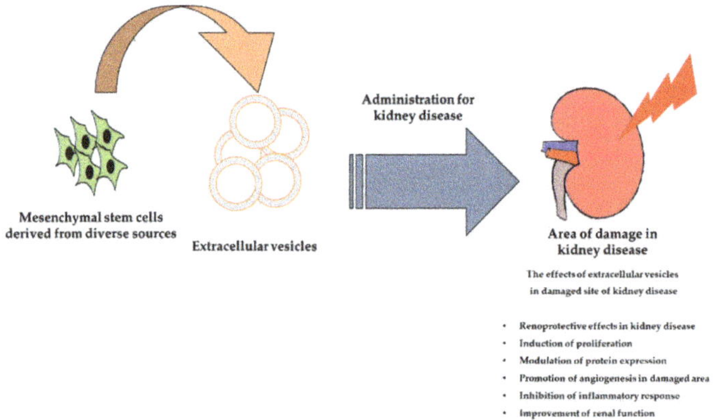

Figure 2. Schematic representation of the therapeutic efficacy of mesenchymal stem cell-derived extracellular vesicles for the treatment of kidney disease.

Renal ischemia/reperfusion injury (IRI) is one of the causes of acute kidney injury. It occurs as a result of a sudden blockage of blood flow to the kidney, with a subsequent restoration of flow and re-oxygenation. It is significantly associated with morbidity and mortality in AKI patients [63]. In addition, AKI is a potential risk factor for progressive CKD [32], but there is currently no effective therapy for AKI. One study has suggested that human adMSC-derived exosomes inhibit the AKI-CKD transition via modulation of SOX9, which is a transcription factor related to the development of kidney disease in mouse model of AKI [33]. The pathogenesis of renal IRI is unclear, but ischemic conditions and the generation of reactive oxygen species can induce inflammation and cell death, which lead to AKI [34]. In an animal model renal IRI, EVs have been shown to incorporate into damaged tubular cells, where they decrease cell death and increase cell proliferation. These results suggest that MSC-derived EVs may protect tubular cells against metabolic stress [36]. In another study, the renal-protective effects of MSC-derived EVs were assessed in an animal model of renal IRI. Treatment with MSC-derived EVs significantly decreased epithelial tubular cell damage and apoptosis and increased cell proliferation and kidney function [35]. The administration of EVs attenuates renal oxidative stress by modulating the expression of the pro-oxidant, NADPH oxidase 2, enhancing renal cell proliferation, and decreasing apoptosis and serum creatinine levels [37]. In addition, some studies have shown that the renoprotective effects of EVs are caused by regulating kidney neovascularization. Treatment with MSC-derived EVs improves renal capillary density and reduces kidney fibrosis via the expression of vascular endothelial growth factor and other angiogenesis-related mRNAs in a rat AKI model [23]. Furthermore, treatment with EVs is reported to reduce inflammation after AKI by reducing macrophage infiltration in the kidney and regulating the levels of chemokines and related immune responses via the actions of miRNAs carried by the EVs [64].

Drug-induced nephrotoxicity is a one of the common causes of AKI, with an incidence as high as 60% [65,66]. Several clinical treatments, such as anti-inflammatory drugs, antibiotics, and contrast agents, are toxic to renal cells and compromise renal function by changing intraglomerular hemodynamics, inducing inflammation, and increasing uric acid deposition [67]. Recent studies have shown that MSC-derived EVs have beneficial effects in the treatment of drug-induced nephropathy. The anticancer drug, cisplatin, can induce nephropathy and lead to an increase in BUN and creatinine levels, oxidative stress, and apoptosis [68,69]. The administration of human umbilical cord (huc) MSC-derived exosomes improves cisplatin-mediated renal damage in AKI rat models and NRK-52E cells [70]. The therapeutic effects of exosomes on cisplatin-induced kidney damage occur via a decrease in oxidative stress and apoptosis and enhanced cell proliferation. In addition, cisplatin-induced nephrotoxicity results in mitochondrial apoptosis and the induction of an inflammatory response in the kidney [71]. The administration of hucMSC-derived exosomes inhibits mitochondrial apoptosis and the release of inflammatory cytokines by inducing autophagy in a cisplatin-induced nephrotoxicity model. In a glycerol-induced AKI model, EVs isolated from MSCs reduce kidney damage [72]. The administration of EVs induces tubular cell proliferation and EVs containing mRNAs, miRNAs, and growth factors, increase cell proliferation, improve kidney function, and promote AKI recovery. Moreover, MSC-derived EVs transfer miRNA to recipient cells and, thereby, affect the expression of pro-inflammatory genes and promote regeneration in AKI models [73].

CKD is a progressive disorder, with complex symptoms and diverse causes. Several factors influence the degree of severity and rate of progression of CKD [74]. Numerous studies have confirmed the efficacy of EVs to treat CKD. Renovascular disease (RVD) is one of the causes of CKD [75]. It is associated with renal injury, poor renal function, and metabolic syndrome [76]. A recent study has demonstrated that MSC-derived EVs improve renal function and structural recovery [77]. In a renal disease model, the administration of MSC-derived EVs improves renal inflammation by decreasing the levels of inflammatory cytokines, such as TNF-α, IL-6, and IL-1-β. Moreover, in this model, EVs ameliorate renal fibrosis and enhance renal function, thus demonstrating renoprotective effects of MSC-derived EVs. Another study has shown that MSC-derived EVs contain a diverse array of pro-angiogenic genes and proteins, which promote angiogenesis and vascular recovery [78]. Moreover, the administration of EVs increases microcirculation and decreases tissue damage in the kidney and improves renal function. The unilateral ureteral obstruction (UUO) model, which induces renal inflammation, apoptosis, and fibrosis, is a popular experimental model to study mechanisms associated with kidney diseases, such as AKI and CKD [79]. Recent studies have tested the efficacy of MSC-derived EVs in the treatment of kidney disease in UUO animal models. EV administration restores epithelial-mesenchymal transition (EMT) morphological changes induced by renal fibrosis, by modulating TGF-β, E-cadherin, and αSMA expression in HK2 cells and improves renal function in animal models [80]. In addition, EVs isolated from kidney-derived MSCs have been shown to ameliorate EMT morphological changes and enhance the proliferation of TGF-β1-treated human umbilical vein epithelial cells and suppress inflammatory cell infiltration and renal fibrosis in UUO mouse models [81]. One clinical trial has investigated the renoprotective efficacy of MSC-derived EVs in patients with CKD. Treatment with MSC-derived EVs resulted in significant recovery of eGFR, creatinine, and BUN levels. EV treatment not only decreased TNF-α levels, but also increased IL-10 levels in CKD patients and this ameliorated the inflammatory immune reaction. Moreover, kidney biopsies revealed that EV administration increased the levels of renal regeneration and differentiation markers [82]. These results suggest that MSC-derived EV therapy decreases inflammation and improves renal function in patients with CKD.

DN is a severe complication of diabetes mellitus and is a major cause of CKD [83]. Treatment with MSC-derived exosomes results in improved renal function and repair of damaged renal tissues by modulating autophagy and fibrotic markers in a diabetic mouse model [84]. MSC-derived EV therapy has been shown to prevent the effects of DN progression and reduce urine volume and albumin excretion. Moreover, EV therapy protects podocytes and tubular epithelial cells from apoptosis and promotes vascular regeneration and cell survival [85] (Table 2).

Table 2. The effects of MSC-derived extracellular vesicles in the treatment of kidney disease.

Pathological Condition	Type of Source	Findings	Reference
Renal ischemic/Reperfusion injury (IRI)	BM-MSC derived exosomes	Inhibition of AKI-CKD transition, modulation of SOX9	[33]
Renal IRI	BM-MSC derived exosomes	Recovery of damaged tubular cells, decrease in cell death, enhancement of cell proliferation, protection for metabolic stress	[36]
Renal IRI	BM-MSC derived exosomes	Decrease in epithelial tubular cell damage and apoptosis, improvement of cell proliferation and kidney function	[35]
AKI	UC-MSC derived exosomes	Enhancement of renal capillary density, reduction of kidney fibrosis, modulation of vascular endothelial growth factor and angiogenesis-related mRNAs	[23]
AKI	UC-MSC derived exosomes	Reduction of inflammation and macrophage infiltration, modulation of chemokine levels and immune response	[64]
Drug-induced nephrotoxicity (DN-AKI)	UC-MSC derived exosomes	Decrease in oxidative stress and apoptosis, improvement in cell proliferation, inhibition of inflammation, induction of autophagy	[70,71]
AKI	BM-MSC derived exosomes	Induction of tubular cell proliferation, improvement of kidney function, promotion of kidney regeneration	[72]
CKD	BM-derived MSC	Reduction of inflammation, amelioration of renal fibrosis, enhancement of renal function	[77]
CKD in unilateral ureteral obstruction (UUO)	BM-MSC derived exosomes	Reduced renal fibrosis and improved renal function	[80]
CKD in UUO	kidney-MSC derived exosomes	Reduction in EMT morphological change, enhancement of cell proliferation, suppression of inflammatory cell infiltration and renal fibrosis	[81]
Clinical trial (CKD)	UC-MSC derived exosomes	Reno-protective efficacy of MSC derived EVs, recovery of eGFR, creatinine, and BUN, reduction of inflammatory immune reaction, renal regeneration	[82]
DN-CKD	BM-MSC derived exosomes	Improvement in renal function, repair of damaged renal tissue, modulation of autophagy	[84]
DN-CKD	Urine-MSC derived exosomes	Prevention of DN progression, reduction of urine volume and albumin excretion, protection of podocytes and tubular epithelial cells, promotion of vascular regeneration and cell survival	[85]

5. Enhancement of MSC Functionality to Improve their Therapeutic Effects in Kidney Disease

MSC-based therapy has been widely studied for the treatment of kidney disease and has been shown to result in improved renal function and the recovery of damaged renal tissues in animal studies and clinical trials [6]. However, MSC-based therapy is limited by the low survival rate of MSCs when used to treat severe kidney disease [86]. Several factors, such as anoikis, ischemia, inflammation, and ROS production reduce the efficacy of MSC-based therapies [87,88]. Some studies have suggested that the preconditioning of MSCs protects them from the harmful environment at site of damage and improves their function. These pretreatment methods include incubation with cytokines or natural or chemical compounds and the application of supporting materials (Figure 3).

Many cytokines and natural/chemical compounds have been shown to have protective effects by enhancing cell survival and proliferation and modulating downstream pathways [89]. Docosahexaenoic acid (DHA) is a necessary omega-3 fatty acid found in blood and in the kidney. 14S,21R-dihydroxy-doxosa 4Z,7Z19Z,12E,16Z,19Z-hexaenoic acid (14S,21R-dHDHA) has been identified as a new DHA-derived lipid mediator and treatment with this compound has been shown to enhance the function of MSCs. In vitro and in IRI mouse models, the usage of this compound is revealed that MSCs treated with 14S,21R-dHDHA show reduced apoptosis and inflammatory responses, and improved renal function [90]. Other studies have shown that the pharmacological agent, S-nitroso N-acetyl penicillamine (SNP), a nitric oxide donor associated with cyto-protective and tissue-protective effects, promotes MSC functionality by increasing cell proliferation and survival in a renal ischemia model [91]. Moreover, the administration of SNP-treated MSCs results in a significant improvement in renal function and increases the expression of pro-survival and pro-angiogenic factors in ischemic renal tissue. Darbepoetin-α (DPO) is an erythropoietic agent that shows similar protective and hematopoietic effects and reduces kidney damage in an animal model of renal IRI [92]. DPO-treated MSCs also improve renal function and kidney structure in an ischemic renal disease model.

Atorvastatin (Ator) has diverse biological activities, including anti-apoptosis, antioxidant, and anti-inflammatory effects [93]. Ator-treated MSCs induced renoprotective effects, including improved renal function and enhanced survival of engrafted MSCs in impaired kidneys in an IRI model. Melatonin, a pineal gland secretory hormone associated with the regulation of circadian rhythms and homeostasis, also enhances the function of MSCs via several biological activities [94–96]. Pretreatment with melatonin significantly increases the survival of MSCs injected into damaged sites and the surviving MSCs improved angiogenesis, increased renal cell proliferation, and enhanced renal function in a renal ischemia model [88]. In addition, in a model of ischemic disease associated with CKD, melatonin pretreatment ameliorated oxidative stress and senescence by enhancing PrP^C-mediated mitochondrial function [97]. In an in vivo model of ischemia, the administration of melatonin-pretreated MSCs increased the secretion of angiogenic cytokines and the survival of engrafted MSCs in CKD-associated ischemic sites. Fucoidan is a sulfated polysaccharide extracted from brown algae and seaweed. It shows diverse biological activities, such as anti-inflammation and antioxidant effects [98]. In a p-cresol-induced CKD model, fucoidan treatment inhibits the senescence of MSCs and increase cell proliferation via FAK-Akt-TWIST signal transduction. In addition, in a murine model of hind limb ischemia associated with CKD, fucoidan-treated MSCs show immunomodulatory activity and enhance cell proliferation, angiogenesis, and recovery of the damaged zone [99].

After administration of MSCs, their effects are limited by a poor environment. Anoikis is a general symptom of kidney disease that is characterized by a deficit of anchorage-dependent attachment to the extracellular matrix [100]. Therefore, to mimic the cellular microenvironment in vivo, a novel strategy is necessary to study the supply of extracellular matrix components. A thermosensitive hydrogel may supply a microenvironment similar to the environment in vivo and increase the survival rate of engrafted cells [101,102]. One study has shown that a chitosan-based hydrogel is a suitable carrier material to deliver MSCs into sites of IR-induced injury in a rat model of AKI. This hydrogel scaffold enhances the retention and survival of transplanted MSCs in harsh conditions. In another study, an IGF-1C domain-modified chitosan hydrogel was synthesized. This hydrogel scaffold was shown to protect cells from H_2O_2 treatment and reduce apoptosis [103] (Table 3).

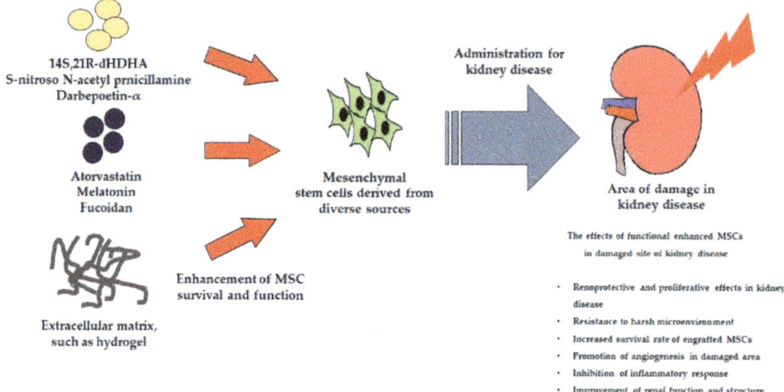

Figure 3. Schematic illustration of the use of active biological factors to enhance MSC functionality for the treatment of kidney disease.

Table 3. Effects of functionally enhanced MSCs in the treatment of kidney disease.

Pathological Condition	Type of Source	Findings	Reference
Renal IRI	14S,21R-dHDHA	Enhancement of MSC function, reduction of apoptosis and inflammatory response, improvement of renal function	[90]
Renal IRI	SNP	Cyto-protective and tissue-protective effects, promotion of MSC functionality (proliferation, survival)	[91]
Renal IRI	DPO	Protective and hematopoietic effects, reduction in kidney damage	[92]
Renal IRI	Ator	Improvement of renal function and survival of engrafted MSCs	[93]
Ischemic disease with CKD	Melatonin	Reduction in oxidative stress and senescence, increase in angiogenesis and injected MSC survival	[97]
CKD	Fucoidan	Inhibition of MSC senescence, increased cell proliferation, enhancement of immunomodulatory activity, recovery of damaged zone	[99]
AKI	chitosan-based hydrogel	Enhancement of transplanted MSC retention and survival, protection of MSC from oxidative stress, reduction of apoptosis	[103]

6. Conclusions

Experimental evidence and clinical trials have demonstrated the feasibility, safety, and efficacy of using MSCs for kidney disease therapy. However, there is still some doubt about the real effects of MSCs on kidney disease. This review has shown that MSCs can be used as therapeutic agents for acute and chronic kidney disease. However, despite the therapeutic potential of MSCs, their use is restricted due to the low survival rate in conditions of inflammation and oxidative stress at sites of injury. In addition, when MSCs are derived from patients with kidney disease for use as autologous MSCs, their function is compromised due to the poor health of the patient. Therefore, novel methods are required to improve the therapeutic efficacy of MSCs under pathophysiological conditions. In this review, we suggest various methods for improving the functionality of MSCs, to enhance their therapeutic potential for kidney disease. The characteristics of MSCs significantly differ depending on their site of origin, their senescence status, and the symptoms of the patient. Therefore, it is also critical to develop optimal methodology to improve the therapeutic efficacy of patient-specific MSCs.

Author Contributions: C.W.Y.: data collection and drafting of manuscript; S.H.L.: organizing the structure of the manuscript, drafting and editing of the manuscript, procurement of funding.

Funding: This work was supported by a National Research Foundation grant funded by the Korean government (NRF-2016R1D1A3B01007727; NRF-2017M3A9B4032528).

Conflicts of Interest: The authors declare no conflicts of interest. The funding body had no role in the study design, data collection or analysis, the decision to publish, or preparation of the manuscript.

References

1. Lentine, K.L.; Kasiske, B.L.; Levey, A.S.; Adams, P.L.; Alberu, J.; Bakr, M.A.; Gallon, L.; Garvey, C.A.; Guleria, S.; Li, P.K.; et al. Summary of kidney disease: Improving global outcomes (kdigo) clinical practice guideline on the evaluation and care of living kidney donors. *Transplantation* **2017**, *101*, 1783–1792. [CrossRef] [PubMed]

2. Fraser, S.D.S.; Roderick, P.J. Kidney disease in the global burden of disease study 2017. *Nat. Rev. Nephrol.* **2019**, *15*, 193–194. [CrossRef] [PubMed]

3. Susantitaphong, P.; Cruz, D.N.; Cerda, J.; Abulfaraj, M.; Alqahtani, F.; Koulouridis, I.; Jaber, B.L.; Acute Kidney Injury Advisory Group of the American Society of Nephrology. World incidence of aki: A meta-analysis. *Clin. J. Am. Soc. Nephrol.* **2013**, *8*, 1482–1493. [CrossRef] [PubMed]

4. English, P.B. Acute renal failure in the dog and cat. *Aust. Vet. J.* **1974**, *50*, 384–392. [CrossRef] [PubMed]

5. Rahman, M.; Shad, F.; Smith, M.C. Acute kidney injury: A guide to diagnosis and management. *Am. Fam. Phys.* **2012**, *86*, 631–639.

6. Aghajani Nargesi, A.; Lerman, L.O.; Eirin, A. Mesenchymal stem cell-derived extracellular vesicles for kidney repair: Current status and looming challenges. *Stem Cell Res. Ther.* **2017**, *8*, 273. [CrossRef]

7. McFetridge, M.L.; Del Borgo, M.P.; Aguilar, M.I.; Ricardo, S.D. The use of hydrogels for cell-based treatment of chronic kidney disease. *Clin. Sci.* **2018**, *132*, 1977–1994. [CrossRef] [PubMed]

8. Chawla, L.S.; Kimmel, P.L. Acute kidney injury and chronic kidney disease: An integrated clinical syndrome. *Kidney Int.* **2012**, *82*, 516–524. [CrossRef]

9. Choi, J.R.; Yong, K.W.; Choi, J.Y. Effects of mechanical loading on human mesenchymal stem cells for cartilage tissue engineering. *J. Cell. Physiol.* **2018**, *233*, 1913–1928. [CrossRef]

10. Wan Safwani, W.K.Z.; Choi, J.R.; Yong, K.W.; Ting, I.; Mat Adenan, N.A.; Pingguan-Murphy, B. Hypoxia enhances the viability, growth and chondrogenic potential of cryopreserved human adipose-derived stem cells. *Cryobiology* **2017**, *75*, 91–99. [CrossRef]

11. Chamberlain, G.; Fox, J.; Ashton, B.; Middleton, J. Concise review: Mesenchymal stem cells: Their phenotype, differentiation capacity, immunological features, and potential for homing. *Stem Cells* **2007**, *25*, 2739–2749. [CrossRef] [PubMed]

12. Bruno, S.; Chiabotto, G.; Camussi, G. Concise review: Different mesenchymal stromal/stem cell populations reside in the adult kidney. *Stem Cells Transl. Med.* **2014**, *3*, 1451–1455. [CrossRef]

13. Choi, J.R.; Pingguan-Murphy, B.; Wan Abas, W.A.; Yong, K.W.; Poon, C.T.; Noor Azmi, M.A.; Omar, S.Z.; Chua, K.H.; Xu, F.; Wan Safwani, W.K. In situ normoxia enhances survival and proliferation rate of human adipose tissue-derived stromal cells without increasing the risk of tumourigenesis. *PLoS ONE* **2015**, *10*, e0115034. [CrossRef] [PubMed]

14. Kramann, R.; Humphreys, B.D. Kidney pericytes: Roles in regeneration and fibrosis. *Semin. Nephrol.* **2014**, *34*, 374–383. [CrossRef] [PubMed]

15. Jia, X.; Pan, J.; Li, X.; Li, N.; Han, Y.; Feng, X.; Cui, J. Bone marrow mesenchymal stromal cells ameliorate angiogenesis and renal damage via promoting pi3k-akt signaling pathway activation in vivo. *Cytotherapy* **2016**, *18*, 838–845. [CrossRef]

16. Casiraghi, F.; Perico, N.; Cortinovis, M.; Remuzzi, G. Mesenchymal stromal cells in renal transplantation: Opportunities and challenges. *Nat. Rev. Nephrol.* **2016**, *12*, 241–253. [CrossRef]

17. Villanueva, S.; Ewertz, E.; Carrion, F.; Tapia, A.; Vergara, C.; Cespedes, C.; Saez, P.J.; Luz, P.; Irarrazabal, C.; Carreno, J.E.; et al. Mesenchymal stem cell injection ameliorates chronic renal failure in a rat model. *Clin. Sci.* **2011**, *121*, 489–499. [CrossRef]

18. Idziak, M.; Pedzisz, P.; Burdzinska, A.; Gala, K.; Paczek, L. Uremic toxins impair human bone marrow-derived mesenchymal stem cells functionality in vitro. *Exp. Toxicol. Pathol.* **2014**, *66*, 187–194. [CrossRef] [PubMed]

19. Yoon, Y.M.; Han, Y.S.; Yun, C.W.; Lee, J.H.; Kim, R.; Lee, S.H. Pioglitazone protects mesenchymal stem cells against p-cresol-induced mitochondrial dysfunction via up-regulation of pink-1. *Int. J. Mol. Sci.* **2018**, *19*, 2898. [CrossRef] [PubMed]

20. Lira, R.; Oliveira, M.; Martins, M.; Silva, C.; Carvalho, S.; Stumbo, A.C.; Cortez, E.; Verdoorn, K.; Einicker-Lamas, M.; Thole, A.; et al. Transplantation of bone marrow-derived mscs improves renal function and na(+)+k(+)-atpase activity in rats with renovascular hypertension. *Cell Tissue Res.* **2017**, *369*, 287–301. [CrossRef]

21. Papazova, D.A.; Oosterhuis, N.R.; Gremmels, H.; van Koppen, A.; Joles, J.A.; Verhaar, M.C. Cell-based therapies for experimental chronic kidney disease: A systematic review and meta-analysis. *Dis. Models Mech.* **2015**, *8*, 281–293. [CrossRef]

22. Peired, A.J.; Sisti, A.; Romagnani, P. Mesenchymal stem cell-based therapy for kidney disease: A review of clinical evidence. *Stem Cells Int.* **2016**, *2016*, 4798639. [CrossRef] [PubMed]

23. Zou, X.; Gu, D.; Xing, X.; Cheng, Z.; Gong, D.; Zhang, G.; Zhu, Y. Human mesenchymal stromal cell-derived extracellular vesicles alleviate renal ischemic reperfusion injury and enhance angiogenesis in rats. *Am. J. Transl. Res.* **2016**, *8*, 4289–4299. [PubMed]

24. Ezquer, F.; Ezquer, M.; Simon, V.; Pardo, F.; Yanez, A.; Carpio, D.; Conget, P. Endovenous administration of bone-marrow-derived multipotent mesenchymal stromal cells prevents renal failure in diabetic mice. *Biol. Blood Marrow Transplant.* **2009**, *15*, 1354–1365. [CrossRef] [PubMed]

25. Fang, Y.; Tian, X.; Bai, S.; Fan, J.; Hou, W.; Tong, H.; Li, D. Autologous transplantation of adipose-derived mesenchymal stem cells ameliorates streptozotocin-induced diabetic nephropathy in rats by inhibiting oxidative stress, pro-inflammatory cytokines and the p38 mapk signaling pathway. *Int. J. Mol. Med.* **2012**, *30*, 85–92.

26. Ezquer, F.; Giraud-Billoud, M.; Carpio, D.; Cabezas, F.; Conget, P.; Ezquer, M. Proregenerative microenvironment triggered by donor mesenchymal stem cells preserves renal function and structure in mice with severe diabetes mellitus. *BioMed Res. Int.* **2015**, *2015*, 164703. [CrossRef]

27. Yu, B.; Zhang, X.; Li, X. Exosomes derived from mesenchymal stem cells. *Int. J. Mol. Sci.* **2014**, *15*, 4142–4157. [CrossRef]

28. Lai, R.C.; Chen, T.S.; Lim, S.K. Mesenchymal stem cell exosome: A novel stem cell-based therapy for cardiovascular disease. *Regen. Med.* **2011**, *6*, 481–492. [CrossRef]

29. Eirin, A.; Riester, S.M.; Zhu, X.Y.; Tang, H.; Evans, J.M.; O'Brien, D.; van Wijnen, A.J.; Lerman, L.O. Microrna and mrna cargo of extracellular vesicles from porcine adipose tissue-derived mesenchymal stem cells. *Gene* **2014**, *551*, 55–64. [CrossRef] [PubMed]

30. Koniusz, S.; Andrzejewska, A.; Muraca, M.; Srivastava, A.K.; Janowski, M.; Lukomska, B. Extracellular vesicles in physiology, pathology, and therapy of the immune and central nervous system, with focus on extracellular vesicles derived from mesenchymal stem cells as therapeutic tools. *Front. Cell. Neurosci.* **2016**, *10*, 109. [CrossRef]

31. Nargesi, A.A.; Lerman, L.O.; Eirin, A. Mesenchymal stem cell-derived extracellular vesicles for renal repair. *Curr. Gene Ther.* **2017**, *17*, 29–42. [CrossRef] [PubMed]

32. Wu, V.C.; Wu, C.H.; Huang, T.M.; Wang, C.Y.; Lai, C.F.; Shiao, C.C.; Chang, C.H.; Lin, S.L.; Chen, Y.Y.; Chen, Y.M.; et al. Long-term risk of coronary events after aki. *J. Am. Soc. Nephrol.* **2014**, *25*, 595–605. [CrossRef] [PubMed]

33. Kumate, J.; Sepulveda-Amor, J.; Valdespino, J.L.; de Mucha, J.; Diaz-Ortega, J.L.; Garcia-Sainz, J.A.; Ruiz-Puente, J.; Jimenez-Paredes, J.; Ruiz-Arriaga, A.; Gutierrez, G.; et al. Mexican contributions to vaccines. *Gac. Med. Mex.* **1988**, *124*, 73–97. [PubMed]

34. Malek, M.; Nematbakhsh, M. Renal ischemia/reperfusion injury; from pathophysiology to treatment. *J. Ren. Inj. Prev.* **2015**, *4*, 20–27. [PubMed]

35. Gatti, S.; Bruno, S.; Deregibus, M.C.; Sordi, A.; Cantaluppi, V.; Tetta, C.; Camussi, G. Microvesicles derived from human adult mesenchymal stem cells protect against ischaemia-reperfusion-induced acute and chronic kidney injury. *Nephrol. Dial. Transplant.* **2011**, *26*, 1474–1483. [CrossRef]

36. Lindoso, R.S.; Collino, F.; Bruno, S.; Araujo, D.S.; Sant'Anna, J.F.; Tetta, C.; Provero, P.; Quesenberry, P.J.; Vieyra, A.; Einicker-Lamas, M.; et al. Extracellular vesicles released from mesenchymal stromal cells modulate mirna in renal tubular cells and inhibit atp depletion injury. *Stem Cells Dev.* **2014**, *23*, 1809–1819. [CrossRef]

37. Zhang, G.; Zou, X.; Miao, S.; Chen, J.; Du, T.; Zhong, L.; Ju, G.; Liu, G.; Zhu, Y. The anti-oxidative role of micro-vesicles derived from human wharton-jelly mesenchymal stromal cells through nox2/gp91(phox) suppression in alleviating renal ischemia-reperfusion injury in rats. *PLoS ONE* **2014**, *9*, e92129. [CrossRef]

38. Squillaro, T.; Peluso, G.; Galderisi, U. Clinical trials with mesenchymal stem cells: An update. *Cell Transplant.* **2016**, *25*, 829–848. [CrossRef]

39. Zeldich, E.; Chen, C.D.; Colvin, T.A.; Bove-Fenderson, E.A.; Liang, J.; Tucker Zhou, T.B.; Harris, D.A.; Abraham, C.R. The neuroprotective effect of klotho is mediated via regulation of members of the redox system. *J. Biol. Chem.* **2014**, *289*, 24700–24715. [CrossRef] [PubMed]

40. Oh, H.J.; Nam, B.Y.; Lee, M.J.; Kim, C.H.; Koo, H.M.; Doh, F.M.; Han, J.H.; Kim, E.J.; Han, J.S.; Park, J.T.; et al. Decreased circulating klotho levels in patients undergoing dialysis and relationship to oxidative stress and inflammation. *Perit. Dial. Int.* **2015**, *35*, 43–51. [CrossRef]

41. Geng, Y.; Zhang, L.; Fu, B.; Zhang, J.; Hong, Q.; Hu, J.; Li, D.; Luo, C.; Cui, S.; Zhu, F.; et al. Mesenchymal stem cells ameliorate rhabdomyolysis-induced acute kidney injury via the activation of m2 macrophages. *Stem Cell Res. Ther.* **2014**, *5*, 80. [CrossRef] [PubMed]

42. Lee, S.J.; Ryu, M.O.; Seo, M.S.; Park, S.B.; Ahn, J.O.; Han, S.M.; Kang, K.S.; Bhang, D.H.; Youn, H.Y. Mesenchymal stem cells contribute to improvement of renal function in a canine kidney injury model. *In Vivo* **2017**, *31*, 1115–1124.

43. Rodrigues, C.E.; Capcha, J.M.; de Braganca, A.C.; Sanches, T.R.; Gouveia, P.Q.; de Oliveira, P.A.; Malheiros, D.M.; Volpini, R.A.; Santinho, M.A.; Santana, B.A.; et al. Human umbilical cord-derived mesenchymal stromal cells protect against premature renal senescence resulting from oxidative stress in rats with acute kidney injury. *Stem Cell Res. Ther.* **2017**, *8*, 19. [CrossRef] [PubMed]

44. Togel, F.; Hu, Z.; Weiss, K.; Isaac, J.; Lange, C.; Westenfelder, C. Administered mesenchymal stem cells protect against ischemic acute renal failure through differentiation-independent mechanisms. *Am. J. Physiol. Ren. Physiol.* **2005**, *289*, F31–F42. [CrossRef]

45. Lai, R.C.; Yeo, R.W.; Lim, S.K. Mesenchymal stem cell exosomes. *Semin. Cell Dev. Biol.* **2015**, *40*, 82–88. [CrossRef]

46. Bellomo, R.; Kellum, J.A.; Ronco, C. Acute kidney injury. *Lancet* **2012**, *380*, 756–766. [CrossRef]

47. Togel, F.E.; Westenfelder, C. Kidney protection and regeneration following acute injury: Progress through stem cell therapy. *Am. J. Kidney Dis.* **2012**, *60*, 1012–1022. [CrossRef] [PubMed]

48. National Kidney, F. K/doqi clinical practice guidelines for chronic kidney disease: Evaluation, classification, and stratification. *Am. J. Kidney Dis.* **2002**, *39* (Suppl. 1), S1–S266.

49. Bruck, K.; Stel, V.S.; Fraser, S.; De Goeij, M.C.; Caskey, F.; Abu-Hanna, A.; Jager, K.J. Translational research in nephrology: Chronic kidney disease prevention and public health. *Clin. Kidney J.* **2015**, *8*, 647–655. [CrossRef]

50. Heywood, J.T.; Fonarow, G.C.; Costanzo, M.R.; Mathur, V.S.; Wigneswaran, J.R.; Wynne, J.; ADHERE Scientific Advisory Committee and Investigators. High prevalence of renal dysfunction and its impact on outcome in 118,465 patients hospitalized with acute decompensated heart failure: A report from the adhere database. *J. Card. Fail.* **2007**, *13*, 422–430. [CrossRef]

51. Tonelli, M.; Riella, M.C. Chronic kidney disease and the aging population. *Kidney Int.* **2014**, *85*, 487–491. [CrossRef]

52. Nugent, R.A.; Fathima, S.F.; Feigl, A.B.; Chyung, D. The burden of chronic kidney disease on developing nations: A 21st century challenge in global health. *Nephron. Clin. Pract.* **2011**, *118*, c269–c277. [CrossRef]

53. Thi Do, D.; Phan, N.N.; Wang, C.Y.; Sun, Z.; Lin, Y.C. Novel regulations of mef2-a, mef2-d, and cacna1s in the functional incompetence of adipose-derived mesenchymal stem cells by induced indoxyl sulfate in chronic kidney disease. *Cytotechnology* **2016**, *68*, 2589–2604. [CrossRef]

54. Meijers, B.K.; Claes, K.; Bammens, B.; de Loor, H.; Viaene, L.; Verbeke, K.; Kuypers, D.; Vanrenterghem, Y.; Evenepoel, P. P-cresol and cardiovascular risk in mild-to-moderate kidney disease. *Clin. J. Am. Soc. Nephrol.* **2010**, *5*, 1182–1189. [CrossRef]

55. Lee, S.R.; Lee, S.H.; Moon, J.Y.; Park, J.Y.; Lee, D.; Lim, S.J.; Jeong, K.H.; Park, J.K.; Lee, T.W.; Ihm, C.G. Repeated administration of bone marrow-derived mesenchymal stem cells improved the protective effects on a remnant kidney model. *Ren. Fail.* **2010**, *32*, 840–848. [CrossRef] [PubMed]

56. Wu, H.J.; Yiu, W.H.; Li, R.X.; Wong, D.W.; Leung, J.C.; Chan, L.Y.; Zhang, Y.; Lian, Q.; Lin, M.; Tse, H.F.; et al. Mesenchymal stem cells modulate albumin-induced renal tubular inflammation and fibrosis. *PLoS ONE* **2014**, *9*, e90883. [CrossRef]

57. Makhlough, A.; Shekarchian, S.; Moghadasali, R.; Einollahi, B.; Hosseini, S.E.; Jaroughi, N.; Bolurieh, T.; Baharvand, H.; Aghdami, N. Safety and tolerability of autologous bone marrow mesenchymal stromal cells in adpkd patients. *Stem Cell Res. Ther.* **2017**, *8*, 116. [CrossRef] [PubMed]

58. Camilleri, E.T.; Gustafson, M.P.; Dudakovic, A.; Riester, S.M.; Garces, C.G.; Paradise, C.R.; Takai, H.; Karperien, M.; Cool, S.; Sampen, H.J.; et al. Identification and validation of multiple cell surface markers of clinical-grade adipose-derived mesenchymal stromal cells as novel release criteria for good manufacturing practice-compliant production. *Stem Cell Res. Ther.* **2016**, *7*, 107. [CrossRef] [PubMed]

59. Saran, R.; Robinson, B.; Abbott, K.C.; Agodoa, L.Y.C.; Bhave, N.; Bragg-Gresham, J.; Balkrishnan, R.; Dietrich, X.; Eckard, A.; Eggers, P.W.; et al. Us renal data system 2017 annual data report: Epidemiology of kidney disease in the united states. *Am. J. Kidney Dis.* **2018**, *71*, A7. [CrossRef]

60. Gallagher, H.; Suckling, R.J. Diabetic nephropathy: Where are we on the journey from pathophysiology to treatment? *Diabetes Obes. Metab.* **2016**, *18*, 641–647. [CrossRef] [PubMed]

61. Abdel Aziz, M.T.; Wassef, M.A.; Ahmed, H.H.; Rashed, L.; Mahfouz, S.; Aly, M.I.; Hussein, R.E.; Abdelaziz, M. The role of bone marrow derived-mesenchymal stem cells in attenuation of kidney function in rats with diabetic nephropathy. *Diabetol. Metab. Syndr.* **2014**, *6*, 34. [CrossRef] [PubMed]

62. Ezquer, M.E.; Ezquer, F.E.; Arango-Rodriguez, M.L.; Conget, P.A. Msc transplantation: A promising therapeutic strategy to manage the onset and progression of diabetic nephropathy. *Biol. Res.* **2012**, *45*, 289–296. [CrossRef]

63. Srisawat, N.; Kellum, J.A. Acute kidney injury: Definition, epidemiology, and outcome. *Curr. Opin. Crit. Care* **2011**, *17*, 548–555. [CrossRef] [PubMed]

64. Zou, X.; Zhang, G.; Cheng, Z.; Yin, D.; Du, T.; Ju, G.; Miao, S.; Liu, G.; Lu, M.; Zhu, Y. Microvesicles derived from human wharton's jelly mesenchymal stromal cells ameliorate renal ischemia-reperfusion injury in rats by suppressing cx3cl1. *Stem Cell Res. Ther.* **2014**, *5*, 40. [CrossRef]

65. Perazella, M.A. Drug-induced renal failure: Update on new medications and unique mechanisms of nephrotoxicity. *Am. J. Med Sci.* **2003**, *325*, 349–362. [CrossRef] [PubMed]

66. Ghane Shahrbaf, F.; Assadi, F. Drug-induced renal disorders. *J. Ren. Inj. Prev.* **2015**, *4*, 57–60. [PubMed]

67. Nash, K.; Hafeez, A.; Hou, S. Hospital-acquired renal insufficiency. *Am. J. Kidney Dis.* **2002**, *39*, 930–936. [CrossRef]

68. Miller, R.P.; Tadagavadi, R.K.; Ramesh, G.; Reeves, W.B. Mechanisms of cisplatin nephrotoxicity. *Toxins* **2010**, *2*, 2490–2518. [CrossRef] [PubMed]

69. Silici, S.; Ekmekcioglu, O.; Kanbur, M.; Deniz, K. The protective effect of royal jelly against cisplatin-induced renal oxidative stress in rats. *World J. Urol.* **2011**, *29*, 127–132. [CrossRef]

70. Zhou, Y.; Xu, H.; Xu, W.; Wang, B.; Wu, H.; Tao, Y.; Zhang, B.; Wang, M.; Mao, F.; Yan, Y.; et al. Exosomes released by human umbilical cord mesenchymal stem cells protect against cisplatin-induced renal oxidative stress and apoptosis in vivo and in vitro. *Stem Cell Res. Ther.* **2013**, *4*, 34. [CrossRef] [PubMed]

71. Wang, B.; Jia, H.; Zhang, B.; Wang, J.; Ji, C.; Zhu, X.; Yan, Y.; Yin, L.; Yu, J.; Qian, H.; et al. Pre-incubation with hucmsc-exosomes prevents cisplatin-induced nephrotoxicity by activating autophagy. *Stem Cell Res. Ther.* **2017**, *8*, 75. [CrossRef] [PubMed]

72. Bruno, S.; Tapparo, M.; Collino, F.; Chiabotto, G.; Deregibus, M.C.; Soares Lindoso, R.; Neri, F.; Kholia, S.; Giunti, S.; Wen, S.; et al. Renal regenerative potential of different extracellular vesicle populations derived from bone marrow mesenchymal stromal cells. *Tissue Eng. Part A* **2017**, *23*, 1262–1273. [CrossRef]

73. Collino, F.; Bruno, S.; Incarnato, D.; Dettori, D.; Neri, F.; Provero, P.; Pomatto, M.; Oliviero, S.; Tetta, C.; Quesenberry, P.J.; et al. Aki recovery induced by mesenchymal stromal cell-derived extracellular vesicles carrying micrornas. *J. Am. Soc. Nephrol.* **2015**, *26*, 2349–2360. [CrossRef] [PubMed]

74. Grange, C.; Iampietro, C.; Bussolati, B. Stem cell extracellular vesicles and kidney injury. *Stem Cell Investig.* **2017**, *4*, 90. [CrossRef] [PubMed]

75. Ritchie, J.; Green, D.; Alderson, H.V.; Chiu, D.; Sinha, S.; Kalra, P.A. Risks for mortality and renal replacement therapy in atherosclerotic renovascular disease compared with other causes of chronic kidney disease. *Nephrology* **2015**, *20*, 688–696. [CrossRef]

76. Zhang, X.; Li, Z.L.; Woollard, J.R.; Eirin, A.; Ebrahimi, B.; Crane, J.A.; Zhu, X.Y.; Pawar, A.S.; Krier, J.D.; Jordan, K.L.; et al. Obesity-metabolic derangement preserves hemodynamics but promotes intrarenal adiposity and macrophage infiltration in swine renovascular disease. *Am. J. Physiol. Ren. Physiol.* **2013**, *305*, F265–F276. [CrossRef]

77. Eirin, A.; Zhu, X.Y.; Puranik, A.S.; Tang, H.; McGurren, K.A.; van Wijnen, A.J.; Lerman, A.; Lerman, L.O. Mesenchymal stem cell-derived extracellular vesicles attenuate kidney inflammation. *Kidney Int.* **2017**, *92*, 114–124. [CrossRef] [PubMed]

78. Eirin, A.; Zhu, X.Y.; Jonnada, S.; Lerman, A.; van Wijnen, A.J.; Lerman, L.O. Mesenchymal stem cell-derived extracellular vesicles improve the renal microvasculature in metabolic renovascular disease in swine. *Cell Transplant.* **2018**, *27*, 1080–1095. [CrossRef]

79. Ucero, A.C.; Benito-Martin, A.; Izquierdo, M.C.; Sanchez-Nino, M.D.; Sanz, A.B.; Ramos, A.M.; Berzal, S.; Ruiz-Ortega, M.; Egido, J.; Ortiz, A. Unilateral ureteral obstruction: Beyond obstruction. *Int. Urol. Nephrol.* **2014**, *46*, 765–776. [CrossRef] [PubMed]

80. He, J.; Wang, Y.; Lu, X.; Zhu, B.; Pei, X.; Wu, J.; Zhao, W. Micro-vesicles derived from bone marrow stem cells protect the kidney both in vivo and in vitro by microrna-dependent repairing. *Nephrology* **2015**, *20*, 591–600. [CrossRef]

81. Choi, H.Y.; Lee, H.G.; Kim, B.S.; Ahn, S.H.; Jung, A.; Lee, M.; Lee, J.E.; Kim, H.J.; Ha, S.K.; Park, H.C. Mesenchymal stem cell-derived microparticles ameliorate peritubular capillary rarefaction via inhibition of endothelial-mesenchymal transition and decrease tubulointerstitial fibrosis in unilateral ureteral obstruction. *Stem Cell Res. Ther.* **2015**, *6*, 18. [CrossRef]

82. Nassar, W.; El-Ansary, M.; Sabry, D.; Mostafa, M.A.; Fayad, T.; Kotb, E.; Temraz, M.; Saad, A.N.; Essa, W.; Adel, H. Umbilical cord mesenchymal stem cells derived extracellular vesicles can safely ameliorate the progression of chronic kidney diseases. *Biomater. Res.* **2016**, *20*, 21. [CrossRef] [PubMed]

83. Martinez-Castelao, A.; Navarro-Gonzalez, J.F.; Gorriz, J.L.; de Alvaro, F. The concept and the epidemiology of diabetic nephropathy have changed in recent years. *J. Clin. Med.* **2015**, *4*, 1207–1216. [CrossRef] [PubMed]

84. Ebrahim, N.; Ahmed, I.A.; Hussien, N.I.; Dessouky, A.A.; Farid, A.S.; Elshazly, A.M.; Mostafa, O.; Gazzar, W.B.E.; Sorour, S.M.; Seleem, Y.; et al. Mesenchymal stem cell-derived exosomes ameliorated diabetic nephropathy by autophagy induction through the mtor signaling pathway. *Cells* **2018**, *7*, 226. [CrossRef] [PubMed]

85. Jiang, Z.Z.; Liu, Y.M.; Niu, X.; Yin, J.Y.; Hu, B.; Guo, S.C.; Fan, Y.; Wang, Y.; Wang, N.S. Exosomes secreted by human urine-derived stem cells could prevent kidney complications from type i diabetes in rats. *Stem Cell Res. Ther.* **2016**, *7*, 24. [CrossRef] [PubMed]

86. Burst, V.R.; Gillis, M.; Putsch, F.; Herzog, R.; Fischer, J.H.; Heid, P.; Muller-Ehmsen, J.; Schenk, K.; Fries, J.W.; Baldamus, C.A.; et al. Poor cell survival limits the beneficial impact of mesenchymal stem cell transplantation on acute kidney injury. *Nephron Exp. Nephrol.* **2010**, *114*, e107–e116. [CrossRef] [PubMed]

87. He, N.; Zhang, L.; Cui, J.; Li, Z. Bone marrow vascular niche: Home for hematopoietic stem cells. *Bone Marrow Res.* **2014**, *2014*, 128436. [CrossRef] [PubMed]

88. Mias, C.; Trouche, E.; Seguelas, M.H.; Calcagno, F.; Dignat-George, F.; Sabatier, F.; Piercecchi-Marti, M.D.; Daniel, L.; Bianchi, P.; Calise, D.; et al. Ex vivo pretreatment with melatonin improves survival, proangiogenic/mitogenic activity, and efficiency of mesenchymal stem cells injected into ischemic kidney. *Stem Cells* **2008**, *26*, 1749–1757. [CrossRef]

89. Manning, B.D.; Toker, A. Akt/pkb signaling: Navigating the network. *Cell* **2017**, *169*, 381–405. [CrossRef] [PubMed]

90. Tian, H.; Lu, Y.; Shah, S.P.; Wang, Q.; Hong, S. 14s,21r-dihydroxy-docosahexaenoic acid treatment enhances mesenchymal stem cell amelioration of renal ischemia/reperfusion injury. *Stem Cells Dev.* **2012**, *21*, 1187–1199. [CrossRef] [PubMed]

91. Masoud, M.S.; Anwar, S.S.; Afzal, M.Z.; Mehmood, A.; Khan, S.N.; Riazuddin, S. Pre-conditioned mesenchymal stem cells ameliorate renal ischemic injury in rats by augmented survival and engraftment. *J. Transl. Med.* **2012**, *10*, 243. [CrossRef]

92. Altun, B.; Yilmaz, R.; Aki, T.; Akoglu, H.; Zeybek, D.; Piskinpasa, S.; Uckan, D.; Purali, N.; Korkusuz, P.; Turgan, C. Use of mesenchymal stem cells and darbepoetin improve ischemia-induced acute kidney injury outcomes. *Am. J. Nephrol.* **2012**, *35*, 531–539. [CrossRef]

93. Cai, J.; Yu, X.; Zhang, B.; Zhang, H.; Fang, Y.; Liu, S.; Liu, T.; Ding, X. Atorvastatin improves survival of implanted stem cells in a rat model of renal ischemia-reperfusion injury. *Am. J. Nephrol.* **2014**, *39*, 466–475. [CrossRef]

94. Fernandez, A.; Ordonez, R.; Reiter, R.J.; Gonzalez-Gallego, J.; Mauriz, J.L. Melatonin and endoplasmic reticulum stress: Relation to autophagy and apoptosis. *J. Pineal Res.* **2015**, *59*, 292–307. [CrossRef] [PubMed]

95. Reiter, R.J.; Mayo, J.C.; Tan, D.X.; Sainz, R.M.; Alatorre-Jimenez, M.; Qin, L. Melatonin as an antioxidant: Under promises but over delivers. *J. Pineal Res.* **2016**, *61*, 253–278. [CrossRef]

96. Mauriz, J.L.; Collado, P.S.; Veneroso, C.; Reiter, R.J.; Gonzalez-Gallego, J. A review of the molecular aspects of melatonin's anti-inflammatory actions: Recent insights and new perspectives. *J. Pineal Res.* **2013**, *54*, 1–14. [CrossRef] [PubMed]

97. Han, Y.S.; Kim, S.M.; Lee, J.H.; Jung, S.K.; Noh, H.; Lee, S.H. Melatonin protects chronic kidney disease mesenchymal stem cells against senescence via prp(c)-dependent enhancement of the mitochondrial function. *J. Pineal Res.* **2019**, *66*, e12535. [CrossRef]

98. Lee, J.H.; Yun, C.W.; Hur, J.; Lee, S.H. Fucoidan rescues p-cresol-induced cellular senescence in mesenchymal stem cells via fak-akt-twist axis. *Mar. Drugs* **2018**, *16*, 121. [CrossRef] [PubMed]

99. Han, Y.S.; Lee, J.H.; Jung, J.S.; Noh, H.; Baek, M.J.; Ryu, J.M.; Yoon, Y.M.; Han, H.J.; Lee, S.H. Fucoidan protects mesenchymal stem cells against oxidative stress and enhances vascular regeneration in a murine hindlimb ischemia model. *Int. J. Cardiol.* **2015**, *198*, 187–195. [CrossRef]

100. Taddei, M.L.; Giannoni, E.; Fiaschi, T.; Chiarugi, P. Anoikis: An emerging hallmark in health and diseases. *J. Pathol.* **2012**, *226*, 380–393. [CrossRef] [PubMed]

101. Christman, K.L.; Vardanian, A.J.; Fang, Q.; Sievers, R.E.; Fok, H.H.; Lee, R.J. Injectable fibrin scaffold improves cell transplant survival, reduces infarct expansion, and induces neovasculature formation in ischemic myocardium. *J. Am. Coll. Cardiol.* **2004**, *44*, 654–660. [CrossRef] [PubMed]

102. Davis, M.E.; Motion, J.P.; Narmoneva, D.A.; Takahashi, T.; Hakuno, D.; Kamm, R.D.; Zhang, S.; Lee, R.T. Injectable self-assembling peptide nanofibers create intramyocardial microenvironments for endothelial cells. *Circulation* **2005**, *111*, 442–450. [CrossRef] [PubMed]

103. Feng, G.; Zhang, J.; Li, Y.; Nie, Y.; Zhu, D.; Wang, R.; Liu, J.; Gao, J.; Liu, N.; He, N.; et al. Igf-1 c domain-modified hydrogel enhances cell therapy for aki. *J. Am. Soc. Nephrol.* **2016**, *27*, 2357–2369. [CrossRef] [PubMed]

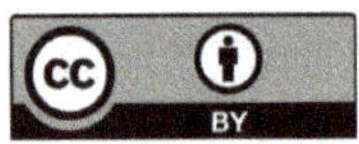

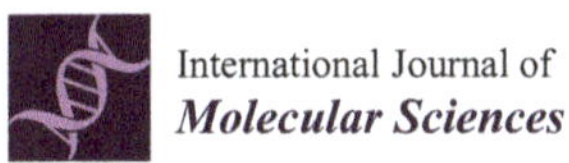

International Journal of
Molecular Sciences

Review

Lysophosphatidic Acid Signaling in Diabetic Nephropathy

Jong Han Lee [1,2], **Donghee Kim** [2], **Yoon Sin Oh** [3] **and Hee-Sook Jun** [1,2,4,*]

1   College of Pharmacy, Gachon University, Incheon 21936, Korea; jhleecw@gachon.ac.kr
2   Lee Gil Ya Cancer and Diabetes Institute, Gachon University, Incheon 21999, Korea; dh2388@gachon.ac.kr
3   Department of Food and Nutrition, Eulji University, Seongnam 13135, Korea; ysoh@eulji.ac.kr
4   Gachon University Gil Medical Center, Gachon Medical and Convergence Institute, Incheon 21565, Korea
*   Correspondence: hsjun@gachon.ac.kr; Tel.: 82-32-899-6056

Received: 6 May 2019; Accepted: 8 June 2019; Published: 11 June 2019

Abstract: Lysophosphatidic acid (LPA) is a bioactive phospholipid present in most tissues and body fluids. LPA acts through specific LPA receptors (LPAR1 to LPAR6) coupled with G protein. LPA binds to receptors and activates multiple cellular signaling pathways, subsequently exerting various biological functions, such as cell proliferation, migration, and apoptosis. LPA also induces cell damage through complex overlapping pathways, including the generation of reactive oxygen species, inflammatory cytokines, and fibrosis. Several reports indicate that the LPA–LPAR axis plays an important role in various diseases, including kidney disease, lung fibrosis, and cancer. Diabetic nephropathy (DN) is one of the most common diabetic complications and the main risk factor for chronic kidney diseases, which mostly progress to end-stage renal disease. There is also growing evidence indicating that the LPA–LPAR axis also plays an important role in inducing pathological alterations of cell structure and function in the kidneys. In this review, we will discuss key mediators or signaling pathways activated by LPA and summarize recent research findings associated with DN.

Keywords: diabetic nephropathy; lysophosphatidic acid; lysophosphatidic acid receptor; chronic kidney injury

---

1. Introduction

Diabetic nephropathy (DN) is a microvascular complication of diabetes and develops in approximately 20–40% patients with diabetes, including type 1 and type 2 diabetes patients [1,2]. It has become the main risk factor for the development of chronic kidney diseases, such that most DN patients progress to end-stage renal disease (ESRD) and require renal replacement in the end [2]. Thus, DN not only increases the health cost for individuals and the society at large but is also a risk factor for morbidity and mortality. Intensive glycemic control is a well-established strategy for the prevention of DN. Despite the efforts for the management of hyperglycemia and hypertension using current therapies, such as angiotensin converting enzyme (ACE) inhibitors and angiotensin II receptor blockers (ARBs) [3,4], the risk of DN progression has still not been reduced. Currently available drugs only delay the progress of the disease, rather than curing it. Therefore, a novel and effective therapeutic approach is urgently needed for patients with DN.

Phospholipids are generally known to be structural components of plasma membranes, but growing evidence indicates that membrane phospholipids also play crucial roles as signaling molecules and exert a wide range of physiological responses. Lysophosphatidic acid (LPA) is a small, naturally occurring glycerophospholipid, which is composed of a glycerol backbone with an ester-linked acyl chain and a phosphate group. It is also produced by the action of various lysophospholipases, including autotaxin (ATX), and phospholipases A1 or A2 (PLA1 and PLA2). LPA acts through specific LPA receptors (LPAR1 to LPAR6) coupled with G protein and is associated with a wide range of cell responses, such as proliferation and migration [5,6], and pathologies of a number of diseases, including fibrosis, cancer, neuronal disorders, and bone metabolism [5,7–10]. Hyperglycemia, advanced glycation end product (AGE), and pro-inflammatory cytokines are considered the three main initial mediators of DN development [11,12]. However, some recent studies also showed that the LPA–LPA receptor axis may play an important role in the pathogenesis of diabetic kidney disease.

In this review article, we review the key mediators and signaling pathways activated by LPA and summarize newly reported signaling pathways modulated by different LPA receptor antagonists in different DN models.

2. Biosynthesis and Degradation of LPA

LPA is the smallest bioactive lysophospholipid (MW 430–480 Da) derived from membrane phospholipids [13] and acts as an extracellular signaling molecule via its receptors, regulating various cellular processes, including cell proliferation, survival, migration, differentiation, remodeling, and cytokine/chemokine secretion [13]. LPA is known to be water soluble and is present in most tissues and biological fluids, such as plasma, saliva, tears, follicular fluid, and cerebrospinal fluid [5,14]. LPA is produced by several enzymes, either in the intracellular or extracellular compartment, as shown in Figure 1. In the intracellular compartment, LPA is naturally synthesized through the action of glycerol-3-phosphate acyltransferase (GPAT) during the process of triglyceride and phospholipid anabolism, which is found mainly in the mitochondria and endoplasmic reticulum of various cell types [15,16]. LPA is also synthesized by the action of intra/extra-cellular PLA1 or PLA2 from phosphatidic acid (PA). Ubiquitously expressed PLA1 and PLA2 in the body hydrolyze the bond between the fatty acid chain and the glycerol backbone at *sn1* (saturated) or *sn2* (unsaturated) positions of PA [17,18]. Membrane phospholipids are major sources for LPA production. Metabolically, they are first converted into lysophospholipids, such as lysophosphatidylethanolamine (LPE), lysophosphatidylcholine (LPC), lysophosphatidylserine (LPS), and then, subsequently cleaved by ATX, also known as ectonucleotidepyrophosphatases/ phosphodiesterases-2. This pathway is considered a determinant for the LPA level in plasma [19,20].

LPA is converted by several classes of enzymes, including lipid phosphate phosphatases (LPPs), LPA acyltransferase, and phospholipases [21–23], as shown in Figure 1. LPPs (LPP1, LPP2, and LPP3) exist extracellularly and intracellularly in the endoplasmic reticulum and Golgi, and dephosphorylate LPA and degrade it into monoacylglycerol (MAG). LPA can also be converted to PA by the action of the acylglycerophosphate acyltransferase (AGPAT) enzyme, also known as LPA acyltransferase [24]. The third alternative pathway for LPA degradation is mediated by the action of lysophospholipases, via formation of glycerol-3-phosphate [25].

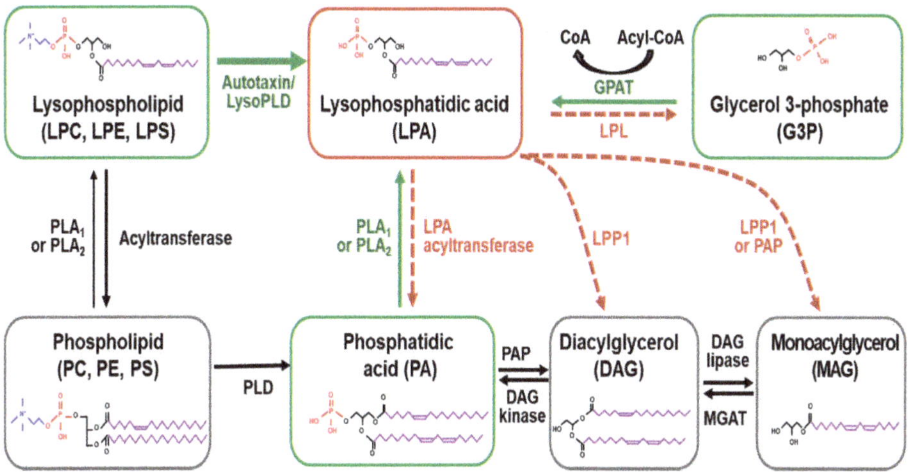

Figure 1. The enzymatic pathways of lysophosphatidic acid (LPA) synthesis and degradation. LPA can be synthesized from different precursors, including lysophospholipids, phosphatidic acid, and glycerol 3-phosphate. The enzymes and pathways involved in LPA production are indicated using green text and a green solid line, respectively. LPA is converted into either monoacylglycerol or phosphatidic acid. The enzymes and pathways involved in LPA conversion are indicated using red text and a red dotted line, respectively. Lysophosphatidylcholine (LPC), lysophosphatidylethanolamine (LPE), lysophosphatidylserine (LPS), lysophospholipase D (Lyso PLD), lysophospholipase (LPL), glycerol 3-phosphate acyltransferase (GPAT), phospholipase C (PLC), phospholipase A1 or A2 (PLA1 and PLA2), diacylglycerol (DAG), monoacylglycerol (MAG), MAG acyltransferase (MGAT), lipid phosphate phosphatase 1 or 2 (LPP1 and LPP2), phosphatidate phosphatase (PAP), phosphatidylcholine (PC), phosphatidylethanolamine (PE), phosphatidylserine (PS), and phospholipase D (PLD).

3. LPA Receptors and Intracellular Signaling Pathways

LPA induces various cellular effects by binding to specific G protein-coupled LPA receptors (LPARs) and activates downstream intracellular signaling pathways, resulting in various physiological and pathophysiological responses [5]. Till now, six LPARs have been identified and classified into A rhodopsin-like G protein-coupled receptors [26]. They can be further grouped into two groups, according to their distinct protein homology, such as LPAR1 to LPAR3 belonging to the endothelial differentiation gene (*Edg*) family, and LPAR4 to LPAR6 belonging to the *P2Y* purinergic gene cluster [6,8]. These receptors have the ability to interact with at least one or more heterotrimeric G subunits, such as Gαi/o, Gαq/11, Gα12/13, and Gs [6]. LPAR1/Edg2 and LPAR2/Edg4 receptors couple with Gαi/o, Gαq/11, and Gα12/13. Once bound together, the complexes transduce extracellular signals into intracellular pathways through molecules, such as the Ras homologous (Rho) protein family of GTPases, phospholipase C (PLC), diacylglycerol (DAG), mitogen-activated protein kinase (MAPK), and phosphatidylinositol 3-kinase (PI3K)-protein kinase B (Akt). Activation of these receptors mostly ends up promoting cell proliferation, survival, and migration [27,28]. LPAR3/Edg7 couples with Gαi/o and Gαq/11, and participates in LPA-induced Ca^{2+} mobilization, PLC, adenylyl-cyclase inhibition, and MAPK activation [28]. LPAR4/GPR23/P2Y9 and LPAR5/GPR92 induce stress fiber formation and neurite retraction through Gα12/13 and downstream Rho/Rho-associated protein kinase (ROCK) pathway [29,30]. LPAR4 is known as the only LPA receptor that can increase intracellular cAMP accumulation by coupling to Gs [29]. LPAR5 interacts with Gαq/11 and increases intracellular Ca^{2+} levels [31]. LPA6/P2Y5 receptor binds to either Gαi/o or Gα12/13, and induces Rho-dependent alteration of cellular morphology [32,33]. In addition, other G protein-coupled receptors, including GPR35 [34] and P2Y10 [35], were also identified as LPARs, which induced Ca^{2+} responses by LPA stimulation.

LPA can also bind to and activate non-GPCR targets, the receptor for advanced glycation end products (RAGE) [36], and the cation channel transient receptor potential vanilloid 1 (TRPV1) [37]. RAGE participates in LPA-induced nicotinamide adenine dinucleotide phosphate (NADPH) oxidase (Nox), reactive oxygen species (ROS) induction, and activation of NF_KB, serum response factor (SRF), PI3K, and Akt [38]. TRPV1 increases intracellular Ca^{2+} levels following LPA stimulation [37]. Another non-GPCR, peroxisome proliferator-activated receptor gamma (PPARγ), is the intracellular receptor for LPA, and is critically important for mediating the effects of LPA on vascular remodeling [39]. Among them, the expression of LPAR1-4 has been detected in renal tissue [40]. Although many LPA receptors and their signaling pathways have been identified, as shown in Figure 2, the functional role of each receptor is poorly understood. Further studies will be required.

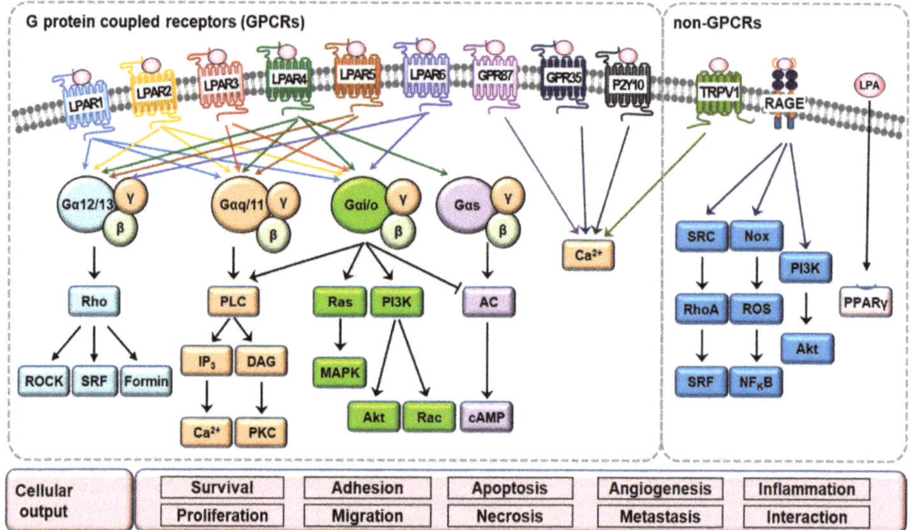

Figure 2. LPA signaling pathways. LPA can induce multiple cellular effects via binding to specific GPCRs, including LPAR1–LPAR6, as well as binding to non-GPCRs, such as transient receptor potential vanilloid 1 (TRPV1), receptor for advanced glycation end products (RAGE), and intracellular peroxisome proliferator-activated receptor gamma (PPARγ). After binding to receptors, LPA activates downstream intracellular signaling pathways, thereby resulting in various physiological and pathophysiological responses, as described in detail in the text.

4. Pathogenesis of DN

4.1. Definition of Chronic Kidney Disease

Kidney disease is a heterogeneous group of disorders affecting kidney structure and function, which can be further classified into two distinct syndromes, acute and chronic kidney disease (CKD) [6]. Acute kidney injury is characterized by rapid diminution of kidney function, resulting in excretion of creatinine [41]. It occurs over several hours or days but not more than three months, whereas chronic kidney injury is in cases of more than three months. Acute kidney injury often leads to the development of chronic kidney failure [41]. Conversely, chronic kidney disease increases the risk of incidence of acute kidney injury [42,43]. Whatever the initial injury, the final pathogenesis of CKD involves renal fibrosis, characterized by excessive extracellular matrix (ECM) accumulation in glomerular and tubular interstitial cells [44,45]. Renal fibrosis changes tissue architecture and function, which leads to kidney dysfunction and failure.

4.2. Glomerulosclerosis

Glomerulosclerosis is hardening of glomeruli in the kidney and is frequently referred to as focal segmental glomerulosclerosis or nodular glomerulosclerosis [46]. The initial pathogenic events start in glomerular endothelium, including the activation and dysfunction of endothelial cells, hemodynamic alterations, as well as loss of glomerular basement membrane (GBM) electrical charge. These alterations subsequently trigger an inflammatory response in the glomerular apparatus, which further affects mesangial cells and induces proliferation and dysfunction of mesangial cells [43,47]. Excessive ECM production is the underlying mechanism for mesangial expansion. Podocytes are the cells located inside the Bowman's capsule of the kidney, which anatomically wrap around capillaries of the glomerulus [48]. The damage in podocytes decreases their number and increases foot process effacement and denudation of GBM. The accumulated damage increases cell death by apoptosis or necrosis, and replacement of glomerular cells by ECM, which, in turn, increases hardening of glomeruli and eventually leads to glomerulosclerosis [16,44].

4.3. Tubular Interstitial Fibrosis

Although the initial glomerular damage and glomerulosclerosis are the major factors for the development of CKDs, the fibrosis in the tubulo-interstitial compartment is also a major contributor [43,49]. Initial glomerular damage increases the leakage of abnormally filtered proteins, including albumin, complement, and cytokines. These proteins and immune effectors or molecules activate tubular cells and initiate an inflammatory response. Simultaneously, different types of inflammatory cells (macrophages, monocytes, lymphocytes, mast cells, and dendritic cells) are recruited from circulation by increasing the expression of chemokines (monocyte chemoattractant protein 1, CCL2/MCP1; regulated upon activation, normal T cell expressed, and secreted, CCL5/RANTES), and adhesion molecules (E and P selectins, intercellular adhesion molecule-1, ICAM-1; vascular cell adhesion molecule-1, VCAM-1) [50]. In particular, the recruited monocytes transdifferentiate into macrophages in the kidney interstitium. Myofibroblasts are responsible for producing fibrillar matrix in the renal interstitium [51]. Under normal conditions, a lower population of myofibroblasts is maintained. However, they are activated, and their number is increased through various ways (proliferation, epithelial mesenchymal transition (EMT), and recruitment of circulating fibrocytes derived from bone marrow cells) in a pathological environment. In addition, accumulation of ECM proteins within the kidney interstitium is the consequence of imbalance between synthesis and degradation of ECM. Thus, the expression of plasminogen activator inhibitor-1 (PAI-1, a specific inhibitor of urokinase-type and tissue-type plasminogen activator (uPA and tPA)) and tissue inhibitor of metalloproteinase 1 (tissue inhibitor matrix metalloproteinase-1, TIMP-1; a specific inhibitor of MMPs) are increased during fibrosis, resulting in the inhibition of ECM degradation [52–54]. Beyond the abovementioned pathological events, hemodynamic alterations also reduce post-glomerular blood flow to peritubular capillaries, which, in turn, leads to hypoxic conditions and damage to tubular epithelium [55].

5. Cellular Signaling Pathways Involved in Pathogenesis of DN

In the diabetic milieu, such as hyperglycemia and dyslipidemia, metabolic alteration increases the production of ROS mainly through the Polyol and/or Nox pathway [56,57]. In addition, an increased intracellular glucose level increases AGE production and ROS by activating the AGEs receptor (RAGE) axis [58]. These abnormal metabolic and physiological consequences directly induce both vascular endothelial cell dysfunction and hemodynamic alterations, including activation of the renin–angiotensin system. Subsequently, this impact triggers a number of cellular signaling cascades, including the protein kinase c (PKC), mitogen-activated protein kinases (MAPKs; p38 and c-Jun N-terminal kinases (JNK)), Janus kinase/signal transducer and activator of transcription protein (JAK/STAT), and transforming growth factor (TGF)-β/Smad, thereby inducing a cellular response via activation of key transcription factors, such as NF-κB [56,57]. In particular, several vasoactive factors (angiotensin II, thromboxane, and endothelin-1) enhance their fibrotic action in diabetic renal diseases via secondary induction of TGF-β expression [56,59].

The Smad signaling pathway has also been reported to be associated with the renal hypertrophy and accumulation of ECM molecules through TGF-β signaling in DN [56,60,61]. Accumulation of AGEs within the glomerular apparatus, mesangial matrix, and tubular cells also directly causes serious alteration of diabetic kidney structure by reacting with plasma proteins and extra vascular proteins. As a consequence, AGEs lead to the transcriptional upregulation of TGF-β1, IL-6, and NF-κB, possibly via activation of PKC and/or oxidative stress [59,62]. PKCs are important players for the onset and progression of DN via hyperglycemia-induced upregulation of vascular endothelial growth factor (VEGF) expression in the mesangial cells [63]. In response to such molecules or signals, chemokines, growth factors, and profibrotic factors are ultimately upregulated in renal cells, such as tubular epithelial cells, podocytes, and mesangial cells, which contribute to cellular injury, progressive fibrosis, and loss of glomerular filtration rate, thereby increasing proteinuria during the development and progression of DN [56,57].

Recently, new molecules or potential signaling pathways have been added to the established pathways, which has made the pathogenesis of DN more complex. However, new observations simultaneously increase the possibility of identifying new targets for the treatment of DN. Interleukin (IL)-33-mediated suppression of the tumorigenicity 2 receptor (ST2) axis is one such pathway, which is very attractive due to its association with inflammatory response. IL-33 was first identified as a member of the IL-1 family in 2005 [64]. IL-33 acts through ST2 [65], which plays an important role in the immunity against pathogens, type 2 inflammation, tissue homeostasis, and repair [66,67]. Soluble ST2 level elevates in the serum of CKD and is associated with the severity of the disease [68], possibly suggesting its role in the development of CKD. However, these studies are very limited.

Sodium–glucose cotransporter (SGLT)-2 may be a potential contributor to CKD. Under normal physiological conditions, urine does not contain glucose, owing to its effective reabsorption by two transporters, SGLT-1 and SGLT-2 [69]. The SGLT-2 transporter is located on the luminal side of the first segment of the proximal tubule in the kidney. It is a high-capacity, low-affinity transporter, but is responsible for the reabsorption of approximately 90% of all filtered glucose [70]. SGLT-2 inhibitor induces glycosuria and natriuresis by blocking reabsorption of glucose and sodium in the proximal tubule [71]. As a consequence, afferent arteriolar vasoconstriction is induced, thereby reducing intraglomerular pressure, decreasing hyperfiltration, and improving renal function [72].

Current evidence also suggests that autophagy is critical in kidney physiology and homeostasis. In the diabetic milieu, increased oxidative stress, inflammation, and mitochondrial dysfunction modulate the autophagy activation and inhibition as well as lead to cellular recycling dysfunction [73]. Reduction of autophagy induces loss of podocytes, damage in proximal tubular cells, and glomerulosclerosis [74,75]. High glucose treatment has activated autophagy in podocytes and protected the podocytes from hyperglycemia-related apoptosis [76]. Similarly, autophagy related 5 (Atg5)-knockout diabetic mice (deficiency of autophagy activation) showed more severe proteinuria and impaired renal function [77,78]. Autophagy also protects mesangial cells from apoptosis induced by TGF-β1 via transforming growth factor β-activated kinase (TAK)1 and PI3K–AKT-dependent pathways [79]. Several studies have consistently indicated that DN is associated with decreased autophagy and increased apoptosis [80–82].

6. Chronic Kidney Injury and LPA–LPAR Axis

CKD has been becoming a major public health problem globally. It involves a progressive loss of kidney function over a period of months or years, which frequently leads to end-stage renal failure [1]. The main risk factors of CKD include high blood pressure, diabetes, cardiac disease, and a family history of kidney failure with genetic problems [83]. The potential role of LPA in the pathogenesis of kidney disease was suggested for the first time following the discovery of a positive correlation between circulation LPA levels and renal dysfunction in patients with kidney disorder at the end of the 1990s [84]. Later on, Grove KJ et al. also reported that the LPA level was elevated in glomeruli of eNOS

(−/−) *db/db* mice, a robust model of DN [85]. Furthermore, LPA induced renal tubulointerstitial fibrosis, a classical hallmark of CKD, in a mouse model of unilateral ureteral obstruction [86]. More recently, LPA was identified as a biomarker of CKD in metabolic screening assay, using plasma samples from CKD patients with diverse etiologies and two different CKD rodent models [87]. Consistent with results of other studies, the LPA and LPC forms (16:0, 18:0, 18:1, and 18:2) were also detected in urine of DN patients [88]. On the contrary, several studies showed similar or reduced LPA levels in the plasma, but an increased urinary LPA level in CKD patients and animal models, suggesting that the local expression levels of LPA and LPARs are more important for the development of CKD [88–90]. LPA regulates various biological responses by binding to G-protein–coupled receptors (LPAR1–LPAR6) [5].

Recently, we and another group reported that the LPAR1 and/or LPAR3 were upregulated in different DN mouse models [91–93]. Treatment with a dual LPAR1/3 antagonist (Ki16425 or BMS002) or AM095 (a novel antagonist of LPAR1) reduced renal injury in the *db/db* mice (leptin receptor-deficient mouse with human type 2 diabetic phenotype) and streptozotocin (STZ)-induced diabetic mice (pancreatic beta cell-destroyed mouse with human type 1 diabetic phenotype) [91–93]. The expression of ATX and LPA production increases and activates the LPAR1-mediated signaling pathway in mesangial cells' exposure to high-glucose media and in the kidney cortex of diabetic *db/db* mice [91]. LPA–LPAR1 activation increases the phosphorylation of glycogen synthase kinase (GSK)3β at serine 9 residue (Ser9) and induces translocation of sterol regulatory element-binding protein (SREBP) 1 into the nucleus [91]. Subsequently, it induces TGF-β expression, which contributes to the development of glomerular injury in *db/db* mice. However, treatment of ki16425 reduces proteinuria, glomerular tuft area and volume, and mesangial matrix expansion by regulating the LPA–GSK3β–SREBP1 axis [91]. In line with our observation, LPAR1 deletion in unilateral ureteral obstruction-induced mice prevents renal fibrosis by suppressing the expression of connective tissue growth factor in proximal tubular epithelial cells [86]. Additionally, Diao et al. reported that LPAR3 deletion affects the spatiotemporal expression of collagen types I, III, IV, and VI in peri-implantation of the mouse uterus [94]. All of these studies suggest that the LPA–LPAR axis regulates renal fibrosis differently for different kidney cell types or different tissues, and that at least two receptors, LPAR1 and LPAR3, might be important contributors to renal fibrosis.

Similarly, Zhang et al. showed improvements in renal function, using a different dual LPAR1/3 antagonist, BMS002, in the endothelial nitric oxide synthase-deficient (eNOS (−/−)) *db/db* mouse [92]. The expressions of ATX, LPAR1, and LPAR3 proteins in these mice significantly increased in the glomerular podocytes and tubular epithelial cells in the renal cortex [92]. Blockading the LPAR1/3 activity ameliorated glomerular injury and reverses kidney dysfunction by reducing podocyte loss and increased the phosphorylation of Akt2 (known to be essential for maintaining podocyte viability and function) [95], which prevented reduction in the glomerular filtration rate and reduced proteinuria without affecting blood pressure [92]. However, the underlying molecular mechanism in their study was not fully addressed and further studies will be needed.

Furthermore, our studies showed that increased LPA levels in STZ-induced diabetic mice increases Toll-like receptor (TLR) 4 expression and directly activates the NF-κB, the master transcription factor responsible for inflammatory cytokine expression. Simultaneously, activated TLR4 also produces ROS through the nicotinamide adenine dinucleotide phosphate (NADPH) oxidase system [93]. All these intracellular changes synergistically activate NF-κB and/or JNK by increasing phosphorylation of p65 and JNK [93]. Ultimately, it leads to renal fibrosis via upregulation of pro-inflammatory cytokines and fibrotic factors, including TGF-β1, TIMP-1, and fibronectin. In contrast, AM095 treatment attenuates DN by downregulation of these signaling pathways in vivo. In mesangial cells, LPA treatment activates these signaling pathways similar to that in mice; however, this degree of activation was reduced by AM095 treatment [93]. We also observed some beneficial effects of AM095 treatment on glycemic control. However, the underlying mechanism should be addressed in future studies.

Mesangial cell proliferation and accumulation in the pathogenesis of DN is a major risk factor contributing to glomerulosclerosis. LPA treatment increased the proliferation of mouse mesangial cells (SV40 MES13), concomitant with the increased expression levels of cyclin D1 and CDK4 and decreased expression of p27^{Kip1}. The expression of Krüppel-like factor 5 (KLF5) was upregulated by activating MAPK and elevating the expression of early growth response 1 (Egr1) in the kidney cortex of *db/db* mice and LPA-treated SV40 MES13 cells. Moreover, LPA significantly increased the activity of Rac1 GTPase in SV40 MES13 cells, and the dominant–negative form of Rac1 blunted the phosphorylation of p38, the upregulation of Egr1, and the LPA-mediated induction of KLF5, indicating that the downstream pathway of Rac1 was involved in LPA-induced mesangial cell proliferation [96]. Taken together, these observations suggested that the Rac1/MAPK/KLF5 signaling pathway is one of the underlying mechanisms contributing to glomerular hyper proliferation during the progression of DN. Recently, Guo et al. showed that LPA activates β-catenin, a downstream mediator of Wnt signaling, in colon cancer cells and KLF5 plays a critical role in β-catenin activation [97]. Several studies directly indicated that the Wnt/β-catenin signaling pathway was implicated in renal fibrosis and apoptosis in CKD models [98,99]. Thus, the regulation of these pathways may provide a potential therapeutic target for the treatment of DN.

Some studies have also suggested that LPA may bind to the receptor for RAGE, a member of the immunoglobulin superfamily [36,100]. Under in vitro conditions, this interaction is essential for LPA-induced ovarian tumor implantation and metastasis, as well as for LPA-mediated proliferation and migration of vascular smooth muscle cells [36]. In addition, LPA failed to activate vascular Akt signaling in mice that were administered soluble RAGE or genetic deletion of RAGE [36]. These observations indicated that RAGE-mediated signal transduction may play an important role in diabetic microvascular complication, including DN. Zaslaysky et al. also revealed that three major LPARs (LPAR1-3) form homo- or hetero-dimers within the LPAR subgroup and hetero-dimers with sphingosine 1 phosphate receptor (S1PR), pH-sensing G protein-coupled receptor (GPR4), and ovarian cancer G-protein coupled receptor-1 (OGR1/GPR68) [101], thereby activating the downstream signaling pathways linked to inflammation and fibrosis. S1PR signaling activation promotes renal fibrosis in the diabetic condition [102–104]. In the terminal ileum of inflammatory bowel diseases, the expression of OGR1/GPR68 positively increases the expression of pro-fibrotic genes and collagen deposition, suggesting the potential involvement of these receptors, signaling for the pathogenesis of DN [105]. However, there is no direct evidence connecting DN pathogenesis with dimer formation between LPARs and these receptors. Another potential LPA receptor is the TRPV1 ion channel [37]. However, there have been no reports demonstrating its role in DN.

7. Conclusions and Future Research Directions

DN is the main risk factor for chronic kidney diseases, which mostly progress to the development of ESRD in the end. The best treatment regimen for DN is kidney replacement; however, it is highly restricted, due to various reasons, such as rare donors and rejection of the transplanted organ. Several medications are currently available for DN, but they are not sufficient for the recovery from kidney injury and restoration of kidney function in DN patients. Alternative drugs are thus required. Accumulated evidence indicates that the LPA–LPAR axis plays an important role in inducing pathological alterations of cell structure and function in the kidneys. Current studies showed that LPAR antagonism using pharmacological inhibitors significantly decreases the abnormality of kidney structure, such as GBM thickness, and increases of renal function, such as reducing proteinuria in different types of diabetic mouse models by regulating several signaling pathways, as shown in Figure 3.

The currently available data suggest that LPA signaling may regulate fibrosis, proliferation, and the inflammatory response in mesangial cells and podocytes or induce apoptosis via the following signaling pathways: 1) PI3K-AKT-GSK3β-TGF-β axis for fibrosis; 2) Rac1GTPase-MAPK-KLF5-CDK4/Cyclin D1 axis for proliferation; 3) TLR4-NADPH oxidase-ROS–NF-$_K$B/MAPK or TLR4-NF-$_K$B/MAPK axis for inflammatory response; 4) PI3K-AKT-GSK3α axis for apoptosis; 5) LPA-RAGE axis for glomerular injury; and 6) Wnt/β-catenin axis for fibrosis and apoptosis. For further details, please see above. LPAR: LPA receptor, RAGE: AGE receptor, Rac1: Ras-related C3 botulinum toxin substrate 1, NADPH:

Nicotinamide adenine dinucleotide phosphate oxidase, TLR4: Toll-like receptor 4, NF-$_K$B: Nuclear factor-$_K$B, KLF5: Krüppel-like factor 5.

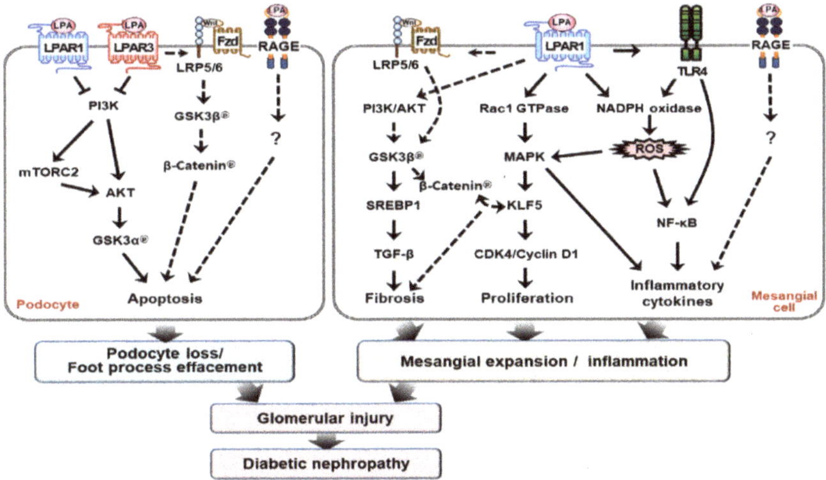

Figure 3. Schematic representation of LPA signaling in diabetic nephropathy models.

However, there are still many unanswered questions. Further studies should be performed in the following directions: Since the kidney consists of heterogeneous cells (such as podocytes, mesangial microvascular endothelial cells, and renal proximal tubule epithelial cells) and the LPAR expression level may be different in different cell types, further studies should first determine the LPAR expression level under different physiological and pathophysiological conditions. In addition, the studies should investigate the effects of LPAR antagonism on each type of kidney cell, using not only pharmacological inhibitors, but also genetically engineered in vivo models. Moreover, there are many different forms of LPA, which exhibit different affinities for each LPAR type. Each LPAR also exhibits various interaction affinities with one or more G protein subunits, thereby promoting different biological effects. These aspects should be further elucidated. Furthermore, the LPA–LPAR-mediated signaling pathway is also modulated by a cross-talk with other signaling pathways, such as epidermal growth factor (EGF) or vasoactive (angiotensin II) receptor-mediated signals [106], which will be defined in future studies. Since LPA regulates local blood flow, systemic blood pressure, and platelet function, and these factors directly play a critical role in renal function [40,107], future studies need to investigate the effect of LPA on the physiological and pathophysiological conditions in the renal vasculature and the tubular system. In addition, there are no studies demonstrating the relationship between the LPA–LPAR axis and the IL-33-ST2 axis and SGLT2 and autophagy. These new avenues should also be investigated in the future. Further understanding of the precise mechanisms underlying LPA action under physiological and pathophysiological conditions may facilitate the development of new therapeutic targets for DN.

Author Contributions: J.H.L. and H.-S.J. collected information and wrote the manuscript; J.H.L, D.K, Y.S.O, and H.-S.J. edited and revised the manuscript; J.H.L. and H.-S.J. approved the final version of the manuscript.

Funding: This work was supported by the Ministry of Education of Korea under a Basic Science Research Program Grant of the National Research Foundation of Korea (NRF-2016R1A2B2013347, NRF-2018R1C1B6000998, NRF-2017R1D1A1B03036210).

Conflicts of Interest: The authors declare no conflict of interest.

Abbreviations

DN	Diabetic nephropathy
ESRD	End-stage renal disease
ACE	Angiotensin converting enzyme
ARBs	Angiotensin II receptor blockers
LPA	Lysophosphatidic acid
ATX	Autotaxin
AGE	Advanced glycation end (product)
GPAT	Glycerol-3-phosphate acyltransferase
PLA1 and PLA2	Phospholipases A1 or A2
PA	Phosphatidic acid
LPE	Lysophosphatidylethanolamine
LPC	Lysophosphatidylcholine
LPS	Lysophosphatidylserine
LPPs	Lipid phosphate phosphatases
MAG	Monoacylglycerol
AGPAT	Acylglycerophosphate acyltransferase
PLC	Phospholipase C
DAG	Diacylglycerol
MAPK	Mitogen-activated protein kinase
PI3K	Phosphatidylinositol 3 kinase
PKB	Protein kinase B
ROCK	Rho-associated protein kinase
RAGE	Receptor for advanced glycation end products
Nox	NADPH oxidase
PPARγ	Peroxisome proliferator-activated receptor γ
CKD	Chronic kidney disease
ECM	Extracellular matrix
GBM	Glomerular basement membrane
EMT	Epithelial mesenchymal transition
CCL2/MCP1	Monocyte chemoattractant protein 1
CCL5/RANTES	Regulated upon activation, normal T cell expressed, and secreted
ICAM-1	Intercellular adhesion molecule-1
VCAM-1	Vascular cell adhesion molecule-1
PAI-1	Plasminogen activator inhibitor-1
uPA and tPA	Urokinase-type and tissue-type plasminogen activator
TIMP-1	Tissue inhibitor matrix metalloproteinase-1
JNK	c-Jun N-terminal kinases
VEGF	Vascular endothelial growth factor
SGLT-2	Sodium–glucose cotransporter-2
GSK3β	Glycogen synthase kinase 3β
SREBP 1	Sterol regulatory element-binding protein1
TGF-β	Transforming growth factor-β
TLR 4	Toll-like receptor 4
NF-κB	Nuclear factor-κB
KLF5	Krüppel-like factor 5
Egr1	Early growth response 1
S1PR	Sphingosine 1 phosphate receptor
GPR4	pH-sensing G protein-coupled receptor
OGR1/GPR68	Ovarian cancer G-protein coupled receptor-1

References

1. Gheith, O.; Farouk, N.; Nampoory, N.; Halim, M.A.; Al-Otaibi, T. Diabetic kidney disease: World wide difference of prevalence and risk factors. *J. Nephropharmacol.* **2016**, *5*, 49–56. [CrossRef] [PubMed]
2. Alicic, R.Z.; Rooney, M.T.; Tuttle, K.R. Diabetic kidney disease: Challenges, progress, and possibilities. *Clin. J. Am. Soc. Nephrol.* **2017**, *12*, 2032–2045. [CrossRef] [PubMed]
3. Dounousi, E.; Duni, A.; Leivaditis, K.; Vaios, V.; Eleftheriadis, T.; Liakopoulos, V. Improvements in the management of diabetic nephropathy. *Rev. Diabet. Stud.* **2015**, *12*, 119–133. [CrossRef] [PubMed]
4. Bash, L.D.; Selvin, E.; Steffes, M.; Coresh, J.; Astor, B.C. Poor glycemic control in diabetes and the risk of incident chronic kidney disease even in the absence of albuminuria and retinopathy: Atherosclerosis risk in communities (ARIC) study. *Arch. Intern. Med.* **2008**, *168*, 2440–2447. [CrossRef] [PubMed]
5. Yung, Y.C.; Stoddard, N.C.; Chun, J. LPA receptor signaling: Pharmacology, physiology, and pathophysiology. *J. Lipid Res.* **2014**, *55*, 1192–1214. [CrossRef] [PubMed]
6. Park, F.; Miller, D.D. Role of lysophosphatidic acid and its receptors in the kidney. *Physiol. Genom.* **2017**, *49*, 659–666. [CrossRef] [PubMed]
7. Aikawa, S.; Hashimoto, T.; Kano, K.; Aoki, J. Lysophosphatidic acid as a lipid mediator with multiple biological actions. *J. Biochem.* **2015**, *157*, 81–89. [CrossRef] [PubMed]
8. Choi, J.W.; Herr, D.R.; Noguchi, K.; Yung, Y.C.; Lee, C.W.; Mutoh, T.; Lin, M.E.; Teo, S.T.; Park, K.E.; Mosley, A.N.; et al. LPA receptors: Subtypes and biological actions. *Annu. Rev. Pharmacol. Toxicol.* **2010**, *50*, 157–186. [CrossRef]
9. Budd, D.C.; Qian, Y. Development of lysophosphatidic acid pathway modulators as therapies for fibrosis. *Future Med. Chem.* **2013**, *5*, 1935–1952. [CrossRef] [PubMed]
10. Chu, X.; Wei, X.; Lu, S.; He, P. Autotaxin-lpa receptor axis in the pathogenesis of lung diseases. *Int. J. Clin. Exp. Med.* **2015**, *8*, 17117–17122. [PubMed]
11. Rhee, S.Y.; Kim, Y.S. The role of advanced glycation end products in diabetic vascular complications. *Diabetes Metab. J.* **2018**, *42*, 188–195. [CrossRef] [PubMed]
12. Rabbani, N.; Thornalley, P.J. Advanced glycation end products in the pathogenesis of chronic kidney disease. *Kidney Int.* **2018**, *93*, 803–813. [CrossRef] [PubMed]
13. Valdes-Rives, S.A.; Gonzalez-Arenas, A. Autotaxin-lysophosphatidic acid: From inflammation to cancer development. *Mediat. Inflamm.* **2017**, *2017*, 9173090. [CrossRef]
14. Aoki, J. Mechanisms of lysophosphatidic acid production. *Semin. Cell Dev. Biol.* **2004**, *15*, 477–489. [CrossRef] [PubMed]
15. Prentki, M.; Madiraju, S.R. Glycerolipid metabolism and signaling in health and disease. *Endocr. Rev.* **2008**, *29*, 647–676. [CrossRef] [PubMed]
16. Mirzoyan, K. The Role of lpa in Kidney Pathologies. Ph.D. Thesis, Université Toulouse 3 Paul Sabatier, Toulouse, France, 2018.
17. Nakajima, K.; Sonoda, H.; Mizoguchi, T.; Aoki, J.; Arai, H.; Nagahama, M.; Tagaya, M.; Tani, K. A novel phospholipase a1 with sequence homology to a mammalian sec23p-interacting protein, p125. *J. Biol. Chem.* **2002**, *277*, 11329–11335. [CrossRef] [PubMed]
18. Richmond, G.S.; Smith, T.K. The role and characterization of phospholipase a1 in mediating lysophosphatidylcholine synthesis in trypanosoma brucei. *Biochem. J.* **2007**, *405*, 319–329. [CrossRef] [PubMed]
19. Aoki, J.; Inoue, A.; Okudaira, S. Two pathways for lysophosphatidic acid production. *Biochim. Biophys. Acta* **2008**, *1781*, 513–518. [CrossRef]
20. Nakanaga, K.; Hama, K.; Aoki, J. Autotaxin—An LPA producing enzyme with diverse functions. *J. Biochem.* **2010**, *148*, 13–24. [CrossRef]
21. Brindley, D.N.; Pilquil, C. Lipid phosphate phosphatases and signaling. *J. Lipid Res.* **2009**, *50* (Suppl. 1), S225–S230. [CrossRef]
22. Saba, J.D. Lysophospholipids in development: Miles apart and edging in. *J. Cell. Biochem.* **2004**, *92*, 967–992. [CrossRef] [PubMed]
23. Kok, B.P.; Venkatraman, G.; Capatos, D.; Brindley, D.N. Unlike two peas in a pod: Lipid phosphate phosphatases and phosphatidate phosphatases. *Chem. Rev.* **2012**, *112*, 5121–5146. [CrossRef] [PubMed]

24. Aguado, B.; Campbell, R.D. Characterization of a human lysophosphatidic acid acyltransferase that is encoded by a gene located in the class iii region of the human major histocompatibility complex. *J. Biol. Chem.* **1998**, *273*, 4096–4105. [CrossRef] [PubMed]

25. Wang, A.; Dennis, E.A. Mammalian lysophospholipases. *Biochim. Biophys. Acta* **1999**, *1439*, 1–16. [CrossRef]

26. Pasternack, S.M.; von Kugelgen, I.; Al Aboud, K.; Lee, Y.A.; Ruschendorf, F.; Voss, K.; Hillmer, A.M.; Molderings, G.J.; Franz, T.; Ramirez, A.; et al. G protein-coupled receptor P2Y5 and its ligand LPA are involved in maintenance of human hair growth. *Nat. Genet.* **2008**, *40*, 329–334. [CrossRef] [PubMed]

27. Fukushima, N.; Kimura, Y.; Chun, J. A single receptor encoded by VZG-1/LPA1/EDG-2 couples to g proteins and mediates multiple cellular responses to lysophosphatidic acid. *Proc. Natl. Acad. Sci. USA* **1998**, *95*, 6151–6156. [CrossRef] [PubMed]

28. Ishii, I.; Contos, J.J.; Fukushima, N.; Chun, J. Functional comparisons of the lysophosphatidic acid receptors, lp(a1)/vzg-1/edg-2, lp(a2)/edg-4, and lp(a3)/edg-7 in neuronal cell lines using a retrovirus expression system. *Mol. Pharmacol.* **2000**, *58*, 895–902. [CrossRef]

29. Lee, C.W.; Rivera, R.; Dubin, A.E.; Chun, J. LPA(4)/GPR23 is a lysophosphatidic acid (LPA) receptor utilizing g(s)-, g(q)/g(i)-mediated calcium signaling and G(12/13)-mediated rho activation. *J. Biol. Chem.* **2007**, *282*, 4310–4317. [CrossRef]

30. Noguchi, K.; Ishii, S.; Shimizu, T. Identification of P2Y9/GPR23 as a novel g protein-coupled receptor for lysophosphatidic acid, structurally distant from the edg family. *J. Biol. Chem.* **2003**, *278*, 25600–25606. [CrossRef]

31. Lee, C.W.; Rivera, R.; Gardell, S.; Dubin, A.E.; Chun, J. GPR92 as a new G12/13- and GQ-coupled lysophosphatidic acid receptor that increases camp, lpa5. *J. Biol. Chem.* **2006**, *281*, 23589–23597. [CrossRef]

32. Yanagida, K.; Masago, K.; Nakanishi, H.; Kihara, Y.; Hamano, F.; Tajima, Y.; Taguchi, R.; Shimizu, T.; Ishii, S. Identification and characterization of a novel lysophosphatidic acid receptor, P2Y5/LPA6. *J. Biol. Chem.* **2009**, *284*, 17731–17741. [CrossRef] [PubMed]

33. Riaz, A.; Huang, Y.; Johansson, S. G-protein-coupled lysophosphatidic acid receptors and their regulation of akt signaling. *Int. J. Mol. Sci.* **2016**, *17*, 215. [CrossRef] [PubMed]

34. Oka, S.; Ota, R.; Shima, M.; Yamashita, A.; Sugiura, T. GPR35 is a novel lysophosphatidic acid receptor. *Biochem. Biophys. Res. Commun.* **2010**, *395*, 232–237. [CrossRef] [PubMed]

35. Murakami, M.; Shiraishi, A.; Tabata, K.; Fujita, N. Identification of the orphan gpcr, p2y(10) receptor as the sphingosine-1-phosphate and lysophosphatidic acid receptor. *Biochem. Biophys. Res. Commun.* **2008**, *371*, 707–712. [CrossRef] [PubMed]

36. Rai, V.; Toure, F.; Chitayat, S.; Pei, R.; Song, F.; Li, Q.; Zhang, J.; Rosario, R.; Ramasamy, R.; Chazin, W.J.; et al. Lysophosphatidic acid targets vascular and oncogenic pathways via rage signaling. *J. Exp. Med.* **2012**, *209*, 2339–2350. [CrossRef] [PubMed]

37. Nieto-Posadas, A.; Picazo-Juarez, G.; Llorente, I.; Jara-Oseguera, A.; Morales-Lazaro, S.; Escalante-Alcalde, D.; Islas, L.D.; Rosenbaum, T. Lysophosphatidic acid directly activates TRPV1 through a c-terminal binding site. *Nat. Chem. Biol.* **2011**, *8*, 78–85. [CrossRef] [PubMed]

38. Bowman, M.A.; Schmidt, A.M. The next generation of rage modulators: Implications for soluble rage therapies in vascular inflammation. *J. Mol. Med.* **2013**, *91*, 1329–1331. [CrossRef] [PubMed]

39. McIntyre, T.M.; Pontsler, A.V.; Silva, A.R.; St Hilaire, A.; Xu, Y.; Hinshaw, J.C.; Zimmerman, G.A.; Hama, K.; Aoki, J.; Arai, H.; et al. Identification of an intracellular receptor for lysophosphatidic acid (LPA): Lpa is a transcellular ppargamma agonist. *Proc. Natl. Acad. Sci. USA* **2003**, *100*, 131–136. [CrossRef]

40. Pradere, J.P.; Gonzalez, J.; Klein, J.; Valet, P.; Gres, S.; Salant, D.; Bascands, J.L.; Saulnier-Blache, J.S.; Schanstra, J.P. Lysophosphatidic acid and renal fibrosis. *Biochim. Biophys. Acta* **2008**, *1781*, 582–587. [CrossRef]

41. Makris, K.; Spanou, L. Acute kidney injury: Definition, pathophysiology and clinical phenotypes. *Clin. Biochem. Rev.* **2016**, *37*, 85–98.

42. Levey, A.S.; Levin, A.; Kellum, J.A. Definition and classification of kidney diseases. *Am. J. Kidney Dis.* **2013**, *61*, 686–688. [CrossRef] [PubMed]

43. Hewitson, T.D.; Holt, S.G.; Smith, E.R. Progression of tubulointerstitial fibrosis and the chronic kidney disease phenotype—Role of risk factors and epigenetics. *Front. Pharmacol.* **2017**, *8*, 520. [CrossRef] [PubMed]

44. Ke, B.; Fan, C.; Yang, L.; Fang, X. Matrix metalloproteinases-7 and kidney fibrosis. *Front. Physiol.* **2017**, *8*, 21. [CrossRef] [PubMed]

45. Xiao, Z.; Chen, C.; Meng, T.; Zhang, W.; Zhou, Q. Resveratrol attenuates renal injury and fibrosis by inhibiting transforming growth factor-β pathway on matrix metalloproteinase 7. *Exp. Biol. Med.* **2016**, *241*, 140–146. [CrossRef] [PubMed]

46. Rosenberg, A.Z.; Kopp, J.B. Focal segmental glomerulosclerosis. *Clin. J. Am. Soc. Nephrol.* **2017**, *12*, 502–517. [CrossRef]

47. Humphreys, B.D. Mechanisms of renal fibrosis. *Annu. Rev. Physiol.* **2018**, *80*, 309–326. [CrossRef]

48. Reiser, J.; Altintas, M.M. Podocytes. *F1000 Res.* **2016**, *5*. [CrossRef]

49. Iwano, M.; Neilson, E.G. Mechanisms of tubulointerstitial fibrosis. *Curr. Opin. Nephrol. Hypertens.* **2004**, *13*, 279–284. [CrossRef]

50. Lee, S.B.; Kalluri, R. Mechanistic connection between inflammation and fibrosis. *Kidney Int. Suppl.* **2010**, S22–S26. [CrossRef]

51. Grgic, I.; Duffield, J.S.; Humphreys, B.D. The origin of interstitial myofibroblasts in chronic kidney disease. *Pediatr. Nephrol.* **2012**, *27*, 183–193. [CrossRef]

52. Ye, Y.; Vattai, A.; Zhang, X.; Zhu, J.; Thaler, C.J.; Mahner, S.; Jeschke, U.; von Schonfeldt, V. Role of plasminogen activator inhibitor type 1 in pathologies of female reproductive diseases. *Int. J. Mol. Sci.* **2017**, *18*, 1651. [CrossRef] [PubMed]

53. Hu, C.; Sun, L.; Xiao, L.; Han, Y.; Fu, X.; Xiong, X.; Xu, X.; Liu, Y.; Yang, S.; Liu, F.; et al. Insights into the mechanisms involved in the expression and regulation of extracellular matrix proteins in diabetic nephropathy. *Curr. Med. Chem.* **2015**, *22*, 2858–2870. [CrossRef] [PubMed]

54. Hodgkins, K.S.; Schnaper, H.W. Tubulointerstitial injury and the progression of chronic kidney disease. *Pediatr. Nephrol.* **2012**, *27*, 901–909. [CrossRef] [PubMed]

55. Singh, D.K.; Winocour, P.; Farrington, K. Mechanisms of disease: The hypoxic tubular hypothesis of diabetic nephropathy. *Nat. Clin. Pract. Nephrol.* **2008**, *4*, 216–226. [CrossRef] [PubMed]

56. Bhattacharjee, N.; Barma, S.; Konwar, N.; Dewanjee, S.; Manna, P. Mechanistic insight of diabetic nephropathy and its pharmacotherapeutic targets: An update. *Eur. J. Pharmacol.* **2016**, *791*, 8–24. [CrossRef] [PubMed]

57. Kawanami, D.; Matoba, K.; Utsunomiya, K. Signaling pathways in diabetic nephropathy. *Histol. Histopathol.* **2016**, *31*, 1059–1067. [PubMed]

58. Kanwar, Y.S.; Wada, J.; Sun, L.; Xie, P.; Wallner, E.I.; Chen, S.; Chugh, S.; Danesh, F.R. Diabetic nephropathy: Mechanisms of renal disease progression. *Exp. Biol. Med.* **2008**, *233*, 4–11. [CrossRef]

59. Nowotny, K.; Jung, T.; Hohn, A.; Weber, D.; Grune, T. Advanced glycation end products and oxidative stress in type 2 diabetes mellitus. *Biomolecules* **2015**, *5*, 194–222. [CrossRef]

60. Sureshbabu, A.; Muhsin, S.A.; Choi, M.E. TGF-β signaling in the kidney: Profibrotic and protective effects. *Am. J. Physiol. Ren. Physiol.* **2016**, *310*, F596–F606. [CrossRef]

61. Chang, A.S.; Hathaway, C.K.; Smithies, O.; Kakoki, M. Transforming growth factor-β1 and diabetic nephropathy. *Am. J. Physiol. Ren. Physiol.* **2016**, *310*, F689–F696. [CrossRef]

62. Volpe, C.M.O.; Villar-Delfino, P.H.; Dos Anjos, P.M.F.; Nogueira-Machado, J.A. Cellular death, reactive oxygen species (ROS) and diabetic complications. *Cell Death Dis.* **2018**, *9*, 119. [CrossRef] [PubMed]

63. Tufro, A.; Veron, D. Vegf and podocytes in diabetic nephropathy. *Semin. Nephrol.* **2012**, *32*, 385–393. [CrossRef] [PubMed]

64. Schmitz, J.; Owyang, A.; Oldham, E.; Song, Y.; Murphy, E.; McClanahan, T.K.; Zurawski, G.; Moshrefi, M.; Qin, J.; Li, X.; et al. IL-33, an interleukin-1-like cytokine that signals via the IL-1 receptor-related protein ST2 and induces t helper type 2-associated cytokines. *Immunity* **2005**, *23*, 479–490. [CrossRef] [PubMed]

65. Gao, Q.; Li, Y.; Li, M. The potential role of IL-33/ST2 signaling in fibrotic diseases. *J. Leukoc. Biol.* **2015**, *98*, 15–22. [CrossRef] [PubMed]

66. Tonacci, A.; Quattrocchi, P.; Gangemi, S. IL33/ST2 axis in diabetic kidney disease: A literature review. *Medicina* **2019**, *55*, 50. [CrossRef] [PubMed]

67. Cao, Q.; Wang, Y.; Niu, Z.; Wang, C.; Wang, R.; Zhang, Z.; Chen, T.; Wang, X.M.; Li, Q.; Lee, V.W.S.; et al. Potentiating tissue-resident type 2 innate lymphoid cells by IL-33 to prevent renal ischemia-reperfusion injury. *J. Am. Soc. Nephrol.* **2018**, *29*, 961–976. [CrossRef]

68. Bao, Y.S.; Na, S.P.; Zhang, P.; Jia, X.B.; Liu, R.C.; Yu, C.Y.; Mu, S.H.; Xie, R.J. Characterization of interleukin-33 and soluble ST2 in serum and their association with disease severity in patients with chronic kidney disease. *J. Clin. Immunol.* **2012**, *32*, 587–594. [CrossRef]

69. Wilding, J.P. The role of the kidneys in glucose homeostasis in type 2 diabetes: Clinical implications and therapeutic significance through sodium glucose co-transporter 2 inhibitors. *Metab. Clin. Exp.* **2014**, *63*, 1228–1237. [CrossRef]

70. Vallon, V.; Thomson, S.C. Targeting renal glucose reabsorption to treat hyperglycaemia: The pleiotropic effects of SGLT2 inhibition. *Diabetologia* **2017**, *60*, 215–225. [CrossRef]

71. Sano, M.; Takei, M.; Shiraishi, Y.; Suzuki, Y. Increased hematocrit during sodium-glucose cotransporter 2 inhibitor therapy indicates recovery of tubulointerstitial function in diabetic kidneys. *J. Clin. Med. Res.* **2016**, *8*, 844–847. [CrossRef]

72. Dekkers, C.C.J.; Gansevoort, R.T.; Heerspink, H.J.L. New diabetes therapies and diabetic kidney disease progression: The role of SGLT-2 inhibitors. *Curr. Diabetes Rep.* **2018**, *18*, 27. [CrossRef] [PubMed]

73. Susztak, K.; Raff, A.C.; Schiffer, M.; Bottinger, E.P. Glucose-induced reactive oxygen species cause apoptosis of podocytes and podocyte depletion at the onset of diabetic nephropathy. *Diabetes* **2006**, *55*, 225–233. [CrossRef] [PubMed]

74. Lin, T.A.; Wu, V.C.; Wang, C.Y. Autophagy in chronic kidney diseases. *Cells* **2019**, *8*, 61. [CrossRef] [PubMed]

75. Tagawa, A.; Yasuda, M.; Kume, S.; Yamahara, K.; Nakazawa, J.; Chin-Kanasaki, M.; Araki, H.; Araki, S.; Koya, D.; Asanuma, K.; et al. Impaired podocyte autophagy exacerbates proteinuria in diabetic nephropathy. *Diabetes* **2016**, *65*, 755–767. [CrossRef]

76. Lenoir, O.; Jasiek, M.; Henique, C.; Guyonnet, L.; Hartleben, B.; Bork, T.; Chipont, A.; Flosseau, K.; Bensaada, I.; Schmitt, A.; et al. Endothelial cell and podocyte autophagy synergistically protect from diabetes-induced glomerulosclerosis. *Autophagy* **2015**, *11*, 1130–1145. [CrossRef] [PubMed]

77. Liu, N.; Xu, L.; Shi, Y.; Zhuang, S. Podocyte autophagy: A potential therapeutic target to prevent the progression of diabetic nephropathy. *J. Diabetes Res.* **2017**, *2017*, 3560238. [CrossRef] [PubMed]

78. Ma, T.; Zhu, J.; Chen, X.; Zha, D.; Singhal, P.C.; Ding, G. High glucose induces autophagy in podocytes. *Exp. Cell Res.* **2013**, *319*, 779–789. [CrossRef]

79. Ding, Y.; Kim, J.K.; Kim, S.I.; Na, H.J.; Jun, S.Y.; Lee, S.J.; Choi, M.E. TGF-β1 protects against mesangial cell apoptosis via induction of autophagy. *J. Biol. Chem.* **2010**, *285*, 37909–37919. [CrossRef]

80. Yasuda-Yamahara, M.; Kume, S.; Tagawa, A.; Maegawa, H.; Uzu, T. Emerging role of podocyte autophagy in the progression of diabetic nephropathy. *Autophagy* **2015**, *11*, 2385–2386. [CrossRef]

81. Ding, Y.; Choi, M.E. Autophagy in diabetic nephropathy. *J. Endocrinol.* **2015**, *224*, R15–R30. [CrossRef]

82. Yamahara, K.; Kume, S.; Koya, D.; Tanaka, Y.; Morita, Y.; Chin-Kanasaki, M.; Araki, H.; Isshiki, K.; Araki, S.; Haneda, M.; et al. Obesity-mediated autophagy insufficiency exacerbates proteinuria-induced tubulointerstitial lesions. *J. Am. Soc. Nephrol.* **2013**, *24*, 1769–1781. [CrossRef] [PubMed]

83. Macisaac, R.J.; Ekinci, E.I.; Jerums, G. Markers of and risk factors for the development and progression of diabetic kidney disease. *Am. J. Kidney Dis.* **2014**, *63*, S39–S62. [CrossRef] [PubMed]

84. Sasagawa, T.; Suzuki, K.; Shiota, T.; Kondo, T.; Okita, M. The significance of plasma lysophospholipids in patients with renal failure on hemodialysis. *J. Nutr. Sci. Vitaminol.* **1998**, *44*, 809–818. [CrossRef] [PubMed]

85. Grove, K.J.; Voziyan, P.A.; Spraggins, J.M.; Wang, S.; Paueksakon, P.; Harris, R.C.; Hudson, B.G.; Caprioli, R.M. Diabetic nephropathy induces alterations in the glomerular and tubule lipid profiles. *J. Lipid Res.* **2014**, *55*, 1375–1385. [CrossRef] [PubMed]

86. Sakai, N.; Chun, J.; Duffield, J.S.; Lagares, D.; Wada, T.; Luster, A.D.; Tager, A.M. Lysophosphatidic acid signaling through its receptor initiates profibrotic epithelial cell fibroblast communication mediated by epithelial cell derived connective tissue growth factor. *Kidney Int.* **2017**, *91*, 628–641. [CrossRef] [PubMed]

87. Zhang, Z.H.; Chen, H.; Vaziri, N.D.; Mao, J.R.; Zhang, L.; Bai, X.; Zhao, Y.Y. Metabolomic signatures of chronic kidney disease of diverse etiologies in the rats and humans. *J. Proteome Res.* **2016**, *15*, 3802–3812. [CrossRef] [PubMed]

88. Saulnier-Blache, J.S.; Feigerlova, E.; Halimi, J.M.; Gourdy, P.; Roussel, R.; Guerci, B.; Dupuy, A.; Bertrand-Michel, J.; Bascands, J.L.; Hadjadj, S.; et al. Urinary lysophopholipids are increased in diabetic patients with nephropathy. *J. Diabetes Its Complicat.* **2017**, *31*, 1103–1108. [CrossRef]

89. Michalczyk, A.; Dolegowska, B.; Heryc, R.; Chlubek, D.; Safranow, K. Associations between plasma lysophospholipids concentrations, chronic kidney disease and the type of renal replacement therapy. *Lipids Health Dis.* **2019**, *18*, 85. [CrossRef]

90. Mirzoyan, K.; Baiotto, A.; Dupuy, A.; Marsal, D.; Denis, C.; Vinel, C.; Sicard, P.; Bertrand-Michel, J.; Bascands, J.L.; Schanstra, J.P.; et al. Increased urinary lysophosphatidic acid in mouse with subtotal

nephrectomy: Potential involvement in chronic kidney disease. *J. Phys. Biochem.* **2016**, *72*, 803–812. [CrossRef]

91. Li, H.Y.; Oh, Y.S.; Choi, J.W.; Jung, J.Y.; Jun, H.S. Blocking lysophosphatidic acid receptor 1 signaling inhibits diabetic nephropathy in db/db mice. *Kidney Int.* **2017**, *91*, 1362–1373. [CrossRef]

92. Zhang, M.Z.; Wang, X.; Yang, H.; Fogo, A.B.; Murphy, B.J.; Kaltenbach, R.; Cheng, P.; Zinker, B.; Harris, R.C. Lysophosphatidic acid receptor antagonism protects against diabetic nephropathy in a type 2 diabetic model. *J. Am. Soc. Nephrol.* **2017**, *28*, 3300–3311. [CrossRef] [PubMed]

93. Lee, J.H.; Sarker, M.K.; Choi, H.; Shin, D.; Kim, D.; Jun, H.S. Lysophosphatidic acid receptor 1 inhibitor, am095, attenuates diabetic nephropathy in mice by downregulation of TLR4/NF-κB signaling and NADPH oxidase. *Biochim. Biophys. Acta. Mol. Basis Dis.* **2019**, *1865*, 1332–1340. [CrossRef] [PubMed]

94. Diao, H.; Aplin, J.D.; Xiao, S.; Chun, J.; Li, Z.; Chen, S.; Ye, X. Altered spatiotemporal expression of collagen types i, iii, iv, and vi in LPAR3-deficient peri-implantation mouse uterus. *Biol. Reprod.* **2011**, *84*, 255–265. [CrossRef] [PubMed]

95. Canaud, G.; Bienaime, F.; Viau, A.; Treins, C.; Baron, W.; Nguyen, C.; Burtin, M.; Berissi, S.; Giannakakis, K.; Muda, A.O.; et al. Akt2 is essential to maintain podocyte viability and function during chronic kidney disease. *Nat. Med.* **2013**, *19*, 1288–1296. [CrossRef] [PubMed]

96. Kim, D.; Li, H.Y.; Lee, J.H.; Oh, Y.S.; Jun, H.S. Lysophosphatidic acid increases mesangial cell proliferation in models of diabetic nephropathy via RAC1/MAPK/KLF5 signaling. *Exp. Mol. Med.* **2019**, *51*, 18. [CrossRef] [PubMed]

97. Guo, L.; He, P.; No, Y.R.; Yun, C.C. Kruppel-like factor 5 incorporates into the β-catenin/TCF complex in response to LPA in colon cancer cells. *Cell. Signal.* **2015**, *27*, 961–968. [CrossRef] [PubMed]

98. Lin, X.; Zha, Y.; Zeng, X.Z.; Dong, R.; Wang, Q.H.; Wang, D.T. Role of the wnt/β-catenin signaling pathway in inducing apoptosis and renal fibrosis in 5/6-nephrectomized rats. *Mol. Med. Rep.* **2017**, *15*, 3575–3582. [CrossRef] [PubMed]

99. Tan, R.J.; Zhou, D.; Zhou, L.; Liu, Y. Wnt/β-catenin signaling and kidney fibrosis. *Kidney Int. Suppl.* **2014**, *4*, 84–90. [CrossRef]

100. Manigrasso, M.B.; Juranek, J.; Ramasamy, R.; Schmidt, A.M. Unlocking the biology of rage in diabetic microvascular complications. *Trends Endocrinol. Metab.* **2014**, *25*, 15–22. [CrossRef]

101. Zaslavsky, A.; Singh, L.S.; Tan, H.; Ding, H.; Liang, Z.; Xu, Y. Homo- and hetero-dimerization of LPA/S1P receptors, OGR1 and GPR4. *Biochimi. Biophys. Acta* **2006**, *1761*, 1200–1212. [CrossRef]

102. Yaghobian, D.; Don, A.S.; Yaghobian, S.; Chen, X.; Pollock, C.A.; Saad, S. Increased sphingosine 1-phosphate mediates inflammation and fibrosis in tubular injury in diabetic nephropathy. *Clin. Exp. Pharmacol. Physiol.* **2016**, *43*, 56–66. [CrossRef] [PubMed]

103. Ishizawa, S.; Takahashi-Fujigasaki, J.; Kanazawa, Y.; Matoba, K.; Kawanami, D.; Yokota, T.; Iwamoto, T.; Tajima, N.; Manome, Y.; Utsunomiya, K. Sphingosine-1-phosphate induces differentiation of cultured renal tubular epithelial cells under rho kinase activation via the S1P2 receptor. *Clin. Exp. Nephrol.* **2014**, *18*, 844–852. [CrossRef] [PubMed]

104. Huang, K.; Liu, W.; Lan, T.; Xie, X.; Peng, J.; Huang, J.; Wang, S.; Shen, X.; Liu, P.; Huang, H. Berberine reduces fibronectin expression by suppressing the S1P-S1P2 receptor pathway in experimental diabetic nephropathy models. *PLoS ONE* **2012**, *7*, e43874. [CrossRef]

105. Hutter, S.; van Haaften, W.T.; Hunerwadel, A.; Baebler, K.; Herfarth, N.; Raselli, T.; Mamie, C.; Misselwitz, B.; Rogler, G.; Weder, B.; et al. Intestinal activation of ph-sensing receptor OGR1 [GPR68] contributes to fibrogenesis. *J. Crohn Colitis* **2018**, *12*, 1348–1358. [CrossRef] [PubMed]

106. Colin-Santana, C.C.; Avendano-Vazquez, S.E.; Alcantara-Hernandez, R.; Garcia-Sainz, J.A. Egf and angiotensin ii modulate lysophosphatidic acid LPA(1) receptor function and phosphorylation state. *Biochim. Biophys. Acta* **2011**, *1810*, 1170–1177. [CrossRef] [PubMed]

107. Xu, K.; Ma, L.; Li, Y.; Wang, F.; Zheng, G.Y.; Sun, Z.; Jiang, F.; Chen, Y.; Liu, H.; Dang, A.; et al. Genetic and functional evidence supports lpar1 as a susceptibility gene for hypertension. *Hypertension* **2015**, *66*, 641–646. [CrossRef]

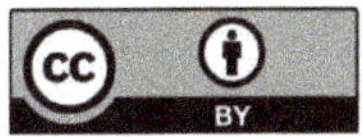

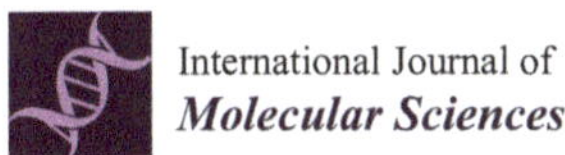 International Journal of
Molecular Sciences

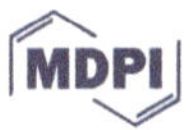

Review

Unraveling the Role of Inflammation in the Pathogenesis of Diabetic Kidney Disease

Keiichiro Matoba [1,*], Yusuke Takeda [1], Yosuke Nagai [1], Daiji Kawanami [2], Kazunori Utsunomiya [3] and Rimei Nishimura [1]

1   Division of Diabetes, Metabolism, and Endocrinology, Department of Internal Medicine, The Jikei University School of Medicine, Tokyo 105-8461, Japan
2   Department of Endocrinology and Diabetes Mellitus, Fukuoka University School of Medicine, Fukuoka 814-0180, Japan
3   Center for Preventive Medicine, The Jikei University School of Medicine, Tokyo 105-8461, Japan
*   Correspondence: matoba@jikei.ac.jp

Received: 10 June 2019; Accepted: 8 July 2019; Published: 10 July 2019

Abstract: Diabetic kidney disease (DKD) remains the leading cause of end-stage renal disease (ESRD) and is therefore a major burden on the healthcare system. Patients with DKD are highly susceptible to developing cardiovascular disease, which contributes to increased morbidity and mortality rates. While progress has been made to inhibit the acceleration of DKD, current standards of care reduce but do not eliminate the risk of DKD. There is growing appreciation for the role of inflammation in modulating the process of DKD. The focus of this review is on providing an overview of the current status of knowledge regarding the pathologic roles of inflammation in the development of DKD. Finally, we summarize recent therapeutic advances to prevent DKD, with a focus on the anti-inflammatory effects of newly developed agents.

Keywords: diabetic kidney disease; diabetic nephropathy; inflammation; signaling cascade

---

1. Introduction

The pandemic of diabetes has become a global health burden. Despite accumulating evidence supporting the prevention of obesity and related metabolic disorders, this knowledge has not translated into action that strongly reduces the prevalence of diabetes, especially in middle- and low-income countries. The International Diabetes Federation (IDF) estimates that diabetes affects 425 million people globally, and the number of diabetic patients will increase to 630 million in 2045.

Such an increase also means that the prevalence of diabetic kidney disease (DKD) continues to rise. DKD is the leading cause of end-stage renal disease (ESRD) and is associated with increased mortality due to cardiovascular disease in subjects with diabetes. Evidence is mounting that albuminuria is not only a hallmark of DKD but also an independent risk factor of coronary disease. The UK Prospective Diabetes Study (UKPDS) demonstrated that annual cardiovascular mortality rates increase to 3%, 4.6%, and 19.2% with the progression to microalbuminuria, macroalbuminuria, and renal failure, respectively [1]. Indeed, patients with DKD are more likely to die from coronary disease than to ever reach ESRD. Due to its high morbidity and mortality, the socioeconomic costs of DKD are staggering. It is therefore urgent that we establish effective and safe therapeutic strategies against DKD in order to improve the prognosis of diabetic patients. To this end, a detailed understanding of the molecular mechanisms that drive DKD is required.

The current understanding of the mechanisms responsible for the progression of DKD recognizes the involvement of metabolic abnormalities (e.g., hyperglycemia, hypertension, and dyslipidemia), hemodynamic changes, renin–angiotensin system (RAS) activation, and oxidative stress. While several approaches have been clinically implemented in order to slow the acceleration of DKD, the current management of DKD is insufficient, both for preventing DKD and for halting its progression.

Given the limitations of therapeutic regimens for inhibiting DKD, there has been an ongoing effort to elucidate the molecular basis responsible for the renal damage and to develop novel drugs. Recent research is characterized by a variety of investigations exploring the inflammatory regulators of DKD. Circulating levels of inflammatory mediators and macrophage infiltration into renal tissue have been found to be increased in both animal models and patients with DKD. Furthermore, adhesion molecules and chemokines are upregulated in diabetic kidneys. These findings highlight the importance of inflammatory mechanisms in facilitating renal damage in the setting of diabetes.

We herein review the inflammatory mediators of diabetes and their contribution to renal injury and describe the potential of anti-diabetic medications as well as drug candidates for inhibiting renal inflammation in the progression of DKD.

2. Inflammatory Mediators in Diabetic Kidney Disease (DKD)

Low-grade inflammation is defined as an activation of the innate immune system response. This is clinically considered an increase in circulating levels of pro-inflammatory cytokines and other mediators that activate the immune system. Chronic low-grade inflammation plays a causal role in the progression of obesity and insulin resistance. Deficits in specific genes critical for inflammation are known to be protective against the initiation and development of metabolic diseases in animal models. Therefore, inflammation is considered to be a trigger rather than a result of chronic underlying conditions.

Inflammation is increasingly postulated to be central to the progression of atherogenic changes and microvascular complications in the setting of diabetes [2]. For example, the activation of inflammatory pathways, especially E-selectin and other adhesion molecules, is linked to the pathogenesis of diabetic retinopathy [3]. These adhesion mediators stimulate the migration of retinal capillary endothelium and angiogenesis in the progression of diabetic retinopathy. In addition, evidence of the role of inflammatory signals in the development of diabetic neuropathy has been shown in experimental models of diabetes [4,5] and in clinical studies [6,7]. Diabetic patients with painful peripheral neuropathy have higher levels of inflammatory markers than subjects without pain, and the elevation of interleukin (IL)-1, IL-6, and tumor necrosis factor α (TNF-α) are correlated with the progression of degenerative changes in the peripheral nerves. The expression of nuclear factor-2 erythroid related factor 2 (Nrf2), a regulator of endogenous anti-oxidant production, is decreased in patients with diabetic peripheral neuropathy, which can result in inflammation, exacerbated oxidative stress, nerve injury, and an insufficient blood supply [8]. As with retinopathy and neuropathy, the infiltration of inflammatory cells and expression of adhesion molecules and cytokines are detected in renal tissue obtained from subjects with DKD.

2.1. Macrophages

Blood monocytes and tissue macrophages are key members of the mononuclear phagocyte system, a component of innate immunity. Recently, intensive research has shown that the influx of macrophages is a prominent feature during the progression of chronic kidney disease [9] and is tightly correlated with the decline in the glomerular filtration rate (GFR), histological changes, and a poor outcome in this condition [10]. Macrophage-derived products, including reactive oxygen species (ROS), pro-inflammatory factors, metalloproteinases, and growth factors, can induce further renal damage in the setting of diabetes. Macrophage-depletion studies in rodent models have shown a causal role for macrophages in the progression of DKD. For instance, the deletion of a macrophage scavenger receptor protected diabetic mice from albuminuria, mesangial matrix expansion, and the overproduction of transforming growth factor β (TGF-β) [11]. The gene expression of pro-inflammatory factors was strongly suppressed in this diabetic mouse model.

Macrophages are classified into classically-activated M1 and alternatively-activated M2 states [12]. M1 macrophages promote the inflammatory process by elaborating pro-inflammatory factors and ROS, whereas M2 macrophages resolve inflammation and induce tissue remodeling with the release of growth factors. In simple inflammatory reactions, such as acute arthritis, macrophages progress linearly through the M1 and M2 phases. However, under chronic inflammatory conditions, such as atherosclerosis and DKD, both M1 and M2 macrophages coexist, and this imbalance in the M1/M2 macrophage phenotype may be a key point of DKD.

Notably, an experimental study showed that macrophages in streptozotocin-induced DKD are predominantly of the M1 phenotype [9,13]. Furthermore, RAW264.7 macrophages switch to the M1 phenotype when cultured in a high-glucose milieu. Consistent with these results, the glomerular expression of inducible nitric oxide and TNF-α is increased in insulin-deficient diabetic mouse models, suggesting the presence of M1 macrophages. The deletion of the Toll-like receptor-2 gene significantly induces a macrophage M1 to M2 polarization shift in the diabetic kidney, attenuates urinary albumin excretion, and protects podocytes from apoptosis and morphological changes [13]. The mechanisms by which M2 macrophages promote kidney repair and attenuate DKD progression are still under debate and merit further investigation.

2.2. Adhesion Molecules and Chemokines

While the precise molecular mechanisms that direct monocyte homing into the sites of renal inflammation are not fully understood, endothelial-leukocyte adhesion molecules, including vascular cell adhesion molecule 1 (VCAM1) and intercellular adhesion molecule 1 (ICAM1), have been considered to play important roles in the initiation of renal inflammation. Several studies provide compelling evidence supporting the importance of these molecules in monocyte recruitment. For example, these adhesion molecules are abundantly expressed in renal biopsy specimens obtained from patients with DKD. Furthermore, circulating levels of VCAM1 and ICAM1 are independently associated with DKD progression [14,15].

VCAM1, also known as CD106, is a transmembrane glycoprotein expressed in activated endothelium under a variety of pathologic conditions, including atherosclerosis and DKD. VCAM1 binds to $\alpha4\beta1$ integrin, which is constitutively expressed on lymphocytes, monocytes, and eosinophils. The renal filtration function declines and urinary albumin excretion levels increase progressively with the elevation in VCAM1 levels in serum [16]. ICAM1, also known as CD54, is expressed structurally on endothelial cells and works as a ligand for lymphocyte function-associated antigen 1 (LFA-1) on monocytes. Its expression is also upregulated in endothelial cells in a diabetic milieu, and genetic polymorphisms in its gene are associated with DKD progression [17]. The deletion of the ICAM1 gene ameliorates renal inflammation in mice [18], indicating that ICAM1 contributes to the pathogenesis of DKD.

After adhering to the endothelium, monocytes migrate through endothelial cells via chemokines. Studies of DKD rodents and in human diabetic kidneys have shown that macrophages infiltrate the renal tissue in response to an upregulation of chemokines, such as monocyte chemoattractant protein 1 (MCP1), also known as CCL2. Nadkarni et al. investigated urinary MCP1 for its associations with the deterioration of the renal function in order to illuminate its potential as a urinary marker of DKD progression [19]. They reported that an increased level of urinary MCP1 was strongly associated with a decline in the renal function in patients with diabetes, suggesting that excreted MCP1 levels may be a useful biomarker for predicting progressive decline in DKD [20].

The induction of MCP1 by inflammatory cytokines in renal cells elicits the initial step of glomerular and tubular inflammation. Although a number of cytokines have been shown to be involved in the production of MCP1, there is compelling evidence that TNF-α functions as a potent inducer of MCP1 expression in the kidney. TNF-α is expressed in adipose tissue and has been implicated in the pathogenesis of insulin resistance and type 2 diabetes. In addition, it has been shown that the serum concentrations and urinary excretion of TNF-α are increased in patients with various kidney diseases, suggesting that excessive TNF-α in the systemic circulation may result in the upregulation of MCP1 in the kidney. Furthermore, elevated serum levels of TNF receptors (TNF-R) 1 or 2 are strongly associated with a risk of renal functional decline or ESRD [7,21]. Niewczas et al. investigated 194 circulating inflammatory factors in patients from three independent cohorts with type 1 and type 2 diabetes and demonstrated an extremely robust kidney risk inflammatory signature, including 17 proteins enriched in TNF-R superfamily members [22], which were associated with a 10-year risk of ESRD.

TNF-α secreted by infiltrated macrophages itself may also stimulate the local production of MCP1 in renal cells. Consequently, manipulating the MCP1 signaling axis offers an opportunity for therapeutic gain. A clinical trial is underway investigating the effectiveness of MCP1 inhibitors in patients with progressive DKD [23]. Treatment with emapticap pegol, a Spiegelmer that specifically binds and inhibits MCP1, was found to be generally safe and well tolerated. In that study, albuminuria was attenuated by treatment with emapticap pegol, and the beneficial effects were maintained even after cessation of the intervention.

Intrarenal amplification of macrophages also plays an important role in the progression of renal disease, including DKD. Colony-stimulating factor 1 (CSF1), also known as macrophage colony-stimulating factor, is a homodimer glycoprotein that governs the survival, proliferation, and differentiation of macrophages. In particular, CSF1 is required for macrophage proliferation throughout the G1 phase of the cell cycle, and this chemokine is constitutively expressed in glomerular mesangial cells, tubular epithelial cells, and endothelial cells. Experimental studies have demonstrated that the deletion of CSF1 in mice leads to the attenuation of macrophage recruitment and proliferation during renal inflammation [24]. Of interest, the implantation of CSF1-generating cells into the kidneys of autoimmune lupus mice incites local macrophage-mediated inflammation [25]. CSF1 is also upregulated in type 2 diabetic db/db mice [26]. Furthermore, the administration of an antibody against the CSF1 receptor attenuates the accumulation of macrophages in rodent models of renal diseases, including unilateral ureteric obstruction, renal allograft rejection, and DKD [27]. Given these findings, it is reasonable to suggest that CSF1 is a critical determinant of the survival and proliferation of macrophages in several kidney diseases.

Dysregulation of the immune system is an important determinant in the initiation of DKD. Studies have provided convincing evidence that T cells, B cells, and NK cells are critical drivers of inflammation. Activated T cells cause renal damage directly via cytotoxic effects and indirectly by the recruitment and activation of macrophages. It is possible that pro-inflammatory cytokines secreted by T cells activate neighboring macrophages and stimulate the production of MCP1 and CSF-1 from glomerular cells. B cells could affect the proliferation of Th17 and the production of pro-inflammatory cytokines in patients with diabetes. Both T cells and B cells were shown to infiltrate glomeruli in a diabetic mouse model of diabetes, however, the evidence for the involvement of B cells and NK cells in DKD is more limited than that for T cells [28].

Overall, these findings provide evidence that immune system components are involved in the initiation of DKD and that adhesion molecules and chemokines play an essential role in the progression of inflammation in DKD.

3. Signaling Cascade Governing Inflammatory Reactions

A variety of upstream mediators (e.g., metabolic changes, altered redox balance, and intestinal dysbiosis) have been shown to be associated with inflammation in renal tissue. Cell death is induced under hyperglycemic conditions and activates the infiltration of macrophages and other immune cells into the kidney. Furthermore, the hyperglycemia-associated generation of advanced glycation end products (AGEs) and engagement of the receptor for AGE (RAGE) with its ligands induces oxidative stress and renal inflammation, resulting in a decline in renal function. Thus, the inhibition of AGE–RAGE signaling seems to be an attractive therapeutic strategy against renal inflammation. Interestingly, recent studies have reported the beneficial effects of RAGE blockade with FPS-ZM1 and RAGE-aptamers in DKD [29]. In addition to hyperglycemia-associated factors, systemic inflammation leads to dysregulation of the microcirculation network in the kidney and contributes to the in-site production of pro-inflammatory factors and ROS. Signaling events during renal inflammation orchestrate widespread transcriptional programs that affect the functions of adhesion molecules and inflammatory immune cells. An accumulating body of evidence exists defining the important roles for several signaling cascades in the control of renal inflammation, which we review below (Figure 1).

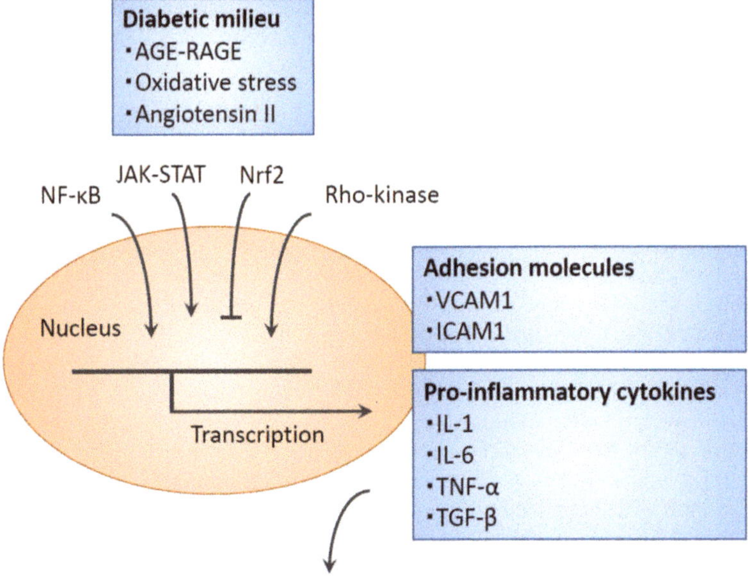

Figure 1. In the diabetic kidney, advanced glycation end products (AGEs) and oxidative stress activate a variety of signaling cascades to induce monocyte infiltration. In addition, chemokines drive inflammation, leading to macrophage-mediated tissue injury. DKD, Diabetic kidney disease; RAGE, receptor for AGE; VCAM1, vascular cell adhesion molecule 1; ICAM1, intercellular adhesion molecule 1; JAK-STAT, Janus kinase/signal transducer and activator of transcription; NF-κB, Nuclear factor Kb; Nrf2, nuclear factor-2 erythroid related factor 2; TNF-α, tumor necrosis factor α; TGF-β, transforming growth factor β.

3.1. Nuclear Factor κB (NF-κB) and Activating Protein 1 (AP1)

Nuclear factor κB (NF-κB) is a family of transcription factors central in regulating inflammatory signals. The complex of NF-κB is a dimer of two members of the Rel family of proteins: p65 and p50. In unstimulated cells, NF-κB is sequestered in the cytoplasm by IκB family proteins, the best characterized of which is IκBα. IκBα phosphorylation leads to its ubiquitination and subsequent proteasome-mediated protein degradation, which exposes its nuclear localization signal. The subsequent recognition of NF-κB by karyopherin β directs it to the nuclear pore complex, where nuclear translocation takes place. In addition, the coactivator p300 can complex with the p65/p50 heterodimer to stabilize the chromatin structure for efficient transcription.

Glucose can activate NF-κB, resulting in increased inflammatory gene expression, in part through oxidative stress, AGEs, protein kinase C, and Mitogen-activated protein kinases (MAPKs) [30]. Increased renal NF-κB levels are detected in the kidneys of diabetic experimental models, and this activates glomerular and tubular cells to induce renal injury [26,31]. Downstream targets of NF-κB include adhesion molecules and pro-inflammatory cytokines (e.g., IL-6, TNF-α, MCP1, RANTES

(Regulated on Activation, Normal T Cell Expressed and Secreted)), which all drive the development of DKD.

Similar to NF-κB, activating protein 1 (AP1) is activated by glucose and oxidative and inflammatory stimuli. AP1 regulates the TGF-β expression in mesangial cells, and the AP1 binding activity was found to be markedly enhanced by high glucose treatment [32]. PPARγ ligands are known to inhibit inflammatory gene expression via the attenuation of AP1, suggesting a potential anti-inflammatory therapeutic strategy by thiazolidine (TZD). Indeed, TZD decreases albuminuria, mesangial expansion, and the expression of TGF-β and osteopontin, a phosphor–glycoprotein adhesion molecule, in mouse models of diabetes [33]. Further clinical and mechanistic studies are required in order to validate the role of AP1 in the pathogenesis of DKD.

3.2. Janus Kinase/Signal Transducer and Activator of Transcription (JAK-STAT)

Experimental work over the past several years has shown the key roles of the Janus kinase/signal transducer and activator of transcription (JAK-STAT) pathway. The JAK-STAT pathway transduces signals from extracellular ligands (e.g., cytokines, chemokines, growth factors, and hormones) directly to the nucleus to activate a variety of cellular responses. Most of these reactions have been extensively studied in lymphoid cells, however, JAK-STAT signals also play critical roles in renal cells, including mesangial cells, podocytes, and tubular epithelial cells [34]. Studies have shown that JAK-STAT signaling is activated in renal tissue in patients with DKD. This pathway is activated by ROS induced by hyperglycemic states and is associated with glomerular hypertrophy [31]. A transcriptomic examination was performed in renal tissues obtained from subjects with early and progressive DKD [35]. In this analysis, all JAK-STAT genes were found to be highly expressed in the glomeruli from patients with early DKD compared with healthy controls. In contrast, tubular JAK-STAT genes were not increased in early DKD but were high in progressive DKD. Notably, the degree of induction of JAK-STAT gene expression was tightly and inversely correlated with the decline in the GFR.

A series of studies indicated that JAK family members JAK1, 2, and 3, as well as STAT1 and STAT3, are induced in DKD. In addition, Zhang et al. showed that the overexpression of JAK2 in podocytes can lead to worse renal damage in mouse models of diabetes [36]. Baricitinib, an oral inhibitor of the JAK family of protein tyrosine kinases that selectively inhibits JAK1 and JAK2, attenuates urinary albumin excretion in diabetic patients. Therefore, inhibiting JAK-STAT signaling may have potential utility for treating DKD and improving health outcomes in patients with diabetes [34].

3.3. Nuclear Factor-2 Erythroid Related Factor (Nrf2)-Keep1

The upregulation of Nrf2-dependent antioxidants attenuates systemic oxidative overload and renal inflammation. Beyond the resolution of oxidative stress, Nrf2 inhibits inflammation by directly regulating the transcription of pro-inflammatory cytokines (e.g., IL-1, IL-6). Kobayashi et al. reported that Nrf2 binds to the regulatory regions of inflammatory genes and thereby induces their transcription in macrophages and alleviates RNA polymerase II recruitment [37]. The pharmacological activation of Nrf2 decreases cytokine production, M1 macrophage accumulation, and the formation of an atherosclerotic plaque lipid core in the experimental model of streptozotocin-induced diabetic mice on an apolipoprotein E-deficient background [38]. Importantly, Nrf2 activation improves the pathological changes in the glomerulus of streptozotocin-injected diabetic mice through a reduction in oxidative stress, TGF-β expression, and extracellular matrix proteins [39]. Furthermore, Nrf2 attenuates mesangial hypertrophy induced by high glucose. Thus, Nrf2 activators have been suggested to prevent DKD. Bardoxolone methyl, one such Nrf2 activator, has been demonstrated in clinical trials to have reno-protective effects in patients with type 2 diabetes [40].

3.4. Rho-Kinase Signaling

A Rho-associated coiled-coil containing protein kinase (Rho-kinase) was initially identified as a regulator of Rho-induced stress fiber formation. Rho-kinase activation results in the phosphorylation of downstream targets, including myosin phosphatase target subunit, which has been demonstrated to mediate a wide array of cellular functions (e.g., cell proliferation, contraction, migration, and transcriptional regulation). Recent experimental studies have implicated Rho-kinase signaling in cardiovascular and kidney disease. Initial insights linking Rho-kinase to diabetes were gleaned from our studies defining Rho-kinase as a regulator of diabetic complications both in the microvasculature and large blood vessels. For example, Rho-kinase inhibition attenuates albuminuria, glomerular matrix expansion [41,42], and infiltration of macrophages [26] in mouse models of DKD. Subsequent analyses in endothelial cells identified Rho-kinase as a key molecule of vascular inflammation [43].

Of note, Rho-kinase mediates the production of MCP1 and monocyte chemotaxis toward glomerular cells. Furthermore, Rho-kinase functions as an important regulator of CSF1 production both in vitro and in vivo. From a transcriptional standpoint, there is evidence for an interaction between Rho-kinase and NF-κB activation. We recently showed that thrombin induces endothelial NF-κB activation through a molecular mechanism involving Rho-kinase [44]. Furthermore, Rho-kinase also plays an important role in the regulation of lysophosphatidic acid-induced endothelial NF-κB activation [45] and has been shown to be associated with neuropeptide-induced NF-κB activation and subsequent IL-8 induction in colonic epithelial cells [46]. Moreover, Rho exchange factor regulates NF-κB activation in monocytes, and the significance of the Rho-kinase/NF-κB axis in the kidney has been shown in mouse models of lipopolysaccharide injection [47]. These data suggest the existence of a mechanistic linkage between Rho-kinase and NF-κB signaling. CSF1 production in the glomerular mesangium is dependent on the NF-κB function, and the inhibition of Rho-kinase significantly inhibits NF-κB-mediated reporter activity via the p38 MAPK pathway. While some studies have demonstrated the direct regulation of Rho-kinase on either IκBα degradation or p65 phosphorylation, an interaction between Rho-kinase and the nuclear translocation of p65 without affecting either IκBα degradation or phosphorylation of p65 has also been reported [26].

Rho-kinase (ROCK) has two isoforms, ROCK1 and ROCK2, that share 65% sequence similarity but have different activation mechanisms. It has become increasingly clear that ROCK1 and ROCK2 play distinctive roles in regulating the cellular function. For instance, Takeda et al. showed the strong contribution of ROCK2 to the induction of E-selectin and MCP1 via NF-κB activation [48]. In vitro, ROCK2 is known to be localized in the nucleus and interacts with p300 acetyltransferase to activate p300-modulated transcription [49]. Taken together, these findings raise the possibility that targeting Rho-kinase may be a new therapeutic target against renal inflammation through a reduction in NF-κB-mediated macrophage accumulation.

4. Targeting Renal Inflammation for Prophylaxis and Therapy

With the discovery that inflammatory mediators are increased in DKD, researchers have begun to focus on therapeutic strategies targeting these inflammatory mediators. Several approaches have been proposed to treat inflammation in DKD, including lifestyle modifications, drugs, and dialysis optimization. As discussed above, the suppression of cytokine signaling with specific inhibitors, antibodies, or aptamers has the potential to reduce the risk of albuminuria and decline in the filtration function, highlighting the important role of these inflammatory mediators in DKD. In addition, novel pharmacological approaches to the management of diabetes have direct or indirect anti-inflammatory actions, the latter potentially attributable to an improvement in the metabolic status.

4.1. Sodium-Glucose Co-Transporter-2 (SGLT2) Inhibitors

SGLT2 inhibitors are now established therapies for treating hyperglycemia in patients with diabetes. By blocking SGLT2 at the proximal tubule, these agents limit the reabsorption of glucose, which in turn induces glycosuria and blood glucose reduction, independent of the insulin action [50]. Treatment with SGLT2 inhibitors leads to sustained systolic and diastolic blood pressure reductions, partially via natriuresis, which also contributes to the improvement of glomerular hyperfiltration and albuminuria through the activation of tubuloglomerular feedback [51].

Secondary outcome analyses in cardiovascular safety trials have shown the potential of SGLT2 inhibition to attenuate the risks of DKD progression and ESRD. For example, the renal composite outcomes (doubling of creatinine, renal replacement therapy, or renal death) decreased by 46% in patients with type 2 diabetes treated with empagliflozin [52]. A similar trend was reported with canagliflozin. The Canagliflozin and Renal Endpoints in Diabetes with Established Nephropathy Clinical Evaluation (CREDENCE) trial was designed to assess the efficacy and safety of canagliflozin versus placebo for reducing clinically important renal and cardiovascular outcomes in patients with diabetes and established kidney disease. This trial was restricted to participants who were taking the maximum tolerated dose of an angiotensin-converting enzyme inhibitor or angiotensin receptor blocker. Compared to a placebo, the reduction in the relative risk of renal-specific composites of ESRD, doubling of the creatinine level, or death from renal causes was greater in the canagliflozin group. An important observation from the CREDENCE trial is that the canagliflozin group also had a lower risk of cardiovascular death, myocardial infarction, or stroke and hospitalization for heart failure than the placebo group. Importantly, this trial showed no imbalance in rates of amputation or bone fracture, and no new safety concerns were identified [53]. Because few drugs are capable of preventing the progressive loss of the kidney function for this population, the current data will provide important evidence supporting the development of diabetes and nephrology guidelines.

Notably, canagliflozin reduces the plasma levels of TNF-R1 (9.2%; $p < 0.001$) and IL-6 (26.6%; $p = 0.010$) compared to glimepiride in patients with diabetes [54]. Similar effects were reported by Garvey et al. [55]. This evidence indicates that canagliflozin reverses molecular processes induced by inflammation. Experimental studies have also suggested the anti-inflammatory effects of SGLT2 inhibitors [56,57]. In diabetic Akita mice, empagliflozin inhibited albuminuria via a reduction in the levels of inflammatory cytokines, including MCP1 and IL-6 [57]. However, whether or not SGLT2 inhibitors can reduce the renal risk in patients with type 1 diabetes is unclear. This point will be investigated in a multicentre international randomized parallel group double-blind placebo-controlled clinical trial of EMPAgliflozin once daily to assess cardio-renal outcomes in patients with chronic KIDNEY disease (EMPA-KIDNEY), which will include patients with type 1 diabetes.

Basic mechanisms to explain anti-inflammatory effects may involve body weight loss and the improvement of obesity-induced insulin resistance. For instance, empagliflozin was shown to modulate energy metabolism by promoting fat utilization, browning of white adipose tissue, and blocking the infiltration of macrophages in high-fat-diet-fed obese mice [58]. Since there is a direct association between fat mass and the amount of pro-inflammatory mediators, a lower fat mass reflects less storage space for pro-inflammatory mediators and thus results in the attenuation of kidney inflammation. In addition, SGLT2 inhibitors may suppress inflammatory responses in the kidney by modulating RAS activity, hemodynamic changes, and changes in the immune system function. The increase in ketone bodies and inhibition of oxidative stress might also have contributed to the beneficial effects on renal inflammation.

Further studies are required in order to assess the inflammatory markers and elucidate the specific contribution of SGLT2 inhibition to the reduction in the DKD risk and associated mortality. When considered alongside very recent observations concerning the SGLT2-mediated oxidative pathway in mesangial cells [59], it will also be interesting to explore whether or not SGLT2 inhibitors affect glomerular inflammation directly.

4.2. Glucagon-Like Peptide 1 (GLP-1) Receptor Agonists and Dipeptidyl Peptidase 4 (DPP-4) Inhibitors

Glucagon-like peptide 1 (GLP-1) is a gut-derived peptide secreted from intestinal L-cells upon meal ingestion, that regulates glucose homeostasis by modulating the pancreatic islet cell function, food intake, and gastrointestinal motility. In addition to pancreatic β cells, GLP-1 receptor is expressed in proximal tubular cells and the kidney vasculature. GLP-1 receptor-mediated natriuresis is induced by the inhibition of sodium-hydrogen exchanger 3 (NHE3), which is located at the brush border of the renal proximal tubule. Mechanistically, GLP-1 receptor agonists (GLP-1RA) promote the phosphorylation of NHE3 at Ser552 and Ser605, which results in a decreased activity of NHE3 and natriuresis. Experimental studies in rodents and humans have shown that the activation of GLP-1 receptor leads to an increase in lithium clearance and pH, indicating the existence of NHE3-mediated regulation. Such proximal natriuresis would be expected to activate tubuloglomerular feedback and afferent vasoconstriction, leading to the downregulation of the renal blood flow and GFR. However, there were no changes in the renal hemodynamics or GFR in subjects with type 2 diabetes treated with GLP-1RA. These data are attributed to the direct nitric oxide-dependent reduction of afferent vascular resistance by GLP-1RA, which might override vasoconstriction induced by tubuloglomerular feedback [60].

GLP-1 receptors are expressed in renal tissue as well as the pancreas, heart, and intestine. Although the exact distribution of GLP-1 receptors in the kidney is not well characterized, clinical studies have shown that treatment with GLP-1RA reduces new-onset macroalbuminuria. These renal benefits may be explained by the known actions of GLP-1RA on metabolic risk factors for DKD, including reductions in blood glucose, blood pressure, and weight. However, several studies in rodents have demonstrated renoprotective effects of GLP-1RA beyond metabolic improvements in models of DKD. Aside from GLP-1RA, DPP-4 inhibitors also exert various extrapancreatic actions. DPP-4 inhibitors can attenuate inflammatory signaling pathways. For example, linagliptin exerts antioxidant and anti-inflammatory actions in endothelium, independent of its glucose-lowering effects [61,62]. In'addition, circulating levels of inflammatory cytokines and markers of inflammation were reduced in diabetic patients treated with sitagliptin or vildagliptin [63]. Experimental studies have demonstrated the renoprotective effects of DPP-4 inhibitors in the models of DKD and nondiabetic glomerular injury [64]. Some of these beneficial actions may be due to elevated GLP-1 levels. However, evidence suggests that the albuminuria-lowering effect of the DPP-4 inhibitor is weak compared to that of GLP-1RA [65,66].

The protective effect of GLP-1RA is mediated at least in part via inhibitory effects on renal inflammation, as well as NHE3-dependent sodium reabsorption [67]. For instance, exenatide was shown to inhibit albuminuria and the influx of glomerular macrophages in type 2 diabetic db/db mice [68]. Albuminuria and mesangial expansion were attenuated by treatment with exenatide in streptozotocin-injected type 1 diabetic rats through a mechanism involving inflammatory cytokines and adhesion molecules [69]. Furthermore, exenatide and dulaglutide reduced the circulating levels of C-reactive protein (CRP) in patients with type 2 diabetes [70]. Studies have shown that GLP-1RA's anti-inflammatory effects are modulated through the prevention of oxidative stress. Subsequent detailed investigations have revealed that liraglutide treatment inhibited albuminuria and nicotinamide adenine dinucleotide phosphate oxidase activity in a KK/Ta-Akita mouse model of type 1 diabetes without altering the blood glucose levels [71]. A more detailed understanding will be required to fully characterize the exact renal tissue distribution of GLP-1 receptors, as well as the associated anti-inflammatory effects and antioxidant mechanisms, in order to explain the renoprotection mediated by GLP-1RA.

4.3. Metformin

Metformin is now widely used for the treatment of type 2 diabetes as a first-line drug. Clinical studies have demonstrated that metformin not only attenuates chronic inflammation through the improvement of metabolic parameters (e.g., hyperglycemia, dyslipidemia), but also has direct anti-inflammatory properties. Metformin regulates miR-34a, a tumor-suppressor microRNA, to inhibit mesangial inflammation under high glucose conditions [72]. By activating AMPK, metformin disrupts the phosphorylation of STAT signaling and attenuates the differentiation of monocytes into macrophages [73].

4.4. Immunosuppressive Agents

Pharmacological modulation of the immune system may have beneficial effects on DKD development. For example, glucocorticoids are known to exert anti-inflammatory and immunosuppressive actions by genomic and nongenomic effects. Glucocorticoids have been extensively used in nephrotic syndrome. Cell-based studies suggest that glucocorticoids may have protective effects on podocyte injury [74]. Mechanistically, glucocorticoids reduce podocyte apoptosis and increase the number of podocyte progenitors via key components of the glucocorticoid receptor complex (e.g., heat shock protein 90, immunophilins FK506 binding protein (FKBP) 51, and FKBP52). However, the risk and potential clinical benefits of glucocorticoids are different for each patient. It is important to consider whether the benefits outweigh the side effects.

Mycophenolate mofetil is an anti-lymphocyte agent with immunosuppressive properties. This drug is clinically used to prevent allograft rejection. Mycophenolic acid, the active metabolite of mycophenolate mofetil, attenuates lymphocyte proliferation by blocking the early phases of the cell cycle. Experimental studies have demonstrated that mycophenolate mofetil decreases proteinuria and glomerulosclerosis through the reduction of macrophage infiltration in rodent models of type 1 and type 2 diabetes [75,76]. Furthermore, podocyte apoptosis and ROS production were attenuated in mycophenolate mofetil-treated diabetic mice [77]. Clinical evidence is required before recommendations can be made for treatment against DKD.

Regulatory T-cells (Tregs) control self-tolerance and allogeneic tolerance, and the dysfunction of Tregs is supposed to mediate the progression of DKD. Recent evidence from the Treg inhibition approach with anti-CD25 antibody emphasizes the importance of Treg in DKD. Treatment with anti-CD25 accelerated kidney damage in db/db mice and the adoptive transfer of Tregs inhibited proteinuria and glomerular hypertrophy [78]. Therefore, Tregs may be an attractive target for the treatment of DKD. Since the transfer of Treg has technical limitations, approaches that enhance endogenous Tregs are likely to be beneficial for DKD patients.

5. Conclusions and Future Perspectives

It is becoming clear that DKD is associated with the increased expression of inflammation-associated mediators. Since the diagnosis of DKD is still difficult due to a lack of reliable biomarkers capable of predicting patient outcomes, especially in the early stages (albuminuria is not specific for diabetic renal damage), the levels of pro-inflammatory cytokines may be a useful marker for making a diagnosis of DKD. From this standpoint, urinary proteomics and peptidomics have gained attention as a study tool for the detection of diagnostic markers of DKD. The urinary omics studies in DKD have revealed several markers, including inflammatory mediators such as MCP1 and TGF-β [79,80]. Whether inflammation is a trigger or a result of a chronic underlying condition is an important topic. Gene manipulation studies on the impact of renal inflammation on DKD development have greatly expanded our knowledge in this field. Furthermore, studies exploring the cause of this pro-inflammatory milieu and the contribution of these pathways to DKD development will strengthen the significance of inflammatory mediators as biomarker of DKD.

Recent systems biological approaches have revealed molecular abnormalities in DKD and have directly led to the identification of potential targets for DKD. A comprehensive transcriptome analysis demonstrated that the top differentially regulated genes in DKD tissue are associated with inflammation and fibrosis [81]. In this assessment, the complement signal was the highest degree of statistical significance in both glomeruli and tubulointerstitium. Studies will be required to determine the pathological significance of the complement system in human DKD.

The cumulative data on the role of inflammation in the pathogenesis of DKD are sufficient to warrant their consideration as therapeutic targets. Targeting inflammatory cytokines or adhesion molecules will offer novel avenues for therapeutic intervention. However, a central challenge remains: how to leverage our comprehension of the inflammatory mechanism in order to establish an intervention that can prevent DKD progression and prolong the lifespan of diabetic patients. Over the past decade, new classes of anti-hyperglycemic drugs with renal benefits have been introduced for the management of diabetes, namely SGLT2 inhibitors and GLP-1RA. These agents seem to have additional pleiotropic anti-inflammatory properties mediated through distinct molecular mechanisms by both direct and indirect actions. A greater understanding of the mechanisms underlying these agents' renal benefits would facilitate the development of novel therapies for DKD and its associated sequelae.

Author Contributions: K.M. wrote the manuscript; Y.T., Y.N., D.K., K.U. and R.N. helped edit the manuscript and revised the manuscript for important intellectual content. All of the authors read and approved the final manuscript.

Acknowledgments: This work was supported by a Grant-in-Aid for Scientific Research from Japan Society for the Promotion of Science (to Keiichiro Matoba and Daiji Kawanami), the Ichiro Kanehara Foundation (to Keiichiro Matoba), the MSD Life Science Foundation (to Keiichiro Matoba), and the Yokoyama Foundation for Clinical Pharmacology (to Keiichiro Matoba).

Conflicts of Interest: Kazunori Utsunomiya has received research support from Terumo, Novo Nordisk Pharma, Taisho Pharmaceutical, Böehringer Ingelheim, Kyowa Hakko Kirin, Sumitomo Dainippon Pharma, and Ono Pharmaceutical as well as speaker honoraria from Tanabe Pharma, Sanofi Kabushiki Kaisya, Sumitomo Dainippon Pharma, Eli Lilly, and Böehringer Ingelheim. Rimei Nishimura has received speaker honoraria from Astellas Pharma, Nippon Boehringer Ingelheim, Eli Lilly Japan Kabushiki Kaisya, Kissei Pharmaceutical, Medtronic Japan, MSD, Novartis Pharma Kabushiki Kaisya, Novo Nordisk Pharma, Sanofi Kabushiki Kaisya, and Takeda Pharmaceutical and contract research fees for collaborative research with the Japan Diabetes Foundation.

References

1. Adler, A.I.; Stevens, R.J.; Manley, S.E.; Bilous, R.W.; Cull, C.A.; Holman, R.R.; UKPDS GROUP. Development and progression of nephropathy in type 2 diabetes: The United Kingdom Prospective Diabetes Study (UKPDS 64). *Kidney Int.* **2003**, *63*, 225–232. [CrossRef] [PubMed]

2. Goldfine, A.B.; Shoelson, S.E. Therapeutic approaches targeting inflammation for diabetes and associated cardiovascular risk. *J. Clin. Invest.* **2017**, *127*, 83–93. [CrossRef] [PubMed]

3. Simo-Servat, O.; Simo, R.; Hernandez, C. Circulating Biomarkers of Diabetic Retinopathy: An Overview Based on Physiopathology. *J. Diabetes Res.* **2016**, *2016*, 5263798. [CrossRef] [PubMed]

4. Paeschke, S.; Paeschke, S.; Baum, P.; Toyka, K.V.; Blüher, M.; Koj, S.; Klöting, N.; Bechmann, I.; Thiery, J.; Kosacka, J.; et al. The Role of Iron and Nerve Inflammation in Diabetes Mellitus Type 2-Induced Peripheral Neuropathy. *Neuroscience* **2019**, *406*, 496–509. [CrossRef] [PubMed]

5. Xu, L.; Lin, X.; Guan, M.; Zeng, Y.; Liu, Y. Verapamil Attenuated Prediabetic Neuropathy in High-Fat Diet-Fed Mice through Inhibiting TXNIP-Mediated Apoptosis and Inflammation. *Oxid Med. Cell Longev.* **2019**, *2019*, 1896041. [CrossRef]

6. Doupis, J.; Lyons, T.E.; Wu, S.; Gnardellis, C.; Dinh, T.; Veves, A. Microvascular reactivity and inflammatory cytokines in painful and painless peripheral diabetic neuropathy. *J. Clin. Endocrinol Metab.* **2009**, *94*, 2157–2163. [CrossRef] [PubMed]

7. Pop-Busui, R.; Ang, L.; Holmes, C.; Gallagher, K.; Feldman, E.L. Inflammation as a Therapeutic Target for Diabetic Neuropathies. *Curr. Diab. Rep.* **2016**, *16*, 29. [CrossRef]

8. Ganesh Yerra, V.; Negi, G.; Sharma, S.S.; Kumar, A. Potential therapeutic effects of the simultaneous targeting of the Nrf2 and NF-kappaB pathways in diabetic neuropathy. *Redox Biol.* **2013**, *1*, 394–397. [CrossRef]

9. Tian, S.; Chen, S.Y. Macrophage polarization in kidney diseases. *Macrophage (Houst)* **2015**, *2*, e679.

10. Klessens, C.Q.F.; Zandbergen, M.; Wolterbeek, R.; Bruijn, J.A.; Rabelink, T.J.; Bajema, I.M.; IJpelaar, D.H.T. Macrophages in diabetic nephropathy in patients with type 2 diabetes. *Nephrol. Dial. Transpl.* **2017**, *32*, 1322–1329. [CrossRef]

11. Usui, H.K.; Shikata, K.; Sasaki, M.; Okada, S.; Matsuda, M.; Shikata, Y.; Ogawa, D.; Kido, Y.; Nagase, R.; Yozai, K.; et al. Macrophage scavenger receptor-a-deficient mice are resistant against diabetic nephropathy through amelioration of microinflammation. *Diabetes* **2007**, *56*, 363–372. [CrossRef] [PubMed]

12. Landis, R.C.; Quimby, K.R.; Greenidge, A.R. M1/M2 Macrophages in Diabetic Nephropathy: Nrf2/HO-1 as Therapeutic Targets. *Curr. Pharm. Des.* **2018**, *24*, 2241–2249. [CrossRef] [PubMed]

13. Devaraj, S.; Tobias, P.; Kasinath, B.S.; Ramsamooj, R.; Afify, A.; Jialal, I. Knockout of toll-like receptor-2 attenuates both the proinflammatory state of diabetes and incipient diabetic nephropathy. *Arterioscler Thromb. Vasc. Biol.* **2011**, *31*, 1796–1804. [CrossRef] [PubMed]

14. Clausen, P.; Jacobsen, P.; Rossing, K.; Jensen, J.S.; Parving, H.H.; Feldt-Rasmussen, B. Plasma concentrations of VCAM-1 and ICAM-1 are elevated in patients with Type 1 diabetes mellitus with microalbuminuria and overt nephropathy. *Diabet Med.* **2000**, *17*, 644–649. [CrossRef] [PubMed]

15. Hojs, R.; Ekart, R.; Bevc, S.; Hojs, N. Markers of Inflammation and Oxidative Stress in the Development and Progression of Renal Disease in Diabetic Patients. *Nephron* **2016**, *133*, 159–162. [CrossRef] [PubMed]

16. Liu, J.J.; Yeoh, L.Y.; Sum, C.F.; Tavintharan, S.; Ng, X.W.; Liu, S.; Lee, S.B.; Tang, W.E.; Lim, S.C.; SMART2D study. Vascular cell adhesion molecule-1, but not intercellular adhesion molecule-1, is associated with diabetic kidney disease in Asians with type 2 diabetes. *J. Diabetes Complicat.* **2015**, *29*, 707–712. [CrossRef] [PubMed]

17. Lim, A.K.; Tesch, G.H. Inflammation in diabetic nephropathy. *Mediators Inflamm.* **2012**, *2012*, 146154. [CrossRef] [PubMed]

18. Okada, S.; Shikata, K.; Matsuda, M.; Ogawa, D.; Usui, H.; Kido, Y.; Nagase, R.; Wada, J.; Shikata, Y.; Makino, H. Intercellular adhesion molecule-1-deficient mice are resistant against renal injury after induction of diabetes. *Diabetes* **2003**, *52*, 2586–2593. [CrossRef]

19. Nadkarni, G.N.; Rao, V.; Ismail-Beigi, F.; Fonseca, V.A.; Shah, S.V.; Simonson, M.S.; Cantley, L.; Devarajan, P.; Parikh, C.R.; Coca, S.G. Association of Urinary Biomarkers of Inflammation, Injury, and Fibrosis with Renal Function Decline: The ACCORD Trial. *Clin. J. Am. Soc. Nephrol.* **2016**, *11*, 1343–1352. [CrossRef]

20. Satirapoj, B.; Dispan, R.; Radinahamed, P.; Kitiyakara, C. Urinary epidermal growth factor, monocyte chemoattractant protein-1 or their ratio as predictors for rapid loss of renal function in type 2 diabetic patients with diabetic kidney disease. *BMC Nephrol.* **2018**, *19*, 246. [CrossRef]

21. Niewczas, M.A.; Gohda, T.; Skupien, J.; Smiles, A.M.; Walker, W.H.; Rosetti, F.; Cullere, X.; Eckfeldt, J.H.; Doria, A.; Mayadas, T.N.; et al. Circulating TNF receptors 1 and 2 predict ESRD in type 2 diabetes. *J. Am. Soc. Nephrol.* **2012**, *23*, 507–515. [CrossRef] [PubMed]

22. Niewczas, M.A.; Pavkov, M.E.; Skupien, J.; Smiles, A.; Md Dom, Z.I.; Wilson, J.M.; Park, J.; Nair, V.; Schlafly, A.; Saulnier, P.J.; et al. A signature of circulating inflammatory proteins and development of end-stage renal disease in diabetes. *Nat. Med.* **2019**, *25*, 805–813. [CrossRef] [PubMed]

23. Menne, J.; Eulberg, D.; Beyer, D.; Baumann, M.; Saudek, F.; Valkusz, Z.; Więcek, A.; Haller, H.; Emapticap Study Group. C-C motif-ligand 2 inhibition with emapticap pegol (NOX-E36) in type 2 diabetic patients with albuminuria. *Nephrol. Dial. Transplant.* **2017**, *32*, 307–315. [CrossRef] [PubMed]

24. Lenda, D.M.; Kikawada, E.; Stanley, E.R.; Kelley, V.R. Reduced macrophage recruitment, proliferation, and activation in colony-stimulating factor-1-deficient mice results in decreased tubular apoptosis during renal inflammation. *J. Immunol.* **2003**, *170*, 3254–3262. [CrossRef] [PubMed]

25. Naito, T.; Yokoyama, H.; Moore, K.J.; Dranoff, G.; Mulligan, R.C.; Kelley, V.R. Macrophage growth factors introduced into the kidney initiate renal injury. *Mol. Med.* **1996**, *2*, 297–312. [CrossRef] [PubMed]

26. Matoba, K.; Kawanami, D.; Tsukamoto, M.; Kinoshita, J.; Ito, T.; Ishizawa, S.; Kanazawa, Y.; Yokota, T.; Murai, N.; Matsufuji, S.; et al. Rho-kinase regulation of TNF-alpha-induced nuclear translocation of NF-kappaB RelA/p65 and M-CSF expression via p38 MAPK in mesangial cells. *Am. J. Physiol. Renal Physiol.* **2014**, *307*, F571–F580. [CrossRef] [PubMed]

27. Lim, A.K.; Ma, F.Y.; Nikolic-Paterson, D.J.; Thomas, M.C.; Hurst, L.A.; Tesch, G.H. Antibody blockade of c-fms suppresses the progression of inflammation and injury in early diabetic nephropathy in obese db/db mice. *Diabetologia* **2009**, *52*, 1669–1679. [CrossRef]

28. Pichler, R.; Afkarian, M.; Dieter, B.P.; Tuttle, K.R. Immunity and inflammation in diabetic kidney disease: Translating mechanisms to biomarkers and treatment targets. *Am. J. Physiol. Renal Physiol.* **2017**, *312*, F716–F731. [CrossRef]

29. Sanajou, D.; Ghorbani Haghjo, A.; Argani, H.; Aslani, S. AGE-RAGE axis blockade in diabetic nephropathy: Current status and future directions. *Eur. J. Pharmacol.* **2018**, *833*, 158–164. [CrossRef]

30. Pérez-Morales, R.E.; Del Pino, M.D.; Valdivielso, J.M.; Ortiz, A.; Mora-Fernández, C.; Navarro-González, J.F. Inflammation in Diabetic Kidney Disease. *Nephron* **2018**, 1–5. [CrossRef]

31. Toth-Manikowski, S.; Atta, M.G. Diabetic Kidney Disease: Pathophysiology and Therapeutic Targets. *J. Diabetes Res.* **2015**, *2015*, 697010. [CrossRef] [PubMed]

32. Weigert, C.; Sauer, U.; Brodbeck, K.; Pfeiffer, A.; Häring, H.U.; Schleicher, E.D. AP-1 proteins mediate hyperglycemia-induced activation of the human TGF-beta1 promoter in mesangial cells. *J. Am. Soc. Nephrol.* **2000**, *11*, 2007–2016. [PubMed]

33. Nicholas, S.B.; Liu, J.; Kim, J.; Ren, Y.; Collins, A.R.; Nguyen, L.; Hsueh, W.A. Critical role for osteopontin in diabetic nephropathy. *Kidney Int.* **2010**, *77*, 588–600. [CrossRef] [PubMed]

34. Tuttle, K.R.; Brosius III, F.C.; Adler, S.G.; Kretzler, M.; Mehta, R.L.; Tumlin, J.A.; Tanaka, Y.; Haneda, M.; Liu, J.; Silk, M.E.; et al. JAK1/JAK2 inhibition by baricitinib in diabetic kidney disease: Results from a Phase 2 randomized controlled clinical trial. *Nephrol. Dial. Transplant.* **2018**, *33*, 1950–1959. [CrossRef] [PubMed]

35. Brosius, F.C.; Ju, W. The Promise of Systems Biology for Diabetic Kidney Disease. *Adv. Chronic Kidney Dis.* **2018**, *25*, 202–213. [CrossRef]

36. Zhang, H.; Nair, V.; Saha, J.; Atkins, K.B.; Hodgin, J.B.; Saunders, T.L.; Myers, M.G.Jr.; Werner, T.; Kretzler, M.; Brosius, F.C. Podocyte-specific JAK2 overexpression worsens diabetic kidney disease in mice. *Kidney Int.* **2017**, *92*, 909–921. [CrossRef]

37. Kobayashi, E.H.; Suzuki, T.; Funayama, R.; Nagashima, T.; Hayashi, M.; Sekine, H.; Tanaka, N.; Moriguchi, T.; Motohashi, H.; Nakayama, K.; et al. Nrf2 suppresses macrophage inflammatory response by blocking proinflammatory cytokine transcription. *Nat. Commun.* **2016**, *7*, 11624. [CrossRef]

38. Lazaro, I.; Lopez-Sanz, L.; Bernal, S.; Oguiza, A.; Recio, C.; Melgar, A.; Jimenez-Castilla, L.; Egido, J.; Madrigal-Matute, J.; Gomez-Guerrero, C. Nrf2 Activation Provides Atheroprotection in Diabetic Mice Through Concerted Upregulation of Antioxidant, Anti-inflammatory, and Autophagy Mechanisms. *Front. Pharmacol.* **2018**, *9*, 819. [CrossRef]

39. Zheng, H.; Whitman, S.A.; Wu, W.; Wondrak, G.T.; Wong, P.K.; Fang, D.; Zhang, D.D. Therapeutic potential of Nrf2 activators in streptozotocin-induced diabetic nephropathy. *Diabetes* **2011**, *60*, 3055–3066. [CrossRef]

40. Pergola, P.E.; Raskin, P.; Toto, R.D.; Meyer, C.J.; Huff, J.W.; Grossman, E.B.; Krauth, M.; Ruiz, S.; Audhya, P.; Christ-Schmidt, H.; et al. Bardoxolone methyl and kidney function in CKD with type 2 diabetes. *N. Engl. J. Med.* **2011**, *365*, 327–336. [CrossRef]

41. Matoba, K.; Kawanami, D.; Okada, R.; Tsukamoto, M.; Kinoshita, J.; Ito, T.; Ishizawa, S.; Kanazawa, Y.; Yokota, T.; Murai, N.; et al. Rho-kinase inhibition prevents the progression of diabetic nephropathy by downregulating hypoxia-inducible factor 1alpha. *Kidney Int.* **2013**, *84*, 545–554. [CrossRef] [PubMed]

42. Kawanami, D.; Matoba, K.; Utsunomiya, K. Signaling pathways in diabetic nephropathy. *Histol. Histopathol.* **2016**, *31*, 1059–1067. [PubMed]

43. Kawanami, D.; Matoba, K.; Okada, R.; Tsukamoto, M.; Kinoshita, J.; Ishizawa, S.; Kanazawa, Y.; Yokota, T.; Utsunomiya, K. Fasudil inhibits ER stress-induced VCAM-1 expression by modulating unfolded protein response in endothelial cells. *Biochem. Biophys. Res. Commun.* **2013**, *435*, 171–175. [CrossRef] [PubMed]

44. Kawanami, D.; Matoba, K.; Kanazawa, Y.; Ishizawa, S.; Yokota, T.; Utsunomiya, K. Thrombin induces MCP-1 expression through Rho-kinase and subsequent p38MAPK/NF-kappaB signaling pathway activation in vascular endothelial cells. *Biochem. Biophys. Res. Commun.* **2011**, *411*, 798–803. [CrossRef] [PubMed]

45. Shimada, H.; Rajagopalan, L.E. Rho kinase-2 activation in human endothelial cells drives lysophosphatidic acid-mediated expression of cell adhesion molecules via NF-kappaB p65. *J. Biol. Chem.* **2010**, *285*, 12536–12542. [CrossRef] [PubMed]

46. Zhao, D.; Kuhnt-Moore, S.; Zeng, H.; Wu, J.S.; Moyer, M.P.; Pothoulakis, C. Neurotensin stimulates IL-8 expression in human colonic epithelial cells through Rho GTPase-mediated NF-kappa B pathways. *Am. J. Physiol. Cell Physiol.* **2003**, *284*, C1397–C1404. [CrossRef] [PubMed]

47. Meyer-Schwesinger, C.; Dehde, S.; von Ruffer, C.; Gatzemeier, S.; Klug, P.; Wenzel, U.O.; Stahl, R.A.; Thaiss, F.; Meyer, T.N. Rho kinase inhibition attenuates LPS-induced renal failure in mice in part by attenuation of NF-kappaB p65 signaling. *Am. J. Physiol. Renal Physiol.* **2009**, *296*, F1088–F1099. [CrossRef] [PubMed]

48. Takeda, Y.; Matoba, K.; Kawanami, D.; Nagai, Y.; Akamine, T.; Ishizawa, S.; Kanazawa, Y.; Yokota, T.; Utsunomiya, K. ROCK2 Regulates Monocyte Migration and Cell to Cell Adhesion in Vascular Endothelial Cells. *Int. J. Mol. Sci.* **2019**, *20*, 1331. [CrossRef]

49. Tanaka, T.; Nishimura, D.; Wu, R.C.; Amano, M.; Iso, T.; Kedes, L.; Nishida, H.; Kaibuchi, K.; Hamamori, Y. Nuclear Rho kinase, ROCK2, targets p300 acetyltransferase. *J. Biol. Chem.* **2006**, *281*, 15320–15329. [CrossRef]

50. Thomas, M.C.; Cherney, D.Z.I. The actions of SGLT2 inhibitors on metabolism, renal function and blood pressure. *Diabetologia* **2018**, *61*, 2098–2107. [CrossRef] [PubMed]

51. Kawanami, D.; Matoba, K.; Takeda, Y.; Nagai, Y.; Akamine, T.; Yokota, T.; Sango, K.; Utsunomiya, K. SGLT2 Inhibitors as a Therapeutic Option for Diabetic Nephropathy. *Int. J. Mol. Sci.* **2017**, *18*, 1083. [CrossRef] [PubMed]

52. Wanner, C.; Inzucchi, S.E.; Lachin, J.M.; Fitchett, D.; von Eynatten, M.; Mattheus, M.; Johansen, O.E.; Woerle, H.J.; Broedl, U.C.; Zinman, B.; et al. Empagliflozin and Progression of Kidney Disease in Type 2 Diabetes. *N. Engl. J. Med.* **2016**, *375*, 323–334. [CrossRef] [PubMed]

53. Perkovic, V.; Jardine, M.J.; Neal, B.; Bompoint, S.; Heerspink, H.J.L.; Charytan, D.M.; Edwards, R.; Agarwal, R.; Bakris, G.; Bull, S.; et al. Canagliflozin and Renal Outcomes in Type 2 Diabetes and Nephropathy. *N. Engl. J. Med.* **2019**, *380*, 2295–2306. [CrossRef] [PubMed]

54. Heerspink, H.J.L.; Perco, P.; Mulder, S.; Leierer, J.; Hansen, M.K.; Heinzel, A.; Mayer, G. Canagliflozin reduces inflammation and fibrosis biomarkers: A potential mechanism of action for beneficial effects of SGLT2 inhibitors in diabetic kidney disease. *Diabetologia* **2019**, *62*, 1154–1166. [CrossRef]

55. Garvey, W.T.; Van Gaal, L.; Leiter, L.A.; Vijapurkar, U.; List, J.; Cuddihy, R.; Ren, J.; Davies, M.J. Effects of canagliflozin versus glimepiride on adipokines and inflammatory biomarkers in type 2 diabetes. *Metabolism* **2018**, *85*, 32–37. [CrossRef]

56. Tahara, A.; Takasu, T.; Yokono, M.; Imamura, M.; Kurosaki, E. Characterization and comparison of SGLT2 inhibitors: Part 3. Effects on diabetic complications in type 2 diabetic mice. *Eur. J. Pharmacol.* **2017**, *809*, 163–171. [CrossRef]

57. Vallon, V.; Gerasimova, M.; Rose, M.A.; Masuda, T.; Satriano, J.; Mayoux, E.; Koepsell, H.; Thomson, SC.; Rieg, T. SGLT2 inhibitor empagliflozin reduces renal growth and albuminuria in proportion to hyperglycemia and prevents glomerular hyperfiltration in diabetic Akita mice. *Am. J. Physiol. Renal Physiol.* **2014**, *306*, F194–F204. [CrossRef]

58. Xu, L.; Nagata, N.; Nagashimada, M.; Zhuge, F.; Ni, Y.; Chen, G.; Mayoux, E.; Kaneko, S.; Ota, T. SGLT2 Inhibition by Empagliflozin Promotes Fat Utilization and Browning and Attenuates Inflammation and Insulin Resistance by Polarizing M2 Macrophages in Diet-induced Obese Mice. *EBioMedicine* **2017**, *20*, 137–149. [CrossRef]

59. Maki, T.; Maeno, S.; Maeda, Y.; Yamato, M.; Sonoda, N.; Ogawa, Y.; Wakisaka, M.; Inoguchi, T. Amelioration of diabetic nephropathy by SGLT2 inhibitors independent of its glucose-lowering effect: A possible role of SGLT2 in mesangial cells. *Sci. Rep.* **2019**, *9*, 4703. [CrossRef]

60. Muskiet, M.H.; Tonneijck, L.; Smits, M.M.; Kramer, M.H.; Diamant, M.; Joles, J.A.; van Raalte, D.H. Acute renal haemodynamic effects of glucagon-like peptide-1 receptor agonist exenatide in healthy overweight men. *Diabetes Obes. Metab.* **2016**, *18*, 178–185. [CrossRef]

61. Kröller-Schön, S.; Knorr, M.; Hausding, M.; Oelze, M.; Schuff, A.; Schell, R.; Sudowe, S.; Scholz, A.; Daub, S.; Karbach, S.; et al. Glucose-independent improvement of vascular dysfunction in experimental sepsis by dipeptidyl-peptidase 4 inhibition. *Cardiovasc Res.* **2012**, *96*, 140–149. [CrossRef]

62. Kanasaki, K. The role of renal dipeptidyl peptidase-4 in kidney disease: Renal effects of dipeptidyl peptidase-4 inhibitors with a focus on linagliptin. *Clin. Sci.* **2018**, *132*, 489–507. [CrossRef] [PubMed]

63. Barbieri, M.; Rizzo, M.R.; Marfella, R.; Boccardi, V.; Esposito, A.; Pansini, A.; Paolisso, G. Decreased carotid atherosclerotic process by control of daily acute glucose fluctuations in diabetic patients treated by DPP-IV inhibitors. *Atherosclerosis* **2013**, *227*, 349–354. [CrossRef]

64. Higashijima, Y.; Tanaka, T.; Yamaguchi, J.; Tanaka, S.; Nangaku, M. Anti-inflammatory role of DPP-4 inhibitors in a nondiabetic model of glomerular injury. *Am. J. Physiol. Renal Physiol.* **2015**, *308*, F878–F887. [CrossRef] [PubMed]

65. Pollock, C.; Stefánsson, B.; Reyner, D.; Rossing, P.; Sjöström, C.D.; Wheeler, D.C.; Langkilde, A.M.; Heerspink, H.J.L. Albuminuria-lowering effect of dapagliflozin alone and in combination with saxagliptin and effect of dapagliflozin and saxagliptin on glycaemic control in patients with type 2 diabetes and chronic kidney disease (DELIGHT): A randomised, double-blind, placebo-controlled trial. *Lancet Diabetes Endocrinol.* **2019**, *7*, 429–441. [PubMed]

66. Rosenstock, J.; Perkovic, V.; Johansen, O.E.; Cooper, M.E.; Kahn, S.E.; Marx, N.; Alexander, J.H.; Pencina, M.; Toto, R.D.; Wanner, C.; et al. Effect of Linagliptin vs Placebo on Major Cardiovascular Events in Adults With Type 2 Diabetes and High Cardiovascular and Renal Risk: The CARMELINA Randomized Clinical Trial. *JAMA.* **2019**, *321*, 69–79. [CrossRef]

67. Kawanami, D.; Matoba, K.; Sango, K.; Utsunomiya, K. Incretin-Based Therapies for Diabetic Complications: Basic Mechanisms and Clinical Evidence. *Int. J. Mol. Sci.* **2016**, *17*, 1223. [CrossRef]

68. Park, C.W.; Kim, H.W.; Ko, S.H.; Lim, J.H.; Ryu, G.R.; Chung, H.W.; Han, S.W.; Shin, S.J.; Bang, B.K.; Breyer, M.D.; et al. Long-term treatment of glucagon-like peptide-1 analog exendin-4 ameliorates diabetic nephropathy through improving metabolic anomalies in db/db mice. *J. Am. Soc. Nephrol.* **2017**, *18*, 1227–1238. [CrossRef]

69. Kodera, R.; Shikata, K.; Kataoka, H.U.; Takatsuka, T.; Miyamoto, S.; Sasaki, M.; Kajitani, N.; Nishishita, S.; Sarai, K.; Hirota, D.; et al. Glucagon-like peptide-1 receptor agonist ameliorates renal injury through its anti-inflammatory action without lowering blood glucose level in a rat model of type 1 diabetes. *Diabetologia* **2011**, *54*, 965–978. [CrossRef]

70. Ferdinand, K.C.; White, W.B.; Calhoun, D.A.; Lonn, E.M.; Sager, P.T.; Brunelle, R.; Jiang, H.H.; Threlkeld, R.J.; Robertson, K.E.; Geiger, M.J. Effects of the once-weekly glucagon-like peptide-1 receptor agonist dulaglutide on

ambulatory blood pressure and heart rate in patients with type 2 diabetes mellitus. *Hypertension* **2014**, *64*, 731–737. [CrossRef]

71. Fujita, H.; Morii, T.; Fujishima, H.; Sato, T.; Shimizu, T.; Hosoba, M.; Tsukiyama, K.; Narita, T.; Takahashi, T.; Drucker, D.J.; et al. The protective roles of GLP-1R signaling in diabetic nephropathy: Possible mechanism and therapeutic potential. *Kidney Int.* **2014**, *85*, 579–589. [CrossRef] [PubMed]

72. Wu, C.; Qin, N.; Ren, H.; Yang, M.; Liu, S.; Wang, Q. Metformin Regulating miR-34a Pathway to Inhibit Egr1 in Rat Mesangial Cells Cultured with High Glucose. *Int. J. Endocrinol.* **2018**, *2018*, 6462793. [CrossRef] [PubMed]

73. Vasamsetti, S.B.; Karnewar, S.; Kanugula, A.K.; Thatipalli, A.R.; Kumar, J.M.; Kotamraju, S. Metformin inhibits monocyte-to-macrophage differentiation via AMPK-mediated inhibition of STAT3 activation: Potential role in atherosclerosis. *Diabetes* **2015**, *64*, 2028–2041. [CrossRef]

74. Guess, A.; Agrawal, S.; Wei, C.C.; Ransom, R.F.; Benndorf, R.; Smoyer, W.E. Dose- and time-dependent glucocorticoid receptor signaling in podocytes. *Am. J. Physiol. Renal Physiol.* **2010**, *299*, F553–F845. [CrossRef] [PubMed]

75. Utimura, R.; Fujihara, C.K.; Mattar, A.L.; Malheiros, D.M.; Noronha, I.L.; Zatz, R. Mycophenolate mofetil prevents the development of glomerular injury in experimental diabetes. *Kidney Int.* **2003**, *63*, 209–216. [CrossRef] [PubMed]

76. Rodríguez-Iturbe, B.; Quiroz, Y.; Shahkarami, A.; Li, Z.; Vaziri, N.D. Mycophenolate mofetil ameliorates nephropathy in the obese Zucker rat. *Kidney Int.* **2005**, *68*, 1041–1047. [CrossRef]

77. Seo, J.W.; Kim, Y.G.; Lee, S.H.; Lee, A.; Kim, D.J.; Jeong, K.H.; Lee, K.H.; Hwang, S.J.; Woo, J.S.; Lim, S.J.; et al. Mycophenolate Mofetil Ameliorates Diabetic Nephropathy in db/db Mice. *Biomed. Res. Int.* **2015**, *2015*, 301627. [CrossRef]

78. Eller, K.; Kirsch, A.; Wolf, A.M.; Sopper, S.; Tagwerker, A.; Stanzl, U.; Wolf, D.; Patsch, W.; Rosenkranz, A.R.; Eller, P. Potential role of regulatory T cells in reversing obesity-linked insulin resistance and diabetic nephropathy. *Diabetes* **2011**, *60*, 2954–2962. [CrossRef] [PubMed]

79. Pena, M.J.; Mischak, H.; Heerspink, H.J. Proteomics for prediction of disease progression and response to therapy in diabetic kidney disease. *Diabetologia* **2016**, *59*, 1819–1831. [CrossRef]

80. Verhave, J.C.; Bouchard, J.; Goupil, R.; Pichette, V.; Brachemi, S.; Madore, F.; Troyanov, S. Clinical value of inflammatory urinary biomarkers in overt diabetic nephropathy: A prospective study. *Diabetes Res. Clin. Pract.* **2013**, *101*, 333–340. [CrossRef]

81. Woroniecka, K.I.; Park, A.S.; Mohtat, D.; Thomas, D.B.; Pullman, J.M.; Susztak, K. Transcriptome analysis of human diabetic kidney disease. *Diabetes* **2011**, *60*, 2354–2369. [CrossRef] [PubMed]

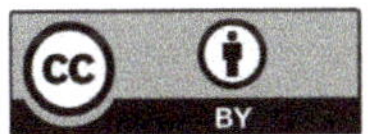

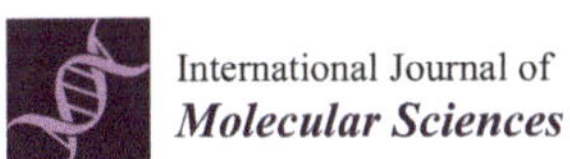

International Journal of
Molecular Sciences

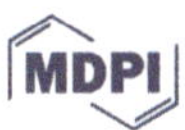

Review

Renal Benefits of SGLT 2 Inhibitors and GLP-1 Receptor Agonists: Evidence Supporting a Paradigm Shift in the Medical Management of Type 2 Diabetes

Vjera Ninčević [1,2], Tea Omanović Kolarić [1,2], Hrvoje Roguljić [1,3], Tomislav Kizivat [4,5], Martina Smolić [1,2] and Ines Bilić Ćurčić [1,6,*]

1   Department of Pharmacology, Faculty of Medicine, Josip Juraj Strossmayer University of Osijek, J. Huttlera 4, 31000 Osijek, Croatia; vnincevic@mefos.hr (V.N.); tomanovic@mefos.hr (T.O.K.); hrvoje.roguljic@mefos.hr (H.R.); martina.smolic@mefos.hr (M.S.)
2   Department of Pharmacology and Biochemistry, Faculty of Dental Medicine and Health, Josip Juraj Strossmayer University of Osijek, Crkvena 21, 31000 Osijek, Croatia
3   Department for Cardiovascular Disease, University Hospital Osijek, 4, 31000 Osijek, Croatia
4   Clinical Institute of Nuclear Medicine and Radiation Protection, University Hospital Osijek, 31000 Osijek, Croatia; tkizivat@mefos.hr
5   Department for Nuclear Medicine and Oncology, Faculty of Medicine, Josip Juraj Strossmayer University of Osijek; J. Huttlera 4, 31000 Osijek, Croatia
6   Department of Diabetes, Endocrinology and Metabolism Disorders, University Hospital Osijek, 31000 Osijek, Croatia
*   Correspondence: ibcurcic@mefos.hr

Received: 30 October 2019; Accepted: 18 November 2019; Published: 20 November 2019

Abstract: Diabetic nephropathy (DN) is one of the most perilous side effects of diabetes mellitus type 1 and type 2 (T1DM and T2DM).). It is known that sodium/glucose cotransporter 2 inhibitors (SGLT 2i) and glucagone like peptide-1 receptor agonists (GLP-1 RAs) have renoprotective effects, but the molecular mechanisms are still unknown. In clinical trials GLP-1 analogs exerted important impact on renal composite outcomes, primarily on macroalbuminuria, possibly through suppression of inflammation-related pathways, however enhancement of natriuresis and diuresis is also one of possible mechanisms of nephroprotection. Dapagliflozin, canagliflozin, and empagliflozin are SGLT2i drugs, useful in reducing hyperglycemia and in their potential renoprotective mechanisms, which include blood pressure control, body weight loss, intraglomerular pressure reduction, and a decrease in urinary proximal tubular injury biomarkers. In this review we have discussed the potential synergistic and/or additive effects of GLP 1 RA and SGLT2 inhibitors on the primary onset and progression of kidney disease, and the potential implications on current guidelines of diabetes type 2 management.

Keywords: diabetic nephropathy; diabetes mellitus; GLP-1 receptor agonists; SGLT2 inhibitors; molecular mechanisms

---

1. Introduction

Diabetic nephropathy (DN) is a complication of diabetes mellitus, both type I and II, caused by changes in microvasculature [1], and which can lead to end-stage renal disease and cardiovascular disease [2,3]. Moreover, it is the leading cause of chronic kidney disease, affecting 30–40% of patients with diabetes mellitus type 1 and 25–40% of patients with diabetes type 2 [4–7].

In its classic definition DN is defined as increased protein excretion in urine [8]. Major representations of diabetes in renal disease include persistent albuminuria, loss of podocytes, glomerular hypertrophy, matrix expansion, and thickening of the glomerular basement membrane [9,10]. The first stages of DN are characterized by microalbuminuria, a small increase in albumin excretion in urine [11–13]. Later stages are defined by macroalbuminuria or proteinuria leading to a decreased glomerular filtration rate [8].

Pathogenesis and progression of diabetic kidney disease are most likely a result of interactions between metabolic and hemodynamic changes which are caused by onset of diabetes [14], but also other factors including genetic predisposition [15], generation of reactive oxygen species (ROS) caused by hyperglycemia [14–16], and inflammation [17].

Studies have shown that diabetic kidney disease can lead to end stage renal disease in 30–40% of diabetes mellitus (DM) patients [18], implying that genetic variations could have impact on the start and progression of DM and the end stage renal disease. Genome-wide studies have been conducted to identify potential candidate genes of importance to DM and diabetic kidney disease [19]. More than fourteen genes have been identified as important to the development of diabetic kidney disease, among which are genes controlling lipid metabolism (*ADIPOQ*), glucose metabolism (*GCKR*), angiogenesis (*EPO promotor* gene), genes related to renal structure and function (*SHROOM3*), inflammation and oxidative stress related genes (*TGF-β1*), renin-angiotensin-aldosterone system related genes (*AGTR1*), and others [15]. Still, the complete effects of these genes and their variants are not completely clear. Results from these studies cannot be replicated among different races indicating race-specific gene polymorphisms or still significant environmental impacts.

Inflammation and chronic high levels of circulating glucose and its end metabolites are main causes of tissue damage in DM by, among other, creating high levels of oxidative and nitrosative stress in kidneys [20,21]. The effects of oxidative stress in other renal diseases like urolithiasis have been described [22]. High production of ROS and nitrosative species (NS) can cause damage to nuclear and mitochondrial DNA, induce apoptosis, and cause endoplasmic reticulum stress, and with this playing a role in cell death pathways such as apoptosis and necrosis in key cell types such as podocytes [20].

Considering the structural changes in diabetic kidney disease, they are similar in both DM1 and DM2, but are more heterogeneous and less predictable in association with clinical presentation in DM2 [23], probably because DM2 has unreliable onset timing, longer exposure to hyperglycemia before diagnosis, older patients, and patients that are treated with renin-angiotensin inhibitors before the onset of diabetes [24].

These structural alterations encompass modifications of several kidney departments. One of the first changes is thickening of the glomerular basal membrane, becoming apparent at 1.5 to 2 years from the diagnosis of DM, and which is closely followed by thickening of the capillary and tubular basement membrane [25–28]. Glomerular changes later include mesangial matrix expansion, loss of endothelial fenestrations, and loss of podocytes with effacement of foot processes [25]. The first signs of mesangial volume expansion are seen after 5–7 years of DM1 onset [27–30]. As DM progresses, segmental mesangiolysis appears and is considered to be connected with the development of micoaneurysms and Kimmelstal–Wilson nodules [31,32]. Subendothelial deposits of proteins forming periodic acid-Schiff-positive and electron-dense deposits accumulate in small arterioles, glomerular capillaries and microaneurysms result in exudative lesions and can cause luminal compromise [25]. Subepithelial deposits similar to subendothelial can be seen in Bowman's capsule and renal tubules. In the later stages of DM, glomerulopathy and interstitial changes grow together to segmental and global sclerosis [25]. Glomerular filtration, albuminuria, and hypertension in DM1 are strongly correlated with mesangial expansion, but to a less degree with glomerular basement membrane width [25].

2. GLP-1 Agonists in Diabetic Nephropathy

2.1. Classes of GLP-1 RA and Mechanism of Action

Glucagon-like peptide-1 (GLP-1) receptor agonists (RAs), an antidiabetic class of drugs, are known for their proven efficacy and safety profile [33]. They can be divided into human originated GLP-1

RAs, synthesized by various modifications of human GLP-1 active fragments, and agents derived from reptile Gila monster venom (exendin-4) [33,34]. Another classification of GLP-1 RAs is based on their pharmacokinetic profile, which divides these drugs into two different groups: short-acting (exenatide twice daily and lixisenatide) and long-acting agonists (once-weekly injected; dulaglutide, liraglutide, semaglutide, albiglutide) [33,34]. The half-lives of GLP-RAs vary between 2–3 h for short-acting agonists and 13 h to 7 days for long-acting agonists [33]. Up-to-date, above-mentioned 6 GLP-1 RAs have been approved for the treatment of patients with type 2 diabetes mellitus (T2DM), and all these drugs are administered by subcutaneous injection [33]. In general, GLP-1 RAs exert various beneficial effects in T2DM: enhancement of glucose-dependent insulin secretion, acceleration of β-cells proliferation and inhibition of β-cells apoptosis, inhibition of motility and gastric emptying, and a stimulation of the sensations of satiety and fullness by direct action on the central nervous system, with reduction in body weight [34–37]. Many other effects are still being investigated, among them reduction in systolic and diastolic blood pressure and improvements in lipid profile [33,38–42]. The main difference between the two groups is the fact that short-acting GLP-1 RAs while delaying gastric emptying, mostly lower postprandial plasma glucose, whereas the long-acting agonists predominantly exhibit insulinotropic and glucagonostatic actions, consequently exerting a much greater effect on fasting glucose concentrations. Various meta-analysis showed that long-acting agonists were more successful in lowering HbA$_{1C}$ compering to short-acting agonists [33,41,43–47]. More specifically, these studies demonstrated that the largest reduction in HbA$_{1c}$ values was associated with dulaglutide and exenatide once weekly, whereas the smallest mean reduction was observed with albiglutide [48]. The same results were observed when comparing the effects on the reduction of body weight [33]. The advantages of liraglutide in comparison with exenatide were: less frequent nausea and vomiting (shorter duration of GI side effects at the beginning of the therapy), more efficacy in lowering glycemic parameters, fasting glucose, and improving the homeostatic model assessment of β cells [34]. Generally, the most often side effects of GLP-1 RA therapy are gastrointestinal events (nausea, vomiting, diarrhea; shorter duration in short-acting agonists because of their lack of substantial effects on gastric emptying), and injection-site reactions (notable for albiglutide and lixisenatide), immunogenicity (exendin-4 derivates are more likely to be associated with the development of antidrug antibodies compared to GLP-1 RAs modified from human GLP-1) [33,49,50]. Nevertheless, these adverse events are rarely serious or persistent, nor the cause of discontinuation of therapy, especially because of the high efficiency of these drugs.

2.2. Potential Nephroprotective Actions of GLP-1 Agonists

Among all the above-mentioned therapeutic effects (lowering glucose, reducing body-weight etc.), GLP-1 RAs exert possible nephroprotective effects in T2DM, which have been demonstrated in various studies. Yin W et al. showed that GLP-1 RAs reduced albuminuria and ameliorated kidney tubules and tubulointerstitial lesions in the diabetic nephropathy rats model [51]. GLP-1 RAs downregulated the expression of tubulointerstitial tumor necrosis factor alpha (TNFα), monocyte chemoattractant protein-1(MCP-1), collagen I, alpha-smooth muscle actin (α-SMA), and fibronectin (FN) which are all reported to play a role in the diabetic nephropathy [51]. Additionally, the level of C-peptide, which was found to inhibit tubulointerstitial fibrosis [52], was increased by GLP-1 RAs and this may be one of the ways of improving tubuluinterstitial and tubular injury in GK rats with diabetic nephropathy [51]. In the study of Kodera et al. various beneficial effects of exendin-4 were showed, with emphasis on the prevention of macrophage infiltration, decrease of protein levels of intercellular adhesion molecul-1 (ICAM-1) and type IV collagen in glomeruli, as well as the decrease of oxidative stress (downregulation of *Nox4* gene expression) and nuclear factor-kB (known for contributing to cross-talk between inflammation and oxidative stress) activation in kidney tissue [53]. Furthermore, liraglutide is capable of inhibiting NAD(P)H oxidase through generation of cAMP, followed by activation of PKA or Epac2 [54–57]. Hendarto et al. confirmed the role of liraglutide in the normalization of oxidative stress markers and expression of renal NAD(P)H oxidase components (Nox4, gp91phox, p22phox, p47phox) in diabetic rats, but independently of lowering plasma glucose levels [58]. Similar results were demonstrated in the mouse model of diabetic nephrophathy with the crucial role of liraglutide in protection against renal oxidative stress and lowering of fibronectin accumulation in glomerular capillary walls [59]. Molecular mechanisms included in these actions are inhibition of NAD(P)H oxidase and activation of cAMP-PKA pathway as already explained [59]. The in vitro beneficial effects of liraglutide were also showed in various studies. Zhao et al. proved that liraglutide enhances cell viability in HK-2 cells (human proximal tubular cells) by downregulating caspase-3 expression [37]. Furthermore, mRNA and protein expression of GLP-1R was significantly enhanced by liraglutide, whereas the expression of the autophagic markers LC3-II and Beclin1 was ameliorated [37]. All these effects were blocked by the GLP-1R antagonist exendin-(9–39) [37]. Additionally, another study on HK2 cells treated with GLP1 RAs showed decrease in the expression of profibrotic factors like fibronectin, α-SMA, collagen I, and TNFα [51]. In the same study GLP-1RAs inhibited the activity of NF-κB and p38MAPK (two significant signaling pathways for kidney fibrosis) via GLP-1R [51]. Various studies confirmed the role of GLP-1RAs in water and electrolyte balance. One of the suggested mechanisms for this effect is inhibition of intestinal sodium–hydrogen exchanger isoform 3 (NHE3) activity [60]. This NHE3 exchanger is located on the renal proximal tubule, and GLP-1RA, by inhibiting its activity, enhance natriuresis and diuresis [61]. Accordingly, when adding GLP-1R blocker exendin-9, a decrease in renal excretion of sodium and water is observed [62]. Furthermore, exendin-9 has been connected with slight decrease in glomerular filtration rate (GFR), although it would be expected to increase GFR by increasing proximal tubular reabsorption, followed by inhibition of tubuloglomerular feedback signals and reduction in afferent arteriolar resistance [62]. However, this implicates another possible positive effect of GLP-1RA on nephroprotection and water/sodium balance [62]. Glomerular hyperfiltration enhanced by GLP-1RAs increases filtration and in the end excretion of electrolytes [61]. Finally, all these studies, which show the beneficial effects of GLP-1RAs in diabetic glomerular, tubulointerstitial, and tubular nephropathy, implicate the possible clinical use of these agents in treatment of diabetic nephropathy.

2.3. Assessment of Nephroprotective Effect of GLP-1 Receptor Agonists in Clinical Trials

Recent clinical trials demonstrate notable evidence of glucagon-like peptide-1 (GLP-1) agonists exerting renal benefits.

Between June 2012 and August 2013 the LIRA–RENAL trial examined the efficacy and safety profile of liraglutide in diabetic patients with moderate renal impairment (defined as eGFR 30–59 mL/min/1.73 m^2) [63]. This double blinded, randomized, placebo-controlled trial included 279 patients with type 2 DM who had HbA1c in the range of 7% to 10%. Addition of liraglutide to background glucose-lowering therapy reduced HbA1c more than placebo treatment (−1.05% vs. −0.38%). During the trial no deterioration of renal function was observed in patients treated with liraglutide in comparison with placebo. Furthermore, albuminuria assessed as the urinary albumin-to-creatinine ratio showed lower increase at week 26 in patients treated with liraglutide, although it was not significantly.

A more extensive and longer study of liraglutide treatment effect on renal outcomes in patients with diabetic nephropathy was the Liraglutide Effect and Action in Diabetes: Evaluation of Cardiovascular Outcome Results (LEADER) trial [64]. The LEADER trial included 9340 patients with type 2 diabetes and a high risk of cardiovascular disease with a median follow-up of 3.84 years. 23.1% of the trial population had mean estimated GFR less than 59 mL per minute per 1.73 m^2; and furthermore, microalbuminuria and macroalbuminuria were present at the baseline (26.3% and 10.5%, respectively). The renal outcome showed a lower rate of occurrence in the liraglutide group in comparison with placebo (5.7% vs. 7.2%). That was primarily the result of lower incidence of new-onset persistent macroalbuminuria in patients treated with liraglutide (3.4% vs. 4.6%). During the follow-up the urinary albumin-to-creatinine ratio growth was slower in liraglutide group while decline of estimated GFR and the rates of renal adverse effects were similar between the two groups. Interestingly, the effect of liraglutide on composite renal outcomes showed no difference in prespecified subgroups of patients with an elevated baseline renal risk, suggesting effectiveness of the liraglutide renal benefit to be an independent factor of stage of chronic kidney disease.

While the LEADER trial included patients with macroalbuminuria from the baseline to the onset of sustained albuminuria in the endpoint, the Evaluation of Lixisenatide in Acute Coronary Syndrome (ELIXA) trial assessed renal outcomes in patients only with normoalbuminuria or microalbuminuria [65]. This randomized, double blinded study primarily examined the effect on cardiovascular outcomes of short-acting GLP1 agonist lixisenatide in 6068 patients with type 2 diabetes and a recent acute coronary syndrome. Beside cardiovascular safety, the addition of lixisenatide to standard therapy showed beneficial impact on renal outcomes. The renoprotective effect manifested as lower rate of increase in urinary albumin-to-creatinine ratio, 34% in the placebo group vs. 24% in lixisenatide group. No significant difference was observed between the two groups in eGFR decline or doubling of serum creatinine, while overall incidence of renal adverse effects was low in both groups. Evidently the difference in pharmacokinetics of GLP-1 analogs, short-acting versus long-acting analogs, has no impact on renal composite outcomes. Somewhat different results were obtained in AWARD-7 study which examined the effect of long acting GLP-1 analog dulaglutide versus insulin glargine on renal outcomes in patients with diabetes type 2 and moderate-to-severe CKD [66]. 577 participants were randomized in three groups, dulaglutide 1.5 mg or 0.75 mg treated groups and insulin glargine group. The decline of eGFR after 52 weeks of treatment with dulaglutide was significantly smaller in dulaglutide treated patients compared to insulin group. The albuminuria decrease was similar between all treatment groups, with a slightly greater decrease of urinary albumin-to-creatinine ratio in dulaglutide treated patients. Although dulaglutide enhanced body loss, whether fat or muscle tissue, the study confirmed the beneficial renal effect of GLP-1 analog as an independent action. In the Trial to Evaluate Cardiovascular and other Long-term Outcomes with Semaglutide in Subjects with Type 2 Diabetes (SUSTAIN-6), the rate of persistent macroalbuminuria was lower in patients receiving semaglutide, than in those receiving placebo [67].

Taken together, GLP-1 analogs as antidiabetic medications show significant influence on renal composite outcomes, primarily on a new onset of macroalbuminuria as shown in Table 1. Numerous previous studies characterized development of albuminuria as an independent predictor of diabetic nephropathy progression with subsequent deterioration of estimated glomerular filtration and development of end stage renal disease [68–70]. Definitely, more intensive glycemic control achieved by addition of GLP-1 agonist to background antidiabetic therapy justifies a decrease of macroalbuminuria incidence in diabetic patients due to a well-known effect of serum high glucose concentration on increased filtration rate of proteins via glomerular capillary membrane and on impaired tubular reabsorption [71]. Another possible mechanism of GLP-1 beneficial renal effect could be suppression of inflammation-related pathways. Preclinical studies have unambiguously demonstrated anti-inflammatory and antioxidative effect of GLP-1 analogs [59,72]. This was also suggested during the LIRA-RENAL trial when lower concentration of inflammation marker hsCRP was obtained in liraglutid treated group in comparison with placebo [63]. Although the mechanism of beneficial renal effect of GLP-1 agonists still remains elusive, it is definitely achieved as a combined effect through glucose lowering treatment and extra-glycemic effects.

Table 1. The pharmacokinetic properties and renal outcomes of clinical trials with GLP-1 receptor agonists.

Drug.	Dose	Half Life (h)	Elimination	Clinical Study	Renal Benefit
Short-acting GLP-1 receptor agonists					
Exenatide	5–10 µg twice-daily s.c.	2.4	Mostly renal	/	/
Lixisenatide	10–20 µg once-daily s.c.	3.0	Mostly renal	ELIXA [65]	Lower rate of increase in urinary albumin-to-creatinine ratio
Long-acting GLP-1 receptor agonists					
Exenatide	2 mg QW s.c.	2.4	Mostly renal		
Liraglutide	0.6 mg, 1.2 mg or 1.8 mg once-daily s.c.	11.6–13.0	Peptidases and renal 6%; feces 5%	LEADER [64]	↓Nephropathy, ↓UACR, ↓RAS hormone, ↓Progression to macroalbuminuria, ↓Doubling of serum creatinine levels, ↓eGFR of ≤45 mL/min per 1.73 m^2, ↓The initiation of renal-replacement therapy, ↓Risk of end-stage renal disease or renal death, ↓Plasma renin concentration, renin activity, angiotensin II
Semaglutide	0.5–1.0 mg once-weekly s.c.	165.0–184.0	Peptidases and renal	SUSTAIN-6 [67]	↓Nephropathy >35%, ↓Progression to macroalbuminuria, ↓Doubling of serum creatinine levels, ↓eGFR of ≤45 mL/min per 1.73 m^2, ↓The initiation of renal-replacement therapy
Dulaglutide	0.75–1.5 mg once-weekly s.c.	~112.8	Peptidases and renal	AWARD VII [66]	Reduced albuminuria, slower decline in renal function
Albiglutide	30–50 mg once-weekly s.c.	~120.0	Peptidases and renal	/	/

Abbrevations: s.c., subcutaneous injection; eGFR, estimated glomerular filtration rate in mL/min/1.73m^2; UACR, urine albumin/creatinine ratio; RAS, renin-angiotensin system; CVR, cardiovascular risk, ↓ decline.

3. SGLT2 Inhibitors in Diabetic Nephropathy

3.1. Mechanism of Action

Sodium/glucose cotransporter 2 (SGLT2) inhibitors are orally administrated hypoglycemic drugs with a novel mechanism of action that is useful across a continuum of diabetes regardless of duration of diabetes, baseline Hba1c or concomitant antidiabetic therapy [73,74]. Glucose reabsorbtion takes place in the proximal tubule via the sodium dependent glucose transporters (SGLT), placed on the apical side of the proximal tubule cell through the basolateral Na, K-ATPase pump [75,76]. SGLT2 is expressed almost entirely in the renal proximal tubules, hence selective inhibition of this protein leads to renal glucose excretion and reduction of plasma glucose levels without influencing other metabolic processes [77]. Sodium glucose cotransporter 2 (SGLT2) is the main luminal glucose transporter placed in the S1 and S2 portions of the proximal tubule (PT) while sodium glucose cotransporter 1 (SGLT1) is placed in the S3 portion and supply fewer than 10% of entire luminal glucose transport [78]. SGLT2 on the apical membrane is connected with GLUT2 on the basolateral part and jointly they reabsorb up to 90% of filtered glucose beneath normoglycaemic conditions [79]. Increased renin angiotensin system (RAS) activity with SGLT2 inhibition is explained by the normal volume depletion with this kind of therapy [80], although a tendency for diminished GFR with SGLT2 inhibition is probably due to enlarged afferent tone over tubuloglomerular feedback [81]. Furthermore, maximal renoprotection from glomerular injury, renal fibrosis, and proteinuria was achieved when luseogliflozin (SGLT2 inhibitor) was combined with the ACE inhibitor, lisinopril [82]. At the early stage of kidney impairment, therapies that prevent the RAS activity are as well indicated, but these approaches are not completely beneficial [83]. One of the possible mechanisms of SGLT2 inhibitors is prevention of glucose influx to the kidney proximal tubular cell responsible for development of diabetic nephropathy [84–86]. Histological variation detected in the glomerulus is the traditional focal point in diabetic nephropathy, but it has become extensively recognized that the changes detected in tubulointerstitial fibrosis and in the tubulointerstitium correspond more firmly with impairment in renal function [79]. Dapagliflozin, canagliflozin, and empagliflozin are SGLT2i drugs, useful in reducing hyperglycemia and improvement of glycemic control. They are used in mild renal impairment and have combined beneficial effects such as the lowering of body weight and blood pressure (BP) [73]. The pharmacokinetic properties of SGLT2 inhibitors demonstrate an excellent oral bioavailability, a rather long elimination half-life permitting once daily administration, a short accumulation index, no active metabolites and restricted renal excretion [87]. Moreover, these drugs share an insignificant risk of drug–drug interactions [88]. The risk for hypoglycemia is low because inhibition of SGLT2 does not increase the excretion of insulin or impede with gluconeogenesis. Additionally, there are some indications that SGLT2 inhibition improves beta cell function, perhaps by reducing glucotoxicity [89,90]. Loss of excess calories mediated by glucose excretion in urine results in weight loss and can alleviate the weight gain induced by another classes of hypoglycemic agents. In patients with hypertension SGLT2 inhibitors lower blood pressure as well, probably due to glucosuria, subsequent natriuresis, and diuresis [91]. Absorption of dapagliflozin after oral administration is fast, reaching peak plasma concentrations in 1–2 h it. The main organs included in the metabolism of this drug are the liver and kidneys, where inactive metabolites are produced by enzyme uridine diphosphate-glucuronosyltransferase-1A9 (UGT1A9). Clearance of dapagliflozin by renal excretion is not significant, and there are no drug–drug interactions [88]. Dapagliflozin is capable of reducing body weight and fat mass, improving glycemic control and lowering blood pressure [92,93]. Following the treatment of T2DM with 5 or 10 mg dapagliflozin, a higher risk of mild to moderate urinary tract infections was observed, but without a final dose correlatin among UTI and glucosuria [94].Pharmacokinetic properties of canagliflozin include immediate absorption after oral administration, 65% oral bioavailability within a dose range of 50–300 mg, and in dose-dependent manner, high potential as 99% is bounded to plasma proteins, especially albumin, and finally it is metabolized generally to inactive metabolites [88,95]. As opposed to other SGLT2i, canagliflozin is also capable of minor inhibition of SGLT1. Canagliflozin postpones intestinal glucose absorption in addition to increasing UGE, followed by lowering of postprandial glucose and insulin levels [96]. Canagliflozin treatment is also associated with an UTI and symptomatic vulvovaginal adverse events in female patients with T2DM [97]. Empagliflozin is quickly absorbed in single oral doses achieving Cmax after 1.0–2.0 h. Drug-drug interactions among empagliflozin and other oral glucose lowering agents, cardiovascular medications or various other drugs with narrow therapeutic index were not observed [88,98]. In a fasting and postprandial state in T2DM patients, following administration of empagliflozin or dapagliflozin, paradoxical increase in endogenous glucose production was demonstrated [99]. Nevertheless, plasma glucose levels in these patients were reduced by empagliflozin [98]. Ferrannini et al. showed moderate association of a 10 and 25 mg empagliflozin dose and increased incidence of genital infections, but without increase in UTIs incidence [100]. The capacity of SGLT2i to decrease the plasma glucose levels is directly proportional to the glomerular filtration rate (GFR) and is reduced in chronic kidney disease (CKD). Nevertheless, research underway indicates that SGLT2i can contribute to nephroprotection in diabetes independently of glycemic control [73,101–103].

3.2. Evidence of Nephroprotection In Vitro and in Animal Models

Cultured human proximal renal tubular cells of patients with type 2 diabetes demonstrate noticeably enlarged levels of SGLT2 mRNA and protein and increased glucose transporter activity [104]. Several experiments using human proximal tubular cells (HK2) showed that SGLT2 inhibition reduced the output of inflammatory and fibrotic markers induced by high glucose levels [73]. The above-mentioned in vitro findings suggest that SGLT2 inhibitors can provide nephroprotection in diabetes by blocking glucose influx to proximal tubule cells [105]. In new preclinical trials, nephroprotection with SGLT2 inhibition has been observed after improvement of glycemic control [82,105–109].

Accordingly, the effect of SGLT2 inhibition on early kidney growth, inflammation, and fibrosis was proposed to result from blood glucose lowering [109]. Thus, blood glucose lowering effect could be responsible for SGLT2i inhibition of inflammation, fibrosis and early renal growth [105]. This hypothesis is supported by several recently published studies conducted in animal models. Inhibition of progression of albuminuria along with drop in plasma glucose by <15 mmol/L was observed in male db/db mice treated with dapagliflozin [107] and females treated with tofogliflozin [109]. Furthermore, Lin et al. showed decrease in albuminuria and glomerulosclerosis followed by improvement of hyperglycemia in male db/db mice treated with empagliflozin [108]. Vallon et al. demonstrated reduction of albuminuria, kidney hypertrophy, and markers of inflammation, proportional to glucose lowering effect in the T1DM model of male Akita mice treated with empagliflozin [105]. The effect of SGLT2 inhibition on diabetic nephropathy, autonomous of blood glucose decrease, was investigated in diabetic eNOS knockout mice [110], while further studies in fat Zucker rats have demonstrated that diabetes enhanced RNA expression of SGLT2 and SGLT1 within the kidney [111]. In addition, proximal tubular cells exposed to the urine of diabetic patients have shown an increase in SGLT2 expression [104]. Diversity of agents have been related to the modification in expression of SGLT1 and 2, including HNF1α and SGK1 [76]. Furthermore, exposure of proximal tubular cells to transforming growth factor β (TGFβ), a profibrotic cytokine, led to upregulation of SGLT2 expression [66].

Interleukin-6 (IL-6) and tumor necrosis factor-α (TNF-α) increased SGLT2 expression in cultured kidney cell lines after exposure for 96–120 h [112], while increase in SGLT2 expression has also been achieved through high glucose-induced pathway exceeding protein kinase A (PKA) and protein kinase C (PKC) reliant pathways [113,114]. Some studies have also shown interaction among the sodium glucose cotransporters and the renin–angiotensin–aldosterone model. For example, losartan decreased SGLT2 expression in diabetic rats in regular or high salt nutrition in animal models [115]. In diabetic rats, enhancement of GLUT2 expression and its translocation to the luminal surface of the proximal tubular cells was observed leading to an increase in glucose reabsorption [78]. One of the potential mechanisms involved in nephroprotection could be linked with a decrease in GLUT 9 expression, a major regulator of urate homeostasis [116–118]. The expression of certain profibrotic genes is diminished with empagliflozin, in line with the effects of first line anti-diabetic agent, metformin in diabetic rat model. Gallo at al. presented that a threshold of blood glucose lowering can be necessary to accomplished complete renoprotection in diabetes, since empagliflozin influenced some markers of fibrosis but had no effect on albuminuria and glomerular sclerosis. So, Gallo et al. suggested that adequate, and stable blood glucose lowering, perhaps with multiple medications, including higher- and/or multiple daily-dosing of SGLT2 inhibition in combination with a RAS blockade, can be necessary to accomplished maximal nephroprotection in diabetes [83].

3.3. Assessment of Nephroprotective Effect of SGLT 2 Inhibitors in Clinical Trials

Presently, short-term studies are available assuring of renal safety with SGLT2i drugs, however there are no long-term data confirming renal benefit [118] SGLT2i decreases albuminuria, the most important renal risk marker in DN [119]. The albuminuria-lowering effects of SGLT2i have been shown in various studies [120,121] but the precise mechanism is still not clear, and it seems to be independent of alterations in eGFR, systolic BP, body weight, or HbA1c [121]. A placebo-controlled study has demonstrated that canagliflozin 100 mg/day diminished albuminuria around 22% [120], likewise empagliflozin 25 mg/day decreased albuminuria roughly 35% relative to placebo in patients with chronic kidney disease and diabetes mellitus type 2 RAS-based drugs such as ACEi or ARBs, and SGLT2i could have complementary but different mechanisms of action, with diverse outcomes to the kidney system and a potential synergistic effect. In a recently published study, the combination of SGLT2i and RAS blockers was associated with additive nephroprotective effect in diabetic nephropathy compared to either medicament alone [106]. Heerspink et al. showed reduction of albuminuria with dapagliflozin 10 mg/day, compared to placebo in patients with hypertension and diabetes already treated with RAS blockers [121].

Decrease of uric acid in serum is another way where SGLT2i may achieve their nephroprotective effect. Elevated levels of uric acid or hyperuricemia, have been demonstrated to hugely correlate with the possibility of renal impairment in diabetes [122–124], and are responsible for microvascular complications in diabetes [125,126]. The beneficial effect of uric acid reduction in serum with SGLT2i can be clinically significant and has been shown in several studies [127–129]. The EMPA-REG outcome study has shown that empagliflozin therapy was associated with improvement in all renal function parameters in patients with estimated glomerular filtration rate of at least 30 mL per minute. Empagliflozin significantly decreased worsening or incident nephropathy, request for renal transplantation or dialysis and doubling of serum creatinine levels compared to placebo, while further analysis showed reduction in albuminuria [67].

In the DECLARE trial there was a 24% reduction with dapagliflozin in a composite renal outcome of a $\geq$40% decrease in estimated glomerular filtration rate (eGFR) (to <60 mL/min/1.73 m^2), end-stage renal disease (ESRD), or death from renal or CV causes compared with placebo [130]. Included patients had eGFR of at least 60 mL/min at baseline, emphasizing the potential role of dapagliflozin not only in treatment but in the prevention of diabetic nephropathy [131,132]. The CANVAS trial showed a 27% reduction in progression of albuminuria, with a 40% reduction in eGFR, need for renal-replacement therapy, or death from renal causes associated with the use of canagliflozin [131]. The CREDENCE study was the first large-scale outcome trial of an SGLT2 inhibitor canagliflozin with primary kidney outcome defined as doubling of serum creatinine, end-stage kidney disease, or death due to cardiovascular or kidney disease. Almost all patients included in the CREDENCE trial (99%) were treated with ACE inhibitors or ARBs compared to other trials (80%) [133], and had eGFR of 30 to <90 mL per minute as shown in Table 2. The trial was stopped early after a planned interim analysis based on positive results since the relative risk of the renal-specific composite outcome was lower by 34% and the relative risk of end-stage kidney disease was lower by 32%. These data demonstrate that renoprotection was accomplished via the whole spectrum of eGFR levels once again establishing nephroprotecitve effect irrispective of baseline kidney function. The nephroprotective effects of SGLT2i could also benefit cardiovascular outcomes by triggering neurohormonal activation and volume wasting [134,135]. Recent meta-analysis demonstrated that SGLT2 inhibitors reduced the risk of dialysis, transplantation, or death due to kidney disease in individuals with type 2 diabetes and provided protection against acute kidney injury, adding additional evidence endorsing SGLT2i therapy as a corner stone of nephroprotection in diabetics [133]. SGLT2i are not presently recommended in patients with an eGFR lower than 45 mL/min per 1.73 m^2, to a large degree because of deficient glycemic effectiveness [136,137]. Proof of renoprotection from the above mentioned trials, due to these limitations, is questionable [138].

Table 2. The pharmacokinetic properties and renal outcomes of clinical trials with SGLT2i.

Drug	Dose (mg)	Half Life (h)	Administration	Clinical Study/Outcome	Renal Benefit
Empagliflozin	10	11.9	Per os, once daily	EMPA-REG OUTCOME [67]/incident or worsening nephropathy and incident albuminuria	↓Nephropathy 39%, ↓Progression to macroalbuminuria, ↓Doubling of serum creatinine levels, ↓the initiation of renal-replacement therapy
Dapagliflozin	10	12.9	Per os, once daily	DECLARE [137]/beneficial effects defined by eGFR status and the attendance or absence of Atherosclerotic cardiovascular illness at baseline	↓eGFR of 40% or more to an eGFR of fewer than 60 mL/min per 1.73 m^2, ↓Combined risk of end-stage renal disease or renal death, ↓Early prevention and decrease in progression of chronic renal disease in patients with T2DM, 31% reduction in the risk of acute renal injury in the dapagliflozin group compared to placebo group
Canagliflozin	100	over 12	Per os, once daily	CANVAS [67,133]/incident albuminuria, incident of renal failure	↓acute ↓acute kidney injury ↓albuminuria ↓eGFR of 40% ↓the initiation of renal-replacementtherapy ↓death from renal causes kidney injury ↓albuminuria ↓eGFR of 40% ↓the initiation of renal-replacementtherapy ↓death from renal causes
				CREDENCE * [133]/patients with established CKD, incident albuminuria, composite of dialysis, transplantation or death due to renal disease	↓Acute kidney injury, Albuminuria, ↓eGFR of 40%, ↓The initiation of renal-replacement therapy, ↓Death from renal causes in acute kidney injury, ↓Doubling of serum creatinine levels ↓Risk of dialysis and transplantation, ↓Risk of end-stage renal, disease or renal death

Abbreviations: eGFR, estimated glomerular filtration rate in mL/min/1.73m², * fewer than 60 mL/min per 1.73m², * use of RASi was obligatory to entry into the CREDENCE trial; DKD, diabetic kidney disease, ↓ decline.

4. Implications of Potential Synergism of GLP 1 RA and SGLT2 Inhibitors on Prevention of Kidney Disease

Although glycemic control along with blood pressure control and blockade of renin–angiotensin–aldosterone system represents a cornerstone of the prevention of new-onset diabetic nephropathy, 30% of diabetic patients will develop significant renal insufficiency [102,139]. Therefore, novel therapeutic measures as well as diabetic polytherapy are a necessity in prevention and treatment of diabetes mellitus associated complications. Recent studies clearly demonstrate the renoprotective effects of GLP-1 receptor agonists primarily achieved through reduction of new onset microalbuminuria [140]. Although the molecular mechanisms of these beneficial effects are not fully clarified some of renal effects of these drugs have been emphasized. GLP1 receptors present in multiple renal cells are responsible for increased glomerular filtration rate, vasodilatation of the afferent arteriole, and enhanced natriuresis [62]. The state of hyperglycaemia causes enhanced reabsorption of Na+ in proximal tubule and reduced delivery of Na+ to the macula densa with consequent vasodilatation of afferent arteriole, glomerular hypertension, and hyperfiltration [4,141]. Both GLP 1 receptor agonists and SGLT2I promote natriuresis within the proximal tubule acting at different sites. Inhibition of SGLT2 co-transporter beside enhanced glucosuria results in increased natiuresis while GLP-1 receptor agonists promote natriuresis through inhibition of NHE3 (sodium hydrogen exchanger-3) transporter in proximale tubule. Increased delivery of Na+ to macula densa due to inhibition of SGLT2 triggers tubuloglomerlar feedback resulting in afferent vasoconstriction, reduced glomerular pressure and a 30–50% decrease in albuminuria [142]. Despite the natriuretic effect, mechanistic studies and clinical trials failed to exhibit renal hemodynamic vasoconstriction in response to GLP-1 RA treatment resulting in overall neutral GFR effect. However, GLP-1 RA treatment of diabetic patients undoubtedly reduces albuminuria probably due to suppression of inflammation-related pathways [139]. Combination of these antihyperglycemic agents characterizes complementary physiological effect on natriuresis while albuminuria reduction is achieved by different mechanisms. Taken together, potential synergistic and/or additive effects of SGLT2I and GLP-1 receptor agonists at renal function implicate direct beneficial impact on progression of diabetic kidney disease (Figure 1.). In addition, renal benefits could be achieved through common extrarenal effects such as weight reduction and lowering of blood pressure. However, to determine whether a synergistic or additive effect is in question, or perhaps a combination of the two, further studies in vitro and in vivo are needed comparing renal molecular mechanisms and clinical outcomes of combined therapy to each monocomponent separately.

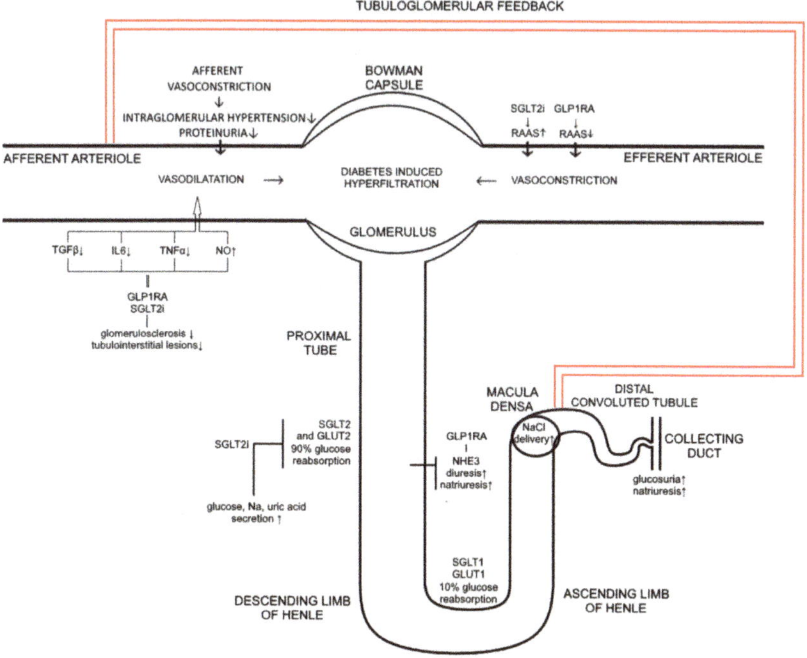

Figure 1. Mechanism of action of SGLT2i and GLP 1RA on kidney. SGLT2i inhibit glucose and sodium transport via SGLT2 and GLUT 2 transporters which are responsible for 90% of glucose reabsorption thus inducing glucosuria, diuresis, natriuresis, and uric acid excretion. At the same time GLP 1RA via NHE3 are also promoting diuresis and natriuresis. Influx of sodium to macula densa is increased thus affecting afferent vasoconstriction causing reduction in intraglomerular pressure and proteinuria through tubuloglomerular feedback. Both, GLP 1RA and SGLT2i induce suppression of inflammatory markers such as TGFβ, IL6, TNFα, decreasing glomerusclerosis and tubulointerstitial lesions and causing afferent vasoconstriction (induction of NO is also involved). GLP 1RA therapy leads to a decrease in RAAS activity causing efferent vasodilatation, while the effect of SGLT2i is quite the opposite, it increases RAAS activity due to natriuresis and volume depletion implying that positive effect on intraglomerular pressure is mediated completely through tubuloglomerular feedback; ↑ increase; ↓ decrease.

5. Conclusions

Both GLP 1 RA and SGLT2i may exhibit direct renoprotective effects through the suppression of inflammatory responses, inhibition of oxidative injury, and prevention of apoptosis as a result of the combined impact of glucose lowering treatment and extra-glycemic effects. Definitely, more intensive glycemic control achieved by addition of GLP-1 agonist and SGLT2i to background antidiabetic therapy justifies a potential benefit on renal function in diabetic patients, however it is obvious that other renoprotective mechanisms exist such as hemodynamic effects, blood pressure control, and body weight loss. Recently, based on the evidence from the trials mentioned above, new European Society of Cardiology (ESC) guidelines in association with European Association for the Study of Diabetes (EASD) position these drugs as the first therapy of choice in patients with diabetes and high cardiovascular risk overthrowing the long-standing paradigm of metformin as the first line therapy in DMT2 [143]. Given the importance of cardiovascular and renal risk reduction in diabetic patients achieved with those therapeutic options, it is only a matter of time before these two classes of drugs will become the gold standard in the treatment of type 2 diabetes.

Author Contributions: V.N. and T.O.K. conceived of and designed the article, and critically revised the manuscript; I.B.Ć. performed critical revision of the manuscript for important intellectual content, obtained funding, and provided administrative, technical and material support; H.R. and T.K. performed literature searches and critical revision of the manuscript for important intellectual content; M.S. performed literature searches, wrote the manuscript, and updated the text of the paper; M.S. performed literature searches and wrote the manuscript.

Funding: APC was funded by University project, VIF-2018-FDMZ-06.

Conflicts of Interest: The authors declare no conflict of interest.

Abbreviations

SGLT2i	sodium glucose lowering transporter2 inhibitors
GLP1 RA	glucagon like peptide 1 receptor agonist
GLUT 2	glucose transporter 2
NHE3	sodium-hydrogen exchanger isoform 3
TGFβ	transforming growth factor β
IL6	interleukin 6
TNFα	transforming nuclear factor α
RAAS	renin–angiotensin–aldosterone system

References

1. Thomas, B. The Global Burden of Diabetic Kidney Disease: Time Trends and Gender Gaps. *Curr. Diabet. Rep.* **2019**, *19*, 18. [CrossRef] [PubMed]
2. Zha, F.; Bai, L.; Tang, B.; Li, J.; Wang, Y.; Zheng, P.; Ji, T.; Bai, S. MicroRNA-503 contributes to podocyte injury via targeting E2F3 in diabetic nephropathy. *J. Cell Biochem.* **2019**, *120*, 12574–12581. [CrossRef] [PubMed]
3. Murea, M.; Ma, L.; Freedman, B.I. Genetic and environmental factors associated with type 2 diabetes and diabetic vascular complications. *Rev. Diabet. Stud.* **2012**, *9*, 6–22. [CrossRef] [PubMed]
4. Abbiss, H.; Maker, G.L.; Trengove, R.D. Metabolomics Approaches for the Diagnosis and Understanding of Kidney Diseases. *Metabolites* **2019**, *9*, 34. [CrossRef] [PubMed]
5. Gross, J.L.; de Azevedo, M.J.; Silveiro, S.P.; Canani, L.H.; Caramori, M.L.; Zelmanovitz, T. Diabetic nephropathy: Diagnosis, prevention, and treatment. *Diabetes Care* **2005**, *28*, 164–176. [CrossRef] [PubMed]
6. Parving, H.H.; Lehnert, H.; Bröchner-Mortensen, J.; Gomis, R.; Andersen, S.; Arner, P. Irbesartan in Patients with Type 2 Diabetes and Microalbuminuria Study Group. The effect of irbesartan on the development of diabetic nephropathy in patients with type 2 diabetes. *N. Engl. J. Med.* **2001**, *345*, 870–878. [CrossRef]
7. Van der Kloet, F.M.; Tempels, F.W.; Ismail, N.; van der Heijden, R.; Kasper, P.T.; Rojas-Cherto, M.; van Doorn, R.; Spijksma, G.; Koek, M.; van der Greef, J.; et al. Discovery of early-stage biomarkers for diabetic kidney disease using ms-based metabolomics (FinnDiane study). *Metabolomics* **2012**, *8*, 109–119. [CrossRef]
8. Zelmanovitz, T.; Gerchman, F.; Balthazar, A.P.; Thomazelli, F.C.; Matos, J.D.; Canani, L.H. Diabetic nephropathy. *Diabet. Metab. Syndr.* **2009**, *1*, 10. [CrossRef]
9. Yoon, J.J.; Park, J.H.; Kim, H.J.; Jin, H.G.; Kim, H.Y.; Ahn, Y.M.; Kim, Y.C.; Lee, H.S.; Lee, Y.J.; Kang, D.G. Improves Glomerular Fibrosis and Renal Dysfunction in Diabetic Nephropathy Model. *Nutrients* **2019**, *11*, 553. [CrossRef]
10. Declèves, A.E.; Sharma, K. New pharmacological treatments for improving renal outcomes in diabetes. *Nat. Rev. Nephrol* **2010**, *6*, 371–380. [CrossRef]
11. Mogensen, C.E.; Christensen, C.K. Predicting diabetic nephropathy in insulin-dependent patients. *N. Engl. J. Med.* **1984**, *311*, 89–93. [CrossRef] [PubMed]
12. Parving, H.H.; Oxenbøll, B.; Svendsen, P.A.; Christiansen, J.S.; Andersen, A.R. Early detection of patients at risk of developing diabetic nephropathy. A longitudinal study of urinary albumin excretion. *Acta Endocrinol. (Copenh)* **1982**, *100*, 550–555. [CrossRef] [PubMed]
13. Viberti, G.C.; Hill, R.D.; Jarrett, R.J.; Argyropoulos, A.; Mahmud, U.; Keen, H. Microalbuminuria as a predictor of clinical nephropathy in insulin-dependent diabetes mellitus. *Lancet* **1982**, *1*, 1430–1432. [CrossRef]
14. Cao, Z.; Cooper, M.E. Pathogenesis of diabetic nephropathy. *J. Diabet. Investig.* **2011**, *2*, 243–247. [CrossRef] [PubMed]

15. Wei, L.; Xiao, Y.; Li, L.; Xiong, X.; Han, Y.; Zhu, X.; Sun, L. The Susceptibility Genes in Diabetic Nephropathy. *Kidney Dis. (Basel)* **2018**, *4*, 226–237. [CrossRef] [PubMed]

16. Mahmoodnia, L.; Aghadavod, E.; Beigrezaei, S.; Rafieian-Kopaei, M. An update on diabetic kidney disease, oxidative stress and antioxidant agents. *J. Renal. Inj. Prev.* **2017**, *6*, 153–157. [CrossRef] [PubMed]

17. Pichler, R.; Afkarian, M.; Dieter, B.P.; Tuttle, K.R. Immunity and inflammation in diabetic kidney disease: Translating mechanisms to biomarkers and treatment targets. *Am. J. Physiol. Ren. Physiol.* **2017**, *312*, F716–F731. [CrossRef]

18. Hill, C.J.; Cardwell, C.R.; Patterson, C.C.; Maxwell, A.P.; Magee, G.M.; Young, R.J.; Matthews, B.; O'Donoghue, D.J.; Fogarty, D.G. Chronic kidney disease and diabetes in the national health service: A cross-sectional survey of the U.K. national diabetes audit. *Diabet. Med.* **2014**, *31*, 448–454. [CrossRef]

19. McDonough, C.W.; Palmer, N.D.; Hicks, P.J.; Roh, B.H.; An, S.S.; Cooke, J.N.; Hester, J.M.; Wing, M.R.; Bostrom, M.A.; Rudock, M.E.; et al. A genome-wide association study for diabetic nephropathy genes in African Americans. *Kidney Int.* **2011**, *79*, 563–572. [CrossRef]

20. Lindblom, R.; Higgins, G.; Coughlan, M.; de Haan, J.B. Targeting Mitochondria and Reactive Oxygen Species-Driven Pathogenesis in Diabetic Nephropathy. *Rev. Diabet. Stud.* **2015**, *12*, 134–156. [CrossRef]

21. Mittal, M.; Siddiqui, M.R.; Tran, K.; Reddy, S.P.; Malik, A.B. Reactive oxygen species in inflammation and tissue injury. *Antioxid. Redox Signal.* **2014**, *20*, 1126–1167. [CrossRef] [PubMed]

22. Kizivat, T.; Smolić, M.; Marić, I.; Tolušić Levak, M.; Smolić, R.; Bilić Čurčić, I.; Kuna, L.; Mihaljević, I.; Včev, A.; Tucak-Zorić, S. Antioxidant Pre-Treatment Reduces the Toxic Effects of Oxalate on Renal Epithelial Cells in a Cell Culture Model of Urolithiasis. *Int. J. Environ. Res. Public Health* **2017**, *14*, 109. [CrossRef] [PubMed]

23. Fioretto, P.; Caramori, M.L.; Mauer, M. The kidney in diabetes: Dynamic pathways of injury and repair. The Camillo Golgi Lecture 2007. *Diabetologia* **2008**, *51*, 1347–1355. [CrossRef] [PubMed]

24. Tervaert, T.W.; Mooyaart, A.L.; Amann, K.; Cohen, A.H.; Cook, H.T.; Drachenberg, C.B.; Ferrario, F.; Fogo, A.B.; Haas, M.; de Heer, E.; et al. Pathologic classification of diabetic nephropathy. *J. Am. Soc. Nephrol.* **2010**, *21*, 556–563. [CrossRef] [PubMed]

25. Alicic, R.Z.; Rooney, M.T.; Tuttle, K.R. Diabetic Kidney Disease: Challenges, Progress, and Possibilities. *Clin. J. Am. Soc. Nephrol.* **2017**, *12*, 2032–2045. [CrossRef] [PubMed]

26. Tyagi, I.; Agrawal, U.; Amitabh, V.; Jain, A.K.; Saxena, S. Thickness of glomerular and tubular basement membranes in preclinical and clinical stages of diabetic nephropathy. *Indian J. Nephrol.* **2008**, *18*, 64–69. [CrossRef]

27. Fioretto, P.; Mauer, M. Histopathology of diabetic nephropathy. *Semin. Nephrol.* **2007**, *27*, 195–207. [CrossRef]

28. Caramori, M.L.; Parks, A.; Mauer, M. Renal lesions predict progression of diabetic nephropathy in type 1 diabetes. *J. Am. Soc. Nephrol.* **2013**, *24*, 1175–1181. [CrossRef]

29. Drummond, K.; Mauer, M.; Group, I.D.N.S. The early natural history of nephropathy in type 1 diabetes: II. Early renal structural changes in type 1 diabetes. *Diabetes* **2002**, *51*, 1580–1587. [CrossRef]

30. Osterby, R.; Tapia, J.; Nyberg, G.; Tencer, J.; Willner, J.; Rippe, B.; Torffvit, O. Renal structures in type 2 diabetic patients with elevated albumin excretion rate. *APMIS* **2001**, *109*, 751–761. [CrossRef]

31. Saito, Y.; Kida, H.; Takeda, S.; Yoshimura, M.; Yokoyama, H.; Koshino, Y.; Hattori, N. Mesangiolysis in diabetic glomeruli: Its role in the formation of nodular lesions. *Kidney Int.* **1988**, *34*, 389–396. [CrossRef] [PubMed]

32. Stout, L.C.; Kumar, S.; Whorton, E.B. Focal mesangiolysis and the pathogenesis of the Kimmelstiel-Wilson nodule. *Hum. Pathol.* **1993**, *24*, 77–89. [CrossRef]

33. Gentilella, R.; Pechtner, V.; Corcos, A.; Consoli, A. Glucagon-like peptide-1 receptor agonists in type 2 diabetes treatment: Are they all the same? *Diabetes Metab Res. Rev.* **2019**, *35*, e3070. [CrossRef] [PubMed]

34. Gallwitz, B. Glucagon-like peptide-1 receptor agonists. In *Handbook of Incretin-Based Therapies in Type 2 Diabetes*; Gough, S., Ed.; Springer International Publishing Switzerland: Cham, Switzerland, 2016; pp. 31–43.

35. Baggio, L.L.; Drucker, D.J. Biology of incretins: GLP-1 and GIP. *Gastroenterology* **2007**, *132*, 2131–2157. [CrossRef]

36. Turton, M.D.; O'Shea, D.; Gunn, I.; Beak, S.A.; Edwards, C.M.; Meeran, K.; Choi, S.J.; Taylor, G.M.; Heath, M.M.; Lambert, P.D.; et al. A role for glucagon-like peptide-1 in the central regulation of feeding. *Nature* **1996**, *379*, 69–72. [CrossRef]

37. Zhao, X.; Liu, G.; Shen, H.; Gao, B.; Li, X.; Fu, J.; Zhou, J.; Ji, Q. Liraglutide inhibits autophagy and apoptosis induced by high glucose through GLP-1R in renal tubular epithelial cells. *Int. J. Mol. Med.* **2015**, *35*, 684–692. [CrossRef]

38. Nauck, M.A.; Duran, S.; Kim, D.; Johns, D.; Northrup, J.; Festa, A.; Brodows, R.; Trautmann, M. A comparison of twice-daily exenatide and biphasic insulin aspart in patients with type 2 diabetes who were suboptimally controlled with sulfonylurea and metformin: A non-inferiority study. *Diabetologia* **2007**, *50*, 259–267. [CrossRef]

39. Buse, J.B.; Bergenstal, R.M.; Glass, L.C.; Heilmann, C.R.; Lewis, M.S.; Kwan, A.Y.; Hoogwerf, B.J.; Rosenstock, J. Use of twice-daily exenatide in Basal insulin-treated patients with type 2 diabetes: A randomized, controlled trial. *Ann. Intern. Med.* **2011**, *154*, 103–112. [CrossRef]

40. Weissman, P.N.; Carr, M.C.; Ye, J.; Cirkel, D.T.; Stewart, M.; Perry, C.; Pratley, R. HARMONY 4: Randomised clinical trial comparing once-weekly albiglutide and insulin glargine in patients with type 2 diabetes inadequately controlled with metformin with or without sulfonylurea. *Diabetologia* **2014**, *57*, 2475–2484. [CrossRef]

41. Wysham, C.; Blevins, T.; Arakaki, R.; Colon, G.; Garcia, P.; Atisso, C.; Kuhstoss, D.; Lakshmanan, M. Efficacy and safety of dulaglutide added onto pioglitazone and metformin versus exenatide in type 2 diabetes in a randomized controlled trial (AWARD-1). *Diabetes Care* **2014**, *37*, 2159–2167. [CrossRef]

42. Nauck, M.; Weinstock, R.S.; Umpierrez, G.E.; Guerci, B.; Skrivanek, Z.; Milicevic, Z. Efficacy and safety of dulaglutide versus sitagliptin after 52 weeks in type 2 diabetes in a randomized controlled trial (AWARD-5). *Diabetes Care* **2014**, *37*, 2149–2158. [CrossRef]

43. Drucker, D.J.; Buse, J.B.; Taylor, K.; Kendall, D.M.; Trautmann, M.; Zhuang, D.; Porter, L.; Group, D.-S. Exenatide once weekly versus twice daily for the treatment of type 2 diabetes: A randomised, open-label, non-inferiority study. *Lancet* **2008**, *372*, 1240–1250. [CrossRef]

44. Blevins, T.; Pullman, J.; Malloy, J.; Yan, P.; Taylor, K.; Schulteis, C.; Trautmann, M.; Porter, L. DURATION-5: Exenatide once weekly resulted in greater improvements in glycemic control compared with exenatide twice daily in patients with type 2 diabetes. *J. Clin. Endocrinol. Metab.* **2011**, *96*, 1301–1310. [CrossRef]

45. Buse, J.B.; Drucker, D.J.; Taylor, K.L.; Kim, T.; Walsh, B.; Hu, H.; Wilhelm, K.; Trautmann, M.; Shen, L.Z.; Porter, L.E.; et al. DURATION-1: Exenatide once weekly produces sustained glycemic control and weight loss over 52 weeks. *Diabetes Care* **2010**, *33*, 1255–1261. [CrossRef]

46. Buse, J.B.; Rosenstock, J.; Sesti, G.; Schmidt, W.E.; Montanya, E.; Brett, J.H.; Zychma, M.; Blonde, L.; Group, L.-S. Liraglutide once a day versus exenatide twice a day for type 2 diabetes: A 26-week randomised, parallel-group, multinational, open-label trial (LEAD-6). *Lancet* **2009**, *374*, 39–47. [CrossRef]

47. Abd El Aziz, M.S.; Kahle, M.; Meier, J.J.; Nauck, M.A. A meta-analysis comparing clinical effects of short- or long-acting GLP-1 receptor agonists versus insulin treatment from head-to-head studies in type 2 diabetic patients. *Diabetes Obes. Metab.* **2017**, *19*, 216–227. [CrossRef]

48. Zaccardi, F.; Htike, Z.Z.; Webb, D.R.; Khunti, K.; Davies, M.J. Benefits and Harms of Once-Weekly Glucagon-like Peptide-1 Receptor Agonist Treatments: A Systematic Review and Network Meta-analysis. *Ann. Intern. Med.* **2016**, *164*, 102–113. [CrossRef]

49. DeFronzo, R.A.; Ratner, R.E.; Han, J.; Kim, D.D.; Fineman, M.S.; Baron, A.D. Effects of exenatide (exendin-4) on glycemic control and weight over 30 weeks in metformin-treated patients with type 2 diabetes. *Diabetes Care* **2005**, *28*, 1092–1100. [CrossRef]

50. Lorenz, M.; Evers, A.; Wagner, M. Recent progress and future options in the development of GLP-1 receptor agonists for the treatment of diabesity. *Bioorg. Med. Chem. Lett.* **2013**, *23*, 4011–4018. [CrossRef]

51. Yin, W.; Xu, S.; Wang, Z.; Liu, H.; Peng, L.; Fang, Q.; Deng, T.; Zhang, W.; Lou, J. Recombinant human GLP-1(rhGLP-1) alleviating renal tubulointestitial injury in diabetic STZ-induced rats. *Biochem. Biophys. Res. Commun.* **2018**, *495*, 793–800. [CrossRef]

52. Hills, C.E.; Al-Rasheed, N.; Willars, G.B.; Brunskill, N.J. C-peptide reverses TGF-beta1-induced changes in renal proximal tubular cells: Implications for treatment of diabetic nephropathy. *Am. J. Physiol. Ren. Physiol.* **2009**, *296*, F614–F621. [CrossRef] [PubMed]

53. Kodera, R.; Shikata, K.; Kataoka, H.U.; Takatsuka, T.; Miyamoto, S.; Sasaki, M.; Kajitani, N.; Nishishita, S.; Sarai, K.; Hirota, D.; et al. Glucagon-like peptide-1 receptor agonist ameliorates renal injury through its anti-inflammatory action without lowering blood glucose level in a rat model of type 1 diabetes. *Diabetologia* **2011**, *54*, 965–978. [CrossRef] [PubMed]

54. Leech, C.A.; Holz, G.G.; Habener, J.F. Signal transduction of PACAP and GLP-1 in pancreatic beta cells. *Ann. N. Y. Acad. Sci.* **1996**, *805*, 81–92. [CrossRef]

55. Holz, G.G. Epac: A new cAMP-binding protein in support of glucagon-like peptide-1 receptor-mediated signal transduction in the pancreatic beta-cell. *Diabetes* **2004**, *53*, 5–13. [CrossRef]

56. Bengis-Garber, C.; Gruener, N. Protein kinase A downregulates the phosphorylation of p47 phox in human neutrophils: A possible pathway for inhibition of the respiratory burst. *Cell Signal.* **1996**, *8*, 291–296. [CrossRef]

57. Savitha, G.; Salimath, B.P. Cross-talk between protein kinase C and protein kinase A down-regulates the respiratory burst in polymorphonuclear leukocytes. *Cell Signal.* **1993**, *5*, 107–117. [CrossRef]

58. Hendarto, H.; Inoguchi, T.; Maeda, Y.; Ikeda, N.; Zheng, J.; Takei, R.; Yokomizo, H.; Hirata, E.; Sonoda, N.; Takayanagi, R. GLP-1 analog liraglutide protects against oxidative stress and albuminuria in streptozotocin-induced diabetic rats via protein kinase A-mediated inhibition of renal NAD(P)H oxidases. *Metabolism* **2012**, *61*, 1422–1434. [CrossRef]

59. Fujita, H.; Morii, T.; Fujishima, H.; Sato, T.; Shimizu, T.; Hosoba, M.; Tsukiyama, K.; Narita, T.; Takahashi, T.; Drucker, D.J.; et al. The protective roles of GLP-1R signaling in diabetic nephropathy: Possible mechanism and therapeutic potential. *Kidney Int.* **2014**, *85*, 579–589. [CrossRef]

60. Gutzwiller, J.P.; Hruz, P.; Huber, A.R.; Hamel, C.; Zehnder, C.; Drewe, J.; Gutmann, H.; Stanga, Z.; Vogel, D.; Beglinger, C. Glucagon-like peptide-1 is involved in sodium and water homeostasis in humans. *Digestion* **2006**, *73*, 142–150. [CrossRef]

61. Rieg, T.; Gerasimova, M.; Murray, F.; Masuda, T.; Tang, T.; Rose, M.; Drucker, D.J.; Vallon, V. Natriuretic effect by exendin-4, but not the DPP-4 inhibitor alogliptin, is mediated via the GLP-1 receptor and preserved in obese type 2 diabetic mice. *Am. J. Physiol. Renal. Physiol.* **2012**, *303*, F963–F971. [CrossRef]

62. Muskiet, M.H.A.; Tonneijck, L.; Smits, M.M.; van Baar, M.J.B.; Kramer, M.H.H.; Hoorn, E.J.; Joles, J.A.; van Raalte, D.H. GLP-1 and the kidney: From physiology to pharmacology and outcomes in diabetes. *Nat. Rev. Nephrol.* **2017**, *13*, 605–628. [CrossRef]

63. Davies, M.J.; Bain, S.C.; Atkin, S.L.; Rossing, P.; Scott, D.; Shamkhalova, M.S.; Bosch-Traberg, H.; Syrén, A.; Umpierrez, G.E. Efficacy and Safety of Liraglutide Versus Placebo as Add-on to Glucose-Lowering Therapy in Patients with Type 2 Diabetes and Moderate Renal Impairment (LIRA-RENAL): A Randomized Clinical Trial. *Diabetes Care* **2016**, *39*, 222–230. [CrossRef]

64. Mann, J.F.E.; Ørsted, D.D.; Buse, J.B. Liraglutide and Renal Outcomes in Type 2 Diabetes. *N. Engl. J. Med.* **2017**, *377*, 2197–2198. [CrossRef]

65. Muskiet, M.H.A.; Tonneijck, L.; Huang, Y.; Liu, M.; Saremi, A.; Heerspink, H.J.L.; van Raalte, D.H. Lixisenatide and renal outcomes in patients with type 2 diabetes and acute coronary syndrome: An exploratory analysis of the ELIXA randomised, placebo-controlled trial. *Lancet Diabetes Endocrinol.* **2018**, *6*, 859–869. [CrossRef]

66. Tuttle, K.R.; Lakshmanan, M.C.; Rayner, B.; Busch, R.S.; Zimmermann, A.G.; Woodward, D.B.; Botros, F.T. Dulaglutide versus insulin glargine in patients with type 2 diabetes and moderate-to-severe chronic kidney disease (AWARD-7): A multicentre, open-label, randomised trial. *Lancet Diabetes Endocrinol.* **2018**, *6*, 605–617. [CrossRef]

67. De Vos, L.C.; Hettige, T.S.; Cooper, M.E. New Glucose-Lowering Agents for Diabetic Kidney Disease. *Adv. Chronic Kidney Dis.* **2018**, *25*, 149–157. [CrossRef] [PubMed]

68. Fuhrman, D.Y.; Schneider, M.F.; Dell, K.M.; Blydt-Hansen, T.D.; Mak, R.; Saland, J.M.; Furth, S.L.; Warady, B.A.; Moxey-Mims, M.M.; Schwartz, G.J. Albuminuria, Proteinuria, and Renal Disease Progression in Children with CKD. *Clin. J. Am. Soc. Nephrol.* **2017**, *12*, 912–920. [CrossRef]

69. Fox, C.S.; Matsushita, K.; Woodward, M.; Bilo, H.J.; Chalmers, J.; Heerspink, H.J.; Lee, B.J.; Perkins, R.M.; Rossing, P.; Sairenchi, T.; et al. Associations of kidney disease measures with mortality and end-stage renal disease in individuals with and without diabetes: A meta-analysis. *Lancet* **2012**, *380*, 1662–1673. [CrossRef]

70. Lorenzo, V.; Saracho, R.; Zamora, J.; Rufino, M.; Torres, A. Similar renal decline in diabetic and non-diabetic patients with comparable levels of albuminuria. *Nephrol. Dial. Transplant.* **2010**, *25*, 835–841. [CrossRef]

71. Marso, S.P.; Bain, S.C.; Consoli, A.; Eliaschewitz, F.G.; Jódar, E.; Leiter, L.A.; Lingvay, I.; Rosenstock, J.; Seufert, J.; Warren, M.L.; et al. Semaglutide and Cardiovascular Outcomes in Patients with Type 2 Diabetes. *N. Engl. J. Med.* **2016**, *375*, 1834–1844. [CrossRef]

72. Muskiet, M.H.; Smits, M.M.; Morsink, L.M.; Diamant, M. The gut-renal axis: Do incretin-based agents confer renoprotection in diabetes? *Nat. Rev. Nephrol.* **2014**, *10*, 88–103. [CrossRef]

73. Panchapakesan, U.; Pegg, K.; Gross, S.; Komala, M.G.; Mudaliar, H.; Forbes, J.; Pollock, C.; Mather, A. Effects of SGLT2 inhibition in human kidney proximal tubular cells—Renoprotection in diabetic nephropathy? *PLoS ONE* **2013**, *8*, e54442. [CrossRef]

74. Katz, P.M.; Leiter, L.A. The Role of the Kidney and SGLT2 Inhibitors in Type 2 Diabetes. *Can. J. Diabetes* **2015**, *39* (Suppl. S5), S167–S175. [CrossRef]

75. Mather, A.; Pollock, C. Glucose handling by the kidney. *Kidney Int. Suppl.* **2011**, *79*, S1–S6. [CrossRef]

76. Mather, A.; Pollock, C. Renal glucose transporters: Novel targets for hyperglycemia management. *Nat. Rev. Nephrol.* **2010**, *6*, 307–311. [CrossRef]

77. Abdul-Ghani, M.A.; DeFronzo, R.A.; Norton, L. Novel hypothesis to explain why SGLT2 inhibitors inhibit only 30-50% of filtered glucose load in humans. *Diabetes* **2013**, *62*, 3324–3328. [CrossRef]

78. Marks, J.; Carvou, N.J.; Debnam, E.S.; Srai, S.K.; Unwin, R.J. Diabetes increases facilitative glucose uptake and GLUT2 expression at the rat proximal tubule brush border membrane. *J. Physiol.* **2003**, *553*, 137–145. [CrossRef]

79. Gilbert, R.E.; Cooper, M.E. The tubulointerstitium in progressive diabetic kidney disease: More than an aftermath of glomerular injury? *Kidney Int.* **1999**, *56*, 1627–1637. [CrossRef]

80. Cherney, D.Z.; Perkins, B.A.; Soleymanlou, N.; Xiao, F.; Zimpelmann, J.; Woerle, H.J.; Johansen, O.E.; Broedl, U.C.; von Eynatten, M.; Burns, K.D. Sodium glucose cotransport-2 inhibition and intrarenal RAS activity in people with type 1 diabetes. *Kidney Int.* **2014**, *86*, 1057–1058. [CrossRef]

81. Vallon, V.; Richter, K.; Blantz, R.C.; Thomson, S.; Osswald, H. Glomerular hyperfiltration in experimental diabetes mellitus: Potential role of tubular reabsorption. *J. Am. Soc. Nephrol.* **1999**, *10*, 2569–2576.

82. Kojima, N.; Williams, J.M.; Slaughter, T.N.; Kato, S.; Takahashi, T.; Miyata, N.; Roman, R.J. Renoprotective effects of combined SGLT2 and ACE inhibitor therapy in diabetic Dahl S rats. *Physiol. Rep.* **2015**, *3*, e12436. [CrossRef]

83. Gallo, L.A.; Ward, M.S.; Fotheringham, A.K.; Zhuang, A.; Borg, D.J.; Flemming, N.B.; Harvie, B.M.; Kinneally, T.L.; Yeh, S.M.; McCarthy, D.A.; et al. Erratum: Once daily administration of the SGLT2 inhibitor, empagliflozin, attenuates markers of renal fibrosis without improving albuminuria in diabetic db/db mice. *Sci. Rep.* **2016**, *6*, 28124. [CrossRef]

84. Johnson, D.W.; Saunders, H.J.; Brew, B.K.; Poronnik, P.; Cook, D.I.; Field, M.J.; Pollock, C.A. TGF-beta 1 dissociates human proximal tubule cell growth and Na(+)-H+ exchange activity. *Kidney Int.* **1998**, *53*, 1601–1607. [CrossRef]

85. Panchapakesan, U.; Pollock, C.A.; Chen, X.M. The effect of high glucose and PPAR-gamma agonists on PPAR-gamma expression and function in HK-2 cells. *Am. J. Physiol Renal Physiol.* **2004**, *287*, F528–F534. [CrossRef]

86. Qi, W.; Chen, X.; Holian, J.; Mreich, E.; Twigg, S.; Gilbert, R.E.; Pollock, C.A. Transforming growth factor-beta1 differentially mediates fibronectin and inflammatory cytokine expression in kidney tubular cells. *Am. J. Physiol. Renal Physiol.* **2006**, *291*, F1070–F1077. [CrossRef]

87. Scheen, A.J. Evaluating SGLT2 inhibitors for type 2 diabetes: Pharmacokinetic and toxicological considerations. *Expert Opin. Drug Metab. Toxicol.* **2014**, *10*, 647–663. [CrossRef]

88. Scheen, A.J. Drug-drug interactions with sodium-glucose cotransporters type 2 (SGLT2) inhibitors, new oral glucose-lowering agents for the management of type 2 diabetes mellitus. *Clin. Pharmacokinet.* **2014**, *53*, 295–304. [CrossRef]

89. Merovci, A.; Mari, A.; Solis-Herrera, C.; Xiong, J.; Daniele, G.; Chavez-Velazquez, A.; Tripathy, D.; Urban McCarthy, S.; Abdul-Ghani, M.; DeFronzo, R.A. Dapagliflozin lowers plasma glucose concentration and improves β-cell function. *J. Clin. Endocrinol. Metab.* **2015**, *100*, 1927–1932. [CrossRef]

90. Del Prato, S. Role of glucotoxicity and lipotoxicity in the pathophysiology of Type 2 diabetes mellitus and emerging treatment strategies. *Diabet. Med.* **2009**, *26*, 1185–1192. [CrossRef]

91. Wilding, J.P.; Blonde, L.; Leiter, L.A.; Cerdas, S.; Tong, C.; Yee, J.; Meininger, G. Efficacy and safety of canagliflozin by baseline HbA1c and known duration of type 2 diabetes mellitus. *J. Diabetes Complic.* **2015**, *29*, 438–444. [CrossRef]

92. Bolinder, J.; Ljunggren, Ö.; Johansson, L.; Wilding, J.; Langkilde, A.M.; Sjöström, C.D.; Sugg, J.; Parikh, S. Dapagliflozin maintains glycaemic control while reducing weight and body fat mass over 2 years in patients with type 2 diabetes mellitus inadequately controlled on metformin. *Diabetes Obes. Metab.* **2014**, *16*, 159–169. [CrossRef]

93. Engeli, S.; Jordan, J. Novel metabolic drugs and blood pressure: Implications for the treatment of obese hypertensive patients? *Curr. Hypertens Rep.* **2013**, *15*, 470–474. [CrossRef]

94. Johnsson, K.M.; Ptaszynska, A.; Schmitz, B.; Sugg, J.; Parikh, S.J.; List, J.F. Urinary tract infections in patients with diabetes treated with dapagliflozin. *J. Diabetes Complic.* **2013**, *27*, 473–478. [CrossRef]

95. Elkinson, S.; Scott, L.J. Canagliflozin: First global approval. *Drugs* **2013**, *73*, 979–988. [CrossRef]

96. Polidori, D.; Sha, S.; Mudaliar, S.; Ciaraldi, T.P.; Ghosh, A.; Vaccaro, N.; Farrell, K.; Rothenberg, P.; Henry, R.R. Canagliflozin lowers postprandial glucose and insulin by delaying intestinal glucose absorption in addition to increasing urinary glucose excretion: Results of a randomized, placebo-controlled study. *Diabetes Care* **2013**, *36*, 2154–2161. [CrossRef]

97. Nyirjesy, P.; Zhao, Y.; Ways, K.; Usiskin, K. Evaluation of vulvovaginal symptoms and Candida colonization in women with type 2 diabetes mellitus treated with canagliflozin, a sodium glucose co-transporter 2 inhibitor. *Curr. Med. Res. Opin.* **2012**, *28*, 1173–1178. [CrossRef]

98. Scheen, A.J. Pharmacokinetic and pharmacodynamic profile of empagliflozin, a sodium glucose co-transporter 2 inhibitor. *Clin. Pharmacokinet.* **2014**, *53*, 213–225. [CrossRef]

99. Ferrannini, E.; Muscelli, E.; Frascerra, S.; Baldi, S.; Mari, A.; Heise, T.; Broedl, U.C.; Woerle, H.J. Metabolic response to sodium-glucose cotransporter 2 inhibition in type 2 diabetic patients. *J. Clin. Invest.* **2014**, *124*, 499–508. [CrossRef]

100. Ferrannini, E.; Berk, A.; Hantel, S.; Pinnetti, S.; Hach, T.; Woerle, H.J.; Broedl, U.C. Long-term safety and efficacy of empagliflozin, sitagliptin, and metformin: An active-controlled, parallel-group, randomized, 78-week open-label extension study in patients with type 2 diabetes. *Diabetes Care* **2013**, *36*, 4015–4021. [CrossRef]

101. Gerich, J.E. Role of the kidney in normal glucose homeostasis and in the hyperglycaemia of diabetes mellitus: Therapeutic implications. *Diabet. Med.* **2010**, *27*, 136–142. [CrossRef]

102. Cherney, D.Z.; Scholey, J.W.; Jiang, S.; Har, R.; Lai, V.; Sochett, E.B.; Reich, H.N. The effect of direct renin inhibition alone and in combination with ACE inhibition on endothelial function, arterial stiffness, and renal function in type 1 diabetes. *Diabetes Care* **2012**, *35*, 2324–2330. [CrossRef] [PubMed]

103. De Nicola, L.; Gabbai, F.B.; Liberti, M.E.; Sagliocca, A.; Conte, G.; Minutolo, R. Sodium/glucose cotransporter 2 inhibitors and prevention of diabetic nephropathy: Targeting the renal tubule in diabetes. *Am. J. Kidney Dis.* **2014**, *64*, 16–24. [CrossRef] [PubMed]

104. Rahmoune, H.; Thompson, P.W.; Ward, J.M.; Smith, C.D.; Hong, G.; Brown, J. Glucose transporters in human renal proximal tubular cells isolated from the urine of patients with non-insulin-dependent diabetes. *Diabetes* **2005**, *54*, 3427–3434. [CrossRef] [PubMed]

105. Vallon, V.; Gerasimova, M.; Rose, M.A.; Masuda, T.; Satriano, J.; Mayoux, E.; Koepsell, H.; Thomson, S.C.; Rieg, T. SGLT2 inhibitor empagliflozin reduces renal growth and albuminuria in proportion to hyperglycemia and prevents glomerular hyperfiltration in diabetic Akita mice. *Am. J. Physiol. Renal Physiol.* **2014**, *306*, F194–F204. [CrossRef] [PubMed]

106. Kojima, N.; Williams, J.M.; Takahashi, T.; Miyata, N.; Roman, R.J. Effects of a new SGLT2 inhibitor, luseogliflozin, on diabetic nephropathy in T2DN rats. *J. Pharmacol. Exp. Ther.* **2013**, *345*, 464–472. [CrossRef] [PubMed]

107. Terami, N.; Ogawa, D.; Tachibana, H.; Hatanaka, T.; Wada, J.; Nakatsuka, A.; Eguchi, J.; Horiguchi, C.S.; Nishii, N.; Yamada, H.; et al. Long-term treatment with the sodium glucose cotransporter 2 inhibitor, dapagliflozin, ameliorates glucose homeostasis and diabetic nephropathy in db/db mice. *PLoS ONE* **2014**, *9*, e100777. [CrossRef] [PubMed]

108. Lin, B.; Koibuchi, N.; Hasegawa, Y.; Sueta, D.; Toyama, K.; Uekawa, K.; Ma, M.; Nakagawa, T.; Kusaka, H.; Kim-Mitsuyama, S. Glycemic control with empagliflozin, a novel selective SGLT2 inhibitor, ameliorates cardiovascular injury and cognitive dysfunction in obese and type 2 diabetic mice. *Cardiovasc. Diabetol.* **2014**, *13*, 148. [CrossRef]

109. Nagata, T.; Fukuzawa, T.; Takeda, M.; Fukazawa, M.; Mori, T.; Nihei, T.; Honda, K.; Suzuki, Y.; Kawabe, Y. Tofogliflozin, a novel sodium-glucose co-transporter 2 inhibitor, improves renal and pancreatic function in db/db mice. *Br. J. Pharmacol.* **2013**, *170*, 519–531. [CrossRef] [PubMed]

110. Gangadharan Komala, M.; Gross, S.; Mudaliar, H.; Huang, C.; Pegg, K.; Mather, A.; Shen, S.; Pollock, C.A.; Panchapakesan, U. Inhibition of kidney proximal tubular glucose reabsorption does not prevent against diabetic nephropathy in type 1 diabetic eNOS knockout mice. *PLoS ONE* **2014**, *9*, e108994. [CrossRef]

111. Tabatabai, N.M.; Sharma, M.; Blumenthal, S.S.; Petering, D.H. Enhanced expressions of sodium-glucose cotransporters in the kidneys of diabetic Zucker rats. *Diabetes Res. Clin. Pract.* **2009**, *83*, e27–e30. [CrossRef]

112. Maldonado-Cervantes, M.I.; Galicia, O.G.; Moreno-Jaime, B.; Zapata-Morales, J.R.; Montoya-Contreras, A.; Bautista-Perez, R.; Martinez-Morales, F. Autocrine modulation of glucose transporter SGLT2 by IL-6 and TNF-α in LLC-PK(1) cells. *J. Physiol. Biochem.* **2012**, *68*, 411–420. [CrossRef] [PubMed]

113. Beloto-Silva, O.; Machado, U.F.; Oliveira-Souza, M. Glucose-induced regulation of NHEs activity and SGLTs expression involves the PKA signaling pathway. *J. Membr. Biol.* **2011**, *239*, 157–165. [CrossRef] [PubMed]

114. Ghezzi, C.; Wright, E.M. Regulation of the human Na+-dependent glucose cotransporter hSGLT2. *Am. J. Physiol. Cell Physiol.* **2012**, *303*, C348–C354. [CrossRef] [PubMed]

115. Osorio, H.; Bautista, R.; Rios, A.; Franco, M.; Santamaría, J.; Escalante, B. Effect of treatment with losartan on salt sensitivity and SGLT2 expression in hypertensive diabetic rats. *Diabetes Res. Clin. Pract.* **2009**, *86*, e46–e49. [CrossRef] [PubMed]

116. Doblado, M.; Moley, K.H. Facilitative glucose transporter 9, a unique hexose and urate transporter. *Am. J. Physiol. Endocrinol. Metab.* **2009**, *297*, E831–E835. [CrossRef] [PubMed]

117. Cain, L.; Shankar, A.; Ducatman, A.M.; Steenland, K. The relationship between serum uric acid and chronic kidney disease among Appalachian adults. *Nephrol. Dial. Transplant.* **2010**, *25*, 3593–3599. [CrossRef]

118. Komala, M.G.; Panchapakesan, U.; Pollock, C.; Mather, A. Sodium glucose cotransporter 2 and the diabetic kidney. *Curr. Opin. Nephrol. Hypertens* **2013**, *22*, 113–119. [CrossRef]

119. De Zeeuw, D.; Remuzzi, G.; Parving, H.H.; Keane, W.F.; Zhang, Z.; Shahinfar, S.; Snapinn, S.; Cooper, M.E.; Mitch, W.E.; Brenner, B.M. Proteinuria, a target for renoprotection in patients with type 2 diabetic nephropathy: Lessons from RENAAL. *Kidney Int.* **2004**, *65*, 2309–2320. [CrossRef]

120. Yale, J.F.; Bakris, G.; Cariou, B.; Yue, D.; David-Neto, E.; Xi, L.; Figueroa, K.; Wajs, E.; Usiskin, K.; Meininger, G. Efficacy and safety of canagliflozin in subjects with type 2 diabetes and chronic kidney disease. *Diabetes Obes. Metab.* **2013**, *15*, 463–473. [CrossRef]

121. Heerspink, H.J.; Johnsson, E.; Gause-Nilsson, I.; Cain, V.A.; Sjöström, C.D. Dapagliflozin reduces albuminuria in patients with diabetes and hypertension receiving renin-angiotensin blockers. *Diabetes Obes. Metab.* **2016**, *18*, 590–597. [CrossRef]

122. Chonchol, M.; Shlipak, M.G.; Katz, R.; Sarnak, M.J.; Newman, A.B.; Siscovick, D.S.; Kestenbaum, B.; Carney, J.K.; Fried, L.F. Relationship of uric acid with progression of kidney disease. *Am. J. Kidney Dis.* **2007**, *50*, 239–247. [CrossRef] [PubMed]

123. Goicoechea, M.; de Vinuesa, S.G.; Verdalles, U.; Ruiz-Caro, C.; Ampuero, J.; Rincón, A.; Arroyo, D.; Luño, J. Effect of allopurinol in chronic kidney disease progression and cardiovascular risk. *Clin. J. Am. Soc. Nephrol.* **2010**, *5*, 1388–1393. [CrossRef] [PubMed]

124. Iseki, K.; Oshiro, S.; Tozawa, M.; Iseki, C.; Ikemiya, Y.; Takishita, S. Significance of hyperuricemia on the early detection of renal failure in a cohort of screened subjects. *Hypertens Res.* **2001**, *24*, 691–697. [CrossRef] [PubMed]

125. Hovind, P.; Rossing, P.; Johnson, R.J.; Parving, H.H. Serum uric acid as a new player in the development of diabetic nephropathy. *J. Ren. Nutr.* **2011**, *21*, 124–127. [CrossRef]

126. Kang, D.H.; Nakagawa, T.; Feng, L.; Watanabe, S.; Han, L.; Mazzali, M.; Truong, L.; Harris, R.; Johnson, R.J. A role for uric acid in the progression of renal disease. *J. Am. Soc. Nephrol.* **2002**, *13*, 2888–2897. [CrossRef]

127. Cefalu, W.T.; Leiter, L.A.; Yoon, K.H.; Arias, P.; Niskanen, L.; Xie, J.; Balis, D.A.; Canovatchel, W.; Meininger, G. Efficacy and safety of canagliflozin versus glimepiride in patients with type 2 diabetes inadequately controlled with metformin (CANTATA-SU): 52 week results from a randomised, double-blind, phase 3 non-inferiority trial. *Lancet* **2013**, *382*, 941–950. [CrossRef]

128. Bailey, C.J.; Gross, J.L.; Pieters, A.; Bastien, A.; List, J.F. Effect of dapagliflozin in patients with type 2 diabetes who have inadequate glycaemic control with metformin: A randomised, double-blind, placebo-controlled trial. *Lancet* **2010**, *375*, 2223–2233. [CrossRef]

129. Wilding, J.P.; Ferrannini, E.; Fonseca, V.A.; Wilpshaar, W.; Dhanjal, P.; Houzer, A. Efficacy and safety of ipragliflozin in patients with type 2 diabetes inadequately controlled on metformin: A dose-finding study. *Diabetes Obes. Metab.* **2013**, *15*, 403–409. [CrossRef]

130. Home, P. Cardiovascular outcome trials of glucose-lowering medications: An update. *Diabetologia* **2019**, *62*, 357–369. [CrossRef]

131. Neal, B.; Perkovic, V.; Matthews, D.R. Canagliflozin and Cardiovascular and Renal Events in Type 2 Diabetes. *N. Engl. J. Med.* **2017**, *377*, 2099. [CrossRef]

132. Mosenzon, O.; Wiviott, S.D.; Cahn, A.; Rozenberg, A.; Yanuv, I.; Goodrich, E.L.; Murphy, S.A.; Heerspink, H.J.L.; Zelniker, T.A.; Dwyer, J.P.; et al. Effects of dapagliflozin on development and progression of kidney disease in patients with type 2 diabetes: An analysis from the DECLARE-TIMI 58 randomised trial. *Lancet Diabetes Endocrinol.* **2019**, *7*, 606–617. [CrossRef]

133. Neuen, B.L.; Young, T.; Heerspink, H.J.L.; Neal, B.; Perkovic, V.; Billot, L.; Mahaffey, K.W.; Charytan, D.M.; Wheeler, D.C.; Arnott, C.; et al. SGLT2 inhibitors for the prevention of kidney failure in patients with type 2 diabetes: A systematic review and meta-analysis. *Lancet Diabetes Endocrinol.* **2019**, *7*, 845–854. [CrossRef]

134. Zinman, B.; Wanner, C.; Lachin, J.M.; Fitchett, D.; Bluhmki, E.; Hantel, S.; Mattheus, M.; Devins, T.; Johansen, O.E.; Woerle, H.J.; et al. Empagliflozin, Cardiovascular Outcomes, and Mortality in Type 2 Diabetes. *N. Engl. J. Med.* **2015**, *373*, 2117–2128. [CrossRef] [PubMed]

135. Schernthaner, G.; Schernthaner-Reiter, M.H.; Schernthaner, G.H. EMPA-REG and Other Cardiovascular Outcome Trials of Glucose-lowering Agents: Implications for Future Treatment Strategies in Type 2 Diabetes Mellitus. *Clin. Ther.* **2016**, *38*, 1288–1298. [CrossRef] [PubMed]

136. Kalra, S.; Singh, V.; Nagrale, D. Sodium-Glucose Cotransporter-2 Inhibition and the Glomerulus: A Review. *Adv. Ther.* **2016**, *33*, 1502–1518. [CrossRef] [PubMed]

137. Heerspink, H.J.L.; Kosiborod, M.; Inzucchi, S.E.; Cherney, D.Z.I. Renoprotective effects of sodium-glucose cotransporter-2 inhibitors. *Kidney Int.* **2018**, *94*, 26–39. [CrossRef]

138. Molitch, M.E.; Adler, A.I.; Flyvbjerg, A.; Nelson, R.G.; So, W.Y.; Wanner, C.; Kasiske, B.L.; Wheeler, D.C.; de Zeeuw, D.; Mogensen, C.E. Diabetic kidney disease: A clinical update from Kidney Disease: Improving Global Outcomes. *Kidney Int.* **2015**, *87*, 20–30. [CrossRef]

139. Cherney, D.Z.I.; Bakris, G.L. Novel therapies for diabetic kidney disease. *Kidney Int. Suppl.* **2018**, *8*, 18–25. [CrossRef]

140. Bloomgarden, Z. The kidney and cardiovascular outcome trials. *J. Diabetes* **2018**, *10*, 88–89. [CrossRef]

141. Yaribeygi, H.; Atkin, S.L.; Katsiki, N.; Sahebkar, A. Narrative review of the effects of antidiabetic drugs on albuminuria. *J. Cell Physiol.* **2019**, *234*, 5786–5797. [CrossRef]

142. León Jiménez, D.; Cherney, D.Z.I.; Bjornstad, P.; Guerra, L.C.; Miramontes González, J.P. Antihyperglycemic agents as novel natriuretic therapies in diabetic kidney disease. *Am. J. Physiol. Renal Physiol.* **2018**, *315*, F1406–F1415. [CrossRef] [PubMed]

143. Cosentino, F.; Grant, P.J.; Aboyans, V.; Bailey, C.J.; Ceriello, A.; Delgado, V.; Federici, M.; Filippatos, G.; Grobbee, D.E.; Hansen, T.B.; et al. 2019 ESC Guidelines on diabetes, pre-diabetes, and cardiovascular diseases developed in collaboration with the EASD. *Eur. Heart J.* **2019**. [CrossRef] [PubMed]

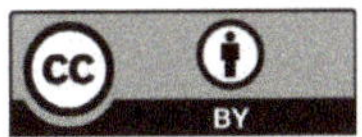

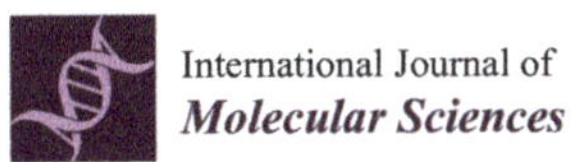
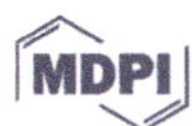

International Journal of
Molecular Sciences

Review

Non-Coding RNAs as New Therapeutic Targets in the Context of Renal Fibrosis

Cynthia Van der Hauwaert [1,2], François Glowacki [1,3], Nicolas Pottier [1,4] and Christelle Cauffiez [1,*]

1   EA 4483-IMPECS-IMPact of Environmental ChemicalS on Human Health, Univ. Lille, 59045 Lille CEDEX, France; cynthia.vanderhauwaert@gmail.com (C.V.d.H.); francois.glowacki@chru-lille.fr (F.G.); nicolas.pottier@univ-lille.fr (N.P.)
2   Département de la Recherche en Santé, CHU Lille, 59037 Lille, France
3   Service de Néphrologie, CHU Lille, 59037 Lille, France
4   Service de Toxicologie et Génopathies, CHU Lille, 59037 Lille, France
*   Correspondence: christelle.cauffiez@univ-lille2.fr

Received: 28 March 2019; Accepted: 20 April 2019; Published: 23 April 2019

Abstract: Fibrosis, or tissue scarring, is defined as the excessive, persistent and destructive accumulation of extracellular matrix components in response to chronic tissue injury. Renal fibrosis represents the final stage of most chronic kidney diseases and contributes to the progressive and irreversible decline in kidney function. Limited therapeutic options are available and the molecular mechanisms governing the renal fibrosis process are complex and remain poorly understood. Recently, the role of non-coding RNAs, and in particular microRNAs (miRNAs), has been described in kidney fibrosis. Seminal studies have highlighted their potential importance as new therapeutic targets and innovative diagnostic and/or prognostic biomarkers. This review will summarize recent scientific advances and will discuss potential clinical applications as well as future research directions.

Keywords: non-coding RNAs; microRNAs; long non-coding RNAs; renal fibrosis; biomarkers; therapeutics targets

---

1. Introduction

Chronic kidney disease (CKD) is increasingly recognized as a major public health concern. CKD prevalence has been estimated to be 8–16% worldwide [1]. In particular, CKD has been evaluated to affect more than 10% of the western population [2]. The common feature of CKD is renal fibrosis, which contributes to the progressive and irreversible decline in renal function and is associated with high morbidity and mortality.

Renal fibrosis, defined as an aberrant wound healing process in response to chronic injury, is characterized by the progressive and persistent accumulation of extracellular matrix components (ECM) in the kidney, ultimately leading to renal failure. As tissue scarring affects all compartments of the kidney, renal fibrosis is typically associated with glomerulosclerosis, arteriosclerosis and tubulointerstitial fibrosis [2]. Disruption of the epithelium and/or endothelium integrity during injury results in the activation of a complex cascade of molecular and cellular events. First, an inflammatory response initiates the release of profibrotic cytokines, chemokines and growth factors, which in turn promotes the proliferative phase of the scarring process characterized in particular by the recruitment and activation of fibroblasts into ECM-secreting myofibroblasts [3,4]. Finally, ECM accumulation results in the formation of a permanent fibrotic scar associated with renal tissue remodeling [5]. Once deposited, ECM components are further cross-linked and acquire resistance properties to degradation, precluding fibrosis resolution [6].

Although histological analysis of renal biopsies represents the gold standard to evaluate fibrosis, indirect biological parameters such as evolution of estimated Glomerular Filtration Rate are widely used in clinical practice for monitoring the progression of fibrotic lesions [7,8]. Furthermore, no specific treatment directly targeting fibrosis is currently approved [2]. Therefore, identifying new therapeutic targets and innovative diagnostic and/or prognostic biomarkers remains critical.

Recently, among the various mechanisms triggering fibrogenesis, non-coding RNAs (ncRNAs) have emerged as important regulators of this deleterious process [9–13].

In this review, we summarize the implication of ncRNAs in renal fibrosis and their potential value as either biomarkers or therapeutic targets, with an emphasis on microRNAs (miRNAs) and long non-coding RNAs (lncRNAs).

2. Non-Coding RNAs

New high-throughput technologies have revolutionized our understanding of the genome. Indeed, transcriptome of higher eukaryotic organism is far more complex than anticipated and contains large amounts of RNA molecules without coding potential (only 2% mRNAs in humans). Besides transfer and ribosomal RNAs that have been known since the 1950s, non-coding RNAs (ncRNAs) form a large and heterogenous class of RNA species involved in the regulation of gene expression. Non-coding RNAs are classified according to their length, localization and/or function into long non-coding RNAs (lncRNAs), microRNAs (miRNAs), small interfering RNAs (siRNAs), small nucleolar RNAs (snoRNAs), small nuclear RNAs (snRNAs) and PIWI-interacting RNAs (piRNAs) (Figure 1) [14–17]. Given that the role of some classes of ncRNAs (including siRNAs, snoRNAs or piRNAs) in kidney fibrosis remains largely unknown, this review will be restricted to miRNAs and lncRNAs.

				Function
RNAs	**Coding RNAs**		**mRNAs**	**Protein expression**
	Non coding RNAs		**rRNAs**	**Protein synthesis**
			tRNAs	**Protein synthesis**
			Long Non coding RNAs	**Regulation of chromatin structure** **Post-transcriptional regulation** **Regulation of transcription**
		Small non coding RNAs	**microRNAs (miRNAs)**	**Regulation of target mRNAs**
			small interfering RNAs (siRNAs)	**Post-transcriptional silencing**
			small nucleolar RNAs (snoRNAs)	**Chemical modifications of other RNAs**
			small nuclear RNAs (snRNAs)	**Maturation of RNAs**
			PIWI-interacting RNAs (piRNAs)	**Silencing of transposon activity during germline development**

Figure 1. Classification and function of non-coding RNAs (ncRNAs).

2.1. microRNAs (miRNAs)

miRNAs are ncRNAs of about 22 nucleotides usually conserved between species and involved in post-transcriptional regulation of gene expression. Currently, about 2700 mature miRNAs have been identified in humans, regulating at least 60% of mRNAs (miRbase v.22.1, October 2018 [18]). As miRNAs are involved in a vast array of physiological processes, such as embryogenesis, cellular homeostasis and differentiation [19]. Their aberrant expression plays a causative role in most complex disorders such as cancer, cardio-vascular diseases and fibro-proliferative disorders [20–23].

About 60% of miRNAs are localized in intergenic regions and possess their own transcriptional unit [24]. Other miRNAs are localized in intron of coding genes and are either co-transcribed with their host genes or under the control of a specific promoter [25,26]. miRNAs are usually transcribed by RNA polymerase II into a primary transcript, termed pri-miRNA. This pri-miRNA is then processed into a pre-miRNA of about 70 nucleotides by a multiproteic complex, called microprocessor and composed of two subunits: The RNAse III endonuclease DROSHA and the RNA binding protein DGCR8 (DiGiorge Critical Region 8). The pre-miRNA is recognized by EXP5 (Exportin 5)-Ran-GTP and exported to the cytoplasm. The last step of maturation is catalyzed by the RNAse III DICER associated with TRBP (TAR RNA binding protein). The PAZ domain (PIWI-AGOZWILLE) of the complex allows the recognition and positioning of DICER, then the RNAse III domain cleaves the pre-miRNA loop, generating a 22-nucleotide miRNA duplex [27]. The association with an Argonaute protein into the RISC (RNA-induced silencing complex) allows the dissociation of the duplex [28]. The passenger strand (termed miRNA*) is then cleaved and released into the cytoplasm for degradation [29] whereas the guide strand, or mature miRNA, persists within RISC [30]. When both strands lead to a mature miRNA, they are identified by the suffix -3p or -5p depending on whether they come from the 3′ or 5′ end of their precursor.

By preferentially binding on specific sequences, called "seed" sequences, which are mainly localized in the mRNA 3′-UTR (UnTranslated Region), mature miRNAs induce the degradation of the target mRNAs if miRNA-mRNA complementarity is perfect. However, this mechanism is minor in animals. Indeed, in the majority of cases, miRNAs regulate the expression levels of their target mRNAs by the recruitment of protein partners responsible for the activation of de-adenylation and de-capping associated with the 5′-to-3′ decay of mRNAs and possibly to translational repression mechanisms [30].

2.2. Long Non-Coding RNAs (lncRNAs)

In the human genome, about 30,000 lncRNA transcripts have been identified to date (GENCODE v29, [31]). LncRNAs, which are defined by being larger than 200 nucleotides, share common features with mRNAs, including being transcribed by RNA polymerase II, capped, cleaved, spliced, and polyadenylated [32,33].

LncRNA members are a heterogeneous family that can be subdivided according to their biogenesis loci into intergenic lncRNAs (lincRNAs), intronic lncRNAs, antisense lncRNAs (aslncRNA or natural antisense transcripts, NATs), bidirectional lncRNAs, and enhancer RNAs (eRNAs) [34–37] (Figure 2). Their functions are still poorly explored due to their subcellular localization [34] and their tissue- and temporal-specific expression [38]. Moreover, the low conservation of lncRNAs between species is a major obstacle to their identification and characterization in animal models [39]. Nevertheless, lncRNAs have been shown to display wide-ranging functions, probably due to their ability to bind to either DNA, RNA or protein. In particular, seminal functional studies have demonstrated their important role in the modulation of gene expression or DNA remodeling in physiological and pathological processes [32].

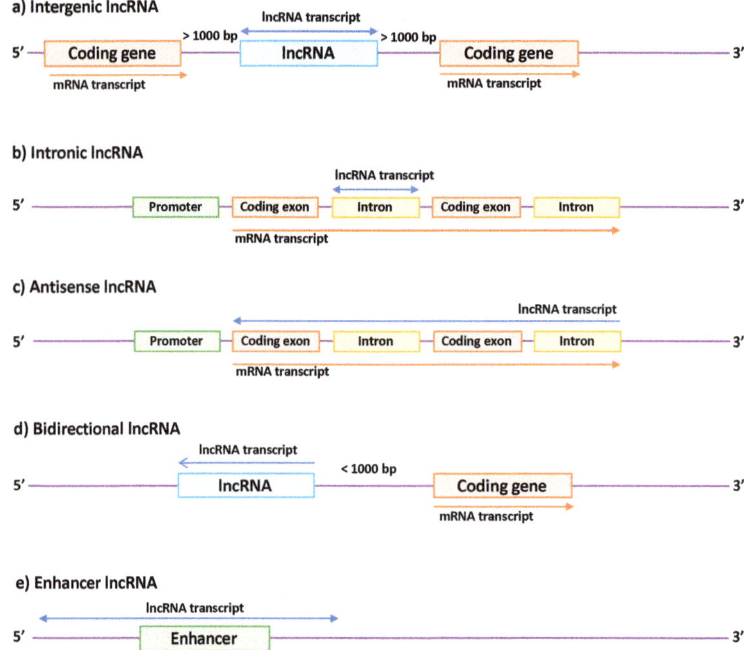

Figure 2. Classification of long non-coding RNAs (lncRNAs) according to their genomic location. (**a**) Intergenic lncRNAs are located between two coding genes; (**b**) intronic lncRNAs are transcribed entirely from introns of protein-coding genes; (**c**) antisense lncRNAs are transcribed from the antisense strand of a coding gene and overlap at least one exon; (**d**) bidirectional lncRNAs are localized within 1 kb of the promoter of a coding gene and oriented in the other direction; (**e**) enhancer lncRNAs are located in enhancer regions associated with a coding gene. Arrows indicate the direction of transcription.

3. miRNAs Implicated in Renal Fibrosis

Among the various classes of ncRNAs, miRNAs have first retained the attention of the scientific community. Many studies that focused on miRNAs in renal fibrosis have been published and allowed the identification of about thirty miRNAs with either an anti-fibrotic or pro-fibrotic effect, also called "fibromiRs" [4,40]. While Table 1 outlines publications highlighting the major role of miRNAs in renal fibrosis, we will describe more precisely the role of few particularly well-characterized miRNAs.

Table 1. Summary of miRNAs involved in renal fibrosis.

Regulation	miRNA	Models	Gene Target	References
Up	miR-21	Renal tissues from kidney transplanted patients Renal tissues from patients with IgA nephropathy Renal tissues from patients with Alport Syndrome UUO mouse model DN mouse model Ichemia reperfusion mouse model RPTEC cells Mesangial cells	PTEN, SMAD7, PPARA, PDCD4, BCL2, PHD2, MKK3, RECK, TIMP3, THSP1, RAB11A	[41–63]
	miR-22	DN rat model RPTEC cells	PTEN	[64]
	miR-135a	Serum and renal tissues from patients with DN DN mouse model Mesangial cells	TRPC1	[65]
	miR-150	renal tissue from patients with lupus nephritis RPTEC cells Mesangial cells	SOCS1	[66]
	miR-155	UUO mouse model RPTEC cells	PDE3A	[67,68]
	miR-184	UUO mouse models RPTEC cells	HIF1AN	[69]
	miR-214	UUO mouse model DN mouse model RPTEC cells Mesangial cells	DKK3, CDH1, PTEN	[70–72]
	miR-215	DN mouse model Mesangial cells	CTNNBIP1	[73]
	miR-216a	DN mouse model Mesangial cells	YBX1	[74]
	miR-324	Rat model of nephropathy (Munich Wistar Fromter rats) RPTEC cells	PREP	[75]
	miR-433	UUO mouse model RPTEC cells	AZIN1	[76]
	miR-1207	RPTEC cells Mesangial cells	G6PD, PMEPAI1, PDK1, SMAD7	[77]

Table 1. *Cont.*

Regulation	miRNA	Models	Gene Target	References
Down	let-7 family	DN mouse model RPTEC cells	HMGA2, TGFBR1	[78,79]
	miR-29 family	UUO mouse model Adenine gavage in mice Chronic renal failure rat model (5/6e nephrectomy) DN mouse model RPTEC cells Endothelial cells Podcytes HEK293 treated with ochratoxin A Renal tissues from kidney transplanted patients	COL, FN1, AGT, ADAM12, ADAM19, PIK3R2	[80–88]
	miR-30	UUO mouse model DN mouse model RPTEC cells	CTGF, KLF11, UCP2	[89–91]
	miR-34 family	UUO mouse model RPTEC cells	NOTCH1/JAG1	[92]
	miR-152	RPTEC cells	HPIP	[93]
	miR-181	UUO mouse model	EGR1	[94]
	miR-194	Ischemia reperfusion mouse model RPTEC cells	RHEB	[95]
	miR-200 family	UUO mouse model Adenine gavage in mice RPTEC cells	ZEB1/2, ETS1	[96–102]
	miR-455	DN rat model RPTEC cells Mesangial cells	ROCK2	[103]
Down/Up (controversial)	miR-192	UUO mouse model DN mouse model IgA nephropathy mouse model RPTEC cells	ZEB1/2	[104–109]

Abbreviations: UUO (ureteral unilateral obstruction); RPTEC (renal proximal tubular epithelial cells); DN (diabetic nephropathy).

3.1. miR-21

A large number of studies have emphasized the role of miR-21 in tissue fibrosis, notably in pulmonary [110], cardiac [111] or renal fibrosis [42]. The miR-21 gene locus is located within the *TMEM49* gene coding for Vacuole Membrane Protein 1 [112]. Interestingly, while miR-21 is one of the most highly expressed miRNAs in the healthy kidney [11], studies suggest that loss of miR-21 has no effect on development or healthy tissue function. This could be explained by its sequestration into an intracellular compartment. Nevertheless, in various stress conditions, miR-21 could be released into the cytoplasm to exert its regulatory functions [42,113]. In different experimental models such as the renal fibrosis (unilateral ureteral obstruction (UUO) mouse model, acute kidney injury (ischemia-reperfusion model) or diabetic nephropathy (*db/db* mice, streptozotocine-induced diabetes)), miR-21 is highly expressed in injured kidney regions [41,42,53,57]. Overexpression of miR-21 was also confirmed in renal allograft biopsies, in renal tissues of patients with IgA nephropathy or with Alport Syndrome exhibiting severe fibrotic injuries, particularly in regions enriched in fibroblasts/myofibroblasts, in the tubular epithelium and glomeruli [58–60]. The deleterious role of miR-21 in renal fibrosis was further explored using miR-21 null mice. Following UUO or ischemia-reperfusion injuries, miR-21$^{-/-}$ mice exhibited less fibrosis. Moreover, authors showed that miR-21 is also involved in lipid metabolism and mitochondrial redox regulation [42]. While only a limited number of miR-21 target genes have been experimentally validated, miR-21 has been demonstrated to be involved in the regulation of critical signaling pathways related to fibrogenesis such as cellular proliferation (PTEN) [61], apoptosis (PDCD4, Bcl2) [43,62,63], regulation of cellular metabolism (PPARα, PHD2) [44–46], inflammation (MKK3) [47,48], ECM components (Reck, TIMP3) [49–52], TGF-β signaling pathway (Smad7) [54], angiogenesis (Reck, THSP-1, PHD2) [46,49,50,55] and autophagy (Rab11a) [56].

3.2. miR-214

miR-214 has been shown to act as a fibromiR in several types of tissue fibrosis, including liver [114] and heart fibrosis [115]. miR-214 has been also consistently associated with renal fibrosis. It is in particular upregulated by the activation of the transcription factor TWIST in response to hypoxia in renal tubular epithelial cells [71]. Moreover, Denby et al., using miR-214 null mice and the UUO model of kidney fibrosis, showed that miR-214 promotes renal fibrosis independently of TGF-β pathway [116]. Similarly, treatment with an antagonist of miR-214 before UUO protected against fibrogenesis without blocking Smad2/Smad3 activation and TGF-β signaling [116]. Other studies have mechanistically linked miR-214 pro-fibrotic function with the targeting of DKK3 (Wnt/β -catenin pathway) [72], CDH1 (EMT) [71] or PTEN (proliferation) [70].

3.3. miR-200 Family

Members of the miR-200 family include five members organized into two clusters, miR-200b/a/429 and miR-200c/141 [117,118]. In animal models of renal fibrosis either induced by UUO or gavage with adenine, miR-200 family members are consistently downregulated [98,99]. Indeed, the anti-fibrotic role of these miRNAs is mainly associated with epithelial differentiation [100] by protecting renal tubular cells from EMT process through the direct regulation of ZEB1/2 (zinc finger E-box-Binding homeobox proteins 1/2) and Ets-1 transcription factors [81,101–103]. Of note, miR-200 family is also involved in TGF-β signaling pathway by modulating TGF-β2 [98].

3.4. miR-29 Family

miR-29 family is composed of three members: miR-29a, miR-29b and miR-29c [119]. Expression of miR-29abc is invariably downregulated during fibrosis and their low expression is associated with the up-regulation of ECM-related genes [80]. In fact, decreased expression of miR-29 family members is a general downstream molecular event of TGF-β signaling, which is essential for the release of ECM components by fibroblasts, as miR-29 family members directly target multiple collagen isoforms and other ECM components [81–83].

In various animal models of renal fibrosis, expression of miR-29 members is downregulated regardless of the cause of injury [84,85]. Interestingly, TGF-β inhibited miR-29 expression not only in renal fibroblasts, but also in mesangial cells, epithelial cells and podocytes [85], suggesting that miR-29abc exert also an anti-fibrotic function in non-fibroblastic renal cells. For example, both Adam12 and Adam19 represent two pro-fibrotic targets of miR-29abc in renal tubular epithelial cells [84]. Similarly, Hu et al. showed that miR-29 targets, in renal tubular epithelial cells, PIK3R2, an effector of PI3K/AKT signaling pathway involved in EMT induced by Angiotensin II [86]. Nevertheless, the precise contribution of miR-29abc during fibrosis in non-stromal cells remains to be clarified, especially as Long et al. reported an increased expression of miR-29c in both podocytes and endothelial cells in a mouse model of diabetic nephropathy [87].

3.5. miR-192

Data regarding the role of miR-192 in renal fibrosis are currently controversial. In fact, miR-192 is upregulated in various mouse models of CKD such as diabetic nephropathy, UUO and IgA nephropathy [105–108]. In line with this, treatment with an antagonist of miR-192 protected against fibrosis through induction of Zeb1/2 in diabetic nephropathy mouse model [105]. By contrast, other studies have reported in vitro in renal cells exposed to TGF-β, in a mouse model of diabetic nephropathy as well as in renal tissue from patients exhibiting severe renal fibrotic lesions a downregulation of miR-192 [108,109]. Overall, data highlighting the versatile role of miR-192 in renal fibrosis represent a relevant example of the complexity of miRNA regulation mechanisms.

4. Long Non-Coding RNAs Implicated in Renal Fibrosis

Even if elucidation of the role of lncRNAs is still ongoing, it is now accepted that besides their involvement in physiological processes such as organ development, immunity or homeostasis, their modulation can occur in chronic multifactorial diseases [35].

In the context of fibrosis, few examples showing their pro-fibrotic role have been documented, such as MALAT1 in cardiac fibrosis, H19 and DNM3os in lung fibrosis, and MALAT1, lnc-LFAR1 and HIF1A-AS1 in liver fibrosis [120–125]. Although studies about lncRNAs and renal fibrosis are quite recent, their number has significantly increased in recent years. In particular, emerging data show that various lncRNAs are involved in renal fibrosis by playing a pro- or anti-fibrotic role (Table 2). Although many studies have shown a deregulation of lncRNA expression, we chose to only focus on mechanistic studies.

Table 2. LncRNAs involved in kidney fibrosis.

Regulation	lncRNA	Models	Functions/Mechanisms	Consequences	References
Up	LOC105375913	Renal tissue of patients with segmental glomeruloscleoris RPTEC cells	Binding to miR-27b and leading to Snail expression	Pro-fibrotic	[126]
	LINC00667	Renal tissue of patients with chronic renal failure Chronic renal failure rat model (partial nephrectomy) RPTEC cells	Binding to Ago2, targeting miR-19b-3p	Pro-fibrotic	[127]
	NEAT1	DN rat model Mesangial cells		Pro-fibrotic and increase of proliferation	[128]
	Lnc-TSI (AP000695.6 or ENST00000429588.1)	RPTEC cells UUO mouse model Ischemia-reperfusion mouse model Renal tissue of patients with IgA nephropathy	Synergic binding to Smad3	Anti-fibrotic	[129]
	HOTAIR	UUO rat model RPTEC cells	Acting as a ceRNA with miR-124: activation of Jagged1/Nocth1 signaling	Pro-fibrotic	[130,131]
	LINC00963	Chronic renal failure rat model (5/6e nephrectomy)	Inhibition of FoxO signaling pathway by targeting FoxO3a	Pro-fibrotic	[132]
	TCONS_00088786	UUO mouse model RPTEC cells	Possibly regulation of miR-132 expression	Pro-fibrotic	[133]
	Errb4-IR (np-5318)	UUO mouse model Anti GBM mouse model RPTEC cells DN mouse model Mesangial cells	Downstream of TGFb/Smad3 pathway by binding Smad7 gene Binding to miR-29b	Pro-fibrotic	[134–136]
	CHCHD4P4	Stone kidney mouse model RPTEC cells		Pro-fibrotic	[137]
	TCONS_00088786	UUO rat model RPTEC cells		Pro-fibrotic	[138]
	TCONS_01496394	UUO rat model RPTEC cells		Pro-fibrotic	[138]
	ASncmtRNA-2	DN mouse model Mesangial cells		Pro-fibrotic	[139]
	LincRNA-Gm4419	DN mouse model Mesangial cells	Activation of NFkB/NLRP3 pathway by interacting with p50	Pro-fibrotic and pro-inflammatory	[140,141]
	H19	UUO mouse model RPTEC cells	Acting as a ceRNA with miR-17 and fibronectin mRNA	Pro-fibrotic	[142]

Table 2. *Cont.*

Regulation	lncRNA	Models	Functions/Mechanisms	Consequences	References
	RP23.45G16.5	UUO mouse model RPTEC cells		Pro-fibrotic	[143]
	AI662270	UUO mouse model RPTEC cells		No significative effect	[143]
	Arid2-IR **(np-28496)**	**UUO mouse model** **RPTEC cells**	**Smad3 binding site in Arid2-IR promoter** **Promoting NF-κB signaling**	**Pro-fibrotic and pro-inflammatory effects**	[144]
	np-17856	UUO mouse model Glomerulonephritis mouse model	Smad3 binding site	Pro-fibrotic and pro-inflammatory	[134]
	NR_033515	**Serum of patients with diabetic nephropathy** **Mesangial cells**	**Targeting miR-743b-5p**	**Pro-fibrotic and promotes proliferation**	[145]
	MALAT1	**DN mouse model** **Podocytes**	**Binding to SRSF1** **Targeting by β-catenin**	**Pro-fibrotic**	[146]
	Gm5524	DN mouse model Podocytes		Autophagy increase and apoptosis decrease	[147]
	WISP1-AS1	RPTEC cells	Modulating ochratoxin-A-induced Egr-1 and E2F activities	Cell viability increase	[148]
Down	Gm15645	DN mouse model Podocytes		Autophagy decrease and apoptosis increase	[147]
	CYP4B1-PS1-001 **(ENSMUST00000118753)**	**DN mouse model** **Mesangial cells**	**Enhancing ubiquitination and degradation of nucleolin**	**Anti-fibrotic and anti-proliferative**	[149,150]
	3110045C21Rik	UUO mouse model RPTEC cells		Anti-fibrotic	[143]
	ENSMUST00000147869	DN mouse model Mesangial cells	Associated with Cyp4a12a	Anti-fibrotic and anti-proliferative	[151]
	lincRNA 1700020I24Rik **(ENSMUSG00000085438)**	**DN mouse model** **Mesangial cells**	**Binding to miR-34a-5p. Inhibition of Sirt1/ HIF-1α signal pathway by targeting miR-34a-5p.**	**Anti-fibrotic**	[152]
	MEG3	**RPTEC cells**		**Anti-fibrotic**	[153]
	ZEB1-AS1	**DN mouse model** **RPTEC cells**	**Promoting Zeb1 expression by binding H3K4 Methyltransferase MLL1**	**Anti-fibrotic**	[154]
	ENST00000453774.1	**Renal tissue of patients with renal fibrosis** UUO mouse model RPTEC cells		**Anti-fibrotic**	[155]

Note: Studies in bold are mechanistic studies. Abbreviations: UUO (ureteral unilateral obstruction); RPTEC (renal proximal tubular epithelial cells); DN (diabetic nephropathy)

4.1. Errb4-IR

LncRNA Errb4-IR (np_5318), located in the ERBB4 intron region between the first and second exons, has been associated with renal fibrosis [134,135]. In the UUO mouse model, Errb4-IR was upregulated and strongly expressed in interstitial fibroblasts and injured tubular epithelial cells. Errb4-IR upregulation was also associated with fibrotic marker expression such as α-SMA or Collagen I. Moreover, in vivo silencing of Errb4-IR in the UUO mouse model significantly decreased fibrotic injuries [135]. Feng et al. also assessed the mechanisms underlying the fibrogenic role of Errb4-IR and showed that, in addition to being induced by TGF-β/Smad3 signaling, Errb4-IR directly targets Smad7, which exerts anti-fibrotic functions [135]. The pathological role of Errb4-IR in renal fibrosis was further confirmed in the context of diabetic nephropathy [136] by demonstrating that Errb4-IR also targets miR-29b, a well-established anti-fibrotic miRNA.

4.2. HOTAIR

HOTAIR (HOX transcript antisense intergenic RNA), embedded in the HOXC locus, is known to drive cancerogenesis [156]. Recently, two studies have demonstrated that HOTAIR is upregulated in renal fibrosis. In the UUO rat model, HOTAIR overexpression was associated with an upregulation of fibrotic and EMT markers as well as with a downregulation of miR-124, a miRNA involved in EMT and acting as a negative regulator of Nocth1 signaling pathway [130,131]. Moreover, lentiviral-mediated overexpression of HOTAIR in UUO rats, led to more severe injuries, such as inflammation, necrosis and collagen deposits, an elevated score of renal fibrosis and an overexpression of fibrotic markers compared to UUO alone. Mechanistically, it has been shown that HOTAIR activates the Notch1/Jagged1 signaling pathway by acting as a ceRNA (competing endogenous RNA—an lncRNA–miRNA duplex which prevents binding miRNA to its target and thus the target inhibition) with miR-124, which targets Notch1 and JAG1, and thereby promotes renal fibrosis [157,158].

4.3. Gm4419

In diabetic nephropathy, lincRNA Gm4419 was found to be involved in renal fibrosis. More precisely, in mesangial cells in high glucose conditions, overexpression of GM4419 was associated with fibrosis, inflammation and cell proliferation. Authors demonstrated that the NF-κB signaling pathway, which plays an important role in fibrogenesis and inflammation [140], was activated by GM4419 by interacting with its subunit p50. Moreover, p50 and GM4419 could have a synergistic effect in the inflammatory pathway [141].

5. New Therapeutic Targets and Innovative Biomarkers

5.1. New Therapeutic Targets

To date, the lack of specific anti-fibrotic therapies remains a critical need in clinical practice. As ncRNAs are involved in many critical pathogenic processes driving renal fibrosis, they represent attractive therapeutic targets. Currently, two strategies can be applied to manipulate ncRNA expression levels: The first relies on restoring the expression of a ncRNA when its level is decreased, the second is related to inhibiting the function of a ncRNA when its expression is increased.

5.1.1. miRNAs as Therapeutic Targets

To restore miRNA function, miRNA mimics or pre-miRNA have been developed. A modified synthetic RNA is introduced into cells as a duplex consisting of one strand identical to the mature miRNA of interest (guide strand) and the second antisense strand with a lower stability [159]. In addition, chemical modifications such as 2'-Fluoro bases have been developed to increase the stability of the guide strand without interfering with the RISC complex [160]. Other modifications include the use of 5'-O-methyl bases on the second strand to limit its incorporation into RISC complex [161]. Finally, addition of cholesterol-like molecules improves the duplex cellular internalization [159]. Although the use of such tools is widely developed for in vitro models, their application in vivo is hampered by delivery [11]. Other approaches involved gene therapy techniques, using notably AAV-mediated miRNA delivery (adeno-associated virus). Indeed, AAVs allow the restoration of the physiological expression level of miRNA with low toxicity and without integration into the genome in a specific tissue or cellular type [159,162].

Such strategies have been successfully applied in preclinical mouse models of tissue fibrosis, including bleomycin-induced lung fibrosis, but still need to be evaluated in the context of kidney fibrosis [163]. The renal tissue is indeed accessible to AAV gene delivery by different routes, including injection through the renal artery, injection into the parenchyma and retrograde injection via the ureter.

Concerning miRNA inhibition, several strategies have been developed, especially antisense oligonucleotides (termed antimiRs) which are widely used in preclinical models of tissue fibrosis and have also entered clinical trials [164]. These molecules are also chemically modified in order to improve their affinity, pharmacokinetics, stability and cellular entrance. The major modifications include the addition on the ribose of particular groups such as 2′O-Methyl, 2′O-Methoxyethyl or 2′-Fluoro and also inclusion of bicyclic structures which lock the ribose into its preferred 3′ endo conformation and increase base-pairing affinity such as methylene bridging group, also known as LNA (locked nucleic acid). Such ribose modifications allow a reduction in the size of antimiRs without loss of affinity and specificity. Finally, backbone modifications such as phosphorothioate linkages or the addition of morpholino structures enhance nuclease resistance [165].

Finally, target site blockers (TSB) inhibit miRNA function by specifically preventing interaction between a miRNA and its target [166,167]. One advantage of this strategy relies on its specificity, as it does not affect expression of the other target genes, and thus reduces the risk of side effects.

In the context of renal fibrosis, proof-of-concept for miRNA targeting has been demonstrated for several fibromiRs. In particular, results indicated that miR-214 antagonism was associated with less fibrotic lesions in the UUO mouse model [116]. In addition, an miR-21 antagonism injection prevented fibrotic injuries in UUO [42], diabetic nephropathy [168] or Alport [169] mouse models. Moreover, Regulus Therapeutics has developed a phase II clinical trial with a miR-21 antagonist in patients with Alport syndrome (RG-012; Regulus Therapeutics Inc.; clinical trial: NCT02855268). This drug candidate has currently received the orphan drug status from the FDA and the European Commission for the treatment of this rare disease.

5.1.2. lncRNAs as Therapeutic Targets

LncRNA deregulation is also viewed as an important driver of renal fibrosis, suggesting their potential value as therapeutic targets. Given their extensive secondary structures and their localization in nuclear and/or cytoplasmic compartments [15,34], pharmacological modulation of lncRNAs is more complex and, until recently, the options for targeting lncRNAs were limited. Moreover, the low conservation of lncRNAs between species is a major obstacle for preclinical validation [39,170]. However, recently, conceptual and technological advances in antisense oligonucleotide therapy offer new pharmacological options to modulate the expression or the function of lncRNAs. For example, the development of technologies including GapmeR-mediated lncRNA silencing, CRISPR inhibition or aptamers directed against lncRNA secondary structure represent novel opportunities to improve lncRNA knowledge and clinical translation [171].

In the context of renal fibrosis, lncRNA modulation remains an almost unexplored area. However, Kato et al. have used GapmeRs, an antisense oligonucleotide technology that induces target degradation in the nuclear compartment by recruiting RNAse H [172], in a mouse model of diabetic nephropathy. Interestingly, injection of such GapmeRs against lnc-MGG induced a decreased expression of profibrotic genes (TGF-β1, Col1a2, Col4a1, Ctgf) and prevented glomerular fibrosis, podocyte death and hypertrophy in diabetic mice [173]. Otherwise, few studies have investigated the opportunity to downregulate lncRNA expression using short hairpin RNAs (shRNAs) by delivery of plasmids or through viral or bacterial vectors in vivo [174]. Indeed, targeting of Errb4-IR was shown to improve renal fibrosis in the *db/db* mouse model [136]. Moreover, in a UUO mouse model, Arid2-IR was also successfully inhibited by a shRNA [144].

6. Biomarkers

Histological examination of biopsied tissue is considered the reference method for the diagnosis and staging of kidney fibrosis [8]. However, as percutaneous tissue sampling of either native kidney or allograft remains associated with patient discomfort, risk for complications, histopathological interpretation variability and high cost [175], the development of alternative non-invasive diagnostic or prognostic biomarkers is an important clinical issue [176]. Interestingly, ncRNAs that have been extensively reported to be dysregulated in fibrotic tissues, have also been detected in a large panel of human biological fluids including serum, plasma and urine [177–179].

6.1. miRNAs

In order to discover relevant biomarkers, miRNA profiling in several biofluids has been performed. Urine is a particularly interesting matrix to explore kidney function, even if miRNAs in urine are less abundant than in plasma or serum, since RNase activity has been reported to be quite high in urine [180]. Cardenas-Gonzalez et al. have screened more than 2000 urinary miRNAs from patients with CKD. In particular, this study demonstrated that downregulation of miR-2861, miR-1915-3p and miR-4532 was associated with a poorer renal function, interstitial fibrosis and tubular atrophy in diabetic nephropathy [181]. Another study profiled more than 1800 miRNAs in urine samples from patients with acute kidney injury. Among the 378 detected miRNAs, 19 were upregulated in patients with acute kidney injury, including miR-21, miR-200c and miR-423 [182]. Sonoda et al. showed that miR-9a, miR-141, miR-200a, miR-200c and miR-429 from exosomes in rat urine were upregulated following ischemia-reperfusion injury [183]. Moreover, Khurana et al. identified nine upregulated miRNAs (let-7c-5p, miR-222–3p, miR-27a-3p, miR-27b-3p, miR-296-5p, miR-31-5p, miR-3687, miR-6769b-5p and miR-877-3p) and seven downregulated miRNAs (miR-133a, miR-133b, miR-15a-5p, miR-181a-5p, miR-34a-5p, miR-181c-5p and miR1-2) in urine exosomes from patients with CKD compared to healthy controls [184]. Finally, other studies showed that dysregulation of urinary miR-29c, miR-21 and miR-200b was correlated with renal fibrotic injuries in patients with CKD or in renal transplanted patients [185–187]. Altogether, these data indicate that detection of miRNAs in the urine could reflect the degree of the renal aggression [188].

Finally, miRNAs were also detectable in serum and, more specifically, in renal transplanted patients serum level expression of miR-21 was found to be associated with the severity of renal fibrosis injuries [58,189,190]. While promising, the clinical use of circulating miRNAs as biomarkers remains tempered by quality control and normalization issues. For example, hemolysis needs to be perfectly avoided since miRNAs can be released from blood cells, thus affecting the amount of detected circulating miRNAs [191]. Furthermore, no standard endogenous control to normalize circulating miRNA levels has been clearly established and this concern is still debated [192,193]. The development of new technologies such as digital PCR (dPCR) are particularly interesting as this approach allows an absolute quantification without internal normalization [194,195].

6.2. lncRNAs

Although the expression of many lncRNAs has been evaluated in the context of fibrosis, their validation as biomarkers is at an earlier stage than miRNAs. Nevertheless, identifying novel lncRNAs as biomarkers is of great interest, since lncRNAs are highly stable in biofluids, especially when they are included in exosomes or in apoptotic bodies [179] and could be present in extracellular vesicles [196]. In renal fibrosis, Sun et al. compared the lncRNA profile in renal tissues and urines of UUO rats. Seven lncRNAs (five upregulated and two downregulated) were similarly modulated in renal tissues and urine. In addition, several conserved Smad3 binding motifs were identified in the sequence of the five upregulated lncRNAs [138]. Altogether, these results raise the possibility of using urinary lncRNAs as non-invasive biomarkers of renal fibrosis. Otherwise, Gao et al. found that in the serum of patients with diabetic nephropathy, the upregulation of lncRNA NR_033515 was correlated with NGAL and KIM1 serum levels, and the severity of the disease [145]. While both of these studies highlighted the potential of lncRNAs as non-invasive biomarkers for renal fibrosis, further studies are clearly required for the robust identification and validation of diagnostic and prognostic biomarkers.

7. Future Directions

NcRNAs, including the well-known miRNAs and the emerging lncRNAs, have been described to be implicated in a large number of physiological and pathological processes (Figure 3). In particular, their modulation between normal and fibrotic renal tissues not only strongly suggests that ncRNAs are involved in the development and the progression of kidney fibrosis, but also that ncRNAs may represent promising biomarkers. However, in contrast to miRNAs, the underlying mechanisms of most of the identified lncRNAs are yet to be determined. Considering both technological advances and rising scientific enthusiasm in lncRNA biology, we foresee that major discoveries will soon be achieved regarding the role of lncRNAs in kidney fibrosis.

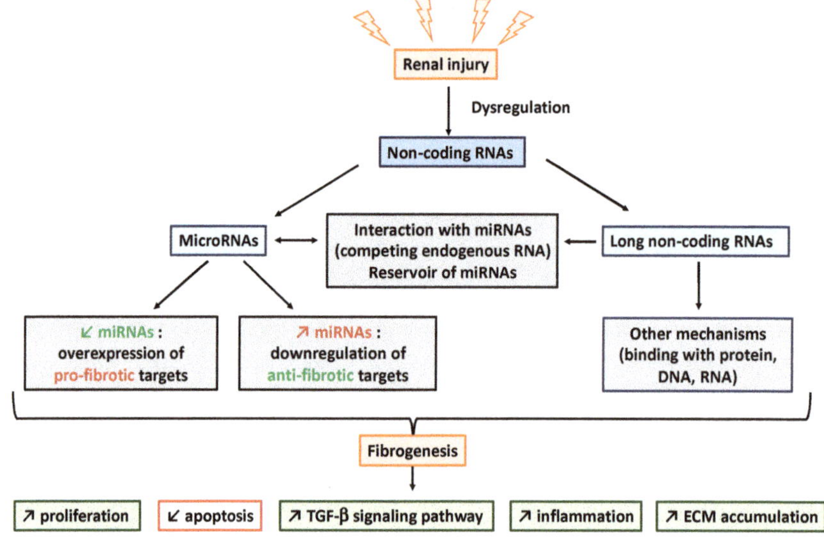

Figure 3. General mechanisms of non-coding RNAs involved in kidney fibrosis.

The proof of concept of ncRNA expression modulation to treat fibroproliferative disorders has been elegantly demonstrated. Clinical translation of these potential new therapeutic targets should be considered a research priority and will undoubtedly represent a gold mine of new therapeutic targets that may lead to the development of novel anti-fibrotics.

Author Contributions: Original draft preparation, C.V.d.H.; writing, C.V.d.H. and C.C.; review and editing, C.V.d.H., C.C., N.P. and F.G.

Funding: The APC was funded by Santélys association.

Conflicts of Interest: The authors declare no conflict of interest.

Abbreviations

AAV	Adeno-associated-virus
ceRNA	Competing endogenous RNA
CKD	Chronic kidney disease
DN	Diabetic nephropathy
ECM	Extracellular matrix
FDA	Food and Drug Administration
HOTAIR	HOX transcript antisense intergenic RNA
lncRNA	Long non-coding RNA
miRNA	microRNA
ncRNA	non-coding RNA
RISC	RNA-induced silencing complex
RPTEC	Renal proximal tubular epithelial cell
shRNA	Short hairpin RNA
UUO	Ureteral unilateral obstruction

References

1. Jha, V.; Garcia-Garcia, G.; Iseki, K.; Li, Z.; Naicker, S.; Plattner, B.; Saran, R.; Wang, A.Y.-M.; Yang, C.-W. Chronic kidney disease: Global dimension and perspectives. *Lancet* **2013**, *382*, 260–272. [CrossRef]
2. Klinkhammer, B.M.; Goldschmeding, R.; Floege, J.; Boor, P. Treatment of renal fibrosis—turning challenges into opportunities. *Adv. Chronic Kidney Dis.* **2017**, *24*, 117–129. [CrossRef]
3. Friedman, S.L.; Sheppard, D.; Duffield, J.S.; Violette, S. Therapy for fibrotic diseases: Nearing the starting line. *Sci. Transl. Med.* **2013**, *5*, 167sr1. [CrossRef]
4. Pottier, N.; Cauffiez, C.; Perrais, M.; Barbry, P.; Mari, B. FibromiRs: Translating molecular discoveries into new anti-fibrotic drugs. *Trends Pharmacol. Sci.* **2014**, *35*, 119–126. [CrossRef] [PubMed]
5. Gurtner, G.C.; Werner, S.; Barrandon, Y.; Longaker, M.T. Wound repair and regeneration. *Nature* **2008**, *453*, 314–321. [CrossRef]
6. Lu, P.; Takai, K.; Weaver, V.M.; Werb, Z. Extracellular matrix degradation and remodeling in development and disease. *Cold Spring Harb. Perspect. Biol.* **2011**, *3*, a005058. [CrossRef]
7. Levey, A.S.; Bosch, J.P.; Lewis, J.B.; Greene, T.; Rogers, N.; Roth, D. A more accurate method to estimate glomerular filtration rate from serum creatinine: A new prediction equation. *Ann. Intern. Med.* **1999**, *130*, 461–470. [CrossRef] [PubMed]
8. Berchtold, L.; Friedli, I.; Vallée, J.-P.; Moll, S.; Martin, P.-Y.; de Seigneux, S. Diagnosis and assessment of renal fibrosis: The state of the art. *Swiss Med. Wkly.* **2017**, *147*, w14442.
9. Chung, A.C.-K.; Lan, H.Y. MicroRNAs in renal fibrosis. *Front. Physiol.* **2015**, *6*, 50. [CrossRef] [PubMed]
10. Van der Hauwaert, C.; Savary, G.; Hennino, M.-F.; Pottier, N.; Glowacki, F.; Cauffiez, C. Implication des microARN dans la fibrose rénale. *Nephrol. Ther.* **2015**, *11*, 474–482. [CrossRef] [PubMed]
11. Gomez, I.G.; Nakagawa, N.; Duffield, J.S. MicroRNAs as novel therapeutic targets to treat kidney injury and fibrosis. *Am. J. Physiol. Renal Physiol.* **2016**, *310*, F931–F944. [CrossRef]
12. Moghaddas Sani, H.; Hejazian, M.; Hosseinian Khatibi, S.M.; Ardalan, M.; Zununi Vahed, S. Long non-coding RNAs: An essential emerging field in kidney pathogenesis. *Biomed. Pharmacother.* **2018**, *99*, 755–765. [CrossRef]
13. Jiang, X.; Zhang, F. Long noncoding RNA: A new contributor and potential therapeutic target in fibrosis. *Epigenomics* **2017**, *9*, 1233–1241. [CrossRef]
14. Cech, T.R.; Steitz, J.A. The noncoding RNA revolution—Trashing old rules to forge new ones. *Cell* **2014**, *157*, 77–94. [CrossRef]
15. Esteller, M. Non-coding RNAs in human disease. *Nat. Rev. Genet.* **2011**, *12*, 861–874. [CrossRef]
16. Ulitsky, I.; Bartel, D.P. lincRNAs: Genomics, evolution, and mechanisms. *Cell* **2013**, *154*, 26–46. [CrossRef]
17. Shi, X.; Sun, M.; Liu, H.; Yao, Y.; Song, Y. Long non-coding RNAs: A new frontier in the study of human diseases. *Cancer Lett.* **2013**, *339*, 159–166. [CrossRef] [PubMed]
18. Kozomara, A.; Birgaoanu, M.; Griffiths-Jones, S. miRBase: From microRNA sequences to function. *Nucleic Acids Res.* **2019**, *47*, D155–D162. [CrossRef]

19. Bartel, D.P. MicroRNAs: Target recognition and regulatory functions. *Cell* **2009**, *136*, 215–233. [CrossRef] [PubMed]
20. Croce, C.M.; Calin, G.A. miRNAs, Cancer, and stem cell division. *Cell* **2005**, *122*, 6–7. [CrossRef]
21. Small, E.M.; Olson, E.N. Pervasive roles of microRNAs in cardiovascular biology. *Nature* **2011**, *469*, 336–342. [CrossRef]
22. Li, G.; Zhou, R.; Zhang, Q.; Jiang, B.; Wu, Q.; Wang, C. Fibroproliferative effect of microRNA-21 in hypertrophic scar derived fibroblasts. *Exp. Cell Res.* **2016**, *345*, 93–99. [CrossRef] [PubMed]
23. Bowen, T.; Jenkins, R.H.; Fraser, D.J. MicroRNAs, transforming growth factor beta-1, and tissue fibrosis. *J. Pathol.* **2013**, *229*, 274–285. [CrossRef]
24. Corcoran, D.L.; Pandit, K.V.; Gordon, B.; Bhattacharjee, A.; Kaminski, N.; Benos, P.V. Features of mammalian microRNA promoters emerge from polymerase II chromatin immunoprecipitation data. *PLoS ONE* **2009**, *4*, e5279. [CrossRef]
25. Baskerville, S.; Bartel, D.P. Microarray profiling of microRNAs reveals frequent coexpression with neighboring miRNAs and host genes. *RNA* **2005**, *11*, 241–247. [CrossRef]
26. Ozsolak, F.; Poling, L.L.; Wang, Z.; Liu, H.; Liu, X.S.; Roeder, R.G.; Zhang, X.; Song, J.S.; Fisher, D.E. Chromatin structure analyses identify miRNA promoters. *Genes Dev.* **2008**, *22*, 3172–3183. [CrossRef] [PubMed]
27. Park, J.-E.; Heo, I.; Tian, Y.; Simanshu, D.K.; Chang, H.; Jee, D.; Patel, D.J.; Kim, V.N. Dicer recognizes the 5′ end of RNA for efficient and accurate processing. *Nature* **2011**, *475*, 201–205. [CrossRef]
28. Su, H.; Trombly, M.I.; Chen, J.; Wang, X. Essential and overlapping functions for mammalian Argonautes in microRNA silencing. *Genes Dev.* **2009**, *23*, 304–317. [CrossRef]
29. Liu, X.; Jin, D.-Y.; McManus, M.T.; Mourelatos, Z. Precursor microRNA-programmed silencing complex assembly pathways in mammals. *Mol. Cell* **2012**, *46*, 507–517. [CrossRef]
30. Jonas, S.; Izaurralde, E. Towards a molecular understanding of microRNA-mediated gene silencing. *Nat. Rev. Genet.* **2015**, *16*, 421–433. [CrossRef] [PubMed]
31. Frankish, A.; Diekhans, M.; Ferreira, A.-M.; Johnson, R.; Jungreis, I.; Loveland, J.; Mudge, J.M.; Sisu, C.; Wright, J.; Armstrong, J.; et al. GENCODE reference annotation for the human and mouse genomes. *Nucleic Acids Res.* **2019**, *47*, D766–D773. [CrossRef]
32. Quinn, J.J.; Chang, H.Y. Unique features of long non-coding RNA biogenesis and function. *Nat. Rev. Genet.* **2016**, *17*, 47–62. [CrossRef]
33. Bunch, H. Gene regulation of mammalian long non-coding RNA. *Mol. Genet. Genomics* **2018**, *293*, 1–15. [CrossRef] [PubMed]
34. Chen, L.-L. Linking long noncoding RNA localization and function. *Trends Biochem. Sci.* **2016**, *41*, 761–772. [CrossRef]
35. Kung, J.T.Y.; Colognori, D.; Lee, J.T. Long noncoding RNAs: Past, present, and future. *Genetics* **2013**, *193*, 651–669. [CrossRef]
36. Derrien, T.; Johnson, R.; Bussotti, G.; Tanzer, A.; Djebali, S.; Tilgner, H.; Guernec, G.; Martin, D.; Merkel, A.; Knowles, D.G.; et al. The GENCODE v7 catalog of human long noncoding RNAs: Analysis of their gene structure, evolution, and expression. *Genome Res.* **2012**, *22*, 1775–1789. [CrossRef]
37. Devaux, Y.; Zangrando, J.; Schroen, B.; Creemers, E.E.; Pedrazzini, T.; Chang, C.-P.; Dorn, G.W.; Thum, T.; Heymans, S.; Cardiolinc Network. Long noncoding RNAs in cardiac development and ageing. *Nat. Rev. Cardiol.* **2015**, *12*, 415–425.
38. Ward, M.; McEwan, C.; Mills, J.D.; Janitz, M. Conservation and tissue-specific transcription patterns of long noncoding RNAs. *J. Hum. Transcript.* **2015**, *1*, 2–9. [CrossRef]
39. Ulitsky, I. Evolution to the rescue: Using comparative genomics to understand long non-coding RNAs. *Nat. Rev. Genet.* **2016**, *17*, 601–614. [CrossRef] [PubMed]
40. Lv, W.; Fan, F.; Wang, Y.; Gonzalez-Fernandez, E.; Wang, C.; Yang, L.; Booz, G.W.; Roman, R.J. Therapeutic potential of microRNAs for the treatment of renal fibrosis and CKD. *Physiol. Genomics* **2018**, *50*, 20–34. [CrossRef] [PubMed]
41. Zarjou, A.; Yang, S.; Abraham, E.; Agarwal, A.; Liu, G. Identification of a microRNA signature in renal fibrosis: Role of miR-21. *Am. J. Physiol. Renal Physiol.* **2011**, *301*, F793–F801. [CrossRef]
42. Chau, B.N.; Xin, C.; Hartner, J.; Ren, S.; Castano, A.P.; Linn, G.; Li, J.; Tran, P.T.; Kaimal, V.; Huang, X.; et al. MicroRNA-21 promotes fibrosis of the kidney by silencing metabolic pathways. *Sci. Transl. Med.* **2012**, *4*, ra18–ra121. [CrossRef]

43. Dong, J.; Zhao, Y.-P.; Zhou, L.; Zhang, T.-P.; Chen, G. Bcl-2 upregulation induced by miR-21 Via a direct interaction is associated with apoptosis and chemoresistance in MIA PaCa-2 pancreatic cancer cells. *Arch. Med. Res.* **2011**, *42*, 8–14. [CrossRef]

44. Zhou, J.; Wang, K.-C.; Wu, W.; Subramaniam, S.; Shyy, J.Y.-J.; Chiu, J.-J.; Li, J.Y.-S.; Chien, S. MicroRNA-21 targets peroxisome proliferators-activated receptor- in an autoregulatory loop to modulate flow-induced endothelial inflammation. *Proc. Natl. Acad. Sci. USA* **2011**, *108*, 10355–10360. [CrossRef]

45. Zhang, K.; Han, L.; Chen, L.; Shi, Z.; Yang, M.; Ren, Y.; Chen, L.; Zhang, J.; Pu, P.; Kang, C. Blockage of a miR-21/EGFR regulatory feedback loop augments anti-EGFR therapy in glioblastomas. *Cancer Lett.* **2014**, *342*, 139–149. [CrossRef]

46. Jiao, X.; Xu, X.; Fang, Y.; Zhang, H.; Liang, M.; Teng, J.; Ding, X. miR-21 Contributes to renal protection by targeting prolyl hydroxylase domain protein 2 in delayed ischaemic preconditioning. *Nephrology* **2017**, *22*, 366–373. [CrossRef]

47. Xu, G.; Zhang, Y.; Wei, J.; Jia, W.; Ge, Z.; Zhang, Z.; Liu, X. MicroRNA-21 promotes hepatocellular carcinoma HepG2 cell proliferation through repression of mitogen-activated protein kinase-kinase 3. *BMC Cancer* **2013**, *13*, 469. [CrossRef]

48. Li, Z.; Deng, X.; Kang, Z.; Wang, Y.; Xia, T.; Ding, N.; Yin, Y. Elevation of miR-21, through targeting MKK3, may be involved in ischemia pretreatment protection from ischemia–reperfusion induced kidney injury. *J. Nephrol.* **2016**, *29*, 27–36. [CrossRef]

49. Zhou, L.; Yang, Z.-X.; Song, W.-J.; Li, Q.-J.; Yang, F.; Wang, D.-S.; Zhang, N.; Dou, K.-F. MicroRNA-21 regulates the migration and invasion of a stem-like population in hepatocellular carcinoma. *Int. J. Oncol.* **2013**, *43*, 661–669. [CrossRef]

50. Zhang, Z.; Li, Z.; Gao, C.; Chen, P.; Chen, J.; Liu, W.; Xiao, S.; Lu, H. miR-21 Plays a pivotal role in gastric cancer pathogenesis and progression. *Lab. Investig.* **2008**, *88*, 1358–1366. [CrossRef]

51. Wang, N.; Zhang, C.; He, J.; Duan, X.; Wang, Y.; Ji, X.; Zang, W.; Li, M.; Ma, Y.; Wang, T.; et al. miR-21 Down-regulation suppresses cell growth, invasion and induces cell apoptosis by targeting FASL, TIMP3, and RECK genes in esophageal carcinoma. *Dig. Dis. Sci.* **2013**, *58*, 1863–1870. [CrossRef]

52. Hu, J.; Ni, S.; Cao, Y.; Zhang, T.; Wu, T.; Yin, X.; Lang, Y.; Lu, H. The angiogenic effect of microRNA-21 targeting TIMP3 through the regulation of MMP2 and MMP9. *PLoS ONE* **2016**, *11*, e0149537. [CrossRef]

53. Zhong, X.; Chung, A.C.K.; Chen, H.Y.; Dong, Y.; Meng, X.M.; Li, R.; Yang, W.; Hou, F.F.; Lan, H.Y. miR-21 Is a key therapeutic target for renal injury in a mouse model of type 2 diabetes. *Diabetologia* **2013**, *56*, 663–674. [CrossRef]

54. Wang, J.-Y.; Gao, Y.-B.; Zhang, N.; Zou, D.-W.; Wang, P.; Zhu, Z.-Y.; Li, J.-Y.; Zhou, S.-N.; Wang, S.-C.; Wang, Y.-Y.; et al. miR-21 Overexpression enhances TGF-β1-induced epithelial-to-mesenchymal transition by target smad7 and aggravates renal damage in diabetic nephropathy. *Mol. Cell. Endocrinol.* **2014**, *392*, 163–172. [CrossRef]

55. Xu, X.; Song, N.; Zhang, X.; Jiao, X.; Hu, J.; Liang, M.; Teng, J.; Ding, X. Renal protection mediated by hypoxia inducible factor-1α depends on proangiogenesis function of miR-21 by targeting thrombospondin 1. *Transplantation* **2017**, *101*, 1811–1819. [CrossRef]

56. Liu, X.; Hong, Q.; Wang, Z.; Yu, Y.; Zou, X.; Xu, L. MiR-21 inhibits autophagy by targeting Rab11a in renal ischemia/reperfusion. *Exp. Cell Res.* **2015**, *338*, 64–69. [CrossRef]

57. Lai, J.Y.; Luo, J.; O'Connor, C.; Jing, X.; Nair, V.; Ju, W.; Randolph, A.; Ben-Dov, I.Z.; Matar, R.N.; Briskin, D.; et al. MicroRNA-21 in glomerular injury. *J. Am. Soc. Nephrol.* **2015**, *26*, 805–816. [CrossRef]

58. Glowacki, F.; Savary, G.; Gnemmi, V.; Buob, D.; Van der Hauwaert, C.; Lo-Guidice, J.-M.; Bouyé, S.; Hazzan, M.; Pottier, N.; Perrais, M.; et al. Increased circulating miR-21 levels are associated with kidney fibrosis. *PLoS ONE* **2013**, *8*, e58014. [CrossRef]

59. Hennino, M.-F.; Buob, D.; Van der Hauwaert, C.; Gnemmi, V.; Jomaa, Z.; Pottier, N.; Savary, G.; Drumez, E.; Noël, C.; Cauffiez, C.; et al. miR-21-5p Renal expression is associated with fibrosis and renal survival in patients with IgA nephropathy. *Sci. Rep.* **2016**, *6*, 27209. [CrossRef]

60. Guo, J.; Song, W.; Boulanger, J.; Xu, E.Y.; Wang, F.; Zhang, Y.; He, Q.; Wang, S.; Yang, L.; Pryce, C.; et al. Dysregulated expression of microRNA-21 and disease related genes in human patients and mouse model of alport syndrome. *Hum. Gene Ther.* **2019**. [CrossRef]

61. Dey, N.; Ghosh-Choudhury, N.; Kasinath, B.S.; Choudhury, G.G. TGFβ-stimulated microrna-21 utilizes PTEN to orchestrate AKT/mTORC1 signaling for mesangial cell hypertrophy and matrix expansion. *PLoS ONE* **2012**, *7*, e42316. [CrossRef]

62. Cheng, Y.; Zhu, P.; Yang, J.; Liu, X.; Dong, S.; Wang, X.; Chun, B.; Zhuang, J.; Zhang, C. Ischaemic preconditioning-regulated miR-21 protects heart against ischaemia/reperfusion injury via anti-apoptosis through its target PDCD4. *Cardiovasc. Res.* **2010**, *87*, 431–439. [CrossRef]

63. Sims, E.K.; Lakhter, A.J.; Anderson-Baucum, E.; Kono, T.; Tong, X.; Evans-Molina, C. MicroRNA 21 targets BCL2 mRNA to increase apoptosis in rat and human beta cells. *Diabetologia* **2017**, *60*, 1057–1065. [CrossRef] [PubMed]

64. Zhang, Y.; Zhao, S.; Wu, D.; Liu, X.; Shi, M.; Wang, Y.; Zhang, F.; Ding, J.; Xiao, Y.; Guo, B. MicroRNA-22 promotes renal tubulointerstitial fibrosis by targeting PTEN and suppressing autophagy in diabetic nephropathy. *J. Diabetes Res.* **2018**, *2018*, 1–11. [CrossRef] [PubMed]

65. He, F.; Peng, F.; Xia, X.; Zhao, C.; Luo, Q.; Guan, W.; Li, Z.; Yu, X.; Huang, F. MiR-135a promotes renal fibrosis in diabetic nephropathy by regulating TRPC1. *Diabetologia* **2014**, *57*, 1726–1736. [CrossRef] [PubMed]

66. Zhou, H.; Hasni, S.A.; Perez, P.; Tandon, M.; Jang, S.-I.; Zheng, C.; Kopp, J.B.; Austin, H.; Balow, J.E.; Alevizos, I.; et al. miR-150 Promotes renal fibrosis in lupus nephritis by downregulating SOCS1. *J. Am. Soc. Nephrol.* **2013**, *24*, 1073–1087. [CrossRef] [PubMed]

67. Xi, W.; Zhao, X.; Wu, M.; Jia, W.; Li, H. Lack of microRNA-155 ameliorates renal fibrosis by targeting PDE3A/TGF-β1/Smad signaling in mice with obstructive nephropathy. *Cell Biol. Int.* **2018**, *42*, 1523–1532. [CrossRef]

68. XIE, S.; CHEN, H.; LI, F.; WANG, S.; GUO, J. Hypoxia-induced microRNA-155 promotes fibrosis in proximal tubule cells. *Mol. Med. Rep.* **2015**, *11*, 4555–4560. [CrossRef] [PubMed]

69. Chen, B. The miRNA-184 drives renal fibrosis by targeting HIF1AN in vitro and in vivo. *Int. Urol. Nephrol.* **2019**, *51*, 543–550. [CrossRef]

70. Bera, A.; Das, F.; Ghosh-Choudhury, N.; Mariappan, M.M.; Kasinath, B.S.; Ghosh Choudhury, G. Reciprocal regulation of miR-214 and PTEN by high glucose regulates renal glomerular mesangial and proximal tubular epithelial cell hypertrophy and matrix expansion. *Am. J. Physiol. Physiol.* **2017**, *313*, C430–C447. [CrossRef]

71. Liu, M.; Liu, L.; Bai, M.; Zhang, L.; Ma, F.; Yang, X.; Sun, S. Hypoxia-induced activation of Twist/miR-214/E-cadherin axis promotes renal tubular epithelial cell mesenchymal transition and renal fibrosis. *Biochem. Biophys. Res. Commun.* **2018**, *495*, 2324–2330. [CrossRef]

72. Zhu, X.; Li, W.; Li, H. miR-214 Ameliorates acute kidney injury via targeting DKK3 and activating of Wnt/β-catenin signaling pathway. *Biol. Res.* **2018**, *51*, 31. [CrossRef]

73. Mu, J.; Pang, Q.; Guo, Y.-H.; Chen, J.-G.; Zeng, W.; Huang, Y.-J.; Zhang, J.; Feng, B. Functional implications of MicroRNA-215 in TGF-β1-induced phenotypic transition of mesangial cells by targeting CTNNBIP1. *PLoS ONE* **2013**, *8*, e58622. [CrossRef]

74. Kato, M.; Wang, L.; Putta, S.; Wang, M.; Yuan, H.; Sun, G.; Lanting, L.; Todorov, I.; Rossi, J.J.; Natarajan, R. Post-transcriptional up-regulation of Tsc-22 by Ybx1, a target of miR-216a, mediates TGF-β-induced collagen expression in kidney cells. *J. Biol. Chem.* **2010**, *285*, 34004–34015. [CrossRef]

75. Macconi, D.; Tomasoni, S.; Romagnani, P.; Trionfini, P.; Sangalli, F.; Mazzinghi, B.; Rizzo, P.; Lazzeri, E.; Abbate, M.; Remuzzi, G.; et al. MicroRNA-324-3p promotes renal fibrosis and is a target of ACE inhibition. *J. Am. Soc. Nephrol.* **2012**, *23*, 1496–1505. [CrossRef]

76. Li, R.; Chung, A.C.K.; Dong, Y.; Yang, W.; Zhong, X.; Lan, H.Y. The microRNA miR-433 promotes renal fibrosis by amplifying the TGF-β/Smad3-Azin1 pathway. *Kidney Int.* **2013**, *84*, 1129–1144. [CrossRef]

77. Alvarez, M.L.; Khosroheidari, M.; Eddy, E.; Kiefer, J. Role of MicroRNA 1207-5P and its host gene, the long non-coding RNA Pvt1, as mediators of extracellular matrix accumulation in the kidney: Implications for diabetic nephropathy. *PLoS ONE* **2013**, *8*, e77468. [CrossRef]

78. Brennan, E.P.; Nolan, K.A.; Börgeson, E.; Gough, O.S.; McEvoy, C.M.; Docherty, N.G.; Higgins, D.F.; Murphy, M.; Sadlier, D.M.; Ali-Shah, S.T.; et al. Lipoxins attenuate renal fibrosis by inducing let-7c and suppressing TGF β R1. *J. Am. Soc. Nephrol.* **2013**, *24*, 627–637. [CrossRef]

79. Wang, B.; Jha, J.C.; Hagiwara, S.; McClelland, A.D.; Jandeleit-Dahm, K.; Thomas, M.C.; Cooper, M.E.; Kantharidis, P. Transforming growth factor-β1-mediated renal fibrosis is dependent on the regulation of transforming growth factor receptor 1 expression by let-7b. *Kidney Int.* **2014**, *85*, 352–361. [CrossRef]

80. Cushing, L.; Kuang, P.; Lü, J. The role of miR-29 in pulmonary fibrosis. *Biochem. Cell Biol.* **2015**, *93*, 109–118. [CrossRef]

81. Meng, X.-M.; Tang, P.M.-K.; Li, J.; Lan, H.Y. TGF-β2/Smad signaling in renal fibrosis. *Front. Physiol.* **2015**, *6*, 82. [CrossRef] [PubMed]

82. Van Rooij, E.; Sutherland, L.B.; Thatcher, J.E.; DiMaio, J.M.; Naseem, R.H.; Marshall, W.S.; Hill, J.A.; Olson, E.N. Dysregulation of microRNAs after myocardial infarction reveals a role of miR-29 in cardiac fibrosis. *Proc. Natl. Acad. Sci. USA* **2008**, *105*, 13027–13032. [CrossRef] [PubMed]

83. Qin, W.; Chung, A.C.K.; Huang, X.R.; Meng, X.-M.; Hui, D.S.C.; Yu, C.-M.; Sung, J.J.Y.; Lan, H.Y. TGF-β/Smad3 signaling promotes renal fibrosis by inhibiting miR-29. *J. Am. Soc. Nephrol.* **2011**, *22*, 1462–1474. [CrossRef] [PubMed]

84. Ramdas, V.; McBride, M.; Denby, L.; Baker, A.H. Canonical transforming growth factor-β signaling regulates disintegrin metalloprotease expression in experimental renal fibrosis via miR-29. *Am. J. Pathol.* **2013**, *183*, 1885–1896. [CrossRef] [PubMed]

85. Wang, B.; Komers, R.; Carew, R.; Winbanks, C.E.; Xu, B.; Herman-Edelstein, M.; Koh, P.; Thomas, M.; Jandeleit-Dahm, K.; Gregorevic, P.; et al. Suppression of microRNA-29 expression by TGF-β1 promotes collagen expression and renal fibrosis. *J. Am. Soc. Nephrol.* **2012**, *23*, 252–265. [CrossRef] [PubMed]

86. Hu, H.; Hu, S.; Xu, S.; Gao, Y.; Zeng, F.; Shui, H. miR-29b Regulates Ang II-induced EMT of rat renal tubular epithelial cells via targeting PI3K/AKT signaling pathway. *Int. J. Mol. Med.* **2018**, *42*, 453–460. [CrossRef] [PubMed]

87. Long, J.; Wang, Y.; Wang, W.; Chang, B.H.J.; Danesh, F.R. MicroRNA-29c is a signature microrna under high glucose conditions that targets sprouty homolog 1, and its in vivo knockdown prevents progression of diabetic nephropathy. *J. Biol. Chem.* **2011**, *286*, 11837–11848. [CrossRef] [PubMed]

88. Hennemeier, I.; Humpf, H.-U.; Gekle, M.; Schwerdt, G. Role of microRNA-29b in the ochratoxin a-induced enhanced collagen formation in human kidney cells. *Toxicology* **2014**, *324*, 116–122. [CrossRef] [PubMed]

89. Ben-Dov, I.Z.; Muthukumar, T.; Morozov, P.; Mueller, F.B.; Tuschl, T.; Suthanthiran, M. MicroRNA sequence profiles of human kidney allografts with or without tubulointerstitial fibrosis. *Transplantation* **2012**, *94*, 1086–1094. [CrossRef]

90. Jiang, L.; Qiu, W.; Zhou, Y.; Wen, P.; Fang, L.; Cao, H.; Zen, K.; He, W.; Zhang, C.; Dai, C.; et al. A microRNA-30e/mitochondrial uncoupling protein 2 axis mediates TGF-β1-induced tubular epithelial cell extracellular matrix production and kidney fibrosis. *Kidney Int.* **2013**, *84*, 285–296. [CrossRef] [PubMed]

91. Wang, J.; Duan, L.; Guo, T.; Gao, Y.; Tian, L.; Liu, J.; Wang, S.; Yang, J. Downregulation of miR-30c promotes renal fibrosis by target CTGF in diabetic nephropathy. *J. Diabetes Complications* **2016**, *30*, 406–414. [CrossRef]

92. Morizane, R.; Fujii, S.; Monkawa, T.; Hiratsuka, K.; Yamaguchi, S.; Homma, K.; Itoh, H. miR-34c Attenuates epithelial-mesenchymal transition and kidney fibrosis with ureteral obstruction. *Sci. Rep.* **2015**, *4*, 4578. [CrossRef]

93. Ning, Y.; Wang, X.; Wang, J.; Zeng, R.; Wang, G. miR-152 Regulates TGF-β1-induced epithelial-mesenchymal transition by targeting HPIP in tubular epithelial cells. *Mol. Med. Rep.* **2018**, *17*, 7973–7979. [CrossRef]

94. Zhang, X.; Yang, Z.; Heng, Y.; Miao, C. MicroRNA-181 exerts an inhibitory role during renal fibrosis by targeting early growth response factor-1 and attenuating the expression of profibrotic markers. *Mol. Med. Rep.* **2019**. [CrossRef]

95. Shen, Y.; Zhao, Y.; Wang, L.; Zhang, W.; Liu, C.; Yin, A. MicroRNA-194 overexpression protects against hypoxia/reperfusion-induced HK-2 cell injury through direct targeting Rheb. *J. Cell. Biochem.* **2019**, *120*, 8311–8318. [CrossRef]

96. Liu, F.; Zhang, Z.-P.; Xin, G.-D.; Guo, L.-H.; Jiang, Q.; Wang, Z.-X. miR-192 Prevents renal tubulointerstitial fibrosis in diabetic nephropathy by targeting Egr1. *Eur. Rev. Med. Pharmacol. Sci.* **2018**, *22*, 4252–4260.

97. Wang, B.; Koh, P.; Winbanks, C.; Coughlan, M.T.; McClelland, A.; Watson, A.; Jandeleit-Dahm, K.; Burns, W.C.; Thomas, M.C.; Cooper, M.E.; et al. miR-200a Prevents renal fibrogenesis through repression of TGF-β2 expression. *Diabetes* **2011**, *60*, 280–287. [CrossRef]

98. Oba, S.; Kumano, S.; Suzuki, E.; Nishimatsu, H.; Takahashi, M.; Takamori, H.; Kasuya, M.; Ogawa, Y.; Sato, K.; Kimura, K.; et al. miR-200b Precursor can ameliorate renal tubulointerstitial fibrosis. *PLoS ONE* **2010**, *5*, e13614. [CrossRef]

99. Howe, E.N.; Cochrane, D.R.; Richer, J.K. The miR-200 and miR-221/222 microRNA families: Opposing effects on epithelial identity. *J. Mammary Gland Biol. Neoplasia* **2012**, *17*, 65–77. [CrossRef]

100. Bai, J.; Xiao, X.; Zhang, X.; Cui, H.; Hao, J.; Han, J.; Cao, N. Erythropoietin inhibits hypoxia–induced epithelial-to-mesenchymal transition via upregulation of miR-200b in HK-2 cells. *Cell. Physiol. Biochem.* **2017**, *42*, 269–280. [CrossRef]

101. Xiong, M.; Jiang, L.; Zhou, Y.; Qiu, W.; Fang, L.; Tan, R.; Wen, P.; Yang, J. The miR-200 family regulates TGF-β1-induced renal tubular epithelial to mesenchymal transition through Smad pathway by targeting ZEB1 and ZEB2 expression. *Am. J. Physiol. Physiol.* **2012**, *302*, F369–F379. [CrossRef]

102. Tang, O.; Chen, X.-M.; Shen, S.; Hahn, M.; Pollock, C.A. MiRNA-200b represses transforming growth factor-β1-induced EMT and fibronectin expression in kidney proximal tubular cells. *Am. J. Physiol. Physiol.* **2013**, *304*, F1266–F1273. [CrossRef]

103. Wu, J.; Liu, J.; Ding, Y.; Zhu, M.; Lu, K.; Zhou, J.; Xie, X.; Xu, Y.; Shen, X.; Chen, Y.; et al. MiR-455-3p suppresses renal fibrosis through repression of ROCK2 expression in diabetic nephropathy. *Biochem. Biophys. Res. Commun.* **2018**, *503*, 977–983. [CrossRef]

104. Putta, S.; Lanting, L.; Sun, G.; Lawson, G.; Kato, M.; Natarajan, R. Inhibiting MicroRNA-192 ameliorates renal fibrosis in diabetic nephropathy. *J. Am. Soc. Nephrol.* **2012**, *23*, 458–469. [CrossRef]

105. Kato, M.; Zhang, J.; Wang, M.; Lanting, L.; Yuan, H.; Rossi, J.J.; Natarajan, R. MicroRNA-192 in diabetic kidney glomeruli and its function in TGF-beta-induced collagen expression via inhibition of E-box repressors. *Proc. Natl. Acad. Sci. USA* **2007**, *104*, 3432–3437. [CrossRef]

106. Chung, A.C.K.; Huang, X.R.; Meng, X.; Lan, H.Y. miR-192 Mediates TGF-β/Smad3-driven renal fibrosis. *J. Am. Soc. Nephrol.* **2010**, *21*, 1317–1325. [CrossRef]

107. Chung, A.C.K.; Dong, Y.; Yang, W.; Zhong, X.; Li, R.; Lan, H.Y. Smad7 suppresses renal fibrosis via altering expression of TGF-β/Smad3-regulated microRNAs. *Mol. Ther.* **2013**, *21*, 388–398. [CrossRef]

108. Krupa, A.; Jenkins, R.; Luo, D.D.; Lewis, A.; Phillips, A.; Fraser, D. Loss of MicroRNA-192 promotes fibrogenesis in diabetic nephropathy. *J. Am. Soc. Nephrol.* **2010**, *21*, 438–447. [CrossRef]

109. Wang, B.; Herman-Edelstein, M.; Koh, P.; Burns, W.; Jandeleit-Dahm, K.; Watson, A.; Saleem, M.; Goodall, G.J.; Twigg, S.M.; Cooper, M.E.; et al. E-cadherin expression is regulated by miR-192/215 by a mechanism that is independent of the profibrotic effects of transforming growth factor-beta. *Diabetes* **2010**, *59*, 1794–1802. [CrossRef]

110. Liu, G.; Friggeri, A.; Yang, Y.; Milosevic, J.; Ding, Q.; Thannickal, V.J.; Kaminski, N.; Abraham, E. miR-21 Mediates fibrogenic activation of pulmonary fibroblasts and lung fibrosis. *J. Exp. Med.* **2010**, *207*, 1589–1597. [CrossRef]

111. Zhou, X.; Xu, H.; Liu, Z.; Wu, Q.; Zhu, R.; Liu, J. miR-21 Promotes cardiac fibroblast-to-myofibroblast transformation and myocardial fibrosis by targeting Jagged1. *J. Cell. Mol. Med.* **2018**, *22*, 3816–3824. [CrossRef]

112. Krichevsky, A.M.; Gabriely, G. miR-21: A small multi-faceted RNA. *J. Cell. Mol. Med.* **2009**, *13*, 39–53. [CrossRef]

113. Androsavich, J.R.; Chau, B.N.; Bhat, B.; Linsley, P.S.; Walter, N.G. Disease-linked microRNA-21 exhibits drastically reduced mRNA binding and silencing activity in healthy mouse liver. *RNA* **2012**, *18*, 1510–1526. [CrossRef]

114. Ma, L.; Yang, X.; Wei, R.; Ye, T.; Zhou, J.-K.; Wen, M.; Men, R.; Li, P.; Dong, B.; Liu, L.; et al. MicroRNA-214 promotes hepatic stellate cell activation and liver fibrosis by suppressing Sufu expression. *Cell Death Dis.* **2018**, *9*, 718. [CrossRef]

115. Sun, M.; Yu, H.; Zhang, Y.; Li, Z.; Gao, W. MicroRNA-214 mediates isoproterenol-induced proliferation and collagen synthesis in cardiac fibroblasts. *Sci. Rep.* **2016**, *5*, 18351. [CrossRef]

116. Denby, L.; Ramdas, V.; Lu, R.; Conway, B.R.; Grant, J.S.; Dickinson, B.; Aurora, A.B.; McClure, J.D.; Kipgen, D.; Delles, C.; et al. MicroRNA-214 antagonism protects against renal fibrosis. *J. Am. Soc. Nephrol.* **2014**, *25*, 65–80. [CrossRef]

117. Humphries, B.; Yang, C. The microRNA-200 family: Small molecules with novel roles in cancer development, progression and therapy. *Oncotarget* **2015**, *6*, 6472–6498. [CrossRef]

118. Korpal, M.; Kang, Y. The emerging role of miR-200 family of microRNAs in epithelial-mesenchymal transition and cancer metastasis. *RNA Biol.* **2008**, *5*, 115–119. [CrossRef]

119. Kriegel, A.J.; Liu, Y.; Fang, Y.; Ding, X.; Liang, M. The miR-29 family: Genomics, cell biology, and relevance to renal and cardiovascular injury. *Physiol. Genomics* **2012**, *44*, 237–244. [CrossRef]

120. Huang, S.; Zhang, L.; Song, J.; Wang, Z.; Huang, X.; Guo, Z.; Chen, F.; Zhao, X. Long noncoding RNA MALAT1 mediates cardiac fibrosis in experimental postinfarct myocardium mice model. *J. Cell. Physiol.* **2019**, *234*, 2997–3006. [CrossRef]

121. Yu, F.; Lu, Z.; Cai, J.; Huang, K.; Chen, B.; Li, G.; Dong, P.; Zheng, J. MALAT1 functions as a competing endogenous RNA to mediate Rac1 expression by sequestering miR-101b in liver fibrosis. *Cell Cycle* **2015**, *14*, 3885–3896. [CrossRef] [PubMed]

122. Zhang, K.; Han, X.; Zhang, Z.; Zheng, L.; Hu, Z.; Yao, Q.; Cui, H.; Shu, G.; Si, M.; Li, C.; et al. The liver-enriched lnc-LFAR1 promotes liver fibrosis by activating TGFβ and Notch pathways. *Nat. Commun.* **2017**, *8*, 144. [CrossRef] [PubMed]

123. Zhang, Q.-Q.; Xu, M.-Y.; Qu, Y.; Hu, J.-J.; Li, Z.-H.; Zhang, Q.-D.; Lu, L.-G. TET3 mediates the activation of human hepatic stellate cells via modulating the expression of long non-coding RNA HIF1A-AS1. *Int. J. Clin. Exp. Pathol.* **2014**, *7*, 7744–7751.

124. Lu, Q.; Guo, Z.; Xie, W.; Jin, W.; Zhu, D.; Chen, S.; Ren, T. The lncRNA H19 mediates pulmonary fibrosis by regulating the miR-196a/COL1A1 axis. *Inflammation* **2018**, *41*, 896–903. [CrossRef]

125. Savary, G.; Dewaeles, E.; Diazzi, S.; Buscot, M.; Nottet, N.; Fassy, J.; Courcot, E.; Henaoui, I.-S.; Lemaire, J.; Martis, N.; et al. The long non-coding RNA DNM3OS is a reservoir of fibromirs with major functions in lung fibroblast response to TGF-β and pulmonary fibrosis. *Am. J. Respir. Crit. Care Med.* **2019**. [CrossRef] [PubMed]

126. Han, R.; Hu, S.; Qin, W.; Shi, J.; Zeng, C.; Bao, H.; Liu, Z. Upregulated long noncoding RNA LOC105375913 induces tubulointerstitial fibrosis in focal segmental glomerulosclerosis. *Sci. Rep.* **2019**, *9*, 716. [CrossRef] [PubMed]

127. Chen, W.; Zhou, Z.-Q.; Ren, Y.-Q.; Zhang, L.; Sun, L.-N.; Man, Y.-L.; Wang, Z.-K. Effects of long non-coding RNA LINC00667 on renal tubular epithelial cell proliferation, apoptosis and renal fibrosis via the miR-19b-3p/LINC00667/CTGF signaling pathway in chronic renal failure. *Cell. Signal.* **2019**, *54*, 102–114. [CrossRef]

128. Huang, S.; Xu, Y.; Ge, X.; Xu, B.; Peng, W.; Jiang, X.; Shen, L.; Xia, L. Long noncoding RNA NEAT1 accelerates the proliferation and fibrosis in diabetic nephropathy through activating Akt/mTOR signaling pathway. *J. Cell. Physiol.* **2019**, *234*, 11200–11207. [CrossRef]

129. Wang, P.; Luo, M.-L.; Song, E.; Zhou, Z.; Ma, T.; Wang, J.; Jia, N.; Wang, G.; Nie, S.; Liu, Y.; et al. Long noncoding RNA *lnc-TSI* inhibits renal fibrogenesis by negatively regulating the TGF-β/Smad3 pathway. *Sci. Transl. Med.* **2018**, *10*, eaat2039. [CrossRef]

130. Liang, Y.-J.; Wang, Q.-Y.; Zhou, C.-X.; Yin, Q.-Q.; He, M.; Yu, X.-T.; Cao, D.-X.; Chen, G.-Q.; He, J.-R.; Zhao, Q. MiR-124 targets Slug to regulate epithelial–mesenchymal transition and metastasis of breast cancer. *Carcinogenesis* **2013**, *34*, 713–722. [CrossRef] [PubMed]

131. Jiang, L.; Lin, T.; Xu, C.; Hu, S.; Pan, Y.; Jin, R. miR-124 Interacts with the Notch1 signalling pathway and has therapeutic potential against gastric cancer. *J. Cell. Mol. Med.* **2016**, *20*, 313–322. [CrossRef]

132. Chen, W.; Zhang, L.; Zhou, Z.-Q.; Ren, Y.-Q.; Sun, L.-N.; Man, Y.-L.; Ma, Z.-W.; Wang, Z.-K. Effects of long non-coding RNA LINC00963 on renal interstitial fibrosis and oxidative stress of rats with chronic renal failure via the foxo signaling pathway. *Cell. Physiol. Biochem.* **2018**, *46*, 815–828. [CrossRef]

133. Zhou, S.-G.; Zhang, W.; Ma, H.-J.; Guo, Z.-Y.; Xu, Y. Silencing of LncRNA TCONS_00088786 reduces renal fibrosis through miR-132. *Eur. Rev. Med. Pharmacol. Sci.* **2018**, *22*, 166–173.

134. Zhou, Q.; Chung, A.C.K.; Huang, X.R.; Dong, Y.; Yu, X.; Lan, H.Y. Identification of novel long noncoding RNAs associated with TGF-β/Smad3-mediated renal inflammation and fibrosis by RNA sequencing. *Am. J. Pathol.* **2014**, *184*, 409–417. [CrossRef]

135. Feng, M.; Tang, P.M.-K.; Huang, X.-R.; Sun, S.-F.; You, Y.-K.; Xiao, J.; Lv, L.-L.; Xu, A.-P.; Lan, H.-Y. TGF-β mediates renal fibrosis via the Smad3-Erbb4-IR long noncoding RNA axis. *Mol. Ther.* **2018**, *26*, 148–161. [CrossRef]

136. Sun, S.F.; Tang, P.M.K.; Feng, M.; Xiao, J.; Huang, X.R.; Li, P.; Ma, R.C.W.; Lan, H.Y. Novel lncRNA Erbb4-IR promotes diabetic kidney injury in *db/db* mice by targeting miR-29b. *Diabetes* **2018**, *67*, 731–744. [CrossRef]

137. Zhang, C.; Yuan, J.; Hu, H.; Chen, W.; Liu, M.; Zhang, J.; Sun, S.; Guo, Z. Long non-coding RNA CHCHD4P4 promotes epithelial-mesenchymal transition and inhibits cell proliferation in calcium oxalate-induced kidney damage. *Braz. J. Med. Biol. Res.* **2017**, *51*, e6536. [CrossRef]

138. Sun, J.; Zhang, S.; Shi, B.; Zheng, D.; Shi, J. Transcriptome identified lncRNAs associated with renal fibrosis in UUO rat model. *Front. Physiol.* **2017**, *8*, 658. [CrossRef]

139. Gao, Y.; Chen, Z.-Y.; Wang, Y.; Liu, Y.; Ma, J.-X.; Li, Y.-K. Long non-coding RNA ASncmtRNA-2 is upregulated in diabetic kidneys and high glucose-treated mesangial cells. *Exp. Ther. Med.* **2017**, *13*, 581–587. [CrossRef]

140. Zhang, H.; Sun, S.-C. NF-κB in inflammation and renal diseases. *Cell Biosci.* **2015**, *5*, 63. [CrossRef]

141. Yi, H.; Peng, R.; Zhang, L.; Sun, Y.; Peng, H.; Liu, H.; Yu, L.; Li, A.; Zhang, Y.; Jiang, W.; et al. LincRNA-Gm4419 knockdown ameliorates NF-κB/NLRP3 inflammasome-mediated inflammation in diabetic nephropathy. *Cell Death Dis.* **2017**, *8*, e2583. [CrossRef]

142. Xie, H.; Xue, J.-D.; Chao, F.; Jin, Y.-F.; Fu, Q.; Xie, H.; Xue, J.-D.; Chao, F.; Jin, Y.-F.; Fu, Q. Long non-coding RNA-H19 antagonism protects against renal fibrosis. *Oncotarget* **2016**, *7*, 51473–51481. [CrossRef]

143. Arvaniti, E.; Moulos, P.; Vakrakou, A.; Chatziantoniou, C.; Chadjichristos, C.; Kavvadas, P.; Charonis, A.; Politis, P.K. Whole-transcriptome analysis of UUO mouse model of renal fibrosis reveals new molecular players in kidney diseases. *Sci. Rep.* **2016**, *6*, 26235. [CrossRef]

144. Zhou, Q.; Huang, X.R.; Yu, J.; Yu, X.; Lan, H.Y. Long noncoding RNA Arid2-IR is a novel therapeutic target for renal inflammation. *Mol. Ther.* **2015**, *23*, 1034–1043. [CrossRef]

145. Gao, J.; Wang, W.; Wang, F.; Guo, C. LncRNA-NR_033515 promotes proliferation, fibrogenesis and epithelial-to-mesenchymal transition by targeting miR-743b-5p in diabetic nephropathy. *Biomed. Pharmacother.* **2018**, *106*, 543–552. [CrossRef]

146. Hu, M.; Wang, R.; Li, X.; Fan, M.; Lin, J.; Zhen, J.; Chen, L.; Lv, Z. LncRNA MALAT1 is dysregulated in diabetic nephropathy and involved in high glucose-induced podocyte injury via its interplay with β-catenin. *J. Cell. Mol. Med.* **2017**, *21*, 2732–2747. [CrossRef]

147. Feng, Y.; Chen, S.; Xu, J.; Zhu, Q.; Ye, X.; Ding, D.; Yao, W.; Lu, Y.; Ye, X.; Ye, X.; et al. Dysregulation of lncRNAs GM5524 and GM15645 involved in high-glucose-induced podocyte apoptosis and autophagy in diabetic nephropathy. *Mol. Med. Rep.* **2018**, *18*, 3657–3664. [CrossRef]

148. Polovic, M.; Dittmar, S.; Hennemeier, I.; Humpf, H.-U.; Seliger, B.; Fornara, P.; Theil, G.; Azinovic, P.; Nolze, A.; Köhn, M.; et al. Identification of a novel lncRNA induced by the nephrotoxin ochratoxin A and expressed in human renal tumor tissue. *Cell. Mol. Life Sci.* **2018**, *75*, 2241–2256. [CrossRef]

149. Wang, M.; Wang, S.; Yao, D.; Yan, Q.; Lu, W. A novel long non-coding RNA CYP4B1-PS1-001 regulates proliferation and fibrosis in diabetic nephropathy. *Mol. Cell. Endocrinol.* **2016**, *426*, 136–145. [CrossRef]

150. Wang, S.; Chen, X.; Wang, M.; Yao, D.; Chen, T.; Yan, Q.; Lu, W. Long non-coding RNA CYP4B1-PS1-001 inhibits proliferation and fibrosis in diabetic nephropathy by interacting with Nucleolin. *Cell. Physiol. Biochem.* **2018**, *49*, 2174–2187. [CrossRef]

151. Wang, M.; Yao, D.; Wang, S.; Yan, Q.; Lu, W. Long non-coding RNA ENSMUST00000147869 protects mesangial cells from proliferation and fibrosis induced by diabetic nephropathy. *Endocrine* **2016**, *54*, 81–92. [CrossRef]

152. Li, A.; Peng, R.; Sun, Y.; Liu, H.; Peng, H.; Zhang, Z. LincRNA 1700020I14Rik alleviates cell proliferation and fibrosis in diabetic nephropathy via miR-34a-5p/Sirt1/HIF-1α signaling. *Cell Death Dis.* **2018**, *9*, 461. [CrossRef]

153. Xue, R.; Li, Y.; Li, X.; Ma, J.; An, C.; Ma, Z. miR-185 Affected the EMT, cell viability and proliferation via DNMT1/MEG3 pathway in TGF-β1-induced renal fibrosis. *Cell Biol. Int.* **2018**. [CrossRef] [PubMed]

154. Wang, J.; Pang, J.; Li, H.; Long, J.; Fang, F.; Chen, J.; Zhu, X.; Xiang, X.; Zhang, D. lncRNA ZEB1-AS1 was suppressed by p53 for renal fibrosis in diabetic nephropathy. *Mol. Ther. Nucleic Acids* **2018**, *12*, 741–750. [CrossRef] [PubMed]

155. Xiao, X.; Yuan, Q.; Chen, Y.; Huang, Z.; Fang, X.; Zhang, H.; Peng, L.; Xiao, P. LncRNA ENST00000453774.1 contributes to oxidative stress defense dependent on autophagy mediation to reduce extracellular matrix and alleviate renal fibrosis. *J. Cell. Physiol.* **2018**, *234*, 9130–9143. [CrossRef]

156. Hajjari, M.; Salavaty, A. HOTAIR: An oncogenic long non-coding RNA in different cancers. *Cancer Biol. Med.* **2015**, *12*, 1–9.

157. Zhou, H.; Gao, L.; Yu, Z.; Hong, S.; Zhang, Z.; Qiu, Z. LncRNA HOTAIR promotes renal interstitial fibrosis by regulating Notch1 pathway via the modulation of miR-124. *Nephrology* **2018**. [CrossRef] [PubMed]

158. Zhou, H.; Qiu, Z.-Z.; Yu, Z.-H.; Gao, L.; He, J.-M.; Zhang, Z.-W.; Zheng, J. Paeonol reverses promoting effect of the HOTAIR/miR-124/Notch1 axis on renal interstitial fibrosis in a rat model. *J. Cell. Physiol.* **2019**. [CrossRef]

159. Van Rooij, E.; Kauppinen, S. Development of microRNA therapeutics is coming of age. *EMBO Mol. Med.* **2014**, *6*, 851–864. [CrossRef]

160. Chiu, Y.-L.; Rana, T.M. siRNA function in RNAi: A chemical modification analysis. *RNA* **2003**, *9*, 1034–1048. [CrossRef] [PubMed]

161. Chen, P.Y.; Weinmann, L.; Gaidatzis, D.; Pei, Y.; Zavolan, M.; Tuschl, T.; Meister, G. Strand-specific 5′-O-methylation of siRNA duplexes controls guide strand selection and targeting specificity. *RNA* **2008**, *14*, 263–274. [CrossRef]

162. Michelfelder, S.; Trepel, M. Adeno-associated viral vectors and their redirection to cell-type specific receptors. *Adv. Genet.* **2009**, *67*, 29–60. [PubMed]

163. Montgomery, R.L.; Yu, G.; Latimer, P.A.; Stack, C.; Robinson, K.; Dalby, C.M.; Kaminski, N.; van Rooij, E. MicroRNA mimicry blocks pulmonary fibrosis. *EMBO Mol. Med.* **2014**, *6*, 1347–1356. [CrossRef] [PubMed]

164. Chakraborty, C.; Sharma, A.R.; Sharma, G.; Doss, C.G.P.; Lee, S.-S. Therapeutic miRNA and siRNA: Moving from bench to clinic as next generation medicine. *Mol. Ther. Nucleic Acids* **2017**, *8*, 132–143. [CrossRef] [PubMed]

165. Lennox, K.A.; Behlke, M.A. Chemical modification and design of anti-miRNA oligonucleotides. *Gene Ther.* **2011**, *18*, 1111–1120. [CrossRef] [PubMed]

166. Louloupi, A.; Ørom, U.A.V. Inhibiting pri-miRNA processing with target site blockers. *Methods Mol. Biol.* **2018**, *1823*, 63–68. [PubMed]

167. Knauss, J.L.; Bian, S.; Sun, T. Plasmid-based target protectors allow specific blockade of miRNA silencing activity in mammalian developmental systems. *Front. Cell. Neurosci.* **2013**, *7*, 163. [CrossRef] [PubMed]

168. Kölling, M.; Kaucsar, T.; Schauerte, C.; Hübner, A.; Dettling, A.; Park, J.-K.; Busch, M.; Wulff, X.; Meier, M.; Scherf, K.; et al. Therapeutic miR-21 silencing ameliorates diabetic kidney disease in mice. *Mol. Ther.* **2017**, *25*, 165–180. [CrossRef]

169. Gomez, I.G.; MacKenna, D.A.; Johnson, B.G.; Kaimal, V.; Roach, A.M.; Ren, S.; Nakagawa, N.; Xin, C.; Newitt, R.; Pandya, S.; et al. Anti–microRNA-21 oligonucleotides prevent Alport nephropathy progression by stimulating metabolic pathways. *J. Clin. Invest.* **2015**, *125*, 141–156. [CrossRef] [PubMed]

170. Creemers, E.E.; van Rooij, E. Function and therapeutic potential of noncoding RNAs in cardiac fibrosis. *Circ. Res.* **2016**, *118*, 108–118. [CrossRef]

171. Bonetti, A.; Carninci, P. From bench to bedside: The long journey of long non-coding RNAs. *Curr. Opin. Syst. Biol.* **2017**, *3*, 119–124. [CrossRef]

172. Hagedorn, P.H.; Pontoppidan, M.; Bisgaard, T.S.; Berrera, M.; Dieckmann, A.; Ebeling, M.; Møller, M.R.; Hudlebusch, H.; Jensen, M.L.; Hansen, H.F.; et al. Identifying and avoiding off-target effects of RNase H-dependent antisense oligonucleotides in mice. *Nucleic Acids Res.* **2018**, *46*, 5366–5380. [CrossRef]

173. Kato, M.; Wang, M.; Chen, Z.; Bhatt, K.; Oh, H.J.; Lanting, L.; Deshpande, S.; Jia, Y.; Lai, J.Y.C.; O'Connor, C.L.; et al. An endoplasmic reticulum stress-regulated lncRNA hosting a microRNA megacluster induces early features of diabetic nephropathy. *Nat. Commun.* **2016**, *7*, 12864. [CrossRef]

174. Li, C.H.; Chen, Y. Targeting long non-coding RNAs in cancers: Progress and prospects. *Int. J. Biochem. Cell Biol.* **2013**, *45*, 1895–1910. [CrossRef]

175. Prasad, N.; Kumar, S.; Manjunath, R.; Bhadauria, D.; Kaul, A.; Sharma, R.K.; Gupta, A.; Lal, H.; Jain, M.; Agrawal, V. Real-time ultrasound-guided percutaneous renal biopsy with needle guide by nephrologists decreases post-biopsy complications. *Clin. Kidney J.* **2015**, *8*, 151–156. [CrossRef]

176. Schwab, S.; Marwitz, T.; Woitas, R.P. The role of prognostic assessment with biomarkers in chronic kidney disease: A narrative review. *J. Lab. Precis. Med.* **2018**, *3*, 12. [CrossRef]

177. Weber, J.A.; Baxter, D.H.; Zhang, S.; Huang, D.Y.; How Huang, K.; Jen Lee, M.; Galas, D.J.; Wang, K. The microRNA spectrum in 12 body fluids. *Clin. Chem.* **2010**, *56*, 1733–1741. [CrossRef]

178. Mitchell, P.S.; Parkin, R.K.; Kroh, E.M.; Fritz, B.R.; Wyman, S.K.; Pogosova-Agadjanyan, E.L.; Peterson, A.; Noteboom, J.; O'Briant, K.C.; Allen, A.; et al. Circulating microRNAs as stable blood-based markers for cancer detection. *Proc. Natl. Acad. Sci. USA* **2008**, *105*, 10513–10518. [CrossRef]

179. Bolha, L.; Ravnik-Glavač, M.; Glavač, D. Long noncoding RNAs as biomarkers in cancer. *Dis. Markers* **2017**, *2017*, 7243968. [CrossRef]

180. Cheng, L.; Sun, X.; Scicluna, B.J.; Coleman, B.M.; Hill, A.F. Characterization and deep sequencing analysis of exosomal and non-exosomal miRNA in human urine. *Kidney Int.* **2014**, *86*, 433–444. [CrossRef]

181. Cardenas-Gonzalez, M.; Srivastava, A.; Pavkovic, M.; Bijol, V.; Rennke, H.G.; Stillman, I.E.; Zhang, X.; Parikh, S.; Rovin, B.H.; Afkarian, M.; et al. Identification, confirmation, and replication of novel urinary microRNA biomarkers in lupus nephritis and diabetic nephropathy. *Clin. Chem.* **2017**, *63*, 1515–1526. [CrossRef] [PubMed]

182. Ramachandran, K.; Saikumar, J.; Bijol, V.; Koyner, J.L.; Qian, J.; Betensky, R.A.; Waikar, S.S.; Vaidya, V.S. Human miRNome profiling identifies microRNAs differentially present in the urine after kidney injury. *Clin. Chem.* **2013**, *59*, 1742–1752. [CrossRef] [PubMed]

183. Sonoda, H.; Lee, B.R.; Park, K.-H.; Nihalani, D.; Yoon, J.-H.; Ikeda, M.; Kwon, S.-H. miRNA Profiling of urinary exosomes to assess the progression of acute kidney injury. *Sci. Rep.* **2019**, *9*, 4692. [CrossRef] [PubMed]

184. Khurana, R.; Ranches, G.; Schafferer, S.; Lukasser, M.; Rudnicki, M.; Mayer, G.; Hüttenhofer, A. Identification of urinary exosomal noncoding RNAs as novel biomarkers in chronic kidney disease. *RNA* **2017**, *23*, 142–152. [CrossRef]

185. Chen, C.; Lu, C.; Qian, Y.; Li, H.; Tan, Y.; Cai, L.; Weng, H. Urinary miR-21 as a potential biomarker of hypertensive kidney injury and fibrosis. *Sci. Rep.* **2017**, *7*, 17737. [CrossRef] [PubMed]

186. Lv, L.-L.; Cao, Y.-H.; Ni, H.-F.; Xu, M.; Liu, D.; Liu, H.; Chen, P.-S.; Liu, B.-C. MicroRNA-29c in urinary exosome/microvesicle as a biomarker of renal fibrosis. *Am. J. Physiol. Physiol.* **2013**, *305*, F1220–F1227. [CrossRef]

187. Zununi Vahed, S.; Omidi, Y.; Ardalan, M.; Samadi, N. Dysregulation of urinary miR-21 and miR-200b associated with interstitial fibrosis and tubular atrophy (IFTA) in renal transplant recipients. *Clin. Biochem.* **2017**, *50*, 32–39. [CrossRef]

188. Zhou, H.; Cheruvanky, A.; Hu, X.; Matsumoto, T.; Hiramatsu, N.; Cho, M.E.; Berger, A.; Leelahavanichkul, A.; Doi, K.; Chawla, L.S.; et al. Urinary exosomal transcription factors, a new class of biomarkers for renal disease. *Kidney Int.* **2008**, *74*, 613–621. [CrossRef]

189. Zununi Vahed, S.; Poursadegh Zonouzi, A.; Ghanbarian, H.; Ghojazadeh, M.; Samadi, N.; Ardalan, M. Upregulated expression of circulating microRNAs in kidney transplant recipients with interstitial fibrosis and tubular atrophy. *Iran. J. Kidney Dis.* **2017**, *11*, 309–318.

190. Muralidharan, J.; Ramezani, A.; Hubal, M.; Knoblach, S.; Shrivastav, S.; Karandish, S.; Scott, R.; Maxwell, N.; Ozturk, S.; Beddhu, S.; et al. Extracellular microRNA signature in chronic kidney disease. *Am. J. Physiol. Renal Physiol.* **2017**, *312*, F982–F991. [CrossRef]

191. Poel, D.; Buffart, T.E.; Oosterling-Jansen, J.; Verheul, H.M.; Voortman, J. Evaluation of several methodological challenges in circulating miRNA qPCR studies in patients with head and neck cancer. *Exp. Mol. Med.* **2018**, *50*, e454. [CrossRef]

192. Nair, V.S.; Pritchard, C.C.; Tewari, M.; Ioannidis, J.P.A. Design and analysis for studying microRNAs in human disease: A primer on -omic technologies. *Am. J. Epidemiol.* **2014**, *180*, 140–152. [CrossRef]

193. Haider, B.A.; Baras, A.S.; McCall, M.N.; Hertel, J.A.; Cornish, T.C.; Halushka, M.K. A critical evaluation of microRNA biomarkers in non-neoplastic disease. *PLoS ONE* **2014**, *9*, e89565. [CrossRef]

194. Ma, J.; Li, N.; Guarnera, M.; Jiang, F. Quantification of plasma miRNAs by digital PCR for cancer diagnosis. *Biomark. Insights* **2013**, *8*, 127–136. [CrossRef]

195. Hindson, C.M.; Chevillet, J.R.; Briggs, H.A.; Gallichotte, E.N.; Ruf, I.K.; Hindson, B.J.; Vessella, R.L.; Tewari, M. Absolute quantification by droplet digital PCR versus analog real-time PCR. *Nat. Methods* **2013**, *10*, 1003–1005. [CrossRef]

196. Mohankumar, S.; Patel, T. Extracellular vesicle long noncoding RNA as potential biomarkers of liver cancer. *Brief. Funct. Genomics* **2016**, *15*, 249–256. [CrossRef]

MDPI

St. Alban-Anlage 66

4052 Basel

Switzerland

Tel. +41 61 683 77 34

Fax +41 61 302 89 18

www.mdpi.com

International Journal of Molecular Sciences Editorial Office

E-mail: ijms@mdpi.com

www.mdpi.com/journal/ijms